Cambridge Prescriber's Guide in Psychiatry

T0201417

"In the past decade or so, not only has there been a better awareness of psychiatric disorders, but increasingly larger numbers of people are seeking help for these conditions. There is indeed a better focus on personalised psychiatry and pharmacological research. With further recent advances in innovations and better medications, practice of clinical psychiatry is changing with greater hope to patients and their families and carers. In this volume, *Cambridge Prescribers Guide in Psychiatry*, authors have brought together key essentials about medications used in treatments in psychiatry in an impressively coherent and comprehensive manner. The authors deserve our thanks and congratulations on an impressive effort to bring together evidence-based information on how to use medicine and drug interventions which will go a long way in improving outcomes for patients and their carers as well as families."

Dinesh Bhugra, CBE
Professor Emeritus, Mental Health & Cultural Diversity, IoPPN
Kings College, London

"Finally, a colourful handbook about medication in use in psychiatry that you could look up quickly in the field like a bird-watcher guide. Modern clinical practice involves a reflective integration of psychopharmacology with psychosocial interventions that depend on a good grasp of the brain mechanism behind the medication used. Filtering and updating information is difficult for the busy clinician, who could find himself stuck in the clinic trying to google a less familiar medication or side effect. It is particularly reassuring to learn that *The Cambridge Prescriber's Guide in Psychiatry* is the product of coordinated crowd-sourcing of clinical students, active clinicians, as well as neuroscience experts. In particular, the unique section on the Art of Psychopharmacology for each medication presents the wisdom of practising clinicians which has hitherto largely been confined to clinical supervision in specialist apprenticeships. This work will find its place in the pockets of busy clinicians and will be a reliable source of information for students, healthcare professionals, patients and carers."

Professor Eric Chen MA(Oxon), MBChB(Edin), MD(Edin). FRCPsych(UK), FHKAM(Psychiatry)
The University of Hong Kong

"*The Cambridge Prescriber's Guide in Psychiatry* will support informed and inclusive decisions about psychiatric medication as the basis of better outcomes for patients. The collaborative authorship combines Cambridgeshire & Peterborough's experienced NHS consultants, psychopharmacologists and pharmacists with the inquiring minds of our student doctors: an innovative example of why it is so rewarding to practise psychiatry in an academic teaching trust environment. *The Cambridge Prescriber's Guide in Psychiatry* will help make that inquisitive, evidence-based approach more widely available to prescribers in mental health care."

Dr Cathy Walsh
Chief Medical Officer
Cambridgeshire and Peterborough NHS Foundation Trust

"From Acamprosate to Zuclopenthixol - *The Cambridge Prescriber's Guide in Psychiatry* is what it says on the tin. Crystal clear information that prescribers need – to not only prescribe safely and effectively in terms of dosing and side effects but also to understand the underlying mechanism of action. Neat colour coded sections with easy to access bullet point lists of key information makes the guide an easy-to-use reference tool and psychopharmaco-pedia rolled in one. Sections on the art of switching and on the mechanism of action of side effects will be appreciated equally by established clinicians as by trainees across the world. The short but pertinent list of references at the end of each medication will also appeal to those with a more academic interest in psychopharmacology. The inclusion of compound medications (e.g. Buprenorphine and Naoloxone) in the guide is especially welcome lending credence to the title of the guide as a Prescriber's guide. I particularly liked The Art of Psychopharmacology and Pearls sections, what I call the 'Wisdom sections'. Overall, the various sections are guaranteed to make every medication choice discussion with the patient an intellectually stimulating encounter and one that should result in a more rational, more safe prescribing practice – win-win for both patients and prescribers."

Subodh Dave
Dean
Royal College of Psychiatrists

Cambridge Prescriber's Guide in Psychiatry

Edited by

Sepehr Hafizi

Cambridgeshire and Peterborough NHS
Foundation Trust and University of Cambridge, Cambridge

Peter B. Jones

University of Cambridge, Cambridge

Stephen M. Stahl

University of California, San Diego

With illustrations by
Nancy Muntner

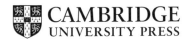

CAMBRIDGE
UNIVERSITY PRESS

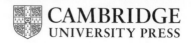

Shaftesbury Road, Cambridge CB2 8EA, United Kingdom

One Liberty Plaza, 20th Floor, New York, NY 10006, USA

477 Williamstown Road, Port Melbourne, VIC 3207, Australia

314–321, 3rd Floor, Plot 3, Splendor Forum, Jasola District Centre, New Delhi – 110025, India

103 Penang Road, #05–06/07, Visioncrest Commercial, Singapore 238467

Cambridge University Press is part of Cambridge University Press & Assessment, a department of the University of Cambridge.

We share the University's mission to contribute to society through the pursuit of education, learning and research at the highest international levels of excellence.

www.cambridge.org
Information on this title: www.cambridge.org/9781108986588

DOI: 10.1017/9781108986335

First published 2024

Printed in the United Kingdom by TJ Books Limited, Padstow Cornwall

A catalogue record for this publication is available from the British Library.

A Cataloging-in-Publication data record for this book is available from the Library of Congress.

ISBN 978-1-108-98658-8 Paperback

Contents

Foreword

With psychiatric conditions being so prevalent and the wide indications of many available medicines, most doctors need to be confident about psychotropic drugs, regardless of whether they prescribe them themselves. But tomorrow's doctors walk a long road from the basic pharmacological principles they learn from the simplicity of the ileum to the complexities of the everyday lives of people seeking help for their mental health. The *Cambridge Prescriber's Guide in Psychiatry* is intended to be an everyday reference to support the clinician, whether physician, psychiatrist or other medical or allied professional involved in helping those who require psychotropic drugs as part of their healthcare. The *Guide* maps the journey from basic pharmacology, through evidence-based prescribing to the "clinical pearls" section which is based on experience and expertise. I am delighted that students from the School of Clinical Medicine at the University of Cambridge have played a central role in compiling the *Guide*. They have sifted, compared and combined the many sources on which prescribers rely to create draft entries, drug-by-drug, to discuss with Associate Editors, mainly senior clinicians from the NHS organisations with which the Clinical School collaborates to provide psychiatric experience for the students. Thus, some of tomorrow's doctors have not only greatly enhanced their learning experience in psychiatry but have contributed to today's clinical practice. All will benefit in terms of their future practice and some, perhaps many, will find that their career path leads to psychiatry.

Professor Paul Wilkinson
Clinical Dean
University of Cambridge School of Clinical Medicine
Honorary Consultant in Child and Adolescent Psychiatry, CPFT

Acknowledgements

The Editors are grateful to the 31 students from the University of Cambridge and the Associate Editors who developed the draft entries with them, and to staff at CUP for their generous support during production.

Dr Hafizi acknowledges salary support from the NIHR Applied Research Collaboration East of England at the Cambridgeshire & Peterborough NHS Foundation Trust during the early stages of the project development through a Fellowship to enhance evidence-based practice. The views expressed are those of the Editors and not necessarily of the funder.

Acknowledgments

Introduction

The *Cambridge Prescriber's Guide in Psychiatry* is intended to complement *Stahl's Essential Psychopharmacology*, and the recently published *Cambridge Textbook of Neuroscience for Psychiatrists*. The former emphasises mechanisms of action and how psychotropic drugs work upon receptors and enzymes in the brain, while the *Cambridge Textbook of Neuroscience for Psychiatrists* reviews the wider understanding of neuroscience in psychiatry and its application to clinical practice. Thus, the *Guide* gives practical neuroscience-based information on how to use psychotropic drugs in clinical practice. We have used the tried, tested and popular format of *Stahl's Prescriber's Guide*, adapting it for a British-English readership and prescribers relying on a UK formulary.

We have taken the unusual step of involving tomorrow's prescribers in the production of the *Guide*: student doctors at the School of Clinical Medicine, University of Cambridge. They reviewed the available pharmacological evidence and existing clinical guidelines according to templates and under the supervision of experienced consultants and pharmacists as Associate Editors; most of these Associate Editors are our clinical colleagues within the Cambridgeshire & Peterborough NHS Foundation Trust (CPFT). This information was then reviewed, cross-checked, and edited further. Through this inter-generational professional partnership, we hope to have excited the students' interest in psychopharmacology and psychiatry while integrating the art of clinical practice with the science of psychopharmacology as seen through fresh eyes.

We cannot include all available information about every drug in a single work, and no attempt is made here to be comprehensive. The *Guide* comprises punchy information and essential facts to help prescribers in everyday practice. Unfortunately, it also means excluding less critical facts and arcane information that may, nevertheless, be useful to the reader. To include everything would make the book too long and dilute the most important information. In deciding what to include and what to omit, the editorial team has drawn upon common sense and many decades of combined clinical experience.

To meet the needs of the clinician and to facilitate future updates of the *Guide*, the opinions of readers are eagerly solicited. Feedback can be emailed to PrescribersGuide@cambridge.org. Any and all suggestions and comments are welcomed.

As in *Stahl's Prescriber's Guide*, the selected drugs are all presented in the same format in order to facilitate rapid access to information. Specifically, each drug is broken down into five sections, each designated by a standard colour background: Therapeutics, Side Effects, Dosing and Use, Special Populations, The Art of Psychopharmacology, followed by Suggested Reading.

Therapeutics covers the brand names in the UK and if the generic form is available; the class of drug; what indications it is prescribed for as in the British National Formulary (BNF) in bold and other common non-BNF indications; how the drug works; how long it takes to work; what to do if it works or if it doesn't work; the best augmenting combinations for partial response or treatment resistance; and the tests (if any) that are required.

Side effects explains how the drug causes side effects; gives a list of notable, life-threatening or dangerous side effects; gives a specific rating for weight gain or sedation; and gives advice about how to handle side effects, including best augmenting agents for side effects.

Dosing and use gives the usual dosing range; dosage forms; how to dose and dosing tips; symptoms of overdose; long-term use; if habit forming, how to stop; pharmacokinetics; drug interactions; when not to use; and other warnings or precautions.

Special populations contains specific information about any possible renal, hepatic, and cardiac impairments, and any precautions to be taken for treating the elderly, children and adolescents, and pregnant and breast-feeding women.

The art of psychopharmacology provides the editorial team's opinions on issues such as the potential advantages and disadvantages of any one drug, the primary target symptoms, and clinical pearls to get the best out of a drug for a specific patient.

The art of switching includes clinical pearls and graphical representations to help guide the switching process that can be particularly problematic unless the relevant pharmacological principles and profiles are considered.

The Medicines and Driving chapter outlines a summary of advice relating to driving for some of the individual drugs and classes of drugs found in the *Guide*.

There is a list of icons used in the *Guide* following this Introduction and at the back of the *Guide* are several indices. The first is an index by drug name, giving both generic names (uncapitalised) and trade names (capitalised and followed by the generic name in parentheses). The second is an index of common uses for the generic drugs included in the *Guide* and is organised by disorder/symptom. Agents that are approved in the BNF for a particular use are shown in bold but additional, evidence-based usage is also included. The third index is organised by drug class and lists all the agents that fall within each class. In addition to these indices there is a list of abbreviations.

We have attempted to make information consistent with what readers may see in other standard sources including the British National Formulary (BNF) British Association of Psychopharmacology condition-specific guidelines, Bumps (best use of medicine in pregnancy), Electronic Medicines Compendium, Martindale: The Complete Drug Reference, Maudsley Prescribing Guidelines, NICE Guidelines, Specialist Pharmacy Service, and The Renal Drug Handbook. Prescribers are encouraged to consult these standard references and comprehensive psychiatry and pharmacology textbooks for more in-depth information. They are also reminded that the Art of Psychopharmacology section is based on the Editors' opinions.

It is strongly advised that readers familiarise themselves with the standard use of these drugs before attempting any of the less frequent uses discussed, such as unusual drug combinations and doses. Reading about both drugs before augmenting one with the other is also strongly recommended. Clinical psychopharmacologists, that includes all prescribers, should regularly track blood pressure, weight, and body mass index for most of their patients. The dutiful clinician will also check out the drug interactions of non-central nervous system (CNS) drugs with those that act in the CNS, including any prescribed by other clinicians with whom they should communicate.

Initiating certain drugs may be for experts only. These might include clozapine and monoamine oxidase (MAO) inhibitors, among others. Off-label uses not included in the BNF, inadequately studied doses or combinations of drugs may also be for the expert only, who can weigh risks and benefits in the presence of sometimes vague and conflicting evidence. Pregnant or nursing women, or individuals with the features of two or more psychiatric illnesses, substance abuse, and/or a concomitant medical illness may be suitable patients for the expert. Controlled substances also require expertise. Use your best judgement as to your level of expertise: we are all learning in this rapidly advancing field and all patients for whom we prescribe represent important n=1 trials from which we can enhance our knowledge. The practice of medicine is often not so much a science as it is an art. It is important to stay within the standards of medical care for the field and within your personal comfort zone. We hope that the medical students involved in compiling the *Guide* will have learned as much about this art as they have done about the science of psychopharmacology; this art includes supporting patients to make informed decisions just as it does expertise in drug prescribing.

Finally, this book is intended to be genuinely helpful for practitioners of psychopharmacology by providing them with the mixture of facts and opinions selected by the Editors. Ultimately, prescribing choices are the reader's responsibility. Every effort has been made in preparing this book to provide accurate and up-to-date information in accord with accepted standards and practice at the time of publication. Nevertheless, the psychopharmacology field is dynamic, and the Editors and publisher make no guarantees that the information contained herein is error-free. Furthermore, the Editors and publisher disclaim any responsibility for the continued currency of this information and disclaim all liability for any and all damages, including direct or consequential damages, resulting from the use of information contained in this book. Doctors recommending and patients using these drugs are strongly advised to consult and pay careful attention to information provided by the manufacturer.

List of icons

 How the drug works, mechanism of action

 Best augmenting agents to add for partial response or treatment resistance

 Life-threatening or dangerous side effects

unusual

not unusual

common

problematic

Weight Gain: Degrees of weight gain associated with the drug, with unusual signifying that weight gain has been reported but is not expected; not unusual signifying that weight gain occurs in a significant minority; common signifying that many experience weight gain and/or it can be significant in amount; and problematic signifying that weight gain occurs frequently, can be significant in amount, and may be a health problem in some patients

unusual

not unusual

common

problematic

Sedation: Degrees of sedation associated with the drug, with unusual signifying that sedation has been reported but is not expected; not unusual signifying that sedation occurs in a significant minority; common signifying that many experience sedation and/or it can be significant in amount; and problematic signifying that sedation occurs frequently, can be significant in amount, and may be a health problem in some patients

 Tips for dosing based on the clinical expertise of the author

 Drug interactions that may occur

 Warnings and precautions regarding use of the drug

 Dosing and other information specific to children and adolescents

 Information regarding use of the drug during pregnancy

Clinical pearls of information based on the clinical expertise of the author

List of icons

 The art of switching

 Suggested reading

List of contributors

Associate Editors

Veronika Dobler StateExamMed, PhD, MRCPsych, PGDipCBT Consultant Child & Adolescent Psychiatrist, Cambridgeshire and Peterborough NHS Foundation Trust

Liliana Galindo MBBS, MRCPsych, Consultant Psychiatrist & Medical Leader in Psychosis, Cambridgeshire and Peterborough NHS Foundation Trust, University of Cambridge

George Griffiths MPharm, PgDip, Cambridgeshire and Peterborough NHS Foundation Trust

Neil Hunt MA, MD, MRCPsych, Consultant Psychiatrist, Cambridge, Affiliated Assistant Professor, University of Cambridge

Mohammad Malkera MBBS, MRCPsych, Consultant Psychiatrist, Liaison Psychiatry, CPFT; Affiliated Assistant Professor, University of Cambridge

Asha Praseedom MBBS, MRCPsych, Consultant Psychiatrist & Associate Clinical Director, Cambridgeshire and Peterborough NHS Foundation Trust

Pranathi Ramachandra MBBS, MRCPsych, Consultant Psychiatrist, Cambridgeshire and Peterborough NHS Foundation Trust

Judy Rubinsztein MBChB, FRCPsych, PhD (Cantab), PGCert MedEd, Affiliated Assistant Professor, University of Cambridge

Shamim Ruhi MBBS, MRCPsych, Consultant Psychiatrist, Norfolk and Suffolk NHS Foundation Trust

Contributors

At the time of writing all contributors were medical students at the University of Cambridge

Lydia Akaje-Macauley

Olivia Baker

Sneha Barai

Sarah Bellis

Maria Eduarda Ferreira Bruco

Alisha Burman

Neil H. J. Cunningham

Fiona Kehinde

Keshini Kulathevanayagam

Katherine M. K. Lee

Jasmine Hughes

Chloe Legard

Lucy Mackie

Lorcán McKeown

Souradip Mookerjee

Juliette Murphy

Sohini Gajanan Pawar

Samuel Perkins

Roxanna Pourkarimi

Samuel Pulman

Innocent Ogunmwonyi

Louise Rockall

Irene Mateos Rodriguez

Tom Ronan

Colette Russell

Aryan Sabir

Pratyasha Saha

Smiji Saji

Lalana A. K. Songra

Tommy Sutton

Ada Ee Der Teo

Ravi Sureshkumar Thakar

Shentong Wang

James Wilkinson

THERAPEUTICS

Brands
- Campral EC

Generic?
Yes

Class
- Neuroscience-based nomenclature: pharmacology domain – glutamate; mode of action – unclear
- Alcohol dependence treatment; glutamate multimodal (Glu-MM)

Commonly Prescribed for
(bold for BNF indication)
- **Maintenance of abstinence in alcohol-dependence** (moderate-severe condition in combination with psychosocial interventions)

How the Drug Works
- Theoretically reduces excitatory glutamate neurotransmission and increases gamma-aminobutyric acid (GABA) to increase abstinence
- Binds to and blocks certain glutamate receptors, including metabotropic glutamate receptors
- Acts as a functional glutamatergic NMDA antagonist
- Because withdrawal of alcohol following chronic administration can lead to excessive glutamate activity and deficient GABA activity, acamprosate can act as "artificial alcohol" to mitigate these effects

How Long Until It Works
- Treatment duration of longer than 6 months suggested
- Has demonstrated efficacy in trials lasting between 13 and 52 weeks

If It Works
- Increases continuous/cumulative abstinence from alcohol

If It Doesn't Work
- Evaluate for and address contributing factors
- Consider switching to another agent, e.g. naltrexone or disulfiram
- Consider augmenting with naltrexone

Best Augmenting Combos for Partial Response or Treatment Resistance
- Naltrexone
- Augmenting therapy may be more effective than monotherapy
- Use in combination with individual psychological interventions (CBT, behavioural therapy, social network/environment-based therapies)

Tests
- Baseline urea and electrolytes, liver function (including gamma-glutamyl transferase)
- Follow-up blood tests: liver function to check on recovery and to increase motivation

SIDE EFFECTS

How Drug Causes Side Effects
- Theoretically, behavioural side effects are due to changes in neurotransmitter concentrations at receptors in parts of the brain and body other than those that cause therapeutic actions
- Gastrointestinal side effects may be related to large doses of a drug that is an amino acid derivative, increasing osmotic absorption in the gastrointestinal tract

Notable Side Effects
- Diarrhoea, nausea
- Anxiety, depression

Common or very common
- GIT: abdominal pain, diarrhoea, flatulence, nausea, vomiting
- Other: sexual dysfunction, skin reactions

Life-Threatening or Dangerous Side Effects
- Suicidal ideation and behaviour (suicidality)

Weight Gain

unusual   not unusual   common   problematic

- Reported but not expected

Acamprosate calcium (Continued)

Sedation

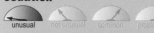
unusual | not unusual | common | problematic

- Reported but not expected

What to Do About Side Effects

- Wait
- Adjust the dose
- If side effects persist, discontinue use

Best Augmenting Agents for Side Effects

- Dose reduction or switching to another agent may be more effective since most side effects cannot be improved with an augmenting agent

DOSING AND USE

Usual Dosage Range

- Adult (body weight <60 kg): 666 mg in the morning, and 333 mg at midday and at night time
- Adult (body weight ≥ 60 kg): 666 mg 3 times per day

Dosage Forms

- Tablet 333 mg

How to Dose

* Maintenance of abstinence in alcohol dependence:
- Patients should begin treatment as soon as possible after achieving detoxification
- Some evidence suggests can be started during detoxification for neuroprotection
- Recommended dose is 666 mg 3 times daily, titration is not required

 Dosing Tips

- Provide psychosocial intervention in combination with acamprosate treatment to increase the chances of success
- Stop if drinking persists 4 to 6 weeks after starting the drug
- Stay under supervision at least monthly for 6 months, then less frequently if taking more than 6 months
- Although absorption of acamprosate is not affected by food, it may aid adherence if patients who regularly eat three meals per day take each dose with a meal
- Adherence with the 3-times-daily dosing can be a problem; having patient focus on frequent oral dosing of drug rather than frequent drinking may be helpful in some patients

Overdose

- Acute overdose can lead to persistent diarrhoea

Long-Term Use

- Should be prescribed for 6 months or longer (licensed for 1 year)
- Has been studied in trials for up to 1 year

Habit Forming

- No

How to Stop

- Taper not necessary

Pharmacokinetics

- Bioavailability reduced when taken with food
- Terminal half-life about 20–33 hours
- Excreted mostly unchanged via kidneys

 Drug Interactions

- Does not inhibit hepatic enzymes, and this is unlikely to affect plasma concentrations of drugs metabolised by those enzymes
- Is not hepatically metabolised and thus is unlikely to be affected by drugs that induce or inhibit hepatic enzymes
- Concomitant administration with naltrexone may increase plasma levels of acamprosate but this does not appear to be clinically significant and dose adjustment is not recommended

 Other Warnings/Precautions

- Monitor patients for emergence of depressed mood or suicidal ideation and behaviour (suicidality)
- Use cautiously in individuals with known psychiatric illness
- Continued alcohol abuse – risk of treatment failure

Do Not Use

- If the patient has severe renal impairment
- If the patient has severe hepatic impairment
- If there is a proven allergy to acamprosate

Renal Impairment
- For moderate impairment, recommended dose is 333 mg 3 times per day
- Contraindicated in severe impairment

Hepatic Impairment
- Dose adjustment not generally necessary
- Avoid in severe liver impairment

Cardiac Impairment
- Limited data available

Elderly
- Some patients may tolerate lower doses better
- Consider monitoring renal function

Children and Adolescents
- Safety and efficacy have not been established

Pregnancy
- Controlled studies have not been conducted in pregnant women
- In animal studies, acamprosate demonstrated teratogenicity in doses approximately equal to the human dose (rat studies) and in doses about 3 times the human dose (rabbit studies)
- Pregnant women needing to stop drinking may consider behavioural therapy before pharmacotherapy
- Not generally recommended for use during pregnancy, especially during first trimester
- Alcohol is a confirmed teratogen and therefore acamprosate use during pregnancy may be considered beneficial in some cases

Breastfeeding
- No evidence of safety
- Long half-life increases the risk of accumulation in the breastfed infant
- Low levels anticipated in milk due to low oral absorption
- Benefit of the mother abstaining from alcohol to the infant may outweigh the risk to the infant of acamprosate

Potential Advantages
- Individuals who have recently abstained from alcohol
- For the chronic, daily drinker
- It works as well as naltrexone for maintenance of abstinence from alcohol

Potential Disadvantages
- Individuals who are not abstinent at time of treatment initiation
- For binge drinkers
- Naltrexone works slightly better for reducing cravings for alcohol and heavy drinking

Primary Target Symptoms
- Alcohol dependence

Pearls
- Because acamprosate serves as "artificial alcohol", it may be less effective in situations in which the individual has not yet abstained from alcohol or suffers a relapse
- Thus, acamprosate may be a preferred treatment if the goal is complete abstinence but may not be preferred if the goal is reduced-risk drinking
- Studies have found that acamprosate works best when used in combination with psychosocial support since the drug facilitates a reduction in alcohol consumption as well as full abstinence
- Over 3 to 12 months it increases the number of people who do not drink at all and the number of days without alcohol
- It appears to work as well as naltrexone for maintenance of abstinence from alcohol, however, naltrexone works slightly better for reducing cravings for alcohol and heavy drinking
- Some evidence suggests that acamprosate is neuroprotective (it protects neurons from damage and death caused by the effects of alcohol withdrawal, and possibly other causes of neurotoxicity)

Suggested Reading

De Witte P, Littleton J, Parot P, et al. Neuroprotective and abstinence-promoting effects of acamprosate: elucidating the mechanism of action. CNS Drugs 2005;19(6):517–37.

Kiefer F, Jahn H, Tarnaske T, et al. Comparing and combining naltrexone and acamprosate in relapse prevention of alcoholism: a double-blind, placebo-controlled study. Arch Gen Psychiatry 2003;60:92–9.

Kranzler HR, Soyka M. Diagnosis and pharmacotherapy of alcohol use disorder: a review. JAMA 2018;320(8):815–24.

Lingford-Hughes AR, Welch S, Peters L, et al. BAP updated guidelines: evidence-based guidelines for the pharmacological management of substance abuse, harmful use, addiction and comorbidity: recommendations from BAP. J Psychopharmacol 2012;26(7):899–952.

Maisel NC, Blodgett JC, Wilbourne PL, Humphreys K, Finney JW. Meta-analysis of naltrexone and acamprosate for treating alcohol use disorders: when are these medications most helpful? Addiction 2013;108(2):275–93.

Mann K, Kiefer F, Spanagel R, et al. Acamprosate: recent findings and future research directions. Alcohol Clin Exp Res 2008;32(7):1105–10.

Mason BJ, Heyser CJ. The neurobiology, clinical efficacy and safety of acamprosate in the treatment of alcohol dependence. Expert Opin Drug Saf 2010;9(1):177–88.

Nutt DJ. Doing it by numbers: a simple approach to reducing the harms of alcohol. J Psychopharmacol 2014;28(1):3–7.

Pilling S, Yesufu-Udechuku A, Taylor C, et al. Diagnosis, assessment, and management of harmful drinking and alcohol dependence: summary of NICE guidance. BMJ 2011;342:d700.

Plosker GL. Acamprosate: a review of its use in alcohol dependence. Drugs 2015;75(11):1255–68.

Agomelatine

THERAPEUTICS

Brands
• Valdoxan

Generic?
Yes

Class
• Neuroscience-based nomenclature: pharmacology domain – melatonin, serotonin; mode of action – agonist and antagonist
• Agonist at melatonin 1 and melatonin 2 receptors
• Antagonist at 5HT2B and 5HT2C receptors

Commonly Prescribed for
(bold for BNF indication)
• **Major depression**
• Generalised anxiety disorder

 How the Drug Works
• Actions at both melatonin and 5HT2C receptors may be synergistic and increase noradrenaline and dopamine neurotransmission in the prefrontal cortex; may resynchronise circadian rhythms that are disturbed in depression
• No influence on extracellular levels of serotonin

How Long Until It Works
• Daytime functioning, anhedonia, and sleep can improve from the first week of treatment
• Onset of full therapeutic actions in depression is usually not immediate, but often delayed 2–4 weeks
• May continue to work for many years to prevent relapse of symptoms

If It Works
• The goal of treatment is complete remission of current symptoms as well as prevention of future relapses
• Treatment most often reduces or even eliminates symptoms, but is not a cure since symptoms can recur after medicine is stopped
• Continue treatment until all symptoms are gone (remission)
• Once symptoms are gone, continue treating for at least 6–9 months for the first episode of depression or >12 months if relapse indicators present
• If >5 episodes and/or 2 episodes in the last few years then need to continue for at least 2 years or indefinitely

If It Doesn't Work
• Many patients have only a partial response where some symptoms are improved but others persist (especially insomnia, fatigue, and problems concentrating)
• Other patients may be non-responders, sometimes called treatment-resistant or treatment-refractory
• Consider increasing dose as early as 2 weeks after initiating treatment if response is insufficient (decision on dose increase has to be balanced with a higher risk of transaminase elevation; dose increases should be made on an individual patient benefit/risk basis and with mandated liver function tests monitoring)
• Consider switching to another agent or adding an appropriate augmenting agent
• Consider psychotherapy
• Consider diagnosis or whether there is a co-morbid condition (e.g. medical illness, substance abuse, etc.)
• Some patients may experience lack of consistent efficacy due to the diagnosis actually being of a bipolar disorder, and require antidepressant discontinuation and consideration of a mood stabiliser or bipolar depression treatment

Best Augmenting Combos for Partial Response or Treatment Resistance
• SSRIs (excluding fluvoxamine), SNRIs, bupropion (use combinations of antidepressants with caution as this may activate bipolar disorder and suicidal ideation or agitation)
• Mood stabilisers or atypical antipsychotics for bipolar depression, psychotic depression, or treatment-resistant depression
• Modafinil, especially for fatigue, sleepiness, and lack of concentration
• Benzodiazepines

Tests
• Liver function tests before initiation of treatment and then at 3, 6, 12, and 24

weeks, and thereafter when clinically indicated
- When increasing the dose, liver function tests should be performed at the same frequency as when initiating treatment
- Liver function tests should be repeated within 48 hours in any patient who develops raised transaminases

SIDE EFFECTS

How Drug Causes Side Effects
- Adverse reactions usually mild to moderate and occur within the first 2 weeks of treatment
- Actions at melatonin receptors and at 5HT2C receptors could contribute to the side effects described below

Notable Side Effects
- Nausea and dizziness

Common or very common
- CNS: anxiety, dizziness, drowsiness, headaches, sleep disorders
- GIT: abdominal pain, constipation, diarrhoea, nausea, vomiting, weight changes
- Other: back pain, fatigue

Uncommon
- Aggression, altered mood, blurred vision, confusion, hyperhidrosis, movement disorders, paraesthesia, skin reactions, suicidal tendencies, tinnitus

Rare or very rare
- Angioedema, facial oedema, hallucination, hepatic disorders, urinary retention

 Life-Threatening or Dangerous Side Effects
- Rare hepatitis, hepatic failure
- Theoretically, rare induction of mania
- Rare activation of suicidal ideation and behaviour (suicidality) (short-term studies did not show an increase in the risk of suicidality with antidepressants compared to placebo beyond age 25)

Weight Gain

- Occurs in significant minority
- In clinical studies, weight changes were similar to those in placebo

- Cases of weight decrease have been reported

Sedation

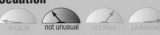
- Somnolence occurs in significant minority
- Generally transient
- May be more likely to cause fatigue than sedation

What to Do About Side Effects
- Wait (unless related to liver)
- Wait
- Stop if transaminase levels reach 3 times the upper limit of normal
- Switch to another drug

Best Augmenting Agents for Side Effects
- Often best to try another antidepressant monotherapy prior to resorting to augmentation strategies to treat side effects
- Many side effects are time-dependent (i.e. they start immediately upon dosing and upon each dose increase, but go away with time)
- Many side effects cannot be improved with an augmenting agent
- Theoretically activation and agitation may represent the induction of a bipolar state, especially a mixed dysphoric state sometimes associated with suicidal ideation, and require the addition of lithium, a mood stabiliser or an atypical antipsychotic, and/or discontinuation of agomelatine

DOSING AND USE

Usual Dosage Range
- Major depression: 25–50 mg/day at bedtime

Dosage Forms
- Tablet 25 mg

How to Dose
- Major depression: initial dose 25 mg/day at bedtime; after 2 weeks can increase to 50 mg/day at bedtime

 Dosing Tips
- If intolerable anxiety, insomnia, agitation, akathisia, or activation occur either upon dosing initiation or discontinuation,

consider the possibility of activated bipolar disorder and switch to a mood stabiliser or an atypical antipsychotic

Overdose
- Drowsiness and stomach pain, fatigue, agitation, anxiety, tension, dizziness, cyanosis, or malaise have been reported

Long-Term Use
- Treatment up to 12 months has been found to decrease rate of relapse

Habit Forming
- No

How to Stop
- No need to taper dose

Pharmacokinetics
- Oral bioavailability generally higher in women versus men
- Half-life 1–2 hours
- Metabolised primarily by CYP450 1A2 – dose adjustments may thus be necessary if smoking status changes

 Drug Interactions
- Use of agomelatine with potent CYP450 1A2 inhibitors (e.g. fluvoxamine) is contraindicated
- Liver metabolism of agomelatine is induced by smoking
- Tramadol increases the risk of seizures in patients taking an antidepressant (class warning)

 Other Warnings/Precautions
- Use with caution in patients with hepatic injury risk factors, such as obesity/overweight/non-alcoholic fatty liver disease, diabetes, patients who drink large quantities of alcohol and/or have alcohol use disorder, or who take medication associated with risk of hepatic injury. Doctors should ask their patients if they have ever had liver problems
- Patients should be informed to seek immediate medical review if they experience symptoms related to liver disorder such as abdominal pain, bruising, dark urine, fatigue, jaundice, light-coloured stools, or pruritus
- Patients should be given a booklet with more information on the risk of hepatic side effects

- Use caution in patients with pre-treatment elevated transaminases (> the upper limit of the normal range and < 3 times the upper limit of the normal range)
- Discontinue treatment if serum transaminases increase to 3 times the upper limit of normal; liver function tests should be performed regularly until serum transaminases return to normal
- Use with caution in patients with bipolar disorder or presenting in a hypomanic or manic state unless treated with concomitant mood-stabilising agent
- Warn patients and their caregivers about the possibility of activating side effects and advise them to report such symptoms immediately
- Monitor patients for activation of suicidal ideation, especially those below the age of 25

Do Not Use
- If patient has hepatic impairment
- If patient has transaminase levels > 3 times the upper limit of normal
- If patient is taking a potent CYP450 1A2 inhibitor (e.g. fluvoxamine, ciprofloxacin)
- If patient is taking MAO inhibitor (MAOI)
- If patient has galactose intolerance, Lapp lactase deficiency, or glucose-galactose malabsorption
- If patient has dementia
- If patient is over 75 years of age
- If there is a proven allergy to agomelatine

SPECIAL POPULATIONS

Renal Impairment
- Drug should be used with caution in moderate to severe impairment

Hepatic Impairment
- Avoid in hepatic impairment or if transaminases exceed 3 times the upper limit of normal

Cardiac Impairment
- Dose adjustment not necessary

Elderly
- Efficacy and safety have been established (< 75 years old)
- Dose adjustment not necessary
- Should not be used in patients aged 75 years and older

Agomelatine (Continued)

- Should not be used in elderly patients with dementia

Children and Adolescents

- Safety and efficacy have not been established and not recommended

Pregnancy

- Controlled studies have not been conducted in pregnant women
- Not generally recommended for use during pregnancy, especially during first trimester
- Must weigh the risk of treatment (first trimester foetal development, third trimester newborn delivery) to the child against the risk of no treatment (recurrence of depression, maternal health, infant bonding) to the mother and child
- For many patients this may mean continuing treatment during pregnancy

Breastfeeding

- Low levels anticipated in milk
- Extremely limited evidence of safety
- Monitor the infant for drowsiness, feeding difficulties and behavioural effects
- Immediate postpartum period is a high-risk time for depression, especially in women who have had prior depressive episodes, antidepressants may need to be reinstituted late in the third trimester or shortly after childbirth to prevent a recurrence during the postpartum period
- Must weigh benefits of breastfeeding with risks and benefits of antidepressant treatment versus nontreatment to both the infant and the mother
- For many patients this may mean continuing treatment during breastfeeding
- Other antidepressants may be preferable, e.g. paroxetine, sertraline, imipramine, or nortriptyline

THE ART OF PSYCHOPHARMACOLOGY

Potential Advantages

- Patients with lack of energy, anhedonia, anxious co-morbidity, and sleep-wake disturbances
- Patients particularly concerned about sexual side effects or weight gain

Potential Disadvantages

- Patients with hepatic impairment

Primary Target Symptoms

- Depressed mood, anhedonia
- Functioning
- Anxiety with depression

Pearls

- Agomelatine tends to be a third-choice antidepressant. It represents a novel approach to depression through a novel pharmacologic profile, agonist at melatonin MT1/MT2 receptors and antagonist at 5HT2C receptors acting synergistically
- This synergy provides agomelatine with a distinctive efficacy profile, different from conventional antidepressants with potentially an early and continuous improvement over time
- Agomelatine improves anhedonia early in treatment
- Improves anxiety in major depressive disorder
- May be fewer withdrawals/discontinuations for adverse events than with other antidepressants
- No significant effect on cardiac parameters such as blood pressure and heart rate
- Some data suggest that agomelatine may be especially efficacious in achieving functional remission
- Agomelatine may improve sleep quality by promoting proper maintenance of circadian rhythms underlying a normal sleep-wake cycle

📖 Suggested Reading

Carvalho AF, Sharma MS, Brunoni AR, et al. The safety, tolerability and risks associated with the use of newer generation antidepressant drugs: a critical review of the literature. Psycother Psychosom 2016;85(5):270–88.

Cipriani A, Furukawa TA, Salanti G, et al. Comparative efficacy and acceptability of 21 antidepressant drugs for the acute treatment of adults with major depressive disorder: a systematic review and network meta-analysis. Lancet 2018;391(10128):1357–66.

Agomelatine (Continued)

DeBodinat C, Guardiola-Lemaitre B, Mocaer E, et al. Agomelatine, the first melatonergic antidepressant: discovery, characterization, and development. Nat Rev Drug Discov 2010;9:628–42.

Goodwin GM, Emsley R, Rembry S, Rouillon F. Agomelatine prevents relapse in patients with major depressive disorder without evidence of a discontinuation syndrome: a 24-week randomized, double-blind, placebo-controlled trial. J Clin Psychiatry 2009;70:1128–37.

Kennedy SH, Avedisova A, Belai'di C, et al. Sustained efficacy of agomelatine 10 mg, 25 mg, and 25–50 mg on depressive symptoms and functional outcomes in patients with major depressive disorder. A placebo-controlled study over 6 months. Neuropsychopharmacol 2016;26(2):378–89.

Stahl SM. Mechanism of action of agomelatine: a novel antidepressant exploiting synergy between monoaminergic and melatonergic properties. CNS Spectrums 2014;19:207–12.

Stahl SM, Fava M, Trivedi M, et al. Agomelatine in the treatment of major depressive disorder. An 8 week, multicenter, randomized, placebo-controlled trial. J Clin Psychiatry 2010;71(5):616–26.

Stein DJ, Picarel-Blanchot F, Kennedy SH. Efficacy of the novel antidepressant agomelatine on anxiety symptoms in major depression. Hum Psychopharmacol 2013;28(2):151–9.

Taylor D, Sparshatt A, Varma S, et al. Antidepressant efficacy of agomelatine: meta-analysis of published and unpublished studies. BMJ 2014;348:g1888 (erratum in BMJ 2014;349:g2496).

Alprazolam

Brands
• Xanax

Generic?
No, not in UK

Class
• Neuroscience-based nomenclature: pharmacology domain – GABA; mode of action – benzodiazepine receptor agonist (non-selective GABA-A receptor positive allosteric modulator – PAM)
• Benzodiazepine (anxiolytic)

Commonly Prescribed for
(bold for BNF indication)
• **Anxiety (short-term use)**
• Generalised anxiety disorder
• Panic disorder
• Other anxiety disorders
• Anxiety associated with depression
• Premenstrual dysphoric disorder
• Irritable bowel syndrome and other somatic symptoms associated with anxiety disorders
• Insomnia
• Acute mania (adjunctive)
• Acute psychosis (adjunctive)
• Catatonia

 ## How the Drug Works
• Binds to benzodiazepine receptors at the GABA-A ligand-gated chloride channel complex
• Enhances the inhibitory effects of GABA
• Boosts chloride conductance through GABA-regulated channels
• Inhibits neuronal activity presumably in amygdala-centred fear circuits to provide therapeutic benefits in anxiety disorders

How Long Until It Works
• Some immediate relief with first dosing is common; can take several weeks with daily dosing for maximal therapeutic benefit

If It Works
• For short-term symptoms of anxiety or muscle spasms – after a few weeks, discontinue use or use on an "as-needed" basis
• For chronic anxiety disorders, the goal of treatment is complete remission of symptoms as well as prevention of future relapses
• For chronic anxiety disorders, treatment most often reduces or even eliminates symptoms, but is not a cure since symptoms can recur after medicine stopped
• For long-term symptoms of anxiety, consider switching to an SSRI or SNRI for long-term maintenance
• Avoid long-term maintenance with a benzodiazepine
• If symptoms re-emerge after stopping a benzodiazepine, consider treatment with an SSRI or SNRI, or consider restarting the benzodiazepine; sometimes benzodiazepines have to be used in combination with SSRIs or SNRIs at the start of treatment for best results

If It Doesn't Work
• Consider switching to another agent or adding an appropriate augmenting agent
• Consider psychotherapy, especially cognitive behavioural psychotherapy
• Consider presence of concomitant substance abuse
• Consider presence of alprazolam abuse
• Consider another diagnosis, such as a co-morbid medical condition

 ## Best Augmenting Combos for Partial Response or Treatment Resistance
• Benzodiazepines are frequently used as augmenting agents for antipsychotics and mood stabilisers in the treatment of psychotic and bipolar disorders
• Benzodiazepines are frequently used as augmenting agents for SSRIs and SNRIs in the treatment of anxiety disorders
• Not generally rational to combine with other benzodiazepines
• Caution if using as an anxiolytic concomitantly with other sedative hypnotics for sleep
• Could consider augmenting alprazolam with either gabapentin or pregabalin for treatment of anxiety disorders

Tests

- In patients with seizure disorders, concomitant medical illness, and/or those with multiple concomitant long-term medications, periodic liver tests and blood counts may be prudent

SIDE EFFECTS

How Drug Causes Side Effects

- Same mechanism for side effects as for therapeutic effects – namely due to excessive actions at benzodiazepine receptors
- Long-term adaptations in benzodiazepine receptors may explain the development of dependence, tolerance, and withdrawal
- Side effects are generally immediate, but immediate side effects often disappear in time

Notable Side Effects

* Sedation, fatigue, depression
* Dizziness, ataxia, slurred speech, weakness
* Forgetfulness, confusion
* Hyperexcitability, nervousness
- Rare hallucinations, mania
* Euphoria-like feelings, with high risk of drug misuse
* High risk of dependence and abuse potential
- Rare hypotension
- Hypersalivation, dry mouth

Common or very common

- CNS: impaired concentration, memory loss, movement disorders
- GIT: constipation, decreased appetite, dry mouth, weight changes
- Other: dermatitis, sexual dysfunction, tolerance and dependence

Uncommon

- Irregular menstruation, urinary incontinence

Frequency not known

- CNS: abnormal thinking, psychosis, suicide
- GIT: gastrointestinal disorder, hepatic disorders
- Other: angioedema, autonomic dysfunction, hyperprolactinaemia, peripheral oedema, photosensitivity reaction

 Life-Threatening or Dangerous Side Effects

- Respiratory depression, especially when taken with CNS depressants in overdose

- Hepatic dysfunction, renal dysfunction, blood dyscrasias

Weight Gain

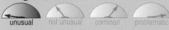

- Reported but not expected

Sedation

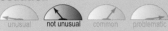

- Occurs in significant minority
- Especially at initiation of treatment or when dose increases
- Tolerance often develops over time

What to Do About Side Effects

- Wait
- Wait
- Wait
- Lower the dose
- Take largest dose at bedtime to avoid sedative effects during the day
- Switch to another agent
- Administer flumazenil if side effects are severe or life-threatening

Best Augmenting Agents for Side Effects

- Many side effects cannot be improved with an augmenting agent

DOSING AND USE

Usual Dosage Range

* Short-term use in anxiety:
- Adult: 750 mcg/day in divided doses – 1.5 mg/day in divided doses, increased as needed up to 3 mg/day in divided doses
- Elderly/debilitated patients: 500 mcg/day in divided doses – 750 mcg/day in divided doses, increased as needed up to 3 mg/day in divided doses

Dosage Forms

- Tablet 250 mcg, 500 mcg

How to Dose

- Short-term use in anxiety:
- Adult: 250–500 mcg 3 times per day, increased as needed up to a total dose of 3 mg/day in divided doses; for debilitated patients use recommended elderly dose

- Elderly: 250 mcg 2–3 times per day, increased as needed up to a total dose of 3 mg/day in divided doses

Dosing Tips

- Use lowest possible effective dose for the shortest period of time (a benzodiazepine-sparing strategy)
- Tolerance will develop to the sedative-hypnotic effects within days of continuous use
- Assess need for continuous treatment regularly
- Risk of dependence may increase with dose and duration of treatment. Consider long-acting benzodiazepines instead
- For inter-dose symptoms of anxiety, can either increase dose or maintain same daily dose but divide into more frequent doses
- Can also use an as-needed occasional "top-up" dose for inter-dose anxiety
- Frequency of dosing in practice is often more than predicted from half-life as duration of biological activity is often shorter than pharmacokinetic terminal half-life
- *Alprazolam is generally dosed twice the dosage of clonazepam
- Alprazolam 1 mg = diazepam 10 mg

Overdose

- Fatalities have been reported both in monotherapy and in conjunction with alcohol; sedation, confusion, poor coordination, diminished reflexes, coma

Long-Term Use

- Risk of dependence, particularly for treatment periods longer than 12 weeks and especially in patients with past or current polysubstance abuse

Habit Forming

- Alprazolam is a Class C/Schedule 4 drug
- Patients may develop dependence and/or tolerance with long-term use

How to Stop

- The fast onset, the peak of the euphoria-like effects and the short duration increase the risk of tolerance, abuse and dependence. Alprazolam is one of the most commonly misused benzodiazepines
- Alprazolam is the sedative drug most commonly sold illegally for recreational use

- Patients with history of seizure may seize upon withdrawal, especially if withdrawal is abrupt
- Taper by 0.5 mg every 3 days to reduce chances of withdrawal effects
- For difficult to taper cases, consider reducing dose much more slowly after reaching 3 mg/day, perhaps by as little as 0.25 mg every week or less
- For other patients with severe problems discontinuing a benzodiazepine, dosing may need to be tapered over many months (i.e. reduce dose by 1% every 3 days by crushing tablet and suspending or dissolving in 100 mL of fruit juice and then disposing of 1 mL while drinking the rest; 3–7 days later, dispose of 2 mL, and so on). This is both a form of very slow biological tapering and a form of behavioural desensitisation
- Be sure to differentiate re-emergence of symptoms requiring reinstitution of treatment from withdrawal symptoms
- Benzodiazepine-dependent anxiety patients and insulin-dependent diabetics are not addicted to their medications. When benzodiazepine-dependent patients stop their medication, disease symptoms can re-emerge, disease symptoms can worsen (rebound), and/or withdrawal symptoms can emerge

Pharmacokinetics

- Metabolised by CYP450 3A4
- Inactive metabolites
- Mean half-life 12–15 hours
- Food does not affect absorption

Drug Interactions

- Increased depressive side effects when taken with other CNS depressants
- Inhibitors of CYP450 3A, such as fluvoxamine, fluoxetine and grapefruit juice may decrease clearance of alprazolam and thereby raise alprazolam plasma levels and enhance sedative side effects; alprazolam dose may need to be lowered
- Thus, azole antifungals (e.g. ketoconazole), macrolide antibiotics and protease inhibitors may also raise alprazolam levels
- Inducers of CYP450 3A, such as carbamazepine, may increase clearance of alprazolam and lower alprazolam plasma levels and possibly reduce therapeutic effects

Other Warnings/Precautions

- Warning regarding the increased risk of CNS-depressant effects when benzodiazepines and opioid medications are used together, including specifically the risk of slowed or difficulty breathing and death
- If alternatives to the combined use of benzodiazepines and opioids are not available, clinicians should limit the dosage and duration of each drug to the minimum possible while still achieving therapeutic efficacy
- Patients and their caregivers should be warned to seek medical attention if unusual dizziness, light-headedness, sedation, slowed or difficulty breathing, or unresponsiveness occur
- Dosage changes should be made in collaboration with prescriber
- History of drug or alcohol abuse often creates greater risk for dependency
- Some depressed patients may experience a worsening of suicidal ideation
- Some patients may exhibit abnormal thinking or behavioural changes similar to those caused by other CNS depressants (i.e. either depressant actions or disinhibiting actions)
- Avoid prolonged use and abrupt cessation
- Use lower doses in debilitated patients and the elderly
- Use with caution in patients with myasthenia gravis; respiratory disease
- Use with caution in patients with personality disorder (dependent/avoidant or anankastic types) as may increase risk of dependence
- Use with great caution in patients with a history of alcohol or drug dependence/abuse, alternatives preferred
- Benzodiazepines may cause a range of paradoxical effects including aggression, antisocial behaviours, anxiety, overexcitement, perceptual abnormalities, and talkativeness. Adjustment of dose may reduce impulses
- Use with caution as alprazolam can cause muscle weakness and organic brain changes

Do Not Use

- If patient has acute pulmonary insufficiency, respiratory depression, significant neuromuscular respiratory weakness, sleep apnoea syndrome, or unstable myasthenia gravis
- Alone in chronic psychosis in adults
- On its own to try to treat depression, anxiety associated with depression, obsessional states or phobic states
- If patient has angle-closure glaucoma
- If there is a proven allergy to alprazolam or any benzodiazepine

SPECIAL POPULATIONS

Renal Impairment

- Increased cerebral sensitivity to benzodiazepines
- Consider dose reduction

Hepatic Impairment

- Caution in mild-moderate impairment
- If treatment is necessary, benzodiazepines with shorter half-life are safer, such as temazepam or oxazepam
- Avoid in severe impairment

Cardiac Impairment

- Benzodiazepines have been used to treat anxiety associated with acute myocardial infarction

Elderly

- Elderly: 250 mcg 2–3 times per day, increased as needed up to 3 mg per day

 Children and Adolescents

- Safety and efficacy not established
- Not indicated for use in children
- Long-term effects of alprazolam in children/adolescents are unknown

 Pregnancy

- Possible increased risk of birth defects when benzodiazepines taken during pregnancy
- Because of the potential risks, alprazolam is not generally recommended as treatment for anxiety during pregnancy, especially during the first trimester
- Drug should be tapered if discontinued
- Infants whose mothers received a benzodiazepine late in pregnancy may experience withdrawal effects

- Neonatal flaccidity has been reported in infants whose mothers took a benzodiazepine during pregnancy
- Seizures, even mild seizures, may cause harm to the embryo/foetus

Breastfeeding

- Some drug is found in mother's breast milk
- Effects of benzodiazepines on infant have been observed and include feeding difficulties, sedation, and weight loss
- Caution should be taken with the use of benzodiazepines in breastfeeding mothers, seek to use low doses for short periods to reduce infant exposure
- Use of short-acting agents, e.g. oxazepam or lorazepam, preferred

THE ART OF PSYCHOPHARMACOLOGY

Potential Advantages

- Rapid onset of action
- Less sedation than some other benzodiazepines

Potential Disadvantages

- Euphoria may lead to abuse
- Abuse especially risky in past or present substance abusers

Primary Target Symptoms

- Panic attacks
- Anxiety

Pearls

- Very high risk of tolerance, dependence, and abuse. "Xanax pills" are one of the most popular prescription drugs sold on the black market worldwide

- Not prescribed in NHS primary care
- Can be a useful adjunct to SSRIs and SNRIs in the treatment of numerous anxiety disorders, but not used as frequently as other benzodiazepines for this purpose
- Not effective for treating psychosis as a monotherapy, but can be used as an adjunct to antipsychotics
- Not effective for treating bipolar disorder as a monotherapy, but can be used as an adjunct to mood stabilisers and antipsychotics
- May both cause depression and treat depression in different patients
- Risk of seizure is greatest during the first 3 days after discontinuation of alprazolam, especially in those with prior seizures, head injuries, or withdrawal from drugs of abuse
- Clinical duration of action may be shorter than plasma half-life, leading to dosing more frequently than 2–3 times per day in some patients
- Adding fluoxetine or fluvoxamine can increase alprazolam levels and make the patient very sleepy unless the alprazolam dose is lowered by half or more
- When using to treat insomnia, remember that insomnia may be a symptom of some other primary disorder itself, and thus warrant evaluation for co-morbid psychiatric and/or medical conditions
- Though not systematically studied, benzodiazepines have been used effectively to treat catatonia and are the initial recommended treatment

---

Suggested Reading

Ait-Daoud N, Hamby AS, Sharma S, et al. A review of alprazolam use, misuse, and withdrawal. J Addict Med 2018;12(1):4–10.

De Vane CL, Ware MR, Lydiard RB. Pharmacokinetics, pharmacodynamics, and treatment issues of benzodiazepines: alprazolam, adinazolam, and clonazepam. Psychopharmacol Bull 1991;27(4):463–73.

Greenblatt DJ, Wright CE. Clinical pharmacokinetics of alprazolam. Therapeutic implications. Clin Pharmacokinet 1993;24(6):453–71.

Jonas JM, Cohon MS. A comparison of the safety and efficacy of alprazolam versus other agents in the treatment of anxiety, panic, and depression: a review of the literature. J Clin Psychiatry 1993;54 Suppl:25–45; discussion 46–8.

Amisulpride

THERAPEUTICS

Brands
• Solian

Generic?
Yes

Class
• Neuroscience-based nomenclature: low-dose amisulpride: pharmacology domain – dopamine; mode of action – presynaptic antagonist; upper-dose amisulpride: pharmacology domain – dopamine; mode of action – antagonist
• Atypical antipsychotic (benzamide; possibly a dopamine stabiliser and dopamine partial agonist)

Commonly Prescribed for
(bold for BNF indication)
• **Acute psychotic episode in schizophrenia**
• **Schizophrenia with predominantly negative symptoms**
• Dysthymia

 How the Drug Works
• Theoretically blocks presynaptic dopamine 2 receptors at low doses
• Theoretically blocks postsynaptic dopamine 2 receptors at higher doses, particularly blocking receptors in the limbic system rather than those in the striatum
∗ May be a partial agonist at dopamine 2 receptors, which would theoretically reduce dopamine output when dopamine concentrations are high and increase dopamine output when dopamine concentrations are low
• Blocks dopamine 3 receptors, which may contribute to its clinical actions
∗ Unlike other atypical antipsychotics, amisulpride does not have potent actions at serotonin 2A, serotonin 1A, histamine H1, or alpha adrenergic receptors
∗ Does have antagonist actions at serotonin 7 receptors and serotonin 2B receptors, which may contribute to antidepressant effects

How Long Until It Works
• Psychotic symptoms can improve within 1 week, but it may take several weeks for full effect on behaviour as well as on cognition and affective stabilisation
• Classically recommended to wait at least 4–6 weeks to determine efficacy of drug, but in practice some patients require up to 16–20 weeks to show a good response, especially on cognitive symptoms

If It Works
• Most often reduces positive symptoms in schizophrenia but does not eliminate them
• Can improve negative symptoms, as well as aggressive, cognitive, and affective symptoms in schizophrenia
• Most patients with schizophrenia do not have a total remission of symptoms but rather a reduction of symptoms by about a third
• Perhaps 5–15% of patients with schizophrenia can experience an overall improvement of >50–60%, especially when receiving stable treatment for >1 year
• Such patients are considered super-responders or "awakeners" since they may be well enough to be employed, live independently, and sustain long-term relationships
• Continue treatment until reaching a plateau of improvement
• After reaching a satisfactory plateau, continue treatment for at least 1 year after first episode of psychosis, but it may be preferable to continue treatment indefinitely to avoid subsequent episodes
• After any subsequent episodes of psychosis, treatment may need to be indefinite

If It Doesn't Work
• Try one of the other atypical antipsychotics (risperidone or olanzapine should be considered first before considering other agents such as quetiapine, aripiprazole, or lurasidone)
• If two or more antipsychotic monotherapies do not work, consider clozapine
• Some patients may require treatment with a typical antipsychotic
• If no atypical antipsychotic is effective, consider higher doses or augmentation with valproate or lamotrigine
• Consider non-concordance and switch to another antipsychotic with fewer side effects or to an antipsychotic that can be given by depot injection
• Consider initiating rehabilitation and psychotherapy such as cognitive remediation
• Consider presence of concomitant drug abuse

Best Augmenting Combos for Partial Response or Treatment Resistance

- Valproic acid (Depakote or Epilim)
- Other mood-stabilising anticonvulsants (carbamazepine, oxcarbazepine, lamotrigine)
- Lithium
- Benzodiazepines
- Augmentation of amisulpride has not been systematically studied

Tests

Before starting an atypical antipsychotic

*Measure weight, BMI, and waist circumference
- Get baseline personal and family history of diabetes, obesity, dyslipidaemia, hypertension, and cardiovascular disease
*Check pulse and blood pressure, fasting plasma glucose or glycosylated haemoglobin (HbA1c), fasting lipid profile, and prolactin levels
- Full blood count (FBC), urea and electrolytes (including creatinine and eGFR), liver function tests (LFTs)
- Assessment of nutritional status, diet, and level of physical activity
- Determine if the patient:
  - is overweight (BMI 25.0–29.9)
  - is obese (BMI ≥30)
  - has pre-diabetes – fasting plasma glucose: 5.5 mmol/L to 6.9 mmol/L or HbA1c: 42 to 47 mmol/mol (6.0 to 6.4%)
  - has diabetes – fasting plasma glucose: >7.0 mmol/L or HbA1c: ≥48 mmol/L (≥6.5%)
  - has hypertension (BP >140/90 mm Hg)
  - has dyslipidaemia (increased total cholesterol, LDL cholesterol, and triglycerides; decreased HDL cholesterol)
- Treat or refer such patients for treatment, including nutrition and weight management, physical activity counselling, smoking cessation, and medical management
- Baseline ECG for: inpatients; those with a personal history or risk factor for cardiac disease

Monitoring after starting an atypical antipsychotic

- FBC annually to detect chronic bone marrow suppression, stop treatment if neutrophils fall below 1.5×10^9/L and refer to specialist care if neutrophils fall below 0.5×10^9/L
- Urea and electrolytes (including creatinine and eGFR) annually
- LFTs annually
- Prolactin levels at 6 months and then annually (amisulpride is likely to increase prolactin levels)
*Weight/BMI/waist circumference, weekly for the first 6 weeks, then at 12 weeks, at 1 year, and then annually
*Pulse and blood pressure at 12 weeks, 1 year, and then annually
*Fasting blood glucose, HbA1c, and blood lipids at 12 weeks, at 1 year, and then annually
*For patients with type 2 diabetes, measure HbA1c at 3–6 month intervals until stable, then every 6 months
*Even in patients without known diabetes, be vigilant for the rare but life-threatening onset of diabetic ketoacidosis, which always requires immediate treatment, by monitoring for the rapid onset of polyuria, polydipsia, weight loss, nausea, vomiting, dehydration, rapid respiration, weakness and clouding of sensorium, even coma
- If HbA1c remains ≥48 mmol/mol (6.5%) then drug therapy should be offered, e.g. metformin
- Treat or refer for treatment or consider switching to another atypical antipsychotic for patients who become overweight, obese, pre-diabetic, diabetic, hypertensive, or dyslipidaemic while receiving an atypical antipsychotic (these problems are relatively less likely with amisulpride)

SIDE EFFECTS

How Drug Causes Side Effects

- By blocking dopamine 2 receptors in the striatum, it can cause motor side effects, especially at high doses
- By blocking dopamine 2 receptors in the pituitary, it can cause elevations in prolactin
- Mechanism of weight gain and possible increased incidence of diabetes and dyslipidaemia with atypical antipsychotics is unknown

Notable Side Effects

*Extrapyramidal symptoms
*Galactorrhoea, amenorrhoea

- Insomnia, sedation, agitation, anxiety
- Constipation
- Rare tardive dyskinesia

Common or very common
- CNS: anxiety, oculogyric crisis
- Other: breast pain, hypersalivation, muscle rigidity, nausea, sexual dysfunction (abnormal orgasm), trismus

Uncommon
- Reduced glycaemic control (hyperglycaemia)

Frequency not known
- CNS: blurred vision, confusion
- CVS: cardiac arrest
- Skin: angioedema, urticaria
- Other: bone disorders, dyslipidaemia, hyponatraemia, nasal congestion, neoplasms, SIADH

 Life-Threatening or Dangerous Side Effects
- Rare seizures
- Dose-dependent QTc prolongation
- Increased risk of death and cerebrovascular events in elderly patients with dementia-related psychosis

Weight Gain

- Occurs in significant minority

Sedation

- Many experience and/or can be significant in amount, especially at high doses

What to Do About Side Effects
- Wait
- Wait
- Wait
- Reduce the dose
- Low-dose benzodiazepine or beta blocker may reduce akathisia
- Take more of the dose at bedtime to help reduce daytime sedation
- Weight loss, exercise programmes, and medical management for high BMIs, diabetes, and dyslipidaemia
- Switch to another antipsychotic (atypical) – quetiapine or clozapine are best in cases of tardive dyskinesia

Best Augmenting Agents for Side Effects
- Dystonia: antimuscarinic drugs (e.g. procyclidine) as oral or IM depending on the severity; botulinum toxin if antimuscarinics not effective
- Parkinsonism: antimuscarinic drugs (e.g. procyclidine)
- Akathisia: beta blocker propranolol (30–80 mg/day) or low-dose benzodiazepine (e.g. 0.5–3.0 mg/day of clonazepam) may help; other agents that may be tried include the 5HT2 antagonists such as cyproheptadine (16 mg/day) or mirtazapine (15 mg at night – caution in bipolar disorder); clonidine (0.2–0.8 mg/day) may be tried if the above ineffective
- Tardive dyskinesia: stop any antimuscarinic, consider tetrabenazine
- Addition of low doses (2.5–5 mg) of aripiprazole can reverse the hyperprolactinaemia/galactorrhoea caused by other antipsychotics
- Addition of aripiprazole (5–15 mg/day) or metformin (500–2000 mg/day) to weight-inducing atypical antipsychotics such as olanzapine and clozapine can help mitigate against weight gain

DOSING AND USE

Usual Dosage Range
- Acute psychotic episode in schizophrenia: 400–1200 mg/day in divided doses
- Schizophrenia with predominantly negative symptom: 50–300 mg/day

Dosage Forms
- Tablet 50 mg, 100 mg, 200 mg, 400 mg
- Oral solution 100 mg/mL

How to Dose
- Acute psychotic episode in schizophrenia: 400–800 mg daily in 2 divided doses, adjusted according to response; max 1.2 g/day
- Schizophrenia with predominantly negative symptoms: 50–300 mg/day

 Dosing Tips
* Efficacy for negative symptoms in schizophrenia may be achieved at lower doses, while efficacy for positive symptoms may require higher doses

Amisulpride (Continued)

- Patients receiving low doses may only need to take the drug once daily
- *Dose-dependent QTc prolongation, so use with caution, especially at higher doses (>800 mg/day)
- *Amisulpride may accumulate in patients with renal insufficiency, requiring lower dosing or switching to another antipsychotic to avoid QTc prolongation in these patients
- Treatment should be suspended if absolute neutrophil count falls below $1.5\text{x}10^9$/L

Overdose

- Fatalities have been reported when overdose combined with other psychotropics; drowsiness, sedation, hypotension, extrapyramidal symptoms, coma

Long-Term Use

- Amisulpride is used for both acute and chronic schizophrenia treatment

Habit Forming

- No

How to Stop

- See Switching section of individual agents for how to stop amisulpride
- Rapid discontinuation may lead to rebound psychosis and worsening of symptoms

Pharmacokinetics

- Elimination half-life about 12 hours
- Excreted largely unchanged

 Drug Interactions

- Can oppose the effects of levodopa, dopamine agonists
- Can increase the effects of antihypertensive drugs
- CNS effects may be increased if used with a CNS depressant
- May enhance QTc prolongation of other drugs capable of prolonging QTc interval
- May increase risk of torsades de pointes when administered with class Ia antiarrhythmics such as quinidine and disopyramide or class III antiarrhythmics such as amiodarone and sotalol
- Since amisulpride is only weakly metabolised, few drug interactions that

could raise amisulpride plasma levels are expected

 Other Warnings/Precautions

- All antipsychotics should be used with caution in patients with angle-closure glaucoma, blood disorders, cardiovascular disease, depression, diabetes, epilepsy and susceptibility to seizures, history of jaundice, myasthenia gravis, Parkinson's disease, photosensitivity, prostatic hypertrophy, severe respiratory disorders
- Use cautiously in patients with alcohol withdrawal or convulsive disorders because of possible lowering of seizure threshold
- If signs of neuroleptic malignant syndrome develop, treatment should be immediately discontinued
- Because amisulpride may dose-dependently prolong QTc interval, use with caution in patients who have bradycardia or who are taking drugs that can induce bradycardia (e.g. beta blockers, calcium channel blockers, clonidine, digitalis)
- Because amisulpride may dose-dependently prolong QTc interval, use with caution in patients who have hypokalaemia and/or hypomagnesaemia or who are taking drugs that can induce hypokalaemia and/or hypo-magnesaemia (e.g. diuretics, stimulant laxatives, intravenous amphotericin B, glucocorticoids, tetracosactide)
- Use only with caution if at all in Lewy body disease, especially at high doses
- Amisulpride should be used with caution in patients with stroke risk factors as randomised clinical trials have observed a three-fold increase of the risk of cerebrovascular events

Do Not Use

- In patients with CNS depression or in a comatose state
- If patient has phaeochromocytoma
- If patient has prolactin-dependent tumour
- If patient is pregnant or nursing
- If patient is taking agents capable of significantly prolonging QTc interval (e.g. pimozide; thioridazine; selected antiarrhythmics such as quinidine, disopyramide, amiodarone, and sotalol; selected antibiotics such as moxifloxacin)

- If there is a history of QTc prolongation or cardiac arrhythmia, recent acute myocardial infarction, decompensated heart failure
- If patient is on intravenous erythromycin, or pentamidine
- In children under 15
- If there is a proven allergy to amisulpride

SPECIAL POPULATIONS

Renal Impairment

- Use with caution; drug may accumulate
- Amisulpride is eliminated by the renal route; in cases of renal insufficiency, the dose should be decreased: reduced to half the normal dose in moderate impairment and to a third of the normal dose in severe impairment
- Consider intermittent treatment or switching to another antipsychotic in very severe impairment

Hepatic Impairment

- Use with caution, but dose adjustment not generally necessary as amisulpride is weakly metabolised by the liver

Cardiac Impairment

- Amisulpride produces a dose-dependent prolongation of QTc interval, which may be enhanced by the existence of bradycardia, hypokalaemia, congenital or acquired long QTc interval, which should be evaluated prior to administering amisulpride
- Use with caution if treating concomitantly with a medication likely to produce prolonged bradycardia, hypokalaemia, slowing of intracardiac conduction, or prolongation of the QTc interval
- Avoid amisulpride in patients with a known history of QTc prolongation, recent acute myocardial infarction, and decompensated heart failure

Elderly

- Treatment of elderly patients is not recommended
- Some patients may be more susceptible to sedative and hypotensive effects
- Although atypical antipsychotics are commonly used for behavioural disturbances in dementia, no agent has been approved for treatment of elderly patients with dementia-related psychosis

- Elderly patients with dementia-related psychosis treated with atypical antipsychotics are at an increased risk of death compared to placebo, and also have an increased risk of cerebrovascular events

Children and Adolescents

- Not licensed for use for children under age 18
- If absolutely required, treatment of adolescents between 15–17 should be under expert supervision
- Acute psychotic episode in schizophrenia: 200–400 mg twice per day, adjusted according to response; max 1.2 g/day
- Schizophrenia with predominantly negative symptoms: 50–300 mg/day
- Amisulpride is absolutely contraindicated in children under 15

Pregnancy

- No specific studies regarding the use of amisulpride in pregnancy
- Increased risks to baby have been reported for antipsychotics as a group although evidence is limited
- There is a risk of abnormal muscle movements and withdrawal symptoms in newborns whose mothers took an antipsychotic during the third trimester; symptoms may include agitation, abnormally increased or decreased muscle tone, tremor, sleepiness, severe difficulty breathing, and difficulty feeding
- Psychotic symptoms may worsen during pregnancy and some form of treatment may be necessary
- Use in pregnancy may be justified if the benefit of continued treatment exceeds any associated risk
- Switching antipsychotics may increase the risk of relapse
- Effects of hyperprolactinaemia on the foetus are unknown
- Olanzapine and clozapine have been associated with maternal hyperglycaemia which may lead to developmental toxicity, risk may also apply for other atypical antipsychotics

Amisulpride (Continued)

Breastfeeding
- Moderate amounts in mother's breast milk
- Extremely limited evidence of safety
- Haloperidol is considered to be the preferred first-generation antipsychotic, and quetiapine the preferred second-generation antipsychotic
- Infants of women who choose to breastfeed should be monitored for possible adverse effects

THE ART OF PSYCHOPHARMACOLOGY
Potential Advantages
- Not as clearly associated with weight gain as some other atypical antipsychotics
- For patients who are responsive to low-dose activation effects that reduce negative symptoms and depression

Potential Disadvantages
- Patients who have difficulty being concordant with twice-daily dosing
- Patients for whom elevated prolactin may not be desired (e.g. possibly pregnant patients; pubescent girls with amenorrhoea; postmenopausal women with low oestrogen who do not take oestrogen replacement therapy)
- Patients with severe renal impairment

Primary Target Symptoms
- Positive symptoms of psychosis
- Negative symptoms of psychosis
- Depressive symptoms

 Pearls

*Efficacy has been particularly well demonstrated in patients with predominantly negative symptoms
*The increase in prolactin caused by amisulpride may cause menstruation to stop
- Some treatment-resistant patients with inadequate responses to clozapine may benefit from amisulpride augmentation of clozapine

- Risks of diabetes and dyslipidaemia not well studied, but does not seem to cause as much weight gain as some other atypical antipsychotics
- Has atypical antipsychotic properties (i.e. antipsychotic action without a high incidence of extrapyramidal symptoms), especially at low doses, but not a serotonin dopamine antagonist
- Mediates its atypical antipsychotic properties via novel actions on dopamine receptors, perhaps dopamine stabilising partial agonist actions on dopamine 2 receptors
- May be more of a dopamine 2 antagonist than aripiprazole, but less of a dopamine 2 antagonist than other atypical or conventional antipsychotics
- Low-dose activating actions may be beneficial for negative symptoms in schizophrenia
- Very low doses may be useful in dysthymia
- Compared to sulpiride, amisulpride has better oral bioavailability and more potency, thus allowing lower dosing, less weight gain, and fewer extrapyramidal symptoms
- Compared to other atypical antipsychotics with potent serotonin 2A antagonism, amisulpride may have more extrapyramidal symptoms and prolactin elevation, but may still be classified as an atypical antipsychotic, particularly at low doses
- Patients have very similar antipsychotic responses to any typical antipsychotic, which is different from atypical antipsychotics where antipsychotic responses of individual patients can occasionally vary greatly from one atypical antipsychotic to another
- Patients with inadequate responses to atypical antipsychotics may benefit from determination of plasma drug levels and, if low, a dosage increase even beyond the usual prescribing limits
- Patients with inadequate responses to atypical antipsychotics may also benefit from a trial of augmentation with a typical antipsychotic or switching to a conventional antipsychotic

- However, long-term polypharmacy with a combination of a typical antipsychotic with an atypical antipsychotic may combine their side effects without clearly augmenting the efficacy of either
- For treatment-resistant patients, especially those with impulsivity, aggression, violence, and self-harm, long-term polypharmacy with 2 atypical antipsychotics or with 1 atypical antipsychotic and 1 conventional antipsychotic may be useful or even necessary while closely monitoring
- In such cases, it may be beneficial to combine 1 depot antipsychotic with 1 oral antipsychotic
- Although a frequent practice by some prescribers, adding two conventional antipsychotics together has little rationale and may reduce tolerability without clearly enhancing efficacy

THE ART OF SWITCHING

 Switching from Oral Antipsychotics to Amisulpride

- It is advisable to begin amisulpride at an intermediate dose and build the dose rapidly over 3–7 days
- Clinical experience has shown that asenapine, quetiapine, and olanzapine should be tapered off slowly over a period of 3–4 weeks, to allow patients to readapt to the withdrawal of blocking cholinergic, histaminergic, and alpha 1 receptors
- Clozapine should always be tapered off slowly, over a period of 4 weeks or more
* Benzodiazepine or anticholinergic medication can be administered during cross-titration to help alleviate side effects such as insomnia, agitation, and/or psychosis

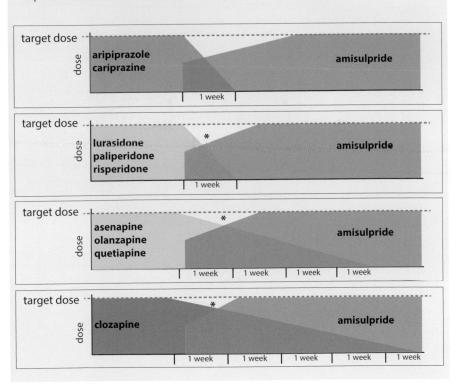

Suggested Reading

Burns T, Bale R. Clinical advantages of amisulpride in the treatment of acute schizophrenia. J Int Med Res 2001;29(6):451–66.

Curran MP, Perry CM. Spotlight on amisulpride in schizophrenia. CNS Drugs 2002;16(3):207–11.

Huhn M, Nikolakopoulou A, Schneider-Thoma J, et al. Comparative efficacy and tolerability of 32 oral antipsychotics for the acute treatment of adults with multi-episode schizophrenia: a systematic review and network meta-analysis. Lancet 2019;394(10202):939–51.

Komossa K, Depping AM, Gaudchau A, et al. Second-generation antipsychotics for major depressive disorder and dysthymia. Cochrane Database Syst Rev 2010;(12):CD008121.

Komossa K, Rummel-Kluge C, Hunder H, et al. Amisulpride versus other atypical antipsychotics for schizophrenia. Cochrane Database Syst Rev 2010;(1):CD006624.

Leucht S, Pitschel-Walz G, Engel RR, et al. Amisulpride, an unusual "atypical" antipsychotic: a meta-analysis of randomized controlled trials. Am J Psychiatry 2002;159(2):180–90.

Pillinger T, McCutcheon RA, Vano L, et al. Comparative effects of 18 antipsychotics on metabolic function in patients with schizophrenia, predictors of metabolic dysregulation, and association with psychopathology: a systematic review and network meta-analysis. Lancet Psychiatry 2020;7(1):64–77.

Amitriptyline hydrochloride

Brands
- Non-proprietary

Generic?
Yes

Class
- Neuroscience-based nomenclature: pharmacology domain – serotonin, norepinephrine; mode of action – multimodal
- Tricyclic antidepressant (TCA)
- Serotonin and noradrenaline reuptake inhibitor

Commonly Prescribed for
(bold for BNF indication)
- **Major depressive disorder (no longer recommended – risk of fatality in overdose)**
- **Neuropathic pain**
- **Prophylaxis for chronic tension headaches**
- **Migraine prophylaxis**
- **Abdominal pain or discomfort (in those who have not responded to laxatives, loperamide or antispasmodics)**
- **Emotional lability in multiple sclerosis (unlicensed)**
- Anxiety
- Insomnia
- Fibromyalgia
- Low back pain/neck pain

 ## How the Drug Works
- Boosts neurotransmitters serotonin and noradrenaline
- Blocks serotonin reuptake pump (serotonin transporter), presumably increasing serotonergic neurotransmission
- Blocks noradrenaline reuptake pump (noradrenaline transporter), presumably increasing noradrenergic neurotransmission
- Presumably desensitises both serotonin 1A receptors and beta adrenergic receptors
- Since dopamine is inactivated by noradrenaline reuptake in the frontal cortex, which largely lacks dopamine transporters, amitriptyline can increase dopamine neurotransmission in this part of the brain

How Long Until It Works
- May have immediate effects in treating insomnia or anxiety

- Onset of therapeutic actions with some antidepressants can be seen within 1–2 weeks, but often delayed 2–4 weeks
- If it is not working within 3–4 weeks for depression, it may require a dosage increase or it may not work at all
- By contrast, for generalised anxiety, onset of response and increases in remission rates may still occur after 8 weeks, and for up to 6 months after initiating dosing
- May continue to work for many years to prevent relapse of symptoms

If It Works
- The goal of treatment is complete remission of current symptoms as well as prevention of future relapses
- Treatment often reduces or even eliminates symptoms, but it is not a cure since symptoms can recur after medicine stopped
- Continue treatment until all symptoms are gone (remission), especially in depression and whenever possible in anxiety disorders
- Once symptoms are gone, continue treating for at least 6–9 months for the first episode of depression or >12 months if relapse indicators present
- If >5 episodes and/or 2 episodes in the last few years then need to continue for at least 2 years or indefinitely
- The goal of treatment of chronic pain conditions such as neuropathic pain, fibromyalgia, headaches, low back pain, and neck pain is to reduce symptoms as much as possible, especially in combination with other treatments
- Treatment of chronic pain conditions such as neuropathic pain, fibromyalgia, headache, low back pain, and neck pain may reduce symptoms, but rarely eliminates them completely, and is not a cure since symptoms can recur after medicine is stopped
- Use in anxiety disorders and chronic pain conditions such as neuropathic pain, fibromyalgia, headache, low back pain, and neck pain may also need to be indefinite, but long-term treatment is not well studied in these conditions

If It Doesn't Work
- It is important to recognise non-response to treatment early on (3–4 weeks)
- Many patients have only a partial response where some symptoms are improved but

others persist (especially insomnia, fatigue, and problems concentrating)
- Other patients may be non-responders, sometimes called treatment-resistant or treatment-refractory
- Some patients who have an initial response may relapse even though they continue treatment
- Consider increasing dose, switching to another agent or adding an appropriate augmenting agent
- Lithium may be added for suicidal patients or those at high risk of relapse
- Consider psychotherapy
- Consider ECT
- Consider evaluation for another diagnosis or for a co-morbid condition (e.g. medical illness, substance abuse, etc.)
- Some patients may experience a switch into mania and so would require antidepressant discontinuation and initiation of a mood stabiliser

Best Augmenting Combos for Partial Response or Treatment Resistance

- Mood stabilisers or atypical antipsychotics for bipolar depression
- Atypical antipsychotics for psychotic depression
- Atypical antipsychotics as first-line augmenting agents (quetiapine MR 300 mg/day or aripiprazole at 2.5–10 mg/day) for treatment-resistant depression
- Atypical antipsychotics as second-line augmenting agents (risperidone 0.5–2 mg/day or olanzapine 2.5–10 mg/day) for treatment-resistant depression
- Mirtazapine at 30–45 mg/day as another second-line augmenting agent (a dual serotonin and noradrenaline combination, but observe for switch into mania, increase in suicidal ideation or serotonin syndrome)
- Although T3 (20–50 mcg/day) is another second-line augmenting agent the evidence suggests that it works best with tricyclic antidepressants
- Other augmenting agents but with less evidence include bupropion (up to 400 mg/day), buspirone (up to 60 mg/day) and lamotrigine (up to 400 mg/day)
- Benzodiazepines if agitation present

- Hypnotics for insomnia
- Augmenting agents reserved for specialist use include: modafinil for sleepiness, fatigue and lack of concentration; stimulants, oestrogens, testosterone
- Lithium is particularly useful for suicidal patients and those at high risk of relapse including with factors such as severe depression, psychomotor retardation, repeated episodes (>3), significant weight loss, or a family history of major depression (aim for lithium plasma levels 0.6–1.0 mmol/L)
- For elderly patients lithium is a very effective augmenting agent
- For severely ill patients other combinations may be tried especially in specialist centres
- Augmenting agents that may be tried include omega-3, SAM-e, L-methylfolate
- Additional non-pharmacological treatments such as exercise, mindfulness, CBT, and IPT can also be helpful
- If present after treatment response (4–8 weeks) or remission (6–12 weeks), the most common residual symptoms of depression include cognitive impairments, reduced energy and problems with sleep
- For chronic pain: gabapentin, other anticonvulsants, or opiates if done by experts while monitoring carefully in difficult cases

Tests

- Baseline ECG is recommended for patients over age 50 as amitriptyline is contraindicated in patients with arrhythmias or heart block
- ECGs may be useful for selected patients (e.g. those with personal or family history of QTc prolongation; cardiac arrhythmia; recent myocardial infarction; decompensated heart failure; or taking agents that prolong QTc interval such as pimozide, thioridazine, selected antiarrhythmics, moxifloxacin etc.)
- *Since tricyclic and tetracyclic antidepressants are frequently associated with weight gain, before starting treatment, weigh all patients and determine if the patient is already overweight (BMI 25.0–29.9) or obese (BMI ≥30)
- Before giving a drug that can cause weight gain to an overweight or obese patient,

consider determining whether the patient already has:

- Pre-diabetes – fasting plasma glucose: 5.5 mmol/L to 6.9 mmol/L or HbA1c: 42 to 47 mmol/mol (6.0 to 6.4%)
- Diabetes – fasting plasma glucose: >7.0 mmol/L or HbA1c: ≥48 mmol/L (≥6.5%)
- Hypertension (BP >140/90 mm Hg)
- Dyslipidaemia (increased total cholesterol, LDL cholesterol, and triglycerides; decreased HDL cholesterol)
- Treat or refer such patients for treatment, including nutrition and weight management, physical activity counselling, smoking cessation, and medical management
* Monitor weight and BMI during treatment
* While giving a drug to a patient who has gained >5% of initial weight, consider evaluating for the presence of pre-diabetes, diabetes, dyslipidaemia, or consider switching to a different antidepressant
- Patients at risk for electrolyte disturbances (e.g. patients aged >60, patients on diuretic therapy) should have baseline and periodic serum potassium and magnesium measurements

SIDE EFFECTS

How Drug Causes Side Effects

- Anticholinergic activity may explain sedative effects, dry mouth, constipation, and blurred vision
- Sedative effects and weight gain may be due to antihistamine properties
- Blockade of alpha adrenergic 1 receptors may explain dizziness, sedation, and hypotension
- Cardiac arrhythmias and seizures, especially in overdose, may be caused by blockade of ion channels

Notable Side Effects

- Anticholinergic side effects
- Increased appetite and weight gain, nausea, diarrhoea, heartburn, unusual taste
- Fatigue, weakness, dizziness, sedation, headache, anxiety, nervousness, restlessness
- Sexual dysfunction (impotence, changes in libido)
- Sweating, rash, itching

Common or very common

- QTc prolongation
- Sedation
- Anticholinergic syndrome (blurred vision, constipation, dry mouth, urinary retention)

Frequency not known

- Blood disorders: agranulocytosis, eosinophilia, leucopenia, thrombocytopenia, bone marrow depression
- CNS/PNS: abnormal sensation, altered mood, anxiety, coma, confusion, delirium, delusions, dizziness, dysarthria, hallucination, headache, impaired concentration, movement disorders, mydriasis, peripheral neuropathy, seizure, sleep disorders, stroke, suicidal tendencies, tinnitus, tremor, vision disorders
- CVS: arrhythmias, cardiac conduction disorders, hypertension, hypotension, myocardial infarction, palpitations, sudden cardiac death, syncope
- Endocrine: galactorrhoea, gynaecomastia
- GIT: abnormal appetite, altered taste, constipation, diarrhoea, dry mouth, epigastric distress, hepatic disorders, nausea, oral disorders, paralytic ileus, vomiting, weight changes
- Other: alopecia, asthenia, breast enlargement, facial oedema, hyperhidrosis, hyperpyrexia, hyponatraemia, neuroleptic malignant syndrome, photosensitivity, sexual dysfunction, SIADH, skin reactions, testicular swelling, urinary disorders, urinary tract dilation, withdrawal syndrome

 Life-Threatening or Dangerous Side Effects

- Paralytic ileus
- Neuroleptic malignant syndrome
- Precipitation of acute angle-closure glaucoma
- Lowered seizure threshold and rare seizures
- QTc prolongation, heart block or sudden death
- Hepatic failure
- Rare induction of mania
- Rare increase in suicidal ideation and behaviours in adolescents and young adults (up to age 25), hence patients should be warned of this potential adverse event

Weight Gain

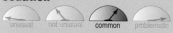

- Many experience and/or can be significant in amount
- Can increase appetite and carbohydrate craving

Sedation

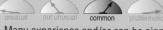

- Many experience and/or can be significant in amount
- Tolerance to sedative effects may develop with long-term use

What to Do About Side Effects

- Wait
- Wait
- Wait
- The risk of side effects is reduced by titrating slowly to the minimum effective dose (every 2–3 days)
- Consider using a lower starting dose in elderly patients
- Manage side effects that are likely to be transient (e.g. drowsiness) by explanation, reassurance and, if necessary, dose reduction and re-titration
- Giving patients simple strategies for managing mild side effects (e.g. dry mouth) may be useful
- For persistent, severe or distressing side effects the options are:
- Dose reduction and re-titration if possible
- Switching to an antidepressant with a lower propensity to cause that side effect
- Non-drug management of the side effect (e.g. diet and exercise for weight gain)

Best Augmenting Agents for Side Effects

- Many side effects cannot be improved with an augmenting agent

DOSING AND USE

Usual Dosage Range

- Depression: 50–150 mg/day
- Neuropathic pain: 10–75 mg/day

Dosage Forms

- Tablet 10 mg, 25 mg, 50 mg
- Oral solution 10 mg/5 mL, 25 mg/5 mL, 50 mg/5 mL

How to Dose

* Depression:
- Adults: initial dose 50 mg/day in 2 divided doses, increased by increments of 25 mg/day on alternate days as needed, max 150 mg/day in 2 divided doses
- Elderly: initial dose 10–25 mg/day, increased as needed up to 100–150 mg/day in 2 divided doses – caution with doses above 100 mg

* Neuropathic pain, Migraine prophylaxis, and Chronic tension-type headache prophylaxis:
- Initial dose 10–25 mg/day (evening), increased as tolerated by increments of 10–25 mg every 3–7 days in 1–2 divided doses; usual dose 25–75 mg/day (evening dose), caution with doses above 100 mg (caution with doses above 75 mg in patients with cardiovascular disease and in the elderly); max 75 mg per dose

* Emotional lability in multiple sclerosis:
- Initial dose 10–25 mg/day; increased as tolerated by increments of 10–25 mg every 1–7 days; max 75 mg/day

* Abdominal pain or discomfort (in patients who have not responded to laxatives, loperamide, or antispasmodics):
- Initial dose 5–10 mg/day (night time); increased by increments of 10 mg at least every 14 days as needed; max 30 mg/day

 Dosing Tips

- If given in a single dose, should generally be administered at bedtime because of its sedative properties
- If given in split doses, largest dose should generally be given at bedtime because of its sedative properties
- If patients experience nightmares, split dose and do not give large dose at bedtime
- Patients treated for chronic pain may only require lower doses

If intolerable anxiety, insomnia, agitation, akathisia, or activation occur either upon dosing initiation or discontinuation, consider the possibility of activated bipolar disorder, and switch to a mood stabiliser or an atypical antipsychotic

Overdose

- Can be fatal; coma, CNS depression, convulsions, hyperreflexia, extensor plantar responses, dilated pupils, cardiac arrhythmias, severe hypotension, ECG changes, hypothermia, respiratory failure, urinary retention

Long-Term Use

- Safe

Habit Forming

- No

How to Stop

- Taper gradually to avoid withdrawal effects
- Even with gradual dose reduction some withdrawal symptoms may appear within the first 2 weeks
- It is best to reduce the dose gradually over 4 weeks or longer if withdrawal symptoms emerge
- If severe withdrawal symptoms emerge during discontinuation, raise dose to stop symptoms and then restart withdrawal much more slowly (over at least 6 months in patients on long-term maintenance treatment)

Pharmacokinetics

- Substrate for CYP450 2D6 and 1A2
- Plasma half-life 9–26 hours
- Metabolised to an active metabolite, nortriptyline, which is predominantly a noradrenaline reuptake inhibitor, by demethylation via CYP450 1A2
- Food does not affect absorption

 Drug Interactions

- Tramadol increases the risk of seizures in patients taking TCAs
- Use of TCAs with anticholinergic drugs may result in paralytic ileus or hyperthermia
- Fluoxetine, paroxetine, bupropion, duloxetine, and other CYP450 2D6 inhibitors may increase TCA concentrations
- Fluvoxamine, a CYP450 1A2 inhibitor, can decrease the conversion of amitriptyline to nortriptyline and increase amitriptyline plasma concentrations
- Cimetidine may increase plasma concentrations of TCAs and cause anticholinergic symptoms
- Phenothiazines or haloperidol may raise TCA blood concentrations
- May alter effects of antihypertensive drugs; may inhibit hypotensive effects of clonidine

- Use of TCAs with sympathomimetic agents may increase sympathetic activity
- Methylphenidate may inhibit metabolism of TCAs
- Activation and agitation, especially following switching or adding antidepressants, may represent the induction of a bipolar state, especially a mixed dysphoric bipolar condition sometimes associated with suicidal ideation, and require the addition of lithium, a mood stabiliser or an atypical antipsychotic, and/or discontinuation of amitriptyline

 Other Warnings/Precautions

- Add or initiate other antidepressants with caution for up to 2 weeks after discontinuing amitriptyline
- Generally, do not use with MAOIs, including 14 days after MAOIs are stopped; do not start an MAOI for at least 5 half-lives (5 to 7 days for most drugs) after discontinuing amitriptyline, but see Pearls
- Use with caution in patients with chronic constipation, prostatic hypertrophy, pyloric stenosis, urinary retention, angle-closure glaucoma
- Use with caution in patients with a history of seizures or epilepsy
- Use with caution in patients with a history of psychosis, bipolar disorder (treatment should be stopped if the patient enters a manic phase) or significant risk of suicide
- Use with caution in patients with cardiovascular disease, hyperthyroidism, phaeochromocytoma
- Use with caution in patients with diabetes
- Use under expert supervision only if patient is taking drugs that inhibit TCA metabolism, including CYP450 2D6 inhibitors
- Use under expert supervision only and at low doses if there is reduced CYP450 2D6 function, such as patients who are poor 2D6 metabolisers
- TCAs can increase QTc interval, especially at toxic doses, which can be attained not only by overdose but also by combining with drugs that inhibit TCA metabolism via CYP450 2D6, potentially causing torsade de pointes-type arrhythmia or sudden death
- Because TCAs can prolong QTc interval, use with caution in patients who have bradycardia or who are taking drugs that can induce bradycardia (e.g. beta blockers,

Amitriptyline hydrochloride (Continued)

calcium channel blockers, clonidine, digitalis)
- Because TCAs can prolong QTc interval, use with caution in patients who have hypokalaemia and/or hypomagnesaemia, or who are taking drugs that can induce hypokalaemia and/or hypo-magnesaemia (e.g. diuretics, stimulant laxatives, intravenous amphotericin B, glucocorticoids, tetracosactide)
- When treating children, carefully weigh the risks and benefits of pharmacological treatment against the risks and benefits of non-treatment with antidepressants and make sure to document this in the patient's chart
- Warn patients and their caregivers about the possibility of activating side effects and advise them to report such symptoms immediately
- Monitor patients for activation of suicidal ideation, especially children and adolescents

Do Not Use
- In patients during a manic phase
- If patient is taking agents capable of significantly prolonging QTc interval (e.g. pimozide, thioridazine, selected antiarrhythmics, moxifloxacin)
- If there is a history of QTc prolongation or cardiac arrhythmia, recent acute myocardial infarction, decompensated heart failure, heart block
- If there is a proven allergy to amitriptyline or nortriptyline

Renal Impairment
- Can be given in usual doses to patients with renal failure

Hepatic Impairment
- Use with caution in mild to moderate impairment; may need to lower dose
- Serum level determination advisable
- Avoid in severe impairment

Cardiac Impairment
- Baseline ECG is recommended
- TCAs have been reported to cause arrhythmias, prolongation of conduction time, orthostatic hypotension, sinus tachycardia, and heart failure, especially in the diseased heart
- Myocardial infarction and stroke have been reported with TCAs
- TCAs produce QTc prolongation, which may be enhanced by the existence of bradycardia, hypokalaemia, congenital or acquired long QTc interval, which should be evaluated prior to administering amitriptyline
- Use with caution if treating concomitantly with a medication likely to produce prolonged bradycardia, hypokalaemia, slowing of intracardiac conduction, or prolongation of the QTc interval
- Avoid TCAs in patients with a known history of QTc prolongation, recent acute myocardial infarction, and decompensated heart failure
- TCAs may cause a sustained increase in heart rate in patients with ischaemic heart disease and may worsen (decrease) heart rate variability, an independent risk of mortality in cardiac populations
- Since SSRIs may improve (increase) heart rate variability in patients following a myocardial infarct and may improve survival as well as mood in patients with acute angina or following a myocardial infarction, these are more appropriate agents for cardiac population than tricyclic/tetracyclic antidepressants
- *Risk/benefit ratio may not justify use of TCAs in cardiac impairment

Elderly
- Baseline ECG is recommended for patients over age 50
- May be more sensitive to anticholinergic, cardiovascular, hypotensive, and sedative effects
- Initial dose 10–25 mg/day in 2 divided doses or once daily at bedtime; if needed increase by 25 mg every 3–7 days; doses over 100 mg/day must be used with caution
- Reduction in the risk of suicidality with antidepressants compared to placebo in adults age 65 and older

 Children and Adolescents
Neuropathic pain:
- Child 2–11 years: initial dose 200–500 mcg/kg/day (max per dose 10 mg) at night,

increased as needed; max 1 mg/kg twice daily on specialist advice
- Child 12–17 years: initial dose 10 mg/day, increased as needed to 75 mg/day at night, dose to be increased gradually, higher doses to be given on specialist advice

Pregnancy
- No strong evidence of TCA maternal use during pregnancy being associated with an increased risk of congenital malformations
- Risk of malformations cannot be ruled out due to limited information on specific TCAs
- Poor neonatal adaptation syndrome and/or withdrawal has been reported in infants whose mothers took a TCA during pregnancy or near delivery
- Maternal use of more than one CNS-acting medication is likely to lead to more severe symptoms in the neonate
- Must weigh the risk of treatment (first trimester foetal development, third trimester newborn delivery) to the child against the risk of no treatment (recurrence of depression, maternal health, infant bonding) to the mother and child
- For many patients this may mean continuing treatment during pregnancy

Breastfeeding
- Small amounts found in mother's breast milk
- Severe sedation and poor feeding reported in infants of mothers taking amitriptyline
- Immediate postpartum period is a high-risk time for depression, especially in women who have had prior depressive episodes, antidepressants may need to be reinstituted late in the third trimester or shortly after childbirth to prevent a recurrence during the postpartum period
- Must weigh benefits of breastfeeding with risks and benefits of antidepressant treatment versus nontreatment to both the infant and the mother
- For many patients this may mean continuing treatment during breastfeeding
- Other antidepressants may be preferable, e.g. imipramine or nortriptyline

Potential Advantages
- Patients with insomnia
- Severe or treatment-resistant depression
- Patients with a wide variety of chronic pain syndromes

Potential Disadvantages
- Paediatric and geriatric patients
- Patients concerned with weight gain
- Cardiac patients

Primary Target Symptoms
- Depressed mood
- Symptoms of anxiety
- Somatic symptoms
- Chronic pain
- Insomnia

Pearls
- Was once one of the most widely prescribed agents for depression
- TCAs are no longer generally considered a first-line treatment option for depression because of their side-effect profile
- Remains one of the most favoured TCAs for treating headache and a wide variety of chronic pain syndromes, including neuropathic pain, fibromyalgia, migraine, neck pain, and low back pain
- *Preference of some prescribers for amitriptyline over other tricyclic/tetracyclic antidepressants for the treatment of chronic pain syndromes is based more upon art and anecdote rather than controlled clinical trials, since many TCAs/tetracylics may be effective for chronic pain syndromes
- *Amitriptyline has been shown to be effective in primary insomnia
- TCAs may aggravate psychotic symptoms
- Alcohol should be avoided because of additive CNS effects
- Underweight patients may be more susceptible to adverse cardiovascular effects
- Children, patients with inadequate hydration, and patients with cardiac disease may be more susceptible to TCA-induced cardiotoxicity than healthy adults
- For the expert only: although generally prohibited, a heroic but potentially dangerous treatment for severely

Amitriptyline hydrochloride (Continued)

treatment-resistant patients is to give a tricyclic/tetracyclic antidepressant other than clomipramine simultaneously with an MAOI for patients who fail to respond to numerous other antidepressants

- If this option is elected, start the MAOI with the tricyclic/tetracyclic antidepressant simultaneously at low doses after appropriate drug washout, then alternately increase doses of these agents every few days to a week as tolerated
- Although very strict dietary and concomitant drug restrictions must be observed to prevent hypertensive crises and serotonin syndrome, the most common side effects of MAOI/tricyclic or tetracyclic combinations may be weight gain and orthostatic hypotension
- Patients on TCAs should be aware that they may experience symptoms such as photosensitivity or blue-green urine

- SSRIs may be more effective than TCAs in women, and TCAs may be more effective than SSRIs in men
- Since tricyclic/tetracyclic antidepressants are substrates for CYP450 2D6, and 7% of the population (especially Whites) may have a genetic variant leading to reduced activity of CYP450 2D6, such patients may not safely tolerate normal doses of tricyclic/tetracyclic antidepressants and may require dose reduction
- Phenotypic testing if available would help to detect this genetic variant prior to dosing with a tricyclic/tetracyclic antidepressant, especially in vulnerable populations such as children, elderly, cardiac populations, and those on concomitant medications
- Patients who seem to have extraordinarily severe side effects at normal or low doses may have this phenotypic CYP450 2D6 variant and require low doses or switching to another antidepressant not metabolised by CYP450 2D6

 Suggested Reading

Cipriani A, Furukawa TA, Salanti G, et al. Comparative efficacy and acceptability of 21 antidepressant drugs for the acute treatment of adults with major depressive disorder: a systematic review and network meta-analysis. Lancet 2018;391(10128):1357–66.

Guaiana G, Barbui C, Hotopf M. Amitriptyline for depression. Cochrane Database Syst Rev 2007;(3):CD004186.

Hauser W, Petzke F, Uceyler N, et al. Comparative efficacy and acceptability of amitriptyline, duloxetine and milnacipran in fibromyalgia syndrome: a systematic review with meta-analysis. Rheumatology (Oxford) 2011;50(3):532–43.

Torrente Castells E, Vazquez Delgado E, Gay Escoda C. Use of amitriptyline for the treatment of chronic tension-type headache. Review of the literature. Med Oral Patol Oral Cir Bucal 2008;13(9):E567–72.

Aripiprazole

Brands
- Abilify
- Arpoya
- Abilify Maintena

Generic?
Yes

Class
- Neuroscience-based nomenclature: pharmacology domain – dopamine, serotonin; mode of action – partial agonist and antagonist
- Dopamine partial agonist (dopamine stabiliser, atypical antipsychotic, third-generation antipsychotic; sometimes included as a second-generation antipsychotic; also a mood stabiliser)

Commonly Prescribed for
(bold for BNF indication)
- **Maintenance of schizophrenia in patients stabilised with oral aripiprazole – CYP450 2D6 poor metabolisers (long-acting injection)**
- **Maintenance of schizophrenia in patients stabilised with oral aripiprazole (long-acting injection)**
- **Schizophrenia (> 15 years)**
- **Treatment and recurrence prevention of mania (up to 12 weeks in adolescents aged >13)**
- **Control of agitation and disturbed behaviour in schizophrenia**
- Bipolar maintenance (monotherapy and adjunct)
- Depression (adjunct)
- Autism-related irritability in children aged 6 to 17
- Tourette syndrome in children aged 6 to 18
- Bipolar depression
- Other psychotic disorders
- Behavioural disturbances in dementias
- Behavioural disturbances in children and adolescents
- Disorders associated with problems with impulse control

How the Drug Works
* Partial agonism at dopamine 2 receptors
- Theoretically reduces dopamine output when dopamine concentrations are high, thus improving positive symptoms and mediating antipsychotic actions
- Theoretically increases dopamine output when dopamine concentrations are low, thus improving cognitive, negative, and mood symptoms
- Actions at dopamine 3 receptors could theoretically contribute to aripiprazole's efficacy
- Partial agonism at serotonin 1A receptors may be relevant at clinical doses
- Blockade of serotonin type 2A receptors may contribute at clinical doses to cause enhancement of dopamine release in certain brain regions, thus reducing motor side effects and possibly improving cognitive and affective symptoms
- Blockade of serotonin type 2 C and 7 receptors as well as partial agonist actions at 5HT1A receptors may contribute to antidepressant actions

How Long Until It Works
- Psychotic and manic symptoms can improve within 1 week, but it may take several weeks for full effect on behaviour as well as on cognition and affective stabilisation
- Classically recommended to wait at least 4–6 weeks to determine efficacy of drug, but in practice some patients require up to 16–20 weeks to show a good response, especially on cognitive symptoms

If It Works
- Most often reduces positive symptoms in schizophrenia but does not eliminate them
- Can improve negative symptoms, as well as aggressive, cognitive, and affective symptoms in schizophrenia
- Most patients with schizophrenia do not have a total remission of symptoms but rather a reduction of symptoms by about a third
- Perhaps 5–15% of patients with schizophrenia can experience an overall improvement of >50–60%, especially when receiving stable treatment for > 1 year
- Such patients are considered super-responders or "awakeners" since they may be well enough to work, live independently, and sustain long-term relationships
- Many bipolar patients may experience a reduction of symptoms by half or more

- Continue treatment until reaching a plateau of improvement
- After reaching a satisfactory plateau, continue treatment for at least 1 year after first episode of psychosis, but it may be preferable to continue treatment indefinitely to avoid subsequent episodes
- After any subsequent episodes of psychosis, treatment may need to be indefinite
- Treatment may not only reduce mania but also prevent recurrences of mania in bipolar disorder

If It Doesn't Work

- If dose is optimised, consider watchful waiting
- If this fails, consider increasing the antipsychotic dose according to tolerability and plasma levels (limited supporting evidence)
- Try one of the other atypical antipsychotics (risperidone or olanzapine should be considered first before considering other agents such as quetiapine, amisulpride or lurasidone)
- If two or more antipsychotic monotherapies do not work, consider clozapine
- Some patients may require treatment with a conventional antipsychotic
- If no first-line atypical antipsychotic is effective, consider time-limited augmentation strategies
- Consider non-concordance and switch to another antipsychotic with fewer side effects or to a depot antipsychotic
- Consider initiating rehabilitation and psychotherapy such as cognitive remediation
- Consider presence of concomitant drug abuse

 Best Augmenting Combos for Partial Response or Treatment Resistance

- Valproic acid (Depakote or Epilim)
- Other mood-stabilising anticonvulsants (carbamazepine, oxcarbazepine, lamotrigine)
- Lithium
- Benzodiazepines

Tests

Before starting an atypical antipsychotic

* Measure weight, BMI, and waist circumference (aripiprazole is not clearly associated with weight gain, but monitoring recommended nonetheless as obesity prevalence is high in this patient group)
- Get baseline personal and family history of diabetes, obesity, dyslipidaemia, hypertension, and cardiovascular disease
* Check pulse and blood pressure, fasting plasma glucose or glycosylated haemoglobin (HbA1c), fasting lipid profile, and prolactin levels
- Full blood count (FBC), urea and electrolytes (including creatinine and eGFR), liver function tests (LFTs)
- Assessment of nutritional status, diet, and level of physical activity
- Determine if the patient:
  - is overweight (BMI 25.0–29.9)
  - is obese (BMI ≥30)
  - has pre-diabetes – fasting plasma glucose: 5.5 mmol/L to 6.9 mmol/L or HbA1c: 42 to 47 mmol/mol (6.0 to 6.4%)
  - has diabetes – fasting plasma glucose: >7.0 mmol/L or HbA1c: ≥48 mmol/L (≥6.5%)
  - has hypertension (BP >140/90 mm Hg)
  - has dyslipidaemia (increased total cholesterol, LDL cholesterol, and triglycerides; decreased HDL cholesterol)
- Treat or refer such patients for treatment, including nutrition and weight management, physical activity counselling, smoking cessation, and medical management
- Baseline ECG for: inpatients; those with a personal history or risk factor for cardiac disease

Children and adolescents:
- As for adults
- Also check history of congenital heart problems, history of dizziness when stressed or on exertion, history of long-QT syndrome, family history of long-QT syndrome, bradycardia, myocarditis, family history of cardiac myopathies, low potassium/low magnesium/low calcium
- Measure weight, BMI, and waist circumference plotted on a growth chart
- Pulse, BP plotted on a percentile chart
- ECG – QTc interval: machine-generated may be incorrect in children as different formula needed if HR <60 or >100

Monitoring after starting an atypical antipsychotic

- FBC annually to detect chronic bone marrow suppression, stop treatment if

neutrophils fall below 1.5x10⁹/L and refer to specialist care if neutrophils fall below 0.5x10⁹/L
- Urea and electrolytes (including creatinine and eGFR) annually
- LFTs annually
- Prolactin levels at 6 months and then annually (aripiprazole is more likely to reduce prolactin levels)
∗Weight/BMI/waist circumference, weekly for the first 6 weeks, then at 12 weeks, at 1 year, and then annually
∗Pulse and blood pressure at 12 weeks, 1 year, and then annually (aripiprazole has less of an effect on blood pressure compared to other antipsychotics and therefore mandatory monitoring of blood pressure is not required)
∗Fasting blood glucose, HbA1c, and blood lipids at 12 weeks, at 1 year, and then annually
∗For patients with type 2 diabetes, measure HbA1c at 3–6 month intervals until stable, then every 6 months
∗Even in patients without known diabetes, be vigilant for the rare but life-threatening onset of diabetic ketoacidosis, which always requires immediate treatment, by monitoring for the rapid onset of polyuria, polydipsia, weight loss, nausea, vomiting, dehydration, rapid respiration, weakness and clouding of sensorium, even coma
- If HbA1c remains ≥48 mmol/mol (6.5%) then drug therapy should be offered, e.g. metformin
- Treat or refer for treatment or consider switching to another atypical antipsychotic for patients who become overweight, obese, pre-diabetic, diabetic, hypertensive, or dyslipidaemic while receiving an atypical antipsychotic (these problems are less likely with aripiprazole)

Children and adolescents:
- As for adults but:
- Weight/BMI/waist circumference, weekly for the first 6 weeks, then at 12 weeks, and then every 6 months, plotted on a growth/percentile chart
- Height every 6 months, plotted on a growth chart
- Pulse and blood pressure at 12 weeks, then every 6 months (aripiprazole has less of an effect on blood pressure compared to other antipsychotics and therefore mandatory monitoring of blood pressure is not required)

- ECG prior to starting and after 2 weeks after dose increase for monitoring of QTc interval. Machine-generated may be incorrect in children as different formula needed if HR <60 or >100
- Prolactin monitoring may not be required, as aripiprazole is not associated with increased prolactin

SIDE EFFECTS

How Drug Causes Side Effects
- By blocking alpha 1 adrenergic receptors, it can cause dizziness, sedation, and hypotension
- Partial agonist actions at dopamine 2 receptors in the striatum can cause motor side effects, such as akathisia
- Partial agonist actions at dopamine 2 receptors can also cause nausea, occasional vomiting, and activating side effects
∗Mechanism of any possible weight gain is unknown; weight gain is not common with aripiprazole and may thus have a different mechanism from atypical antipsychotics for which weight gain is common or problematic
∗Mechanism of any possible increased incidence of diabetes or dyslipidaemia is unknown; early experience suggests these complications are not clearly associated with aripiprazole and if present may therefore have a different mechanism from that of atypical antipsychotics associated with an increased incidence of diabetes and dyslipidaemia

Notable Side Effects
∗Dizziness, insomnia, akathisia, activation, agitation, movement disorders, parkinsonism
∗Nausea, vomiting
- Orthostatic hypotension, occasionally during initial dosing
- Constipation
- Headache, asthenia, sedation
- Theoretical risk of tardive dyskinesia

Common or very common
- CNS: anxiety, headache, visual disturbances
- Endocrine: diabetes mellitus
- GIT: abnormal appetite, gastrointestinal discomfort, hypersalivation, nausea
- Other: fatigue

Uncommon
- CNS: depression
- Endocrine: hyperglycaemia
- GIT: hiccups
- Other: sexual dysfunction

Frequency not known
- CNS: aggression, generalised tonic-clonic seizure, pathological gambling, speech problems, suicidality
- CVS: cardiac arrest, chest pain, high BP, syncope
- Endocrine: diabetes (hyperosmolar coma, ketoacidosis)
- GIT: diarrhoea, dysphagia, hepatic disorders, pancreatitis, weight loss
- Resp: aspiration pneumonia
- Urinary: incontinence
- Other: alopecia, hyperhidrosis, hyponatraemia, laryngospasm, musculoskeletal stiffness, myalgia, oropharyngeal spasm, peripheral oedema, photosensitivity, rhabdomyolysis, serotonin syndrome, temperature dysregulation, thrombocytopenia

 Life-Threatening or Dangerous Side Effects
- Rare impulse control problems
- Rare neuroleptic malignant syndrome (much reduced risk compared to conventional antipsychotics)
- Rare seizures
- Agranulocytosis
- Neonatal withdrawal syndrome
- Diabetic hyperosmolar coma
- Sudden death
- Rhabdomyolysis
- Oropharyngeal spasm
- Increased risk of death and cerebrovascular events in elderly patients with dementia-related psychosis

Weight Gain

- Reported in a few patients, especially those with low BMIs, but not expected
- Less frequent and less severe than for most other antipsychotics
- May be more risk of weight gain in children than in adults

Sedation

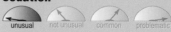

- Reported in a few patients but not expected
- May be less than for some other antipsychotics, but never say never
- Can be activating

What To Do About Side Effects
- Wait
- Wait
- Wait
- Low-dose benzodiazepine or beta blocker may reduce akathisia
- Take more of the dose at bedtime to help reduce daytime sedation
- Weight loss, exercise programmes, and medical management for high BMIs, diabetes, and dyslipidaemia
- Switch to another antipsychotic (atypical) – quetiapine or clozapine are best in cases of tardive dyskinesia

Best Augmenting Agents for Side Effects
- Dystonia: antimuscarinic drugs (e.g. procyclidine) as oral or IM depending on the severity; botulinum toxin if antimuscarinics not effective
- Parkinsonism: antimuscarinic drugs (e.g. procyclidine)
- Akathisia: beta blocker propranolol (30–80 mg/day) or low-dose benzodiazepine (e.g. 0.5–3.0 mg/day of clonazepam) may help; other agents that may be tried include the 5HT2 antagonists such as cyproheptadine (16 mg/day) or mirtazapine (15 mg at night – caution in bipolar disorder); clonidine (0.2–0.8 mg/day) may be tried if the above ineffective
- Tardive dyskinesia: stop any antimuscarinic, consider tetrabenazine

DOSING AND USE

Usual Dosage Range
- 10–30 mg/day for schizophrenia and mania
- 2.5–10 mg/day for augmenting SSRIs/SNRIs in depression
- 5–15 mg/day for autism (should only be used for challenging behaviour that is not improved by supportive or psychosocial interventions)
- 5–20 mg/day for Tourette syndrome

- 300–400 mg every month (minimum of 26 days between injections) with long-acting injection Maintena for schizophrenia, and (by mouth) 10–20 mg/day continued for 14 consecutive days after the first injection

Dosage Forms

- Tablet 5 mg, 10 mg, 15 mg, 30 mg
- Orodispersible tablet 10 mg, 15 mg, 30 mg
- Oral solution 1 mg/mL
- Injection 7.5 mg/mL
- Long-acting injection (Abilify Maintena) 400 mg powder and solvent for prolonged-release suspension for injection or as 400 mg powder and solvent for prolonged-release suspension for injection in pre-filled syringe

How to Dose

* Schizophrenia in adults:
- Orally 10–15 mg/day; usual dose 15 mg/day (max per dose 30 mg/day)

* Mania in adults:
- Orally 15 mg/day, increased as needed up to 30 mg/day

* Control of agitation and disturbed behaviour in schizophrenia in adults:
- IM injection initial dose 5.25–15 mg (usually 9.75 mg) for 1 dose, followed by 5.25–15 mg after 2 hours as needed, max 3 injections in 24 hours; max combined oral and parenteral dose 30 mg in 24 hours

* Long-acting injection in maintenance treatment of schizophrenia in adults:
- Abilify Maintena – establish tolerability with oral aripiprazole first; administer initial injection of 400 mg (300 mg for CYP450 2D6 poor metabolisers) along with overlapping 14-day dosing of oral aripiprazole

* Schizophrenia in children aged 15–17 years:
- Orally 2 mg/day for 2 days, increased to 5 mg/day for 2 days, then increased to 10 mg/day, then increased by increments of 5 mg as needed; max 30 mg/day

* Mania in children aged 13–17 years:
- Orally 2 mg/day for 2 days, increased to 5 mg/day for 2 days, then increased to 10 mg/day, increased by increments of 5 mg as needed up to max dose, max treatment duration 12 weeks, doses above 10 mg/day only in exceptional cases; max 30 mg/day

* Depression (adjunct):
- 2.5–5 mg/day; can increase by 5 mg/day at weekly intervals; max dose 15 mg/day

* Autism:
- 2 mg/day; can increase by 5 mg/day at weekly intervals; max dose 15 mg/day

* Tourette syndrome (patients weighing < 50 kg):
- 2 mg/day; after 2 days increase to 5 mg/day; after another week can increase to 10 mg/day as needed

* Tourette syndrome (patients weighing > 50 kg):
- 2 mg/day; after 2 days increase to 5 mg/day; after another 5 days can increase to 10 mg/day; can increase by 5 mg/day at weekly intervals; max dose 20 mg/day

- Oral solution: solution doses can be substituted for tablet doses on a mg-per-mg basis up to 25 mg; patients receiving 30-mg tablet should receive 25-mg solution

Dosing Tips

* For some, less may be more: frequently, patients not acutely psychotic may benefit from lower doses (e.g. 2.5–10 mg/day) in order to minimise side effects including akathisia and activation

- For others, more may be more: rarely, patients may need to be dosed higher than 30 mg/day for optimum efficacy

- Consider administering 1–5 mg as the oral solution for children and adolescents, as well as for adults very sensitive to side effects

* Although studies suggest patients switching to aripiprazole from another antipsychotic can do well with rapid switch or with cross-titration, clinical experience suggests many patients may do best by adding either an intermediate or full dose of aripiprazole to the maintenance dose of the first antipsychotic for at least several days and possibly as long as 3 or 4 weeks prior to slow down-titration of the first antipsychotic. See also the Switching section below, after Pearls

- Rather than raise the dose above these levels in acutely agitated patients requiring acute antipsychotic actions, consider augmentation with a benzodiazepine or conventional antipsychotic, either orally or IM

- Rather than raise the dose above these levels in partial responders, consider augmentation with a mood-stabilising anticonvulsant, such as valproate or lamotrigine

- Children and elderly should generally be dosed at the lower end of the dosage spectrum
- Due to its very long half-life, aripiprazole will take longer to reach steady state when initiating dosing, and longer to wash out when stopping dosing, than other atypical antipsychotics
- Treatment should be suspended if absolute neutrophil count falls below 1.5×10^9/L

Overdose

- No fatalities have been reported
- Important signs and symptoms may include lethargy, increased blood pressure, tachycardia, nausea, vomiting and diarrhoea
- More concerning signs and symptoms include somnolence, transient loss of consciousness and extrapyramidal symptoms

Long-Term Use

- Approved to delay relapse in long-term treatment of schizophrenia
- Approved for long-term maintenance in bipolar disorder
- Often used for long-term maintenance in various behavioural disorders

Habit Forming

- No

How to Stop

- See Switching section of individual agents for how to stop aripiprazole
- Rapid discontinuation could theoretically lead to rebound psychosis and worsening of symptoms, but less likely with aripiprazole due to its long half-life

Pharmacokinetics

- Metabolised primarily by CYP450 2D6 and 3A4
- Mean elimination half-life 75 hours (aripiprazole) and 94 hours (major metabolite dehydro-aripiprazole)
- Food does not affect absorption
- In poor metabolisers aripiprazole half-life is about 146 hours

 Drug Interactions

- Ketaconazole and possibly other CYP450 3A4 inhibitors such as fluvoxamine, and fluoxetine may increase plasma levels of aripiprazole
- Carbamazepine and possibly other inducers of CYP450 3A4 may decrease plasma levels of aripiprazole
- Quinidine and possibly other inhibitors of CYP450 2D6 such as paroxetine, fluoxetine, and duloxetine may increase plasma levels of aripiprazole
- Aripiprazole may enhance the effects of antihypertensive drugs
- Aripiprazole may antagonise levodopa, dopamine agonists
- Monitoring blood concentration of aripiprazole may be helpful in certain circumstances, such as with suspected drug interactions where the blood concentration of aripiprazole may increase

 Other Warnings/Precautions

- All antipsychotics should be used with caution in patients with angle-closure glaucoma, blood disorders, cardiovascular disease, depression, diabetes, epilepsy and susceptibility to seizures, history of jaundice, myasthenia gravis, Parkinson's disease, photosensitivity, prostatic hypertrophy, severe respiratory disorders
- There have been reports of problems with impulse control in patients taking aripiprazole, including compulsive gambling, shopping, binge eating, and sexual activity; use caution when prescribing to patients at high risk for impulse-control problems (e.g. patients with bipolar disorder, impulsive personality, obsessive-compulsive disorder, substance use disorders) and monitor all patients for emergence of these symptoms; dose should be lowered or discontinued if impulse-control problems manifest
- Use with caution in patients with cerebrovascular disease
- Use with caution in patients with conditions that predispose to hypotension (dehydration, overheating)
- Dysphagia has been associated with antipsychotic use, and aripiprazole should be used cautiously in patients at risk for aspiration pneumonia
- When transferring from oral to depot therapy, the dose by mouth should be reduced gradually

Do Not Use

- In patients with CNS depression or in a comatose state
- In patients with phaeochromocytoma
- If there is a proven allergy to aripiprazole

SPECIAL POPULATIONS

Renal Impairment

- Dose adjustment not necessary

Hepatic Impairment

- Use with caution in severe impairment (oral dosing preferred)

Cardiac Impairment

- Use in patients with cardiac impairment has not been studied, so use with caution because of risk of orthostatic hypotension

Elderly

- Dose adjustment generally not necessary, but some elderly patients may tolerate lower doses better
- Although atypical antipsychotics are commonly used for behavioural disturbances in dementia, no agent has been approved for treatment of elderly patients with dementia-related psychosis
- Elderly patients with dementia-related psychosis treated with atypical antipsychotics are at an increased risk of death compared to placebo, and also have an increased risk of cerebrovascular events

Children and Adolescents

- Approved for use in schizophrenia (ages 15–17), manic episodes (ages 13–17, max duration of treatment 12 weeks), used off-licence for irritability associated with autism (ages 6–17), and treatment of Tourette syndrome (ages 6–18)
- First-line antipsychotic in children is risperidone
- Clinical experience and early data suggest aripiprazole may be safe and effective for behavioural disturbances in children and adolescents, especially at lower doses

Before you prescribe:

- Do not offer antipsychotic medication when transient or attenuated psychotic symptoms or other mental state changes associated with distress, impairment, or help-seeking behaviour are not sufficient for a diagnosis of psychosis or schizophrenia. Consider individual CBT with or without family therapy and other treatments recommended for anxiety, depression, substance use, or emerging personality disorder
- For first-episode psychosis (FEP) antipsychotic medication should only be started by a specialist following a comprehensive multidisciplinary assessment and in conjunction with recommended psychological interventions (CBT, family therapy)
- As first-line treatment: allow patient to choose from aripiprazole, olanzapine or risperidone. As second-line treatment switch to alternative from list
- For bipolar disorder: if bipolar disorder is suspected in primary care in children or adolescents refer them to a specialist service
- Aripiprazole is recommended as an option for treating moderate to severe manic episodes in adolescents with bipolar disorder, within its marketing authorisation (that is, up to 12 weeks of treatment for moderate to severe manic episodes in bipolar disorder in adolescents aged 13 and older)
- Choice of antipsychotic medication should be an informed choice depending on individual factors and side-effect profile (metabolic, cardiovascular, extrapyramidal, hormonal, other)
- Where a child or young person presents with self-harm and suicidal thoughts the immediate risk management may take first priority
- All children and young people with FEP/bipolar should be supported with sleep management, anxiety management, exercise and activation schedules, and healthy diet
- Autism-related irritability in children aged 6 to 17: there are many reasons for challenging behaviours in autism spectrum disorders (ASD) and consideration should be given to possible physical, psychosocial, environmental or ASD-specific causes (e.g. sensory processing difficulties, communication). These should be addressed first. Consider behavioural interventions and family support. Pharmacological treatment can be offered alongside the above. It may be prudent to

Aripiprazole (Continued)

periodically discontinue the prescriptions if symptoms are well controlled, as irritability can change as the patient goes through neurodevelopmental changes

- Tourette syndrome in children aged 6 to 18: transient tics occur in up to 20% of children. Tourette syndrome occurs in 1% of children. Tics wax and wane over time and are variably exacerbated by external factors such as stress, inactivity, fatigue. Tics are a lifelong disorder, but often get better over time. As many as 65% of young people with Tourette syndrome have only mild tics in adult life. Psychoeducation and evidence-based psychological interventions (habit reversal therapy – HRT or exposure and response prevention – ERP) should be offered first. Pharmacological treatment may be considered in conjunction with psychological interventions where tics result in significant impairment or psychosocial consequences and/or where psychological interventions have been ineffective. If co-morbid with ADHD other choices (clonidine/guanfacine) may be better options to avoid polypharmacy
- A risk management plan is important prior to start of medication because of the possible increase in suicidal ideation and behaviours in adolescents and young adults

Practical notes:

- Carefully weigh the risks and benefits of pharmacological treatment against the risks and benefits of non-treatment and make sure to document this in the patient's chart
- Monitor weight, weekly for the first 6 weeks, then at 12 weeks, and then every 6 months (plotted on a growth chart)
- Monitor height every 6 months (plotted on a growth chart)
- Monitor waist circumference every 6 months (plotted on a percentile chart)
- Monitor pulse and blood pressure (plotted on a percentile chart) at 12 weeks and then every 6 months
- Monitor fasting blood glucose, HbA1c, blood lipid and prolactin levels at 12 weeks and then every 6 months
- Monitor for activation of suicidal ideation at the beginning of treatment. Inform parents or guardians of this risk so they can help observe child or adolescent patients
- If it does not work: review child's/young person's profile, consider new/changing contributing individual or systemic factors such as peer or family conflict. Consider drug/substance misuse. Consider dose adjustment before switching or augmentation. Be vigilant of polypharmacy especially in complex and highly vulnerable children/adolescents
- Consider non-concordance by parent or child, consider non-concordance in adolescents, address underlying reasons for non-concordance
- Children are more sensitive to most side effects:
- There is an inverse relationship between age and incidence of EPS
- Exposure to antipsychotics during childhood and young age is associated with a three-fold increase of diabetes mellitus
- Treatment with all atypical antipsychotics has been associated with changes in most lipid parameters
- Weight gain correlates with time on treatment. Any childhood obesity is associated with obesity in adults
- Aripiprazole is least associated with weight gain, changes in lipid parameters, sedation, and prolactin increase amongst atypicals
- Dose adjustments may be necessary in the presence of interacting drugs
- Re-evaluate the need for continued treatment regularly
- Provide Medicines for Children leaflet for aripiprazole for schizophrenia-bipolar-disorder-and-tics

Pregnancy

- Very limited data for the use of aripiprazole in pregnancy
- In animal studies, aripiprazole demonstrated developmental toxicity, including possible teratogenic effects, at doses higher than the maximum recommended human dose
- Increased risks to baby have been reported for antipsychotics as a group although evidence is limited
- There is a risk of abnormal muscle movements and withdrawal symptoms in newborns whose mothers took an antipsychotic during the third trimester; symptoms may include agitation, abnormally increased or decreased muscle tone, tremor, sleepiness, severe difficulty breathing, and difficulty feeding

- Psychotic symptoms may worsen during pregnancy and some form of treatment may be necessary
- Use in pregnancy may be justified if the benefit of continued treatment exceeds any associated risk
- Switching antipsychotics may increase the risk of relapse
- Antipsychotics may be preferable to anticonvulsant mood stabilisers if treatment is required for mania during pregnancy
- Olanzapine and clozapine have been associated with maternal hyperglycaemia which may lead to developmental toxicity, risk may also apply for other atypical antipsychotics
- Depot antipsychotics should only be used when there is a good response to the depot and a history of non-concordance with oral medication

Breastfeeding

- Small amounts in mother's breast milk
- Risk of accumulation in infant due to long half-life
- Haloperidol is considered to be the preferred first-generation antipsychotic, and quetiapine the preferred second-generation antipsychotic
- Infants of women who choose to breastfeed should be monitored for possible adverse effects

THE ART OF PSYCHOPHARMACOLOGY

Potential Advantages

- Some cases of psychosis and bipolar disorder refractory to treatment with other antipsychotics
* Patients concerned about gaining weight and patients who are already obese or overweight
* Patients with diabetes
* Patients with dyslipidaemia (especially elevated triglycerides)
- Patients requiring rapid onset of antipsychotic action without dosage titration
* Patients who wish to avoid sedation

Potential Disadvantages

- Patients in whom sedation is desired
- May be more difficult to dose for children, elderly, or "off-label" uses

Primary Target Symptoms

- Positive symptoms of psychosis
- Negative symptoms of psychosis
- Cognitive symptoms
- Unstable mood and depression
- Aggressive symptoms

Pearls

* Off-label use as an adjunct treatment for depression (e.g. to SSRIs, SNRIs)
- May work better in 2–10 mg/day range than at higher doses for augmenting SSRIs/SNRIs in treatment-resistant unipolar depression
- Frequently used for bipolar depression as augmenting agent to lithium, valproate, and/or lamotrigine
* Well accepted in clinical practice when wanting to avoid weight gain, because it causes less weight gain than most other antipsychotics
* Well accepted in clinical practice when wanting to avoid sedation, because less sedation than most other antipsychotics at all doses
* Can even be activating, which can be reduced by lowering the dose or starting at a lower dose
- If sedation is desired, a benzodiazepine can be added short-term at the initiation of treatment until symptoms of agitation and insomnia are stabilised or intermittently as needed
* May not have diabetes or dyslipidaemia risk, but monitoring is still indicated
- Anecdotal reports of utility in treatment-resistant cases of psychosis
- Has a very favourable tolerability profile in clinical practice
- Favourable tolerability profile leading to "off-label" uses for many indications other than schizophrenia (e.g. bipolar disorder, including hypomanic, mixed, rapid cycling, and depressed phases; treatment-resistant depression; anxiety disorders)
- A short-acting intramuscular formulation is available as well as long-acting injection
- Lacks D1 antagonist, anticholinergic, and antihistamine properties, which may explain relative lack of sedation or cognitive side effects in most patients
- High affinity of aripiprazole for D2 receptors means that combining with other D2 antagonist antipsychotics could reverse their actions and thus often makes sense not to combine with typical antipsychotics

Aripiprazole (Continued)

- Addition of low doses (2.5–5 mg) of aripiprazole can reverse the hyperprolactinaemia/galactorrhoea caused by other antipsychotics
- Addition of aripiprazole to weight-inducing atypical antipsychotics such as olanzapine and clozapine can help mitigate against weight gain
- A clozapine-aripiprazole combination in schizophrenia has been shown to reduce the rates of re-admission to hospital
- Abilify Maintena (long-acting injection) may be particularly well suited to early-onset psychosis/first-episode psychosis to reduce re-admissions and to enhance adherence with relatively low side-effect burden
- Abilify Maintena (long-acting injection) – a loading dose of 800 mg may be used in patients that have previously responded to Abilify Maintena (long-acting injection)

ARIPIPRAZOLE LONG-ACTION INJECTION
Abilify Maintena Properties

Vehicle	Water
Median Tmax	7 days (gluteal), 4 days (deltoid)
T1/2 with multiple dosing	29.9–46.5 days
Time to steady state	About 20 weeks
Able to be loaded	Yes
Dosing schedule (maintenance)	300–400 mg per month
Injection site	Intramuscular gluteal or deltoid
Needle gauge	21 (gluteal, obese patient), 22 (gluteal; deltoid, obese patient), 23 (deltoid)
Dosage forms	400 mg (400 mg powder and solvent for prolonged-release suspension for injection or as 400 mg powder and solvent for prolonged-release suspension for injection in pre-filled syringe)
Injection volume	200 mg/mL

Usual Dosage Range
- 300–400 mg/month

How to Dose
- Not recommended for patients who have not first demonstrated tolerability to oral aripiprazole
- Loading possible with 2x separate injections of 400 mg IM in two different muscles (1 deltoid + 1 gluteal, or 2 deltoid, not 2 gluteal) and one dose of oral 20 mg aripiprazole
- Otherwise 1x 400 mg IM injection with oral coverage with 10–20 mg aripiprazole for 14 days
- Conversion from oral to long-acting injection: administer initial 400 mg injection along with an overlapping 14-day dosing of oral aripiprazole
- Abilify Maintena should be administered once monthly as a single injection (no sooner than 26 days after the previous injection)
- If there are adverse reactions with the 400 mg dosage, reduction of the dose to 300 mg once monthly should be considered
- The safety and efficacy of Abilify Maintena in the treatment of schizophrenia in patients 65 years of age or older has not been established

 ### Dosing Tips
- With long-acting injection, the absorption rate constant is slower than the elimination rate constant, thus resulting in "flip-flop" kinetics – i.e. time to steady state is a function of absorption rate, while concentration at steady state is a function of elimination rate
- The rate-limiting step for plasma drug levels for long-acting injection is not drug metabolism, but rather slow absorption from the injection site
- In general, 5 half-lives of any medication are needed to achieve 97% of steady-state levels
- The long half-life of depot/long-acting injection antipsychotics means that one must either adequately load the dose (if possible) or provide oral supplementation
- The failure to adequately load the dose leads either to prolonged cross-titration from oral antipsychotic or to sub-therapeutic antipsychotic plasma levels for weeks or months in patients who are not receiving (or adhering to) oral supplementation
- Because plasma antipsychotic levels increase gradually over time, dose requirements may ultimately decrease; if

possible obtaining periodic plasma levels can be beneficial to prevent unnecessary plasma level creep
- The time to get a blood level for patients receiving long-acting injections is the morning of the day they will receive their next injection
- Advantages: refrigeration not required
- Disadvantages: requires oral coverage
- Downward dose adjustment is needed for poor CYP450 2D6 metabolisers and patients taking strong CYP450 2D6 or 3A4 inhibitors; avoid use with strong CYP450 3A4 inducers, as this can lead to sub-therapeutic plasma levels

Maintenance dose adjustments of Abilify Maintena in patients who are taking

concomitant strong CYP2D6 inhibitors, strong CYP3A4 inhibitors, and/or CYP3A4 inducers for more than 14 days
Adjusted dose – patients taking 400 mg of Abilify Maintena:
Strong CYP2D6 or strong CYP3A4 inhibitors: 300 mg
Strong CYP2D6 and strong CYP3A4 inhibitors: 200 mg
CYP3A4 inducers: avoid use

Adjusted dose – patients taking 300 mg of Abilify Maintena:
Strong CYP2D6 or strong CYP3A4 inhibitors: 200 mg
Strong CYP2D6 and strong CYP3A4 inhibitors: 160 mg
CYP3A4 inducers: avoid use

THE ART OF SWITCHING

Switching from Oral Antipsychotics to Aripiprazole Long-Acting Injection Formulation

Aripiprazole (Abilify Maintena) Kinetics

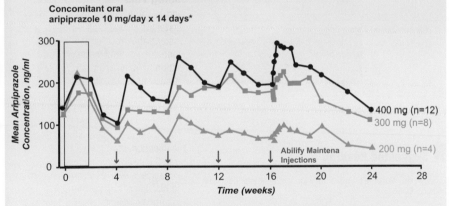

- Discontinuation of oral antipsychotic can begin following oral coverage of 14 days
- How to discontinue oral formulations:
  - Down-titration is not required for: amisulpride, aripiprazole, cariprazine
  - 1-week down-titration is required for: lurasidone, risperidone
  - 3–4-week down-titration is required for: asenapine, olanzapine, quetiapine
  - 4+-week down-titration is required for: clozapine
  - For patients taking benzodiazepine or anticholinergic medication, this can be continued during cross-titration to help alleviate side effects such as insomnia, agitation, and/or psychosis. Once the patient is stable on long-acting injection, these can be tapered one at a time as appropriate

Aripiprazole (Continued)

Switching from Oral Antipsychotics to Aripiprazole

- It is advisable to begin aripiprazole at an intermediate dose and build the dose up rapidly over 3–7 days
- Asenapine, quetiapine or olanzapine should be tapered off slowly over a period of 3–4 weeks, to allow patients to readapt to the withdrawal of blocking cholinergic, histaminergic, and alpha 1 receptors
- Clozapine should always be tapered off slowly, over a period of 4 weeks or more
- *Benzodiazepine or anticholinergic medication can be administered during cross-titration to help alleviate side effects such as insomnia, agitation, and/or psychosis

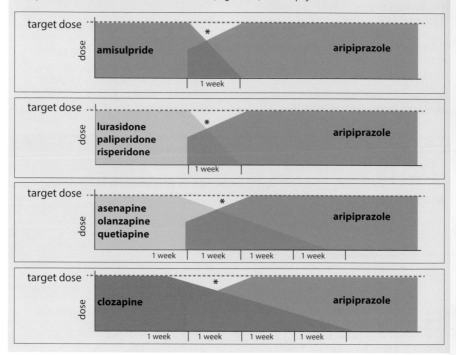

Suggested Reading

El-Sayeh HG, Morganti C. Aripiprazole for schizophrenia. Cochrane Database Syst Rev 2006;(2):CD004578.

Huhn M, Nikolakopoulou A, Schneider-Thoma J, et al. Comparative efficacy and tolerability of 32 oral antipsychotics for the acute treatment of adults with multi-episode schizophrenia: a systematic review and network meta-analysis. Lancet 2019;394(10202):939–51.

Kane JM, Sanchez R, Perry PP, et al. Aripiprazole intramuscular depot as maintenance treatment in patients with schizophrenia: a 52-week, multicenter, randomized, double-blind, placebo-controlled study. J Clin Psychiatry 2012;73(5):617–24.

Marcus RN, McQuade RD, Carson WH, et al. The efficacy and safety of aripiprazole as adjunctive therapy in major depressive disorder: a second multicenter, randomized, double-blind, placebo-controlled study. J Clin Psychopharmacol 2008;28(2):156–65.

Montastruc F, Nie R, Loo S, et al. Association of aripiprazole with the risk for psychiatric hospitalization, self-harm, or suicide. AMA Psychiatry 2019;76(4):409–17.

Nasrallah HA. Atypical antipsychotic-induced metabolic side effects: insights from receptor-binding profiles. Mol Psychiatry 2008;13(1):27–35.

Patel MX, Sethi FN, Barnes TR, et al. Joint BAP NAPICU evidence-based consensus guidelines for the clinical management of acute disturbance: de-escalation and rapid tranquillisation. J Psychopharmacol 2018;32(6):601–40.

Pillinger T, McCutcheon RA, Vano L, et al. Comparative effects of 18 antipsychotics on metabolic function in patients with schizophrenia, predictors of metabolic dysregulation, and association with psychopathology: a systematic review and network meta-analysis. Lancet Psychiatry 2020;7(1):64–77.

Asenapine

Brands
• Sycrest

Generic?
No, not in UK

Class
• Neuroscience-based nomenclature: pharmacology domain – dopamine, serotonin, norepinephrine; mode of action – antagonist
• Atypical antipsychotic (serotonin-dopamine antagonist; second-generation antipsychotics; also a mood stabiliser)

Commonly Prescribed for
(bold for BNF indication)
• **Monotherapy/combination therapy for treatment of moderate-severe manic episodes in adults with bipolar disorder**
• Control of mania in young people
• Schizophrenia, acute and maintenance (adults)
• Other psychotic disorders
• Bipolar maintenance
• Bipolar depression
• Treatment-resistant depression
• Behavioural disturbances in dementia
• Disorders associated with problems with impulse control

 ## How the Drug Works
• Blocks dopamine 2 receptors, reducing positive symptoms of psychosis and stabilising affective symptoms
• Blocks serotonin 2A receptors, causing enhancement of dopamine release in certain brain regions and thus reducing motor side effects and possibly improving cognitive and affective symptoms
∗Serotonin 2C, serotonin 7, and alpha 2 antagonist properties may contribute to antidepressant actions

How Long Until It Works
• For acute mania, effects should occur within a few weeks
• Psychotic symptoms can improve within 1 week, but it may take several weeks for full effect on behaviour as well as on cognition
• For schizophrenia classically recommended to wait at least 4–6 weeks to determine efficacy of drug, but in practice some patients may require up to 16–20 weeks to show a good response, especially on cognitive symptoms

If It Works
• Many bipolar patients may experience a reduction of symptoms by half or more
• Treatment is used to reduce acute mania but may be used off-label to prevent recurrences of mania in bipolar disorder, otherwise may need a switch to another atypical antipsychotic or mood-stabilising agent such as lithium or valproate
• Most often reduces positive symptoms in schizophrenia but does not eliminate them
• Can improve negative symptoms, as well as aggressive, cognitive, and affective symptoms in schizophrenia
• Most patients with schizophrenia do not have a total remission of symptoms but rather a reduction of symptoms by about a third
• Perhaps 5–15% of patients with schizophrenia can experience an overall improvement of >50–60%, especially when receiving stable treatment for > 1 year
• Such patients are considered super-responders or "awakeners" since they may be well enough to be employed, live independently, and sustain long-term relationships
• Continue treatment until reaching a plateau of improvement
• After reaching a satisfactory plateau, continue treatment for at least 1 year after first episode of psychosis, but it may be preferable to continue treatment indefinitely to avoid subsequent episodes
• After any subsequent episodes of psychosis, treatment may need to be indefinite
• Even for first episodes of psychosis, it may be preferable to continue treatment indefinitely to avoid subsequent episodes

If It Doesn't Work
• Check that the patient is not swallowing the tablet, but is allowing it to dissolve sublingually
• Optimise dose first and observe for improvements over time
• If this does not work, then can increase the dose of the antipsychotic according to

side effects and levels of drug in plasma (supporting evidence for this is limited)

- For mania consider switching to another atypical agent such as risperidone, olanzapine, or quetiapine, a conventional antipsychotic such as haloperidol, or a mood stabiliser such as lithium or valproate
- For mania if there is partial response only then can consider adding a mood stabiliser such as lithium or valproate
- For schizophrenia try one of the other atypical antipsychotics (risperidone or olanzapine should be considered first before considering other agents such as quetiapine, amisulpride, aripiprazole, or lurasidone)
- In schizophrenia if two or more antipsychotic monotherapies do not work, consider clozapine
- Some patients may require treatment with a conventional antipsychotic
- If no first-line atypical antipsychotic is effective, consider time-limited augmentation strategies
- Consider non-concordance and switch to another antipsychotic with fewer side effects or to an antipsychotic that can be given by depot injection
- Consider initiating rehabilitation and psychotherapy such as cognitive remediation
- Consider presence of concomitant drug abuse

Best Augmenting Combos for Partial Response or Treatment Resistance

- Valproic acid (Depakote or Epilim)
- Other mood-stabilising anticonvulsants (carbamazepine, oxcarbazepine, lamotrigine)
- Lithium
- Benzodiazepines

Tests

Before starting an atypical antipsychotic

* Measure weight, BMI, and waist circumference (asenapine is not clearly associated with weight gain, but monitoring recommended nonetheless as obesity prevalence is high in this patient group)
- Get baseline personal and family history of diabetes, obesity, dyslipidaemia, hypertension, and cardiovascular disease

* Check pulse and blood pressure, fasting plasma glucose or glycosylated haemoglobin (HbA1c), fasting lipid profile, and prolactin levels
- Full blood count (FBC), urea and electrolytes (including creatinine and eGFR), liver function tests (LFTs)
- Assessment of nutritional status, diet, and level of physical activity
- Determine if the patient:
  - is overweight (BMI 25.0–29.9)
  - is obese (BMI ≥30)
  - has pre-diabetes – fasting plasma glucose: 5.5 mmol/L to 6.9 mmol/L or HbA1c: 42 to 47 mmol/mol (6.0 to 6.4%)
  - has diabetes – fasting plasma glucose: >7.0 mmol/L or HbA1c: ≥48 mmol/L (≥6.5%)
  - has hypertension (BP >140/90 mm Hg)
  - has dyslipidaemia (increased total cholesterol, LDL cholesterol, and triglycerides; decreased HDL cholesterol)
- Treat or refer such patients for treatment, including nutrition and weight management, physical activity counselling, smoking cessation, and medical management
- Baseline ECG for: inpatients; those with a personal history or risk factor for cardiac disease

Monitoring after starting an atypical antipsychotic

- FBC annually to detect chronic bone marrow suppression, stop treatment if neutrophils fall below 1.5x10⁹/L and refer to specialist care if neutrophils fall below 0.5x10⁹/L
- Urea and electrolytes (including creatinine and eGFR) annually
- LFTs annually
- Prolactin levels at 6 months and then annually (asenapine may increase prolactin levels)
* Weight/BMI/waist circumference, weekly for the first 6 weeks, then at 12 weeks, at 1 year, and then annually
* Pulse and blood pressure at 12 weeks, 1 year, and then annually
* Fasting blood glucose, HbA1c, and blood lipids at 12 weeks, at 1 year, and then annually
* For patients with type 2 diabetes, measure HbA1c at 3–6 month intervals until stable, then every 6 months
* Even in patients without known diabetes, be vigilant for the rare but life-threatening onset of diabetic ketoacidosis, which always requires immediate treatment,

by monitoring for the rapid onset of polyuria, polydipsia, weight loss, nausea, vomiting, dehydration, rapid respiration, weakness and clouding of sensorium, even coma
- If HbA1c remains ⩾48 mmol/mol (6.5%) then drug therapy should be offered, e.g. metformin
- Treat or refer for treatment or consider switching to another atypical antipsychotic for patients who become overweight, obese, pre-diabetic, diabetic, hypertensive, or dyslipidaemic while receiving an atypical antipsychotic (these problems may occur with asenapine)

SIDE EFFECTS

How Drug Causes Side Effects
- By blocking alpha 1 adrenergic receptors, it can cause dizziness, sedation, and hypotension
- By blocking dopamine 2 receptors in the striatum, it can cause motor side effects
- By blocking dopamine 2 receptors in the pituitary, it can theoretically cause elevations in prolactin
- Mechanism of weight gain and increased incidence of diabetes and dyslipidaemia with atypical antipsychotics is unknown

Notable Side Effects
∗Sedation, dizziness
- Oral hypoaesthesia
- Application site reactions: oral ulcers, blisters, peeling/sloughing, inflammation
∗Extrapyramidal symptoms, akathisia
∗May increase risk for diabetes and dyslipidaemia
- Rare tardive dyskinesia (much reduced risk compared to conventional antipsychotics)
- Orthostatic hypotension

Common or very common
- GIT: altered taste, increased appetite, nausea, oral disorders
- Other: anxiety, fatigue, increased muscle rigidity

Uncommon
- CVS: bundle branch block, syncope
- Other: dysarthria, dysphagia, hyperglycaemia, sexual dysfunction

Rare or very rare
- Accommodation disorder, rhabdomyolysis

☠ Life-Threatening or Dangerous Side Effects
- Type 1 hypersensitivity reactions (anaphylaxis, angioedema, low blood pressure, rapid heart rate, swollen tongue, difficulty breathing, wheezing, rash)
- Hyperglycaemia, in some cases extreme and associated with ketoacidosis or hyperosmolar coma or death, has been reported in patients taking atypical antipsychotics
- Increased risk of death and cerebrovascular events in elderly patients with dementia-related psychosis
- Rare neuroleptic malignant syndrome (much reduced risk compared to conventional antipsychotics)
- Rare seizures

Weight Gain

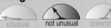

unusual   not unusual   common   problematic

- Occurs in a significant minority
- May be less than for some antipsychotics, more than for others

Sedation

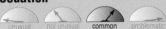

unusual   not unusual   common   problematic

- Many experience and/or can be significant in amount

What To Do About Side Effects
- Wait
- Wait
- Wait
- Reduce the dose
- Low-dose benzodiazepine or beta blocker may reduce akathisia
- Take more of the dose at bedtime to help reduce daytime sedation
- Weight loss, exercise programmes, and medical management for high BMIs, diabetes, and dyslipidaemia
- Switch to another antipsychotic (atypical) – quetiapine or clozapine are best in cases of tardive dyskinesia

Best Augmenting Agents for Side Effects
- Dystonia: antimuscarinic drugs (e.g. procyclidine) as oral or IM depending

on the severity; botulinum toxin if antimuscarinics not effective

- Parkinsonism: antimuscarinic drugs (e.g. procyclidine)
- Akathisia: beta blocker propranolol (30–80 mg/day) or low-dose benzodiazepine (e.g. 0.5–3.0 mg/day of clonazepam) may help; other agents that may be tried include the 5HT2 antagonists such as cyproheptadine (16 mg/day) or mirtazapine (15 mg at night – caution in bipolar disorder); clonidine (0.2–0.8 mg/day) may be tried if the above ineffective
- Tardive dyskinesia: stop any antimuscarinic, consider tetrabenazine
- Addition of low doses (2.5–5 mg) of aripiprazole can reverse the hyperprolactinaemia/galactorrhoea caused by other antipsychotics
- Addition of aripiprazole (5–15 mg/day) or metformin (500–2000 mg/day) to weight-inducing atypical antipsychotics such as olanzapine and clozapine can help mitigate against weight gain

DOSING AND USE

Usual Dosage Range
- 10–20 mg/day in 2 divided doses

Dosage Forms
- Sublingual tablet 5 mg, 10 mg

How to Dose
- 5 mg twice per day, increased as needed to 10 mg twice per day, adjusted according to response

 Dosing Tips
- Asenapine is not absorbed after swallowing (<2% bioavailable orally) and thus must be administered sublingually (35% bioavailable), as swallowing would render asenapine inactive
- Patients should be instructed to place the tablet under the tongue and allow it to dissolve completely, which will occur in seconds; tablet should not be divided, crushed, chewed, or swallowed
- Patients may not eat or drink for 10 minutes following sublingual administration so that the drug in the oral cavity can be absorbed locally and not washed into the stomach (where it would not be absorbed)

- Once daily use seems theoretically possible because the half-life of asenapine is about 24 hours, but this has not been extensively studied and may be limited by the need to expose the limited sublingual surface area to a limited amount of sublingual drug dosage
- Some patients may respond to doses greater than 20 mg/day but no single administration should be greater than 10 mg, thus necessitating 3 or 4 separate daily doses
- Due to rapid onset of action, can be used as a rapid-acting "prn" or "as needed" dose for agitation or transient worsening of psychosis or mania instead of an injection
- Treatment should be suspended if absolute neutrophil count falls below 1.5×10^9/L

Overdose
- Agitation and confusion, akathisia, orofacial dystonia, sedation, and asymptomatic ECG findings (bradycardia, supraventricular complexes, intraventricular conduction delay)

Long-Term Use
- Not studied, but long-term maintenance treatment is often necessary for schizophrenia and bipolar disorder

Habit Forming
- No

How to Stop
- Down-titration, over 2–4 weeks when possible, especially when simultaneously beginning a new antipsychotic while switching (i.e. cross-titration)
- Rapid discontinuation could theoretically lead to rebound psychosis and worsening of symptoms

Pharmacokinetics
- Half-life 24 hours
- Inhibits CYP450 2D6
- Substrate for CYP450 1A2
- Optimal bioavailability is with sublingual administration (about 35%); if food or liquid is consumed within 10 minutes of administration bioavailability decreases to 28%; bioavailability decreases to 2% if swallowed

Drug Interactions

- May increase effects of antihypertensive agents
- May antagonise levodopa, dopamine agonists
- CYP450 1A2 inhibitors (e.g. fluvoxamine) can raise asenapine levels
- Via CYP450 2D6 inhibition, asenapine could theoretically interfere with the analgesic effects of codeine, and increase the plasma levels of some beta blockers, paroxetine and atomoxetine

 Other Warnings/Precautions

- All antipsychotics should be used with caution in patients with angle-closure glaucoma, blood disorders, cardiovascular disease, depression, diabetes, epilepsy and susceptibility to seizures, history of jaundice, myasthenia gravis, Parkinson's disease, photosensitivity, prostatic hypertrophy, severe respiratory disorders
- Use with caution in patients with Lewy body dementia
- Use with caution in patients with conditions that predispose to hypotension (dehydration, overheating)
- Dysphagia has been associated with antipsychotic use, and asenapine should be used cautiously in patients at risk for aspiration pneumonia
- Caution with moderate hepatic impairment

Do Not Use

- Avoid in severe hepatic impairment
- If there is a proven allergy to asenapine

SPECIAL POPULATIONS

Renal Impairment

- Use with caution if eGFR less than 15 mL/minute/1.73 m^2, but generally dose adjustment not necessary

Hepatic Impairment

- Caution with moderate hepatic impairment
- Avoid in severe hepatic impairment

Cardiac Impairment

- Use with caution due to risk of orthostatic hypotension

Elderly

- Some patients may tolerate lower doses better
- Although atypical antipsychotics are commonly used for behavioural disturbances in dementia, no agent has been approved for treatment of elderly patients with dementia-related psychosis
- Elderly patients with dementia-related psychosis treated with atypical antipsychotics are at an increased risk of death compared to placebo, and have an increased risk of cerebrovascular events

 Children and Adolescents

- Asenapine is not currently licensed in young people
- A 3-week double-blind placebo-controlled study showed asenapine was superior to placebo at controlling mania in young people, with a significant difference as early as day 4. However, many adverse effects were reported, including weight gain, metabolic changes (increase in fasting insulin, lipids, glucose) as well as oral hypoesthesia, sedation, somnolence, and paraesthesia

 Pregnancy

- Controlled studies have not been conducted in pregnant women
- There is a risk of abnormal muscle movements and withdrawal symptoms in newborns whose mothers took an antipsychotic during the third trimester; symptoms may include agitation, abnormally increased or decreased muscle tone, tremor, sleepiness, severe difficulty breathing, and difficulty feeding
- In animal studies, asenapine increased post-implantation loss and decreased pup weight and survival at doses similar to or less than recommended clinical doses; there was no increase in the incidence of structural abnormalities
- Symptoms may worsen during pregnancy and some form of treatment may be necessary
- Use in pregnancy may be justified if the benefit of continued treatment exceeds any associated risk

- Switching antipsychotics may increase the risk of relapse
- Antipsychotics may be preferable to anticonvulsant mood stabilisers if treatment is required for mania during pregnancy
- Olanzapine and clozapine have been associated with maternal hyperglycaemia which may lead to developmental toxicity, risk may also apply for other atypical antipsychotics

Breastfeeding

- Small amounts expected in mother's breast milk
- Risk of accumulation in infant due to long half-life
- Haloperidol is considered to be the preferred first-generation antipsychotic, and quetiapine the preferred second-generation antipsychotic
- Infants of women who choose to breastfeed should be monitored for possible adverse effects

THE ART OF PSYCHOPHARMACOLOGY

Potential Advantages

- Patients requiring rapid onset of antipsychotic action without dosage titration

Potential Disadvantages

- Patients who are less likely to be adherent

Primary Target Symptoms

- Positive symptoms of psychosis
- Negative symptoms of psychosis
- Cognitive symptoms
- Unstable mood (both depression and mania)
- Aggressive symptoms

Pearls

- Asenapine's chemical structure is related to the antidepressant mirtazapine and it shares many of the same pharmacologic binding properties of mirtazapine plus many others
- Not approved for depression, but binding properties suggest potential use in treatment-resistant and bipolar depression
- Sublingual administration may require prescribing asenapine to better adherent patients or those who have someone who can supervise drug administration
- Patients with inadequate responses to atypical antipsychotics may benefit from determination of plasma drug levels and, if low, a dosage increase even beyond the usual prescribing limits
- Patients with inadequate responses to atypical antipsychotics may also benefit from a trial of augmentation with a conventional antipsychotic or switching to a conventional antipsychotic
- However, long-term polypharmacy with a combination of a conventional antipsychotic with an atypical antipsychotic may combine their side effects without clearly augmenting the efficacy of either
- For treatment-resistant patients, especially those with impulsivity, aggression, violence, and self-harm, long-term polypharmacy with 2 atypical antipsychotics or with 1 atypical antipsychotic and 1 conventional antipsychotic may be useful or even necessary while closely monitoring
- In such cases, it may be beneficial to combine 1 depot antipsychotic with 1 oral antipsychotic
- Although a frequent practice by some prescribers, adding 2 conventional antipsychotics together has little rationale and may reduce tolerability without clearly enhancing efficacy

THE ART OF SWITCHING

Switching from Oral Antipsychotics to Asenapine

- With aripiprazole and amisulpride, immediate stop is possible; begin asenapine at middle dose
- With risperidone and lurasidone: begin asenapine gradually, titrating over at least 2 weeks to allow patients to become tolerant to the sedating effect

*May need to taper clozapine slowly over 4 weeks or longer

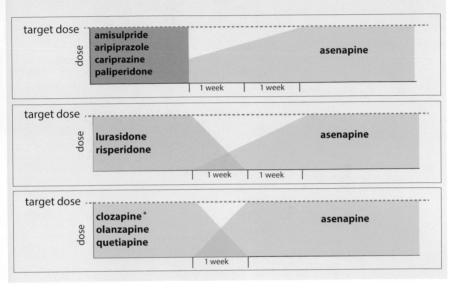

 Suggested Reading

Citrome L. Asenapine for schizophrenia and bipolar disorder: a review of the efficacy and safety profile for this newly approved sublingually absorbed second generation antipsychotic. Int J Clin Pract 2009;63(12):1762–84.

Huhn M, Nikolakopoulou A, Schneider-Thoma J, et al. Comparative efficacy and tolerability of 32 oral antipsychotics for the acute treatment of adults with multi-episode schizophrenia: a systematic review and network meta-analysis. Lancet 2019;394(10202):939–51.

Leucht S, Cipriani A, Spineli L, et al. Comparative efficacy and tolerability of 15 antipsychotic drugs in schizophrenia: a multiple-treatments meta-analysis. Lancet 2013;382(9896):951–62.

Pillinger T, McCutcheon RA, Vano L, et al. Comparative effects of 18 antipsychotics on metabolic function in patients with schizophrenia, predictors of metabolic dysregulation, and association with psychopathology: a systematic review and network meta-analysis. Lancet Psychiatry 2020;7(1):64–77.

Shahid M, Walker GB, Zorn SH, et al. Asenapine: a novel psychopharmacologic agent with a unique human receptor signature. J Psychopharmacol 2009;23(1):65–73.

Stepanova E, Grant B, Findling RL. Asenapine treatment in pediatric patients with bipolar I disorder or schizophrenia: a review. Paediatr Drugs 2018;20(2):121–34.

Tarazi F, Stahl SM. Iloperidone, asenapine and lurasidone: a primer on their current status. Exp Opin Pharmacother 2012;13(13):1911–22.

Atomoxetine

Brands
- ATOMAID
- Strattera

Generic?
Yes

Class
- Neuroscience-based nomenclature: pharmacology domain – norepinephrine; mode of action – reuptake inhibitor
- Selective noradrenaline reuptake inhibitor (SNRI)

Commonly Prescribed for
(bold for BNF indication)
- **Attention deficit hyperactivity disorder (ADHD) in children over 6 years and in adults**

 How the Drug Works
- Boosts neurotransmitter noradrenaline and may also increase dopamine in prefrontal cortex
- Blocks pre-synaptic noradrenaline reuptake pumps, also known as noradrenaline transporters
- Presumably this increases noradrenergic neurotransmission
- Since dopamine is inactivated by noradrenaline reuptake in frontal cortex, which largely lacks dopamine transporters, atomoxetine can also increase dopamine neurotransmission in this part of the brain

How Long Until It Works
- *Onset of therapeutic actions in ADHD can be seen in 4–6 weeks
- Therapeutic actions may continue to improve for 8–12 weeks so it is important to ensure that sufficient time has passed before drawing conclusions on efficacy

If It Works
- The goal of treatment of ADHD is reduction of symptoms of inattentiveness, motor hyperactivity, and/or impulsiveness that disrupt social, school, and/or occupational functioning
- Continue treatment until all symptoms are under control or improvement is stable and then continue treatment indefinitely as long as improvement persists
- Re-evaluate the need for treatment periodically
- Treatment for ADHD begun in childhood may need to be continued into adolescence and adulthood if continued benefit is documented

If It Doesn't Work
- Inform patient it may take several weeks for full effects to be seen
- Consider adjusting dose or switching to another formulation or another agent. It is important to consider if maximal dose has been achieved before deciding there has not been an effect and switching
- Consider behavioural therapy or cognitive behavioural therapy if appropriate – to address issues such as social skills with peers, problem-solving, self-control, active listening and dealing with and expressing emotions
- Consider the possibility of non-concordance and counsel patients and parents
- Consider evaluation for another diagnosis or for a co-morbid condition (e.g. bipolar disorder, substance abuse, medical illness, etc.)
- In children consider other important factors, such as ongoing conflicts, family psychopathology, adverse environment, for which alternate interventions might be more appropriate (e.g. social care referral, trauma-informed care)
- *Some ADHD patients and some depressed patients may experience lack of consistent efficacy due to activation of latent or underlying bipolar disorder, and require either augmenting with a mood stabiliser or switching to a mood stabiliser

 Best Augmenting Combos for Partial Response or Treatment Resistance
- *Best to attempt other monotherapies prior to augmenting
- There is limited evidence supporting either the efficacy or safety of combination therapy
- SSRIs, SNRIs, or mirtazapine for treatment-resistant depression (use combinations

Atomoxetine (Continued)

of antidepressants with atomoxetine with caution as this may theoretically activate bipolar disorder and suicidal ideation)
- Mood stabilisers or atypical antipsychotics for co-morbid bipolar disorder
- For the expert, may combine with modafinil, methylphenidate, or amfetamine for ADHD

Tests
- Pulse, blood pressure, appetite, weight, height, and mental health symptoms should be recorded at start of therapy, following each change in dose, and at least every 6 months after this. In children weight, height, pulse and BP should be recorded on percentile charts
- Monitor for appearance or worsening of anxiety, depression or tics

SIDE EFFECTS

How Drug Causes Side Effects
- Noradrenaline increases in parts of the brain and body and at receptors other than those that cause therapeutic actions (e.g. unwanted actions of noradrenaline on acetylcholine release causing decreased appetite, increased heart rate and blood pressure, dry mouth, urinary retention, etc.)
- Most side effects are immediate, but often go away with time
- Lack of enhancing dopamine activity in limbic areas theoretically explains atomoxetine's lack of abuse potential

Notable Side Effects
*Psychotic or manic symptoms (e.g. hallucinations, delusional thinking, mania, or agitation) in children and adolescents without a history of psychotic illness or mania
*May exacerbate pre-existing or manic symptoms
*Patients and carers should be informed about the potential risk of increased suicidal thinking and behaviours and advised to report any clinical worsening including increased suicidal thinking or behaviours, irritability, agitation, or depression
*Monitor for appearance or worsening of anxiety, depression or tics

Adults:

Common or very common
- CNS/PNS: abnormal sensations, altered mood, anxiety, depression, dizziness, drowsiness, headaches, jitteriness, sleep disorders, tremor
- CVS: arrhythmias, palpitations, vasodilatation
- GIT: abdominal discomfort, altered taste, constipation, decreased appetite, decreased weight, dry mouth, flatulence, thirst, nausea
- Other: asthenia, chills, genital pain, hyperhidrosis, menstrual irregularities, prostatitis, sexual dysfunction, skin reactions, urinary disorders

Uncommon
- CNS/PNS: abnormal behaviour, blurred vision, suicidal behaviour, tics
- CVS: chest pain, syncope, QT prolongation
- Other: dysponea, feeling cold, hypersensitivity, muscle spasms, peripheral coldness

Rare or very rare
- CNS: hallucinations, psychosis, seizures
- GIT: hepatic disorders
- Other: Raynaud's phenomenon

Children and adolescents:

Common or very common
- CNS/PNS: altered mood, anxiety, depression, dizziness, drowsiness, headaches, mydriasis, sleep disorders, tics
- CVS: chest pain
- GIT: abdominal discomfort, constipation, decreased appetite, decreased weight, nausea, vomiting
- Other: asthenia, skin reactions

Uncommon
- CNS/PNS: abnormal behaviour, abnormal sensations, blurred vision, seizures, suicidal behaviour, hallucinations, tremor, psychosis
- CVS: arrhythmias, palpitations, QT interval prolongation, syncope
- Other: dysponea, hyperhidrosis, hypersensitivity

Rare or very rare
- Hepatic disorders, genital pain, Raynaud's phenomenon, sex organ dysfunction, urinary disorders

Life-Threatening or Dangerous Side Effects

- Increased heart rate (≥20 beats per minute in 6–12% adults and children)
- Hypertension (≥15–20 mm Hg in 6–12% adults and children)
- Suicidal behaviour (uncommon)
- Sudden cardiac death (unknown frequency)

Weight Gain

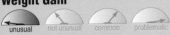

- Reported but not expected
- Patients may experience weight loss

Sedation

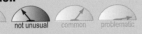

- Occurs in a significant minority, particularly in children

What to Do About Side Effects

- Wait
- Wait
- Wait
- Side effects can usually be managed by symptomatic management and/or dose reduction
- If weight loss is a clinical concern suggest taking medication, with or after food and high calorie food or snacks early morning
- If child or young person on ADHD medication shows sustained resting tachycardia (more than 120 beats per minute), arrhythmia or systolic blood pressure > 95th percentile (or a clinically significant increase) measured on 2 occasions, reduce their dose and refer for paediatric review
- If a child with ADHD develops new seizures or worsening of existing seizures, review their ADHD medication and stop any medication that might be contributing to the seizures. After investigation, cautiously reintroduce ADHD medication if it is unlikely to be the cause of the seizures
- If sleep becomes a problem: assess sleep at baseline. Monitor changes in sleep pattern (e.g. with a sleep diary). Adjust medication accordingly. Advise on sleep hygiene as appropriate. Prescription of melatonin may be helpful to promote sleep onset, where behavioural and environmental adjustments have not been effective
- For patients with ADHD experiencing acute psychosis or mania: stop the ADHD medications; only consider restarting ADHD medication (the original or new) after resolution of the episode based on the balance between benefits vs risks for that individual patient
- If giving once daily, can change to split dose twice daily
- If atomoxetine is sedating, take at night to reduce daytime drowsiness
- In a few weeks, switch or add other drugs

Best Augmenting Agents for Side Effects

- For urinary hesitancy, give an alpha 1 blocker such as tamsulosin
- Often best to try another monotherapy prior to resorting to augmentation strategies to treat side effects
- Many side effects are dose-dependent (i.e. they increase as dose increases, or they re-emerge until tolerance redevelops)
- Many side effects are time-dependent (i.e. they start immediately upon dosing and upon each dose increase, but go away with time)
- Activation and agitation may represent the induction of a bipolar state, especially a mixed dysphoric bipolar condition sometimes associated with suicidal ideation, and require the addition of lithium, a mood stabiliser or an atypical antipsychotic, and/or discontinuation of atomoxetine

DOSING AND USE

Usual Dosage Range

- Children up to 70 kg: 0.5–1.2 mg/kg/day
- Adults: 40–100 mg/day

Dosage Forms

- Capsule 10 mg, 18 mg, 25 mg, 40 mg, 60 mg, 80 mg, 100 mg
- Oral solution 4 mg/mL (300 mL bottle)

Atomoxetine (Continued)

How to Dose

- For children and adults 70 kg or less: initial dose 0.5 mg/kg/day; after 7 days can increase to 1.2 mg/kg/day either once in the morning or divided (last dose no later than early evening); max dose 1.8 mg/kg/day or 120 mg/day (whichever is less)
- For adults and children over 70 kg: initial dose 40 mg/day; after 7 days can increase to 80 mg/day (children) or 80–100 mg/day (adults) once in the morning or divided (last dose no later than early evening); max daily dose 120 mg

*Dosing above 100 mg/day in children and 120 mg/day in adults not licensed

 Dosing Tips

*Efficacy with once-daily dosing despite short half-life suggests therapeutic effects persist beyond direct pharmacologic effects, unlike stimulants whose effects are generally closely correlated with plasma drug levels
- Once-daily dosing may increase gastrointestinal side effects
- Lower starting dose allows detection of those patients who may be especially sensitive to side effects such as tachycardia and increased blood pressure
- Patients especially sensitive to the side effects of atomoxetine may include those individuals deficient in CYP450 2D6, the enzyme that metabolises atomoxetine
- In such individuals, drug should be titrated slowly to tolerability and effectiveness
- Other individuals may require up to 1.8 mg/kg total daily dose

Overdose

- No fatalities have been reported as monotherapy; sedation, agitation, hyperactivity, abnormal behaviour, gastrointestinal symptoms

Long-Term Use

- Safe

Habit Forming

- No

How to Stop

- Taper not necessary

- Re-evaluation of the need for continued therapy beyond 1 year should be performed, particularly when the patient has reached a stable and satisfactory response

Pharmacokinetics

- Metabolised by CYP450 2D6
- Half-life about 3.6 hours in extensive metabolisers and 21 hours in poor metabolisers
- Food does not affect absorption

 Drug Interactions

- Plasma concentrations of atomoxetine may be increased by drugs that inhibit CYP450 2D6 (e.g. paroxetine, fluoxetine), so atomoxetine dose may need to be reduced if co-administered
- Co-administration of atomoxetine with high-dose salbutamol may lead to increases in heart rate and blood pressure
- QT prolonging drugs (such as neuroleptics, class IA and III anti-arrhythmics, moxifloxacin, erythromycin, methadone, mefloquine, tricyclic antidepressants, or lithium), drugs that cause electrolyte imbalance (such as thiazide diuretics), and drugs that inhibit CYP2D6 may increase risk of QT-interval prolongation
- Co-administration with methylphenidate does not increase cardiovascular side effects beyond those seen with methylphenidate alone
- Avoid use with MAOIs, including 14 days after MAOIs are stopped

 Other Warnings/Precautions

- Growth (height and weight) should be monitored during treatment with atomoxetine; for patients who are not growing or gaining weight satisfactorily, interruption of treatment should be considered
- Clinical data do not suggest a deleterious effect of atomoxetine on cognition or sexual maturation; however, the amount of available long-term data is limited. Therefore, patients requiring long-term therapy should be carefully monitored

- Use with caution in patients with hypertension, tachycardia, cardiovascular disease, or cerebrovascular disease
- Use with caution in patients displaying aggressive behaviour, emotional lability, hostility, mania, or psychosis
- Increased risk of sudden death has been reported in children with structural cardiac abnormalities, QT-interval prolongation, or other serious heart conditions
- Use with caution in patients with a history of seizures
- Use with caution in patients susceptible to acute angle-closure glaucoma, urinary retention, and prostatic hypertrophy
- Rare reports of hepatotoxicity; although causality has not been established, atomoxetine should be discontinued in patients who develop jaundice or laboratory evidence of liver injury. Do not restart
- CYP450 2D6 poor metabolisers (non-functional CYP450 2D6 enzyme genotype) have a several-fold higher exposure to atomoxetine and therefore higher risk of adverse events. For patients with a known poor metaboliser genotype, a lower starting dose and slower up-titration of the dose may be considered
- Use with caution with antihypertensive drugs
- When treating children, carefully weigh the risks and benefits of pharmacological treatment against the risks and benefits of nontreatment and make sure to document this in the patient's chart
- Warn patients and their caregivers about the possibility of activating side effects and advise them to report such symptoms immediately
- Monitor patients for activation of suicidal ideation, especially children and adolescents

Do Not Use

- If patient has phaeochromocytoma or history of phaeochromocytoma
- If patient has severe cardiovascular or cerebrovascular disorders that might deteriorate with clinically important increases in heart rate and blood pressure
- If patient is taking an MAOI
- If there is a proven allergy to atomoxetine

Renal Impairment

- Dose adjustment not generally necessary, but may exacerbate hypertension in end-stage renal disease

Hepatic Impairment

- For patients with moderate liver impairment, dose should be reduced to 50% of normal dose
- For patients with severe liver impairment, dose should be reduced to 25% of normal dose

Cardiac Impairment

- Use with caution because atomoxetine can increase heart rate and blood pressure
- Do not use in patients with structural cardiac abnormalities or QT-interval prolongation

Elderly

- The use of atomoxetine in patients over 65 has not been systematically evaluated

 Children and Adolescents

Before you prescribe:
- Diagnosis of ADHD should only be made by specialist psychiatrist, paediatrician or appropriately qualified healthcare professional and after full clinical and psychosocial assessment in different domains, full developmental and psychiatric history, observer reports across different settings and opportunity to speak to the child and carer on their own
- Children and adolescents with untreated anxiety, PTSD and mood disorders, or those who do not have a psychiatric diagnosis but social or environmental stressors, may present with anger, irritability, motor agitation, and concentration problems
- Consider undiagnosed learning disability or specific learning difficulties, and sensory impairments that may potentially cause or contribute to inattention and restlessness, especially in school
- ADHD-specific advice on symptom management and environmental adaptations should be offered to all families and teachers, including reducing distractions, seating, shorter periods of focus, movement breaks and teaching assistants

Atomoxetine (Continued)

- For children >5 years and young people with moderate ADHD pharmacological treatment should be considered if they continue to show significant impairment in at least one setting after symptom management and environmental adaptations have been implemented
- For severe ADHD, behavioural symptom management may not be effective until pharmacological treatment has been established

Practical notes:

- Approved to treat ADHD in children over age 6 years
- Second-line treatment in children who cannot tolerate stimulants
- Atomoxetine can be considered as a first line when a drug diversion is a risk
- Offer the same medication choices to people with ADHD and anxiety disorder, tic disorder or autism spectrum disorder as other people with ADHD
- Monitor patients face-to-face regularly, particularly during the first several weeks of treatment
- Monitor for activation of suicidal ideation at the beginning of treatment
- Insomnia is common, but sedation can occur in a significant minority. If this is the case switch to evening dose
- Consider a course of cognitive behavioural therapy (CBT) for young people with ADHD who have benefited from medication but whose symptoms are still causing a significant impairment in at least one domain, addressing the following areas: social skills with peers, problem-solving, self-control, active listening skills, dealing with and expressing feelings
- Re-evaluate the need for continued treatment regularly
- Medication for ADHD for a child under 5 years should only be considered on specialist advice from an ADHD service with expertise in managing ADHD in young children (ideally a tertiary service). Use of medicines for treating ADHD is off-label in children aged <5
- The safety and efficacy of atomoxetine in children under 6 have not been evaluated and so should not be used
- Sudden death in children and adolescents with serious heart problems has been reported
- Do not use in children with structural cardiac abnormalities or other serious cardiac problems

- Provide the Medicines for Children leaflet: Atomoxetine for attention deficit hyperactivity disorder (ADHD)

Pregnancy

- Two population-based cohort studies described a possible association with spontaneous abortion and decreased Apgar scores, however, data may be confounded by underlying maternal condition and also data was overlapping across ADHD medications
- Theoretical risks of poor neonatal adaptation syndrome, neonatal withdrawal effects and persistent pulmonary hypertension of the newborn (PPHN) due to similarities with SSRIs
- Use in pregnancy may be justified if the benefit of continued treatment exceeds any associated risk
- *For women of childbearing potential, atomoxetine should generally be discontinued before anticipated pregnancies

Breastfeeding

- Unknown if atomoxetine is secreted in human breast milk, but all psychotropics assumed to be secreted in breast milk
- Possible risk of accumulation in infant due to long half-life in slow metaboliser
- Infants of women who choose to breastfeed while on atomoxetine should be monitored for possible adverse effects
- If irritability, sleep disturbance, or poor weight gain develop in nursing infant, may need to discontinue drug or bottle feed

THE ART OF PSYCHOPHARMACOLOGY

Potential Advantages
- No known abuse potential

Potential Disadvantages
- Slower onset of action versus stimulant drugs

Primary Target Symptoms
- Concentration, attention span
- Motor hyperactivity
- Depressed mood

Pearls

*Unlike other agents approved for ADHD, atomoxetine does not have abuse potential and is not a scheduled substance
- Atomoxetine has been shown to not only reduce symptoms in ADHD, but also improve scores on a quality-of-life scale over a 6-month period
- Atomoxetine can be used as an alternative treatment for ADHD, if psychosis develops during treatment with first-line stimulant drugs
- Atomoxetine has a "carry-on licence" for patients who continue to have been on atomoxetine since childhood, but still need continued treatment into adulthood
*Despite its name as a selective noradrenaline reuptake inhibitor, atomoxetine enhances both dopamine and noradrenaline in frontal cortex, presumably accounting for its therapeutic actions on attention and concentration
- Since dopamine is inactivated by noradrenaline reuptake in frontal cortex, which largely lacks dopamine transporters, atomoxetine can increase dopamine as well as noradrenaline in this part of the brain, presumably causing therapeutic actions in ADHD
- Since dopamine is inactivated by dopamine reuptake in nucleus accumbens, which largely lacks noradrenaline transporters, atomoxetine does not increase dopamine in this part of the brain, presumably explaining why atomoxetine lacks abuse potential
- Atomoxetine's known mechanism of action as a selective noradrenaline reuptake inhibitor suggests its efficacy as an antidepressant
- Pro-noradrenergic actions may be theoretically useful for the treatment of chronic pain
- Atomoxetine's mechanism of action and its potential antidepressant actions suggest it has the potential to destabilise latent or undiagnosed bipolar disorder, similar to the known actions of proven antidepressants; thus, administer with caution to ADHD patients who may also have bipolar disorder
- Unlike stimulants, atomoxetine may not exacerbate tics in Tourette syndrome patients with co-morbid ADHD
- Urinary retention in men over 50 with borderline urine flow has been observed with other agents with potent noradrenaline reuptake blocking properties (e.g. reboxetine), so administer atomoxetine with caution to these patients
- Atomoxetine was originally called tomoxetine but the name was changed to avoid potential confusion with tamoxifen, which might lead to errors in drug dispensing

 Suggested Reading

Cortese S, Newcorn JH, Coghill D. A practical, evidence-informed approach to managing stimulant-refractory attention deficit hyperactivity disorder (ADHD). CNS Drugs 2021;35(10):1035–51.

Garnock-Jones KP, Keating GM. Atomoxetine: a review of its use in attention-deficit hyperactivity disorder in children and adolescents. Paediatr Drugs 2009;11(3):203–26.

Kelsey DK, Sumner CR, Casat CD, et al. Once daily atomoxetine treatment for children with attention deficit hyperactivity behavior including an assessment of evening and morning behavior: a double-blind, placebo-controlled trial. Pediatrics 2004;114(1):e1–8.

Michelson D, Adler L, Spencer T, et al. Atomoxetine in adults with ADHD: two randomized, placebo-controlled studies. Biol Psychiatry 2003;53(2):112–20.

Michelson D, Buitelaar JK, Danckaerts M, et al. Relapse prevention in pediatric patients with ADHD treated with atomoxetine: a randomized, double-blind, placebo-controlled study. J Am Acad Child Adolesc Psychiatry 2004;43(7):896–904.

Stiefel G, Besag FMC. Cardiovascular effects of methylphenidate, amphetamines, and atomoxetine in the treatment of attention-deficit hyperactivity disorder. Drug Saf 2010;33(10):821–42.

Benperidol

Brands
• Anquil

Generic?
No, not in UK

Class
• Conventional antipsychotic (neuroleptic, butyrophenone, dopamine 2 antagonist, antiemetic)

Commonly Prescribed for
(bold for BNF indication)
• **Control of deviant antisocial sexual behaviour**
• Schizophrenia

 How the Drug Works
• Blocks dopamine 2 receptors, reducing positive symptoms of psychosis

How Long Until It Works
• Further research is required to guide the length of an adequate trial of treatment
• Psychotic symptoms can improve within 1 week, but it may take several weeks for full effect on behaviour

If It Works
For deviant antisocial sexual behaviour:
• Effectiveness has not been adequately characterised
• There are no widely available guidelines for its use in this context
For schizophrenia:
• Most often reduces positive symptoms in schizophrenia but does not eliminate them
• Most patients with schizophrenia do not have a total remission of symptoms but rather a reduction of symptoms by about a third
• Continue treatment in schizophrenia until reaching a plateau of improvement
• After reaching a satisfactory plateau, continue treatment for at least a year after first episode of psychosis in schizophrenia
• For second and subsequent episodes of psychosis in schizophrenia, treatment may need to be indefinite

If It Doesn't Work
For deviant antisocial sexual behaviour:
• There are no widely available guidelines for its use in this context
For schizophrenia:
• Consider trying one of the first-line atypical antipsychotics (risperidone, olanzapine, quetiapine, aripiprazole, paliperidone, amisulpride)
• Consider trying another conventional antipsychotic
• If two or more antipsychotic monotherapies do not work, consider clozapine

 Best Augmenting Combos for Partial Response or Treatment Resistance
For schizophrenia:
• Augmentation of conventional antipsychotics has not been systematically studied
• Addition of a mood-stabilising anticonvulsant such as valproate, carbamazepine, or lamotrigine may be helpful
• Addition of a benzodiazepine, especially short-term for agitation

Tests
Baseline
∗ Measure weight, BMI, and waist circumference
• Get baseline personal and family history of diabetes, obesity, dyslipidaemia, hypertension, and cardiovascular disease
• Check for personal history of drug-induced leucopenia/neutropenia
∗ Check pulse and blood pressure, fasting plasma glucose or glycosylated haemoglobin (HbA1c), fasting lipid profile, and prolactin levels
• Full blood count (FBC)
• Assessment of nutritional status, diet, and level of physical activity
• Determine if the patient:
  • is overweight (BMI 25.0–29.9)
  • is obese (BMI ≥30)
  • has pre-diabetes – fasting plasma glucose: 5.5 mmol/L to 6.9 mmol/L or HbA1c: 42 to 47 mmol/mol (6.0 to 6.4%)
  • has diabetes – fasting plasma glucose: >7.0 mmol/L or HbA1c: ≥48 mmol/L (≥6.5%)
  • has hypertension (BP >140/90 mm Hg)

- has dyslipidaemia (increased total cholesterol, LDL cholesterol, and triglycerides; decreased HDL cholesterol)
- Treat or refer such patients for treatment, including nutrition and weight management, physical activity counselling, smoking cessation, and medical management
- Baseline ECG for: inpatients; those with a personal history or risk factor for cardiac disease

Monitoring

- Monitor weight and BMI during treatment
- Consider monitoring fasting triglycerides monthly for several months in patients at high risk for metabolic complications and when initiating or switching antipsychotics
- While giving a drug to a patient who has gained >5% of initial weight, consider evaluating for the presence of pre-diabetes, diabetes, or dyslipidaemia, or consider switching to a different antipsychotic
- Patients with low white blood cell count (WBC) or history of drug-induced leucopenia/neutropenia should have full blood count (FBC) monitored frequently during the first few months and benperidol should be discontinued at the first sign of decline of WBC in the absence of other causative factors
- Monitor prolactin levels and for signs and symptoms of hyperprolactinaemia
- Manufacturer advises regular blood counts and liver function tests during long-term treatment

SIDE EFFECTS

How Drug Causes Side Effects

- By blocking dopamine 2 receptors in the striatum, it can cause motor side effects
- By blocking dopamine 2 receptors in the pituitary, it can cause elevations in prolactin
- By blocking dopamine 2 receptors excessively in the mesocortical and mesolimbic dopamine pathways, especially at high doses, it can cause worsening of negative and cognitive symptoms (neuroleptic-induced deficit syndrome)
- By blocking alpha 1 adrenergic receptors, it can cause dizziness, sedation, and hypotension
- Mechanism of weight gain and any possible increased incidence of diabetes

or dyslipidaemia with conventional antipsychotics is unknown

Notable Side Effects

- High incidence of parkinsonism
- High incidence of hyperprolactinaemia with or without galactorrhoea, gynaecomastia, or oligomenorrhoea/amenorrhoea
- Akathisia, anticholinergic side effects, dose-dependent hypotension
- Transient abnormalities of liver function
- Subjective feeling of being mentally slowed down, dizzy, headache, or paradoxical excitement, agitation, or insomnia

Frequency not known

- CNS/PNS: confusion, depression, headache, oculogyric crisis, psychiatric disorder
- CVS: cardiac arrest, hypertension
- GIT: decreased appetite, dyspepsia, hepatic disorders, hypersalivation, nausea, weight change
- Other: blood disorder, hyperhidrosis, muscle rigidity, oedema, oligomenorrhoea, paradoxical drug reaction, pruritus, temperature regulation disorders

 Life-Threatening or Dangerous Side Effects

- Rare neuroleptic malignant syndrome
- Rare tardive dyskinesia
- Rare seizures
- Rare jaundice, agranulocytosis, leucopenia
- Increased risk of death and cerebrovascular events in elderly patients with dementia-related psychosis

Weight Gain

- Reported but not expected

Sedation

- Occurs in significant minority

What To Do About Side Effects

- Wait
- Wait
- Wait
- Reduce the dose

- Low-dose benzodiazepine or beta blocker may reduce akathisia
- Take more of the dose at bedtime to help reduce daytime sedation
- Weight loss, exercise programmmes, and medical management for high BMIs, diabetes, and dyslipidaemia
- Switch to another antipsychotic (atypical) – quetiapine or clozapine are best in cases of tardive dyskinesia

Best Augmenting Agents for Side Effects

- Dystonia: antimuscarinic drugs (e.g. procyclidine) as oral or IM depending on the severity; botulinum toxin if antimuscarinics not effective
- Parkinsonism: antimuscarinic drugs (e.g. procyclidine)
- Akathisia: beta blocker propranolol (30–80 mg/day) or low-dose benzodiazepine (e.g. 0.5–3.0 mg/day of clonazepam) may help; other agents that may be tried include the 5HT2 antagonists such as cyproheptadine (16 mg/day) or mirtazapine (15 mg at night – caution in bipolar disorder); clonidine (0.2–0.8 mg/day) may be tried if the above ineffective
- Tardive dyskinesia: stop any antimuscarinic, consider tetrabenazine

DOSING AND USE

Usual Dosage Range
- 0.25–1.5 mg per day

Dosage Forms
- Tablet 250 mcg
- Oral suspension available by special order from manufacturer

How to Dose
- 0.25–1.5 mg/day in divided doses, adjusted according to response, for debilitated patients, use elderly dose (initial dose 0.125–0.75 mg/day in divided doses, adjusted according to response)

 Dosing Tips
- Due to short half-life, divided dosing is important to maintain plasma level
- Little evidence to guide prescribing of benperidol in schizophrenia or deviant antisocial sexual behaviour

Overdose
- The most prominent effects are extrapyramidal symptoms such as oculogyric crisis, salivation, muscle rigidity, akinesia, and akathisia
- Drowsiness or paradoxical excitement may occur
- Treatment is supportive and symptomatic, with anti-Parkinson medications used as required

Long-Term Use
- Some side effects may be irreversible (e.g. tardive dyskinesia)

Habit Forming
- No

How to Stop
- Slow down-titration is advised as acute withdrawal symptoms (nausea, vomiting, and insomnia) may occur if abrupt cessation of high-dose antipsychotic therapy

Pharmacokinetics
- Half-life about 6–10 hours

 Drug Interactions
- May decrease the effects of levodopa, dopamine agonists
- Reduced effectiveness when given with antimuscarinic medications
- When given with antiepileptic drugs there may be a lower seizure threshold
- May increase risk of hypotension with antihypertensive drugs, anaesthetics and opioids
- Additive effects may occur if used with CNS depressants
- Some pressor agents (e.g. adrenaline) may interact with benperidol to lower blood pressure
- Benperidol and anticholinergic agents together may increase intraocular pressure
- Increased CNS effects when combined with methyldopa
- The effects of sodium benzoate or sodium phenylbutyrate may be reduced
- Usage with lithium may cause neurotoxicity
- Usage with amantadine, metoclopramide, tetrabenazine or lithium increases the risk of extrapyramidal side effects

• Reduced plasma levels with smoking, alcohol consumption, phenobarbital, carbamazepine, phenytoin, rifampicin, and primidone
• Increased plasma levels with fluoxetine, buspirone, and ritonavir

 Other Warnings/Precautions

• All antipsychotics should be used with caution in patients with angle-closure glaucoma, blood disorders, cardiovascular disease, depression, diabetes, epilepsy and susceptibility to seizures, history of jaundice, myasthenia gravis, Parkinson's disease, photosensitivity, prostatic hypertrophy, severe respiratory disorders
• Caution in liver disease or renal failure
• Caution in patients with risk factors for stroke
• If signs of neuroleptic malignant syndrome develop, treatment should be immediately discontinued

Do Not Use

• If there is CNS depression
• If the patient is in a comatose state
• If the patient has phaeochromocytoma
• If there is a proven allergy to benperidol

SPECIAL POPULATIONS

Renal Impairment

• Due to risk of increased cerebral sensitivity, start with small doses in severe renal impairment

Hepatic Impairment

• Caution advised

Cardiac Impairment

• Caution advised in cardiac disease due to the risk of QT interval prolongation and arrhythmias

Elderly

• Initial dose 0.125–0.75 mg/day in divided doses

 Children and Adolescents

• Not indicated for use or recommended in children and adolescents

 Pregnancy

• Controlled studies have not been conducted in pregnant women
• Increased risks to baby have been reported for antipsychotics as a group although evidence is limited
• There is a risk of abnormal muscle movements and withdrawal symptoms in newborns whose mothers took an antipsychotic during the third trimester; symptoms may include agitation, abnormally increased or decreased muscle tone, tremor, sleepiness, severe difficulty breathing, and difficulty feeding
• Indication limits use in pregnancy

Breastfeeding

• Benperidol is secreted in human breast milk
• No evidence of safety
• Indication limits use in breastfeeding

THE ART OF PSYCHOPHARMACOLOGY

Potential Advantages

• For use in control of deviant antisocial sexual behaviour

Potential Disadvantages

• Most potent D2 receptor blocker, thus high risk of extrapyramidal side effects
• Patients with tardive dyskinesia or who wish to avoid tardive dyskinesia and extrapyramidal symptoms
• Vulnerable populations such as children or elderly
• Patients with notable cognitive or mood symptoms

Primary Target Symptoms

• Deviant antisocial sexual behaviour
• Positive symptoms of schizophrenia

 Pearls

• Benperidol is a potent antipsychotic
• It is very little used as an antipsychotic nowadays
• Not clearly effective for improving cognitive or affective symptoms of schizophrenia
• Patients have a very similar antipsychotic response when treated with any of the

conventional antipsychotics, which is different from atypical antipsychotics where antipsychotic responses of individual patients can occasionally vary greatly from one atypical to another
- Patients with inadequate responses to atypical antipsychotics may benefit from a trial of augmentation with a conventional antipsychotic such as benperidol or from switching to a conventional antipsychotic such as benperidol
- However, long-term polypharmacy with a combination of a conventional antipsychotic such as benperidol with an atypical antipsychotic may combine their side effects without clearly augmenting the efficacy of either
- For treatment-resistant patients, especially those with impulsivity, aggression, violence, and self-harm, long-term polypharmacy with 2 atypical antipsychotics and 1 conventional antipsychotic may be useful or even necessary while closely monitoring
- In such cases, it may be beneficial to combine 1 depot antipsychotic with 1 oral antipsychotic

 Suggested Reading

Khan O, Ferriter M, Huband N, et al. Pharmacological interventions for those who have sexually offended or are at risk of offending. Cochrane Database Syst Rev 2015(2):CD007989.

Leucht S, Hartung B. Benperidol for schizophrenia. Cochrane Database Syst Rev 2005(2):CD003083.

Buprenorphine

Brands

- Temgesic
- Tephine
- Natzon
- Subutex
- Espranor

see index for additional brand names

Generic?

Yes

Class

- Neuroscience-based nomenclature: pharmacology domain – opioid; mode of action – partial agonist
- Mu opioid receptor partial agonist; kappa and delta opioid receptor antagonist

Commonly Prescribed for

(bold for BNF indication)

- **Adjunct in treatment of opioid dependence**
- **Moderate-severe pain**
- **Premedication**
- **Intra-operative analgesia**

 ## How the Drug Works

- Buprenorphine is a partial agonist at mu opioid receptors and an antagonist at kappa opioid receptors
- Buprenorphine's activity in opioid maintenance treatment is due to its slowly reversible properties with the mu opioid receptors which, over a prolonged period, might minimise the need of addicted patients for drugs
- Binds with strong affinity to the mu opioid receptor, preventing exogenous opioids from binding there and thus preventing the pleasurable effects of opioid consumption
- Because buprenorphine is a partial agonist, it can cause immediate withdrawal in a patient currently taking opioids (i.e. reduces receptor stimulation in the presence of a full agonist), but can relieve withdrawal if a patient is already experiencing it (i.e. increases receptor stimulation in the absence of a full agonist)

How Long Until It Works

- Each sublingual tablet takes about 5–10 minutes to disintegrate and be absorbed

- It begins working on withdrawal soon after the tablet is dissolved
- Effects on reducing opioid use disorder/ dependence can take many months of treatment

If It Works

- It reduces the symptoms of opioid dependency such as cravings and withdrawal by acting on receptors without producing the euphoric effects. This helps patients abstain from other opioids to which they are addicted
- Reduces the effects of additional opioid use because of high receptor binding affinity (known as a "blocking" effect)
- Reduces the rewarding effects of opioid consumption

If It Doesn't Work

- Evaluate reasons for poor response and address any contributing factors
- Consider switching to alternative agent such as methadone

 ## Best Augmenting Combos for Partial Response or Treatment Resistance

- Augmentation with behavioural, educational, and/or supportive therapy in groups or as an individual is key to successful treatment
- Buprenorphine can be prescribed in combination with naloxone to decrease the potential for abuse or diversion

Tests

- Documented viral hepatitis status is recommended before commencing therapy for opioid dependence
- Buprenorphine levels can be tested for using a urine drug screening kit, not commonly available outside of addiction services (note – buprenorphine <u>cannot</u> be tested for in standard multiple urine drug testing kits in the same way as methadone or heroin)
- Baseline liver function tests (LFTs) should be done before commencing therapy, and regularly throughout treatment

SIDE EFFECTS

How Drug Causes Side Effects
• Binding at mu and kappa opioid receptors

Notable Side Effects
• Headache, constipation, nausea
• Oral hypoaesthesia, glossodynia
• Orthostatic hypotension
• Physical euphoria

Common or very common
• Anxiety, cough suppression, decreased appetite, decreased libido, depression, diarrhoea, dyspnoea, pruritis, syncope, tremor
Sublingual use:
• Fatigue, sedation, sleep disorders

Uncommon
Sublingual use:
• CNS/PNS: abnormal coordination, coma, depersonalisation, diplopia, paraesthesia, psychosis, seizure, slurred speech, tinnitus
• Other: apnoea, atrioventricular block, conjunctivitis, cyanosis, dyspepsia, hypertension, pallor, urinary disorder

Rare or very rare
Sublingual use:
• Angioedema, bronchospasm

Frequency not known
Sublingual use:
• Haemorrhage, hepatic disorders, impaired circulation, increased CSF pressure, oral disorders

Life-Threatening or Dangerous Side Effects
• Angioedema
• Respiratory depression
• Hepatotoxicity
• Arrhythmias

Weight Gain

unusual   not unusual   common   problematic

• Not expected

Sedation

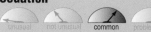
unusual   not unusual   common   problematic

• Many experience and/or can be significant in amount

What To Do About Side Effects
• Wait
• Reduce dose
• Switch to another agent

Best Augmenting Agents for Side Effects
• Most side effects cannot be improved with an augmenting agent

DOSING AND USE

Usual Dosage Range
• Adjunct in the treatment of opioid dependence: 12–24 mg/day

Dosage Forms
• Sublingual tablet 200 mcg, 400 mcg, 2 mg, 8 mg
• Oral lyophilisate 2 mg, 8 mg
• Solution for injection 300 mcg/mL
• Prolonged-release solution for injection 8 mg/0.16 mL, 16 mg/0.32 mL, 24 mg/0.48 mL, 32 mg/0.64 mL, 64 mg/0.18 mL, 96 mg/0.27 mL, 128 mg/0.36 mL
• Transdermal patch 5 mcg/hour, 10 mcg/hour, 15 mcg/hour, 20 mcg/hour, 35 mcg/hour, 52.5 mcg/hour, 70 mcg/hour
• Implant 74.2 mg

How to Dose
∗Adjunct in the treatment of opioid dependence:
• Sublingual tablet: initial dose 0.8–4 mg as a single dose on day 1, adjusted by increments of 2–4 mg/day if continuing evidence of withdrawal present and no evidence of intoxication; max 32 mg/day
• Oral lyophilisate: initial dose 2 mg/day, followed by 2–4 mg as needed on day 1, adjusted by increments of 2–6 mg/day if continuing evidence of withdrawal present and no evidence of intoxication; max 18 mg/day
• Doses above 8 mg buprenorphine should not be given on the first day in non-specialist setting
• Observe patient for at least 2 hours with the initial dose, then arrange 1–2 visits in the first week. During stabilisation patient reviews should be once per week; during maintenance patient reviews should be every 2–4 weeks

- Lower doses may be used for patients not in withdrawal or with co-morbid conditions (medical or psychiatric) and on other medications
- Subcutaneous implantation (adults 18–65; stable and not requiring > 8 mg/day of sublingual buprenorphine): 296.8 mg, dose consists of 4 implants (each containing 74.2 mg) to be left in place for 6 months, sublingual buprenorphine should be discontinued 12 to 24 hours before insertion of implant; consult product literature for supplemental sublingual buprenorphine, treatment discontinuation, and re-treatment

 ## Dosing Tips

- Clear evidence of daily opioid use (including drug testing) and withdrawal symptoms are mandatory before starting a prescription for buprenorphine
- In order to reduce the risk of precipitated withdrawal the first dose of buprenorphine should be administered when the patient is experiencing opioid withdrawal symptoms
- Oral lyophilisates should be placed on the tongue and allowed to dissolve. Patients should be advised not to swallow for 2 minutes and not to consume food or drink for at least 5 minutes after administration
- Espranor oral lyophilisate has different bioavailability to other buprenorphine products and is not interchangeable with them – consult product literature before switching between products
- For patients addicted to short-acting opioids such as heroin, the first dose cannot be taken less than 6 hours after the patient last used opioids
- For patients addicted to long-acting opioids such as methadone the dose of methadone should be reduced to a max of 30 mg/day before starting buprenorphine. This is because buprenorphine may precipitate symptoms of withdrawal in patients dependent on methadone. The first dose cannot be taken less than 24 hours after the patient last used methadone
- For sublingual tablets, with doses of methadone >10 mg/day, buprenorphine can be started at 4 mg/day and titrated as needed; with doses of methadone <10 mg/day, buprenorphine can be started at 2 mg/day
- Due to its long-acting nature buprenorphine can be given in divided doses and the dose

reviewed promptly in the event of intoxication. Duration of action is related to dose: low doses (e.g. 2 mg) are effective for up to 12 hours, while higher doses (e.g. 16–32 mg) are effective for between 48 to 72 hours
- A flexible dosing regime under supervision is required for at least 3 months, until concordance is confirmed
- If doses higher than 16 mg required, the dose should be increased only under advice from addiction specialists
- The transdermal patches are used for treatment of patients with moderate to severe chronic cancer pain
- The formulations of transdermal patches should not be confused — they are available as 72-hourly, 96-hourly and 7-day patches
- In the treatment of opioid use disorder buprenorphine is an agonist/antagonist, meaning that it relieves withdrawal symptoms from other opioids and induces some euphoria, but also blocks the ability for many other opioids, including heroin, to cause an effect
- Unlike full agonists like heroin or methadone, buprenorphine has a ceiling effect, such that taking more medicine will not increase the effects of the drug
- Buprenorphine alone is often used to initiate treatment, while buprenorphine with naloxone is preferred for stabilisation and maintenance treatment
- Buprenorphine not licensed for use in children under 6 years old

Overdose

- Can be fatal (less common than with methadone); may present with apnoea, cardiovascular collapse, drowsiness, miosis, nausea, vomiting, respiratory depression, sedation
- Management includes general supportive measures including cardiac and respiratory systems, and resuscitation if necessary. Naloxone is recommended despite only having a modest effect against buprenorphine, but the long half-life of buprenorphine should be taken into consideration

Long-Term Use

- Use the lowest dose needed for as short a duration as possible, particularly if the patient is also taking other medications that may interact, such as benzodiazepines

- Maintenance treatment may be required; typical maintenance period is up to 2 years

Habit Forming

- Yes
- Buprenorphine is a Class C/Schedule 3 drug

How to Stop

- Patients may experience a mild withdrawal syndrome if buprenorphine is stopped abruptly
- Once the patient is stable, titrate down gradually to a lower maintenance dose and if appropriate, eventually discontinue
- Patients should be monitored following termination of treatment because of the potential for relapse

Pharmacokinetics

- Time of onset 40–80 minutes
- Peak of action 1.5–2 hours
- Buprenorphine is metabolised by CYP450 3A4 to form N-dealkylbuprenorphine, a mu opioid agonist with weak intrinsic activity
- Half-life of sublingual buprenorphine 20–25 hours
- Half-life of transdermal buprenorphine 30 hours
- After-effects 1–3 days

 Drug Interactions

- Opioids can increase the risk of precipitating withdrawal
- Concomitant use with CNS depressants (e.g. alcohol or benzodiazepines) can increase the risk of respiratory depression; consider dose reduction of either or both
- Increased risk of CNS excitation or depression when taken with non-selective irreversible MAOIs (isocarboxazid, phenelzine, tranylcypromine): avoid the combination
- Nalmefene can reduce the efficacy of buprenorphine if taken concomitantly: avoid the combination
- Plasma concentrations of buprenorphine may be increased by drugs that inhibit CYP450 3A4 (e.g. clarithromycin, erythromycin, diltiazem, itraconazole, ketoconazole, ritonavir, verapamil, goldenseal, and grapefruit juice), so

buprenorphine dose may need to be reduced if co-administered
- Plasma concentrations of buprenorphine may be reduced by drugs that induce CYP450 3A4, so buprenorphine dose may need to be increased if co-administered

 Other Warnings/Precautions

- Attempts by patients to overcome blockade of opioid receptors by taking large amounts of exogenous opioids could lead to opioid intoxication or even fatal overdose
- Although the risk is lower, buprenorphine can be abused in a manner similar to other opioids
- Use with caution in patients with compromised respiratory function
- Risk of respiratory depression is increased with concomitant use of CNS depressants – if patients are on other respiratory sedatives then lower doses should be used and the patient monitored for intoxication and respiratory depression
- Can cause severe, possibly fatal respiratory depression in children who are accidentally exposed to it
- Withdrawal symptoms can occur when switching from methadone to buprenorphine
- Buprenorphine may increase intracholedochal pressure and should be administered with caution to patients with dysfunction of the biliary tract
- Concurrent alcohol and illicit drug use should be considered when prescribing buprenorphine due to the higher risk of overdose associated with polysubstance misuse
- Use with caution in debilitated patients and those with myxoedema or hypothyroidism, adrenal cortical insufficiency (e.g. Addison's disease); CNS depression; toxic psychoses; prostatic hypertrophy or urethral stricture; acute alcoholism; delirium tremens; or kyphoscoliosis
- Buprenorphine should be used with caution in patients with impaired consciousness

Do Not Use

- If the patient is naive to opioid use
- If short-acting opioid used within the last 6 hours or long-acting opioid within the last 24 hours

- If the patient has severe respiratory impairment
- In comatose patients
- In patients with a head injury, intracranial lesions, and other circumstances when CSF pressure may be increased
- If patient has paralytic ileus
- If there is a proven allergy to buprenorphine

SPECIAL POPULATIONS

Renal Impairment
- Reduce dose and avoid in severe impairment otherwise increased cerebral sensitivity and opioid effects increased and prolonged

Hepatic Impairment
- In patients with moderate-severe impairment, plasma levels of buprenorphine can be higher and half-life longer; thus these patients should be monitored for signs and symptoms of toxicity/overdose
- For severe impairment, the dose should be reduced
- Before starting any therapy with buprenorphine it is recommended to check and document hepatitis virus status

Cardiac Impairment
- Cardiac side effects may occur

Elderly
- Reduced doses recommended

Children and Adolescents
- Safety and efficacy have not been established – not recommended for use in children and adolescents below the age of 15 years
- For moderate to severe pain: to be used with caution in the age group 15–18 years due to lack of evidence
- Sublingual tablets and IM or intravenous injections not licensed for use in children less than 6 years of age

Pregnancy
- Limited safety data for the use of buprenorphine in pregnancy
- In animal studies, adverse events have been observed at clinically relevant doses; no clear teratogenic effects were seen
- Neonatal withdrawal has been reported following use of opioids during pregnancy
- Use of opioids during pregnancy, especially close to delivery, presents a risk of respiratory depression in the neonate
- Women dependent on opioids should be encouraged to use maintenance treatment
- Detoxification increases risk of relapse, but if requested is best managed in the second trimester (contraindicated during first trimester)
- Withdrawal during first trimester increases risk of spontaneous abortion
- Withdrawal during third trimester increases risk of foetal stress and stillbirth

Breastfeeding
- Small amounts found in mother's breast milk
- Considered safe for short-term use
- Infants of women who choose to breastfeed while on buprenorphine should be monitored for possible adverse effects

THE ART OF PSYCHOPHARMACOLOGY

Potential Advantages
- Patients with mild to moderate physical dependence

Potential Disadvantages
- Patients unable to tolerate mild withdrawal symptoms

Primary Target Symptoms
- Opioid dependence

Pearls
- Buprenorphine is a semisynthetic opioid
- Associated with less stigma than methadone
- Better adherence than with methadone
- Substantially more nausea than other opioids
- Easy to administer with flexible dosing
- Ease of discontinuation
- In the treatment of opioid use disorder buprenorphine is an agonist/antagonist, meaning that it relieves withdrawal symptoms from other opioids and induces some euphoria, but also blocks the ability for many other opioids, including heroin, to cause an effect

Buprenorphine (Continued)

 **Switching**

- Monitor for withdrawal symptoms when switching from methadone to buprenorphine as these can be precipitated. To avoid this, initiate buprenorphine when signs of withdrawal begin to appear (but not less than 24 hours after last dose of methadone)
- Methadone dose should be reduced to 30 mg/day before starting buprenorphine, then titrate as appropriate

 Suggested Reading

Bentzley BS, Barth KS, Back SE, et al. Discontinuation of buprenorphine maintenance therapy: perspectives and outcomes. J Subst Abuse Treat 2015;52:48–57.

Bonhomme J, Shim RS, Gooden R, et al. Opioid addiction and abuse in primary care practice: a comparison of methadone and buprenorphine as treatment options. J Natl Med Assoc 2012;104(7–8):342–50.

Gowing L, Ali R, White JM, et al. Buprenorphine for managing opioid withdrawal. Cochrane Database Syst Rev 2017;2(2):CD002025.

Krans EE, Bogan D, Richardson D, et al. Factors associated with buprenorphine versus methadone use in pregnancy. Subst Abus 2016;37(4):550–7.

Li X, Shorter D, Kosten T. Buprenorphine prescribing: to expand or not to expand. J Psychiatr Pract 2016;22(3):183–92.

Whelan PJ, Remski K. Buprenorphine vs methadone treatment: a review of evidence in both developed and developing worlds. J Neurosci Rural Pract 2012;3(1):45–50.

Buprenorphine with naloxone

Brands
• Suboxone

Generic?
Yes

Class
• Neuroscience-based nomenclature: buprenorphine: pharmacology domain – opioid; mode of action – partial agonist; naloxone: pharmacology domain – opioid; mode of action – antagonist
• mu opioid receptor partial agonist combined with pure mu opioid receptor antagonist

Commonly Prescribed for
(bold for BNF indication)
• **Adjunct in the treatment of opioid dependence (under expert supervision)**

 How the Drug Works

• Buprenorphine is a partial agonist at mu opioid receptors and an antagonist at kappa opioid receptors
• Buprenorphine's activity in opioid maintenance treatment is due to its slowly reversible properties with the mu opioid receptors which, over a prolonged period, might minimise the need of addicted patients for drugs
• Binds with strong affinity to the mu opioid receptor, preventing exogenous opioids from binding there and thus preventing the pleasurable effects of opioid consumption
• Because buprenorphine is a partial agonist, it can cause immediate withdrawal in a patient currently taking opioids (i.e. reduces receptor stimulation in the presence of a full agonist), but can relieve withdrawal if a patient is already experiencing it (i.e. increases receptor stimulation in the absence of a full agonist)
• Buprenorphine is also an antagonist at the kappa opioid receptor
• Naloxone acts as a pure antagonist at mu opioid receptors
• When naloxone is administered intravenously to opioid-dependent patients, it produces marked opioid antagonist effects and opioid withdrawal, thereby deterring intravenous abuse
• When naloxone is administered orally or sublingually to patients experiencing opioid withdrawal, naloxone exhibits little or no pharmacological effect because of its almost complete first-pass metabolism
• The combination helps to decrease the potential for abuse or diversion

How Long Until It Works
• It begins working on withdrawal soon after the tablet is dissolved
• Its effects on reducing opioid use disorder/ dependence can take many months of treatment

If It Works
• It reduces the symptoms of opioid dependency such as cravings and withdrawal by acting on receptors without producing the euphoric effects. This helps patients abstain from other opioids to which they are addicted
• Reduces the effects of additional opioid use because of high receptor binding affinity (known as a "blocking" effect)
• Reduces the rewarding effects of opioid consumption
• It reduces the mortality of opioid use disorder by 50% (by reducing the risk of overdose on full-agonist opioids such as heroin or fentanyl)

If It Doesn't Work
• Evaluate reasons for poor response and address any contributing factors
• Consider switching to alternative agent such as methadone

 Best Augmenting Combos for Partial Response or Treatment Resistance
• Augmentation with behavioural, educational, and/or supportive therapy in groups or as an individual is key to successful treatment

Tests
• Documented viral hepatitis status is recommended before commencing therapy for opioid dependence

- Buprenorphine levels can be tested for using a urine drug screening kit, not commonly available outside of addiction services (note – buprenorphine cannot be tested for in standard multiple urine drug testing kits in the same way as methadone or heroin)
- Baseline liver function tests (LFTs) should be done before commencing therapy, and regularly throughout treatment

SIDE EFFECTS

How Drug Causes Side Effects
- Action at mu and kappa opioid receptors

Notable Side Effects
- Headache, constipation, nausea
- Oral hypoaesthesia, glossodynia
- Orthostatic hypotension

Common or very common
Sublingual use:
- Fatigue, headache, sleep disorders (insomnia or drowsiness), symptoms of withdrawal (headache, hyperhidrosis), nausea, vomiting

Uncommon
Sublingual use:
- CNS/PNS: abnormal coordination, coma, depersonalisation, diplopia, paraesthesia, psychosis, seizure, slurred speech, tinnitus
- CVS: atrioventricular block/arrhythmia, hypertension, hypotension
- GIT: dyspepsia
- Other: apnoea, conjunctivitis, cyanosis, pallor, urinary disorders

Rare or very rare
Sublingual use:
- Angioedema, bronchospasm

Frequency unknown
Sublingual use:
- Haemorrhagic diathesis, hepatic disorders, oral disorders

 Life-Threatening or Dangerous Side Effects
- Angioedema
- Respiratory depression
- Hepatotoxicity
- Arrhythmias

Weight Gain
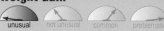
- Weight loss more likely

Sedation
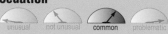
- Many experience and/or can be significant in amount

What To Do About Side Effects
- Wait
- Reduce dose
- Switch to another agent

Best Augmenting Agents for Side Effects
- Most side effects cannot be improved with an augmenting agent

DOSING AND USE

Usual Dosage Range
- 4–24 mg/day

Dosage Forms
- Sublingual tablet: buprenorphine 2 mg/naloxone 500 mcg, buprenorphine 8 mg/naloxone 2 mg, buprenorphine 16 mg/naloxone 4 mg
- Sublingual film: buprenorphine 2 mg/naloxone 500 mcg, buprenorphine 8 mg/naloxone 2 mg

How to Dose
- Initial dose 4 mg/day, this may be repeated up to twice on day 1 depending on patient requirement, then adjusted accordingly for maintenance, the total weekly dose can be divided and given every other day or 3 times per week
- Important to consult product literature for maintenance treatment
- Suboxone sublingual film can also be administered buccally
- Max dose is 24 mg in 24 hours

 Dosing Tips
- Clear evidence of daily opioid use (including drug testing) and withdrawal symptoms are mandatory before

commencing a prescription for buprenorphine

- The first dose of buprenorphine should be administered when the patient is experiencing opioid withdrawal symptoms to reduce the risk of precipitated withdrawal
- For patients addicted to short-acting opioids such as heroin, the first dose cannot be taken less than 6 hours after the patient last used opioids
- For patients addicted to long-acting opioids such as methadone the dose of methadone should be reduced to a max of 30 mg/day before starting buprenorphine. This is because buprenorphine may precipitate symptoms of withdrawal in patients dependent on methadone. The first dose cannot be taken less than 24 hours after the patient last used methadone
- Only buprenorphine with naloxone should be used for unsupervised administration, unless the patient has a proven allergy to naloxone
- Suboxone sublingual tablet and sublingual film are not bioequivalent, thus if a switch is required, then the patient should be monitored for symptoms of overdose or withdrawal
- For Suboxone sublingual films, up to 2 films may be used at the same time if required to make up the prescribed dose, placed on opposite sides of the mouth. A third film may be administered if required once the first 2 films have dissolved
- In the treatment of opioid use disorder buprenorphine is an agonist/antagonist, meaning that it relieves withdrawal symptoms from other opioids and induces some euphoria, but also blocks the ability for many other opioids, including heroin, to cause an effect
- Unlike full agonists like heroin or methadone, buprenorphine has a ceiling effect, such that taking more medicine will not increase the effects of the drug
- Buprenorphine alone is often used to initiate treatment, while buprenorphine with naloxone is preferred for stabilisation and maintenance treatment
- Buprenorphine not licensed for use in children under 6 years old

Overdose

- Buprenorphine alone can cause overdose which is only partially reversible by naloxone. It may present with apnoea, cardiovascular collapse, drowsiness, miosis, nausea, vomiting, respiratory depression, sedation
- It is difficult to overdose on buprenorphine with naloxone if it is injected intravenously due to the effects of naloxone. The addition of naloxone is meant to deter intravenous abuse
- Overdose usually occurs if the drug is mixed with other CNS depressants, e.g. benzodiazepines

Long-Term Use

- Use the lowest dose needed for as short a duration as possible, particularly if the patient is also taking other medications that may interact, such as benzodiazepines
- Maintenance treatment may be required; typical maintenance period is up to 2 years

Habit Forming

- Yes
- Buprenorphine is a Class C/Schedule 3 drug

How to Stop

- Patients may experience a mild withdrawal syndrome if buprenorphine is stopped abruptly
- Once the patient is stable, titrate down gradually to a lower maintenance dose and if appropriate, eventually discontinue
- Patients should be monitored following termination of treatment because of the potential for relapse

Pharmacokinetics

- Buprenorphine: time of onset 40–80 minutes; peak of action 1.5–2 hours
- Buprenorphine is metabolised by CYP450 3A4 to form N-dealkylbuprenorphine, a mu opioid agonist with weak intrinsic activity
- Half-life of sublingual buprenorphine 20–25 hours
- Following sublingual administration, plasma naloxone concentrations are low and decline quickly
- Elimination half-life of naloxone is 2–12 hours

Buprenorphine with naloxone (Continued)

 Drug Interactions

- Opioids can increase the risk of precipitating withdrawal
- Concomitant use with CNS depressants (e.g. alcohol or benzodiazepines) can increase the risk of respiratory depression; consider dose reduction of either or both
- Increased risk of CNS excitation or depression when taken with non-selective irreversible MAOIs (isocarboxazid, phenelzine, tranylcypromine): avoid the combination
- Nalmefene can reduce the efficacy of buprenorphine if taken concomitantly: avoid the combination
- Plasma concentrations of buprenorphine may be increased by drugs that inhibit CYP450 3A4 (e.g. clarithromycin, erythromycin, diltiazem, itraconazole, ketoconazole, ritonavir, verapamil, goldenseal, and grapefruit juice), so buprenorphine dose may need to be reduced if co-administered
- Plasma concentrations of buprenorphine may be reduced by drugs that induce CYP450 3A4, so buprenorphine dose may need to be increased if co-administered

⚠ **Other Warnings/Precautions**

- Although the risk is lower, buprenorphine can be abused in a manner similar to other opioids
- Use with caution in patients with compromised respiratory function
- Risk of respiratory depression is increased with concomitant use of CNS depressants – if patients are on other respiratory sedatives then lower doses should be used and the patient monitored for intoxication and respiratory depression
- Can cause severe, possibly fatal respiratory depression in children who are accidentally exposed to it
- Withdrawal symptoms can occur when switching from methadone to buprenorphine
- Buprenorphine may increase intracholedochal pressure and should be administered with caution to patients with dysfunction of the biliary tract

- Concurrent alcohol and illicit drug consumption must be considered when prescribing buprenorphine due to the increased risk of overdose associated with polysubstance misuse
- Use with caution in debilitated patients and those with myxoedema or hypothyroidism, adrenal cortical insufficiency (e.g. Addison's disease); CNS depression; toxic psychoses; prostatic hypertrophy or urethral stricture; acute alcoholism; delirium tremens; or kyphoscoliosis
- Buprenorphine should be used with caution in patients with impaired consciousness

Do Not Use

- If the patient is naive to opioid use
- If short-acting opioid used within the last 6 hours or long-acting opioid within the last 24 hours
- If the patient has severe respiratory impairment
- In comatose patients
- In patients with a head injury, intracranial lesions, and other circumstances when CSF pressure may be increased
- If patient has paralytic ileus
- If there is a proven allergy to buprenorphine
- If there is a proven allergy to naloxone

Renal Impairment

- Reduce dose and avoid in severe impairment otherwise increased cerebral sensitivity and opioid effects increased and prolonged

Hepatic Impairment

- In patients with moderate-severe impairment, plasma levels of buprenorphine can be higher and half-life longer; thus these patients should be monitored for signs and symptoms of toxicity/overdose
- For severe impairment, the dose should be reduced
- Before starting any therapy with buprenorphine it is recommended to check and document hepatitis virus status

Cardiac Impairment

- Cardiac side effects may occur

Elderly
• Reduced doses recommended

Children and Adolescents
• Safety and efficacy have not been established – not recommended for use in children and adolescents below the age of 15 years
• For moderate to severe pain: to be used with caution in the age group 15–18 years due to lack of evidence
• Sublingual tablets not licensed for use in children under 6 years; IM/intravenous use: injection not licensed for use in children under 6 months

Pregnancy
• Limited safety data for the use of buprenorphine in pregnancy
• In animal studies, adverse events have been observed at clinically relevant doses; no clear teratogenic effects were seen
• Neonatal withdrawal has been reported following use of opioids during pregnancy
• Use of opioids during pregnancy, especially close to delivery, presents a risk of respiratory depression in the neonate
• Women dependent on opioids should be encouraged to use maintenance treatment
• Detoxification increases risk of relapse, but if requested is best managed in the second trimester (contraindicated during first trimester)
• Withdrawal during first trimester increases risk of spontaneous abortion
• Withdrawal during third trimester increases risk of foetal stress and stillbirth

Breastfeeding
• Small amounts of buprenorphine found in mother's breast milk
• Low levels of naloxone expected in mother's breast milk
• No evidence of safety of naloxone
• Infants of women who choose to breastfeed while on buprenorphine should be monitored for possible adverse effects

Potential Advantages
• Patients with mild to moderate physical dependence
• The addition of naloxone helps to reduce abuse by triggering withdrawal symptoms if the drug is injected intravenously
• There is a ceiling effect to the opioid-like symptoms even with further dose increase, which reduces the risk of misuse

Potential Disadvantages
• Patients unable to tolerate mild withdrawal symptoms
• Must be used under supervision

Primary Target Symptoms
• Opioid addiction, where abuse of treatment medication is likely

Pearls
• Buprenorphine is a semisynthetic opioid
• Associated with less stigma than methadone
• Better adherence than with methadone
• Substantially more nausea than other opioids
• Easy to administer with flexible dosing
• Ease of discontinuation
• In the treatment of opioid use disorder buprenorphine is an agonist/antagonist, meaning that it relieves withdrawal symptoms from other opioids and induces some euphoria, but also blocks the ability for many other opioids, including heroin, to cause an effect
• May show reduced abuse potential
• Reduces the mortality of opioid use disorder by 50%

THE ART OF SWITCHING

Switching
• Monitor for withdrawal symptoms when switching from buprenorphine or methadone to buprenorphine with naloxone as these can be precipitated. To avoid this, initiate buprenorphine with naloxone when signs of withdrawal begin to appear (but not less than 24 hours after last dose of methadone)
• Methadone dose should be reduced to 30 mg/day before starting buprenorphine with naloxone, then titrate as appropriate

Suggested Reading

Heo Y-A, Scott LJ. Buprenorphine/Naloxone (Zubsolv ®): a review in opioid dependence. CNS Drugs 2018;32(9):875–82.

Hu T, Nijmeh L, Pyle A. Buprenorphine–naloxone. CMAJ 2018;190(47):E1389.

Kelty E, Cumming C, Troeung L, et al. Buprenorphine alone or with naloxone: which is safer? J Psychopharmacol 2018;32(3):344–52.

Sordo L, Barrio G, Bravo MJ, et al. Mortality risk during and after opioid substitution treatment: systematic review and meta-analysis of cohort studies. BMJ 2017;357:j1550.

Ziaaddini H, Heshmati S, Chegeni M, et al. Comparison of buprenorphine and buprenorphine/naloxone in detoxification of opioid-dependent men. Addict Health 2018;10(4):269–75.

Bupropion hydrochloride

THERAPEUTICS

Brands
- Zyban

Generic?
No, not in UK

Class
- Neuroscience-based nomenclature: pharmacology domain – norepinephrine, dopamine; mode of action – reuptake inhibitor (norepinephrine transporter, dopamine transporter), releaser (norepinephrine, dopamine)
- NDRI (norepinephrine dopamine reuptake inhibitor); antidepressant; smoking cessation treatment

Commonly Prescribed for
(bold for BNF indication)
- **To help with smoking cessation in nicotine-dependence (in combination with motivational support)**
- Major depressive disorder (as augmenting agent)
- Seasonal affective disorder
- Bipolar depression
- Attention deficit hyperactivity disorder (ADHD)
- Sexual dysfunction

How the Drug Works
- Boosts neurotransmitters noradrenaline and dopamine
- Blocks noradrenaline reuptake pump (noradrenaline transporter), presumably increasing noradrenaline neurotransmission
- Since dopamine is inactivated by noradrenaline reuptake in frontal cortex, which largely lacks dopamine transporters, bupropion can increase dopamine neurotransmission in this part of the brain
- Blocks dopamine reuptake pump (dopamine transporter), presumably increasing dopaminergic neurotransmission

How Long Until It Works
- Can be added to SSRIs to treat partial responders
- Onset of therapeutic actions with some antidepressants can be seen within 1–2 weeks, but often delayed 2–4 weeks

- If it is not working within 3–4 weeks as augmenting agent for depression, it may require a dosage increase or it may not work at all
- May continue to work for many years to prevent relapse of symptoms

If It Works
- The goal of treatment is complete remission of current symptoms as well as prevention of future relapses
- Treatment most often reduces or even eliminates symptoms, but is not a cure since symptoms can recur after medicine is stopped
- Continue treatment until all symptoms are gone (remission), especially in depression and whenever possible in anxiety disorders
- Once symptoms are gone, continue treating for at least 6–9 months for the first episode of depression or >12 months if relapse indicators present
- If >5 episodes and/or 2 episodes in the last few years then need to continue for at least 2 years or indefinitely

If It Doesn't Work
- Important to recognise non-response to treatment early on (3–4 weeks)
- Many patients have only a partial response where some symptoms are improved, but others persist (especially insomnia, fatigue, and problems concentrating)
- Other patients may be non-responders, sometimes called treatment-resistant or treatment-refractory
- Some patients who have an initial response may relapse even though they continue treatment
- Consider increasing dose or switching to another augmenting agent
- Lithium may be added for suicidal patients or those at high risk of relapse
- Consider psychotherapy
- Consider ECT
- Consider evaluation for another diagnosis or for a co-morbid condition (e.g. medical illness, substance abuse, etc.)
- Some patients may experience a switch into mania and so would require antidepressant discontinuation and initiation of a mood stabiliser, although this may be a less frequent problem with bupropion than with other antidepressants

Bupropion hydrochloride (Continued)

⚖️ Best Augmenting Combos for Partial Response or Treatment Resistance

Alternative augmenting agents as follows:
- Mood stabilisers or atypical antipsychotics for bipolar depression
- Atypical antipsychotics for psychotic depression
- Atypical antipsychotics as first-line augmenting agents (quetiapine MR 300 mg/day or aripiprazole at 2.5–10 mg/day) for treatment-resistant depression
- Atypical antipsychotics as second-line augmenting agents (risperidone 0.5–2 mg/day or olanzapine 2.5–10 mg/day) for treatment-resistant depression
- Mirtazapine at 30–45 mg/day as another second-line augmenting agent (a dual serotonin and noradrenaline combination, but observe for switch into mania, increase in suicidal ideation or serotonin syndrome)
- Although T3 (20–50 mcg/day) is another second-line augmenting agent the evidence suggests that it works best with tricyclic antidepressants
- Other augmenting agents but with less evidence include buspirone (up to 60 mg/day) and lamotrigine (up to 400 mg/day)
- Benzodiazepines if agitation present
- Hypnotics or trazodone for insomnia
- Augmenting agents reserved for specialist use include: modafinil for sleepiness, fatigue and lack of concentration; stimulants, oestrogens, testosterone
- Lithium is particularly useful for suicidal patients and those at high risk of relapse including with factors such as severe depression, psychomotor retardation, repeated episodes (>3), significant weight loss, or a family history of major depression (aim for lithium plasma levels 0.6–1.0 mmol/L)
- For depressed elderly patients lithium is a very effective augmenting agent
- For severely ill depressed patients other combinations may be tried especially in specialist centres
- Augmenting agents that may be tried include omega-3, SAM-e, L-methylfolate
- Additional non-pharmacological treatments such as exercise, mindfulness, CBT, and IPT can also be helpful

- If present after treatment response (4–8 weeks) or remission (6–12 weeks), the most common residual symptoms of depression include cognitive impairments, reduced energy and problems with sleep

Tests
- Recommended to assess blood pressure at baseline and periodically during treatment

SIDE EFFECTS

How Drug Causes Side Effects
- Side effects are probably caused in part by actions of norepinephrine and dopamine in brain areas with undesired effects (e.g. insomnia, tremor, agitation, headache, dizziness)
- Side effects are probably also caused in part by actions of norepinephrine in the periphery with undesired effects (e.g. sympathetic and parasympathetic effects such as dry mouth, constipation, nausea, anorexia, sweating)
- Most side effects are immediate but often go away with time

Notable Side Effects
- Dry mouth, constipation, nausea, weight loss, anorexia, myalgia
- Insomnia, dizziness, headache, agitation, anxiety, tremor, abdominal pain, tinnitus
- Sweating, rash
- Hypertension

Common or very common
- CNS/PNS: anxiety, dizziness, headache, impaired concentration, insomnia (reduced by avoiding dose at bedtime), tremor
- GIT: abdominal pain, altered taste, constipation, dry mouth, gastrointestinal disorder, nausea, vomiting
- Other: fever, hyperhidrosis, hypersensitivity, skin reactions

Uncommon
- CNS: confusion, tinnitus, visual impairment
- CVS: chest pain, tachycardia, vasodilation
- Other: asthenia, decreased appetite

Rare or very rare
- CNS/PNS: abnormal behaviour, delusions, depersonalisation, hallucination, irritability, memory loss, movement disorders, paraesthesia, parkinsonism, seizure, sleep disorders

- Other: angioedema, arthralgia, bronchospasm, dyspnoea, hepatic disorders, muscle complaints, palpitations, postural hypotension, Stevens-Johnson syndrome, syncope, urinary disorder

 Life-Threatening or Dangerous Side Effects

- Rare seizures (higher incidence for immediate-release than for sustained-release; risk increases with doses above the recommended maximums; risk increases for patients with predisposing factors)
- Anaphylactoid/anaphylactic reactions and Stevens-Johnson syndrome have been reported
- Hypomania (more likely in bipolar patients but perhaps less common than with some other antidepressants)
- Psychosis
- Increase in suicidal tendencies

Weight Gain

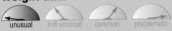

- Reported but not expected
- *Patients may experience weight loss

Sedation

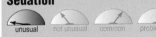

- Reported but not expected

What to Do About Side Effects

- Wait
- Wait
- Wait
- Keep dose as low as possible
- Take no later than mid-afternoon to avoid insomnia
- Switch to another drug

Best Augmenting Agents for Side Effects

- Often best to try another antidepressant monotherapy prior to resorting to augmentation strategies to treat side effects
- Trazodone or a hypnotic for drug-induced insomnia
- Mirtazapine for insomnia, agitation, and gastrointestinal side effects
- Benzodiazepines or buspirone for drug-induced anxiety, agitation

- Many side effects are dose-dependent (i.e. they increase as dose increases, or they re-emerge until tolerance redevelops)
- Many side effects are time-dependent (i.e. they start immediately upon dosing and upon each dose increase, but go away with time)
- Increased activation or agitation may represent the induction of a bipolar state, especially a mixed dysphoric bipolar condition sometimes associated with suicidal ideation, and require the addition of lithium, a mood stabiliser or an atypical antipsychotic, and/or discontinuation of bupropion

DOSING AND USE

Usual Dosage Range

- Bupropion hydrochloride MR: 150–300 mg once daily

Dosage Forms

- Modified-release (MR) tablet 150 mg

How to Dose

- *Depression:
- Initial dose 150 mg/day in the morning; can increase to 300 mg/day after 4 days
- *Nicotine addiction:
- Initial dose 150 mg/day, increase to 150 mg twice per day after at least 3 days; max dose 300 mg/day; bupropion treatment should begin 1–2 weeks before smoking is discontinued

 Dosing Tips

- When used for bipolar depression, it is usually as an augmenting agent to mood stabilisers, lithium, and/or atypical antipsychotics
- For smoking cessation, may be used in conjunction with nicotine replacement therapy
- Do not break or chew MR tablets as this will alter modified-release properties
- The more anxious and agitated the patient, the lower the starting dose, the slower the titration, and the more likely the need for a concomitant agent such as trazodone or a benzodiazepine
- If intolerable anxiety, insomnia, agitation, akathisia or activation occur either upon dosing initiation or discontinuation,

consider the possibility of activated bipolar disorder and switch to a mood stabiliser or an atypical antipsychotic

Overdose
- Rarely lethal; seizures, cardiac disturbances, hallucinations, loss of consciousness

Long-Term Use
- For smoking cessation, treatment for up to 6 months has been found effective
- For depression, treatment up to 1 year has been found to decrease rate of relapse

Habit Forming
- No, but can be abused by individuals who crush and then snort or inject

How to Stop
- Tapering is prudent to avoid withdrawal effects, but no well-documented tolerance, dependence, or withdrawal reactions

Pharmacokinetics
- Food does not affect absorption
- Inhibits CYP450 2D6
- Parent half-life 11–21 hours
- Metabolites half-life range 20–37 hours
- Excretion: urine 87%, faeces 10%

 Drug Interactions
- Tramadol increases the risk of seizures in patients taking an antidepressant
- Can increase TCA levels; use with caution with TCAs or when switching from a TCA to bupropion
- Use with caution with MAOIs, including 14 days after MAOIs are stopped (for the expert)
- There is increased risk of hypertensive reaction if bupropion is used in conjunction with MAOIs or other drugs that increase norepinephrine
- There may be an increased risk of hypertension if bupropion is combined with nicotine replacement therapy
- Via CYP450 2D6 inhibition, bupropion could theoretically interfere with the analgesic actions of codeine, and increase the plasma levels of some beta blockers and of atomoxetine
- Via CYP450 2D6 inhibition, bupropion could theoretically increase concentrations of thioridazine and cause dangerous cardiac arrhythmias

- Risk of serotonin syndrome if bupropion combined with serotonergic agents

 Other Warnings/Precautions
- Use cautiously with other drugs that increase seizure risk (TCAs, lithium, phenothiazines, thioxanthenes, some antipsychotics)
- Bupropion should be used with caution in patients taking levodopa or amantadine, as these agents can potentially enhance dopamine neurotransmission and be activating
- Do not use if patient has severe insomnia
- When treating children, carefully weigh the risks and benefits of pharmacological treatment against the risks and benefits of nontreatment and make sure to document this in the patient's chart
- Warn patients and their caregivers about the possibility of activating side effects and advise them to report such symptoms immediately
- Monitor patients for activation of suicidal ideation, especially children and adolescents
- Discontinuing smoking may lead to pharmacokinetic or pharmacodynamic changes in other drugs the patient is taking, which could potentially require dose adjustment
- Use with caution in alcohol abuse, diabetes, in the elderly, history of head trauma or predisposition to seizures (prescribe only if benefit clearly outweighs risk)

Do Not Use
- In patients in acute alcohol or benzodiazepine withdrawal
- In patients with bipolar disorder or eating disorders
- In patients with a CNS tumour or history of seizures
- In patients with severe hepatic cirrhosis
- If there is a proven allergy to bupropion

Renal Impairment
- Reduce dose to 150 mg/day

Hepatic Impairment
- Reduce dose to 150 mg/day in mild-moderate impairment
- Avoid in severe cirrhosis

Cardiac Impairment
- Limited available data
- Evidence of rise in supine blood pressure
- Use with caution

Elderly
- 150 mg/day for between 7 to 9 weeks, start treatment 1 to 2 weeks before the target stop date, discontinue bupropion if abstinence not reached at 7 weeks; max 150 mg/day
- Increased risk for accumulating bupropion and its metabolites due to decreased clearance

Children and Adolescents
- Not licensed for those less than 18 years of age
- May be used for ADHD in children or adolescents by specialists

Pregnancy
- Available human data does not indicate increased risk of congenital malformations overall or of cardiovascular malformations
- Not associated with intrauterine death, preterm delivery or low birth weight
- Case studies indicate possible association with specific cardiac malformations
- One study found an association between bupropion use during pregnancy and ADHD in the child although data confounded by other factors
- In animal studies, no clear evidence of teratogenicity has been observed; however, slightly increased incidences of foetal malformations and skeletal variations were observed in rabbit studies at doses approximately equal to and greater than the maximum recommended human doses, and greater and decreased foetal weights were observed in rat studies at doses greater than the maximum recommended human doses
- Not routinely recommended for use during pregnancy
- Pregnant women wishing to stop smoking may consider behavioural therapy before pharmacotherapy
- Must weigh the risk of treatment (first trimester foetal development, third trimester newborn delivery) to the child against the risk of no treatment (recurrence of depression, maternal health, infant bonding) to the mother and child

Breastfeeding
- Small amounts are found in mother's breast milk
- Case reports of seizures in the infant
- Immediate postpartum period is a high-risk time for depression, especially in women who have had prior depressive episodes, antidepressants may need to be reinstituted late in the third trimester or shortly after childbirth to prevent a recurrence during the postpartum period
- Must weigh benefits of breastfeeding with risks and benefits of antidepressant treatment versus nontreatment to both the infant and the mother
- For some patients this may mean continuing treatment during breastfeeding

THE ART OF PSYCHOPHARMACOLOGY
Potential Advantages
- Depression with psychomotor retardation
- Atypical depression
- Bipolar depression
- Patients concerned about sexual dysfunction
- Patients concerned about weight gain

Potential Disadvantages
- Patients experiencing weight loss associated with their depression
- Patients who are excessively activated

Primary Target Symptoms
- Depressed mood
- Sleep disturbance, especially hypersomnia
- Cravings associated with nicotine withdrawal
- Cognitive functioning

Pearls
* May be effective if only partial response with an SSRI
- Less likely to produce hypomania than some other antidepressants
* May improve cognitive slowing/pseudodementia
* Reduces hypersomnia and fatigue
- Approved to help reduce craving during smoking cessation
- Anecdotal use in attention deficit disorder

Bupropion hydrochloride (Continued)

- May cause sexual dysfunction only infrequently
- May exacerbate tics
- Bupropion may not be as effective in anxiety disorders as many other antidepressants
- Increased risk of seizures was observed when bupropion immediate-release was dosed at especially high levels to low body weight patients with active anorexia nervosa. However, patients with normal BMI without additional risk factors for seizures may benefit from bupropion MR under expert supervision, with close monitoring and discussion of the potential risks with the patient

- The active enantiomer of the principal active metabolite [(+)-6-hydroxy-bupropion] is in clinical development as a novel antidepressant
- The combination of bupropion and naltrexone (Mysimba) has demonstrated efficacy as a treatment for obesity and is being evaluated for its cardiovascular benefits
- Phase II trials of the combination of bupropion and zonisamide for the treatment of obesity have been completed
- While bupropion demonstrates some potential for misuse, this is less than for other commonly used stimulants, due to features of its pharmacology

 Suggested Reading

Cipriani A, Furukawa TA, Salanti G, et al. Comparative efficacy and acceptability of 21 antidepressant drugs for the acute treatment of adults with major depressive disorder: a systematic review and network meta-analysis. Lancet 2018;391(10128):1357–66.

Clayton AH. Extended-release bupropion: an antidepressant with a broad spectrum of therapeutic activity? Expert Opin Pharmacother 2007;8(4):457–66.

Ferry L, Johnston JA. Efficacy and safety of bupropion SR for smoking cessation: data from clinical trials and five years of postmarketing experience. Int J Clin Pract 2003;57(3):224–30.

Foley KF, DeSanty KP, Kast RE. Bupropion: pharmacology and therapeutic applications. Expert Rev Neurother 2006;6(9):1249–65.

Jefferson JW, Pradko JF, Muir KT. Bupropion for major depressive disorder: pharmacokinetic and formulation considerations. Clin Ther 2005;27(11):1685–95.

Masters AR, Gufford BT, Lu JB, et al. Chiral plasma pharmacokinetics and urinary excretion of bupropion and metabolites in healthy volunteers. J Pharmacol Exp Ther 2016;358(2):230–8.

Naglich AC, Brown ES, Adinoff B. Systematic review of preclinical, clinical, and post-marketing evidence of bupropion misuse potential. Am J Drug Alcohol Abuse 2019;45(4):341–54.

Papakostas GI, Nutt DJ, Hallett LA, et al. Resolution of sleepiness and fatigue in major depressive disorder: a comparison of bupropion and the selective serotonin reuptake inhibitors. Biol Psychiatry 2006;60(12):1350–5.

Ross S, Williams D. Bupropion: risks and benefits. Expert Opin Drug Saf 2005;4(6):995–1003.

Buspirone hydrochloride

THERAPEUTICS

Brands
• Non-proprietary

Generic?
Yes

Class
• Neuroscience-based nomenclature: pharmacology domain – serotonin; mode of action – partial agonist
• Anxiolytic (azapirone; serotonin 1A partial agonist; serotonin stabiliser)

Commonly Prescribed for
(bold for BNF indication)
• **Anxiety (short-term use)**
• Management of anxiety disorders
• Mixed anxiety and depression
• Treatment-resistant depression (augmentation)

 ### How the Drug Works
• Binds to serotonin 1A receptors
• Partial agonist actions postsynaptically may theoretically diminish serotonergic activity and contribute to anxiolytic actions
• Presynaptic agonist actions at presynaptic somatodendritic serotonin autoreceptors may theoretically enhance serotonergic activity and contribute to antidepressant actions

How Long Until It Works
• Generally takes within 2–4 weeks to achieve efficacy
• If it is not working within 6–8 weeks, it may require a dosage increase or it may not work at all

If It Works
• The goal of treatment is complete remission of current symptoms as well as prevention of future relapses
• Treatment most often reduces or even eliminates symptoms, but is not a cure since symptoms can recur after medicine is stopped
• Chronic anxiety disorders may require long-term maintenance with buspirone to control symptoms

If It Doesn't Work
• Consider switching to another agent (a benzodiazepine, pregabalin or an antidepressant)

 ### Best Augmenting Combos for Partial Response or Treatment Resistance
• Sedative hypnotic for insomnia
• Buspirone (up to 60 mg/day) can itself be used as an augmenting agent for antidepressants (SSRI/SNRI) in treatment-resistant depression

Tests
• None for healthy individuals

SIDE EFFECTS

How Drug Causes Side Effects
• Serotonin partial agonist actions in parts of the brain and body and at receptors other than those that cause therapeutic actions

Notable Side Effects
٭ Dizziness, headache, nervousness, sedation, excitement
• Nausea
• Restlessness

Common or very common
• CNS: anger, anxiety, confusion, depression, dizziness, drowsiness, headache, impaired concentration, movement disorders, paraesthesia, sleep disorders, tinnitus, tremor, vision disorders
• CVS: chest pain, tachycardia
• GIT: abdominal pain, constipation, diarrhoea, dry mouth, nausea, vomiting
• Other: cold sweat, fatigue, laryngeal pain, musculoskeletal pain, nasal congestion, skin reactions

Rare or very rare
• CNS/PNS: depersonalisation, emotional lability, hallucination, memory loss, parkinsonism, psychosis, seizure
• CVS: syncope
• Other: serotonin syndrome, urinary retention

 ### Life-Threatening or Dangerous Side Effects
• Rare cardiac symptoms

Buspirone hydrochloride (Continued)

Weight Gain

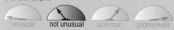

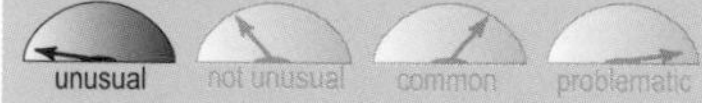

unusual | not unusual | common | problematic

• Reported but not expected

Sedation

unusual | not unusual | common | problematic

• Occurs in a significant minority

What To Do About Side Effects

• Wait
• Wait
• Wait
• Lower the dose
• Give total daily dose divided into 3, 4, or more doses
• Switch to another agent

Best Augmenting Agents for Side Effects

• Many side effects cannot be improved with an augmenting agent

DOSING AND USE

Usual Dosage Range

• Anxiety (short-term use): 15–30 mg/day in divided doses

Dosage Forms

• Tablet 5 mg, 7.5 mg, 10 mg

How to Dose

*Anxiety (short-term use):
• Initial dose 5 mg 2–3 times per day, increased at intervals of 2–3 days as needed up to 45 mg/day; usual dose 15–30 mg/day in divided doses

 Dosing Tips

• Requires dosing 2–3 times per day for full effect
• Absorption is affected by food, so administration with or without food should be consistent

Overdose

• Non-lethal with single agent overdose; sedation, dizziness, small pupils, nausea, vomiting

Long-Term Use

• Limited data suggest that it is safe

Habit Forming

• No

How to Stop

• Taper generally not necessary

Pharmacokinetics

• Metabolised primarily by CYP450 3A4
• Apparent plasma half-life for elimination of parent drug is 2–11 hours
• Absorption affected by food

 Drug Interactions

• Use with caution with MAOIs including for at least 14 days after stopping MAOIs (for the expert)
• CYP450 3A4 inhibitors (e.g. fluoxetine, fluvoxamine) may reduce clearance of buspirone and raise its plasma levels, so the dose of buspirone may need to be lowered when given concomitantly with these agents
• CYP450 3A4 inducers (e.g. carbamazepine) may increase clearance of buspirone and so the dose of buspirone may need to be raised
• Buspirone may increase plasma concentrations of haloperidol
• Buspirone may raise the levels of nordiazepam (active metabolite of diazepam), which may result in increased symptoms of dizziness, headache, or nausea

 Other Warnings/Precautions

• Use with caution in patients with angle-closure glaucoma
• Buspirone does not alleviate symptoms of benzodiazepine withdrawal
• Use with caution in patients with myasthenia gravis
• A patient on a benzodiazepine needs to have the benzodiazepine gradually withdrawn; best to do this before starting buspirone

Do Not Use

• If patient has epilepsy
• If there is a proven allergy to buspirone

SPECIAL POPULATIONS

Renal Impairment
- Use with caution – reduce dose
- Avoid in severe renal impairment due to the risk of accumulation of metabolites

Hepatic Impairment
- Use with caution
- Avoid in severe hepatic failure
- Titrate individual dose carefully in cirrhosis

Cardiac Impairment
- Buspirone has been used to treat hostility in patients with cardiac impairment

Elderly
- Some patients may tolerate lower doses better

Children and Adolescents
- Not licensed for use in children and adolescents
- Safety profile in children encourages use

Pregnancy
- Limited human data
- Controlled studies have not been conducted in pregnant women
- Animal studies have not shown adverse effects
- Not generally recommended in pregnancy, but may be safer than some other options

Breastfeeding
- Some drug is expected in mother's breast milk
- Trace amounts may be present in nursing children whose mothers are on buspirone
- Case report of possible seizure-like activity in infant of mother taking buspirone, carbamazepine and fluoxetine
- If child becomes irritable or sedated, breastfeeding or drug may need to be discontinued

THE ART OF PSYCHOPHARMACOLOGY

Potential Advantages
- Safety profile
- Lack of dependence, withdrawal
- Lack of sexual dysfunction or weight gain

Potential Disadvantages
- May take 4 weeks for beneficial effects to be observed whereas benzodiazepines have an immediate effect

Primary Target Symptoms
- Anxiety

Pearls
- *Buspirone does not appear to cause dependence and shows virtually no withdrawal symptoms
- May have less severe side effects than benzodiazepines
- *Buspirone generally lacks sexual dysfunction
- Buspirone may reduce sexual dysfunction associated with GAD or serotonergic antidepressants
- Sedation more likely at dose above 20 mg/day
- May be less effective against anxiety for some patients versus benzodiazepines
- Generally reserved as an augmenting agent in the treatment of anxiety
- Can be used as an augmenting agent in the management of treatment-resistant depression

Buspirone hydrochloride (Continued)

 Suggested Reading

Apter JT, Allen LA. Buspirone: future directions. J Clin Psychopharmmacol 1999;19(1);86–93.

Caldiroli A, Capuzzi E, Tagliabue I, et al. Treatment-resistant major depression: a comprehensive review. Int J Mol Sci 2021;22(23):13070.

Garakani A, Murrough JW, Freire RC, et al. Pharmacotherapy of anxiety disorders: current and emerging treatment options. Front Psychiatry 2020;11:595584.

Mahmood I, Sahajwalla C. Clinical pharmacokinetics and pharmacodynamics of buspirone, an anxiolytic drug. Clin Pharmacokinet 1999;36(4):277–87.

Pecknold JC. A risk-benefit assessment of buspirone in the treatment of anxiety disorders. Drug Saf 1997;16(2):118–32.

Sramek JJ, Hong WW, Hamid S, et al. Meta-analysis of the safety and tolerability of two dose regimens of buspirone in patients with persistent anxiety. Depress Anxiety 1999;9(3):131–4.

Carbamazepine

THERAPEUTICS

Brands
- Tegretol
- Tegretol Prolonged Release

Generic?
Yes (not for modified-release formulation)

Class
- Neuroscience-based nomenclature: pharmacology domain – glutamate; mode of action – channel blocker
- Anticonvulsant, antineuralgic for chronic pain, voltage-sensitive sodium channel antagonist; glutamate, voltage-gated sodium and calcium channel blocker (Glu-CB)

Commonly Prescribed for
(bold for BNF indication)
- **Seizures: primary generalised tonic-clonic; focal and secondary generalised tonic-clonic; focal and generalised tonic-clonic**
- **Prophylaxis of bipolar disorder unresponsive to lithium – in adults**
- **Trigeminal neuralgia – in adults**
- **Diabetic neuropathy (unlicensed)**
- **Adjunct in acute alcohol withdrawal (unlicensed)**
- Bipolar depression
- Acute mania
- Psychosis, schizophrenia (adjunctive)

 How the Drug Works
- ＊Acts as a use-dependent blocker of voltage-sensitive sodium channels
- ＊Interacts with the open channel conformation of voltage-sensitive sodium channels
- ＊Interacts at a specific site of the alpha pore-forming subunit of voltage-sensitive sodium channels
- Inhibits release of glutamate

How Long Until It Works
- May take several weeks to months to optimise an effect on mood stabilisation
- Should reduce seizures by 2 weeks
- For acute mania, effects should occur within a few weeks

If It Works
- The goal of treatment is complete remission of symptoms (e.g. seizures, mania, pain)
- Continue treatment until all symptoms are gone or until improvement is stable and then continue treating indefinitely as long as improvement persists
- Continue treatment indefinitely to avoid recurrence of mania and seizures
- Treatment of chronic neuropathic pain most often reduces, but does not eliminate pain and is not a cure since symptoms usually recur after medicine stopped

If It Doesn't Work (for bipolar disorder)
- ＊Many patients have only a partial response where some symptoms are improved, but others persist or continue to wax and wane without stabilisation of mood
- Other patients may be non-responders, sometimes called treatment-resistant or treatment-refractory
- Consider increasing dose, switching to another agent or adding an appropriate augmenting agent
- Consider adding psychotherapy
- For bipolar disorder, consider the presence of non-concordance and counsel patient
- Switch to another mood stabiliser with fewer side effects or to modified-release carbamazepine
- Consider evaluation for another diagnosis or for a co-morbid condition (e.g. medical illness, substance abuse, etc.)

 Best Augmenting Combos for Partial Response or Treatment Resistance
- Lithium
- Atypical antipsychotics (especially risperidone, olanzapine, quetiapine, and aripiprazole)
- Valproate (carbamazepine can decrease valproate levels)
- Lamotrigine (carbamazepine can decrease lamotrigine levels)
- ＊Antidepressants (with caution because antidepressants can destabilise mood in some patients, including induction of rapid cycling or suicidal ideation; in particular

consider bupropion; also SSRIs, SNRIs, others; generally avoid TCAs, MAOIs)

Tests

✳Before starting: full blood count, liver, kidney, and thyroid function tests

✳Before starting: individuals with ancestry across broad areas of Asia should consider screening for the presence of the HLA-B*1502 allele; those with HLA-B*1502 should not be treated with carbamazepine

• During treatment: full blood count, liver and kidney tests to be repeated every 6 months. Weight/BMI should be monitored

• Consider monitoring sodium levels because of possibility of hyponatraemia

SIDE EFFECTS

How Drug Causes Side Effects

• CNS side effects theoretically due to excessive actions at voltage-sensitive sodium channels

• Major metabolite (carbamazepine-10, 11 epoxide) may be the cause of many side effects

• Mild anticholinergic effects may contribute to sedation, blurred vision

Notable Side Effects

✳Dizziness, drowsiness, dry mouth, fatigue, gastrointestinal (including nausea, diarrhoea), oedema

• Movement disorders, blurred vision

✳Blood dyscrasia including benign leucopenia (transient; in up to 10%), eosinophilia, thrombocytopenia

• Hyponatraemia

✳Rash

• Side effects such as headache, ataxia, drowsiness, nausea and vomiting, blurred vision, dizziness and allergic skin reactions are dose-related and are more common at the start of treatment and in the elderly

Common or very common

• Blood disorders: eosinophilia, leucopenia, thrombocytopenia

• CNS: dizziness, drowsiness, headache, movement disorders, vision disorders

• GIT: dry mouth, gastrointestinal discomfort, increased weight, nausea, vomiting

• Other: fluid imbalance, hyponatraemia, oedema, skin reactions

Uncommon

• CNS/PNS: eye disorders, tic, tremor

• GIT: constipation, diarrhoea

Rare or very rare

• Blood disorders: agranulocytosis, anaemia, haemolytic anaemia, hypogammaglobulinaemia, leucocytosis, red cell abnormalities

• CNS/PNS: aggression, anxiety, aseptic meningitis, confusion, depression, hallucinations, hearing impairment, hyperacusia, nervous system disorder, paraesthesia, paresis, peripheral neuropathy, psychosis, speech impairment, tinnitus

• CVS: arrhythmias, cardiac conduction disorders, circulatory collapse, congestive heart failure, coronary artery disease aggravated, embolism and thrombosis, hypertension, hypotension, syncope

• Endocrine: galactorrhoea, gynaecomastia, hirsutism

• GIT: altered taste, decreased appetite, hepatic disorders, oral disorders, pancreatitis, vanishing bile duct syndrome

• Resp: dyspnoea, pneumonia, pneumonitis

• Genitourinary: abnormal spermatogenesis, albuminuria, azotaemia, haematuria, renal impairment, sexual dysfunction, tuberointerstitial nephritis, urinary disorders

• Other: alopecia, angioedema, arthralgia, bone disorders, bone marrow disorders, conjunctivitis, erythema nodosum, fever, folate deficiency, hyperhidrosis, hypersensitivity, lens opacity, lymphadenopathy, muscle complaints, muscle weakness, neuroleptic malignant syndrome, photosensitivity reaction, pseudolymphoma, severe cutaneous adverse reactions (SCARs), systemic lupus erythematosus (SLE), vasculitis

Frequency not known

• CNS: memory loss, suicidal behaviours

• Other: bone fracture, colitis, nail loss, reactivation of herpes virus 6

 Life-Threatening or Dangerous Side Effects

✳Rare aplastic anaemia, agranulocytosis (unusual bleeding or bruising, mouth sores, infections, fever, sore throat)

✳Rare severe dermatologic reactions (purpura, Stevens-Johnson syndrome)

• Rare cardiac problems

- Rare induction of psychosis or mania
* SIADH (syndrome of inappropriate antidiuretic hormone secretion) with hyponatraemia
- Increased frequency of generalised convulsions (in patients with atypical absence seizures)
- Rare activation of suicidal ideation and behaviour (suicidality)

Weight Gain

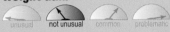

- Occurs in significant minority

Sedation

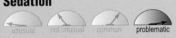

- Frequent and can be significant in amount
- Some patients may not tolerate it
- Dose-related
- Can wear off with time, but commonly does not wear off at high doses
- CNS side effects significantly lower with modified-release formulation

What to Do About Side Effects

- Wait
- Wait
- Wait
- Take with food or split dose to avoid gastrointestinal effects
- Take at night to reduce daytime sedation
- Switch to another agent or to modified-release carbamazepine

Best Augmenting Agents for Side Effects

- Many side effects cannot be improved with an augmenting agent

DOSING AND USE

Usual Dosage Range

- Seizures: 100–2,000 mg/day in divided doses
- Trigeminal neuralgia: 100–1,600 mg/day in divided doses
- Prophylaxis of bipolar disorder unresponsive to lithium: 400–1,600 mg/day in divided doses
- Adjunct in acute alcohol withdrawal: 200–800 mg/day in divided doses
- Diabetic neuropathy: 100–1,600 mg/day in divided doses

Dosage Forms

- Tablet 100 mg, 200 mg, 400 mg
- Modified-release tablet 200 mg, 400 mg
- Oral suspension 100 mg/5 mL (300 mL)
- Suppository 125 mg, 250 mg

How to Dose

Adults:

* Seizures:
- Immediate-release: initial oral dose 100–200 mg 1–2 times per day, increased by increments of 100–200 mg every 2 weeks; usual dose 0.8–1.2 g/day in divided doses; increased as needed up to 1.6–2 g/day in divided doses
- Modified-release: initial oral dose 100–400 mg/day in 1–2 divided doses, increased by increments of 100–200 mg every 2 weeks; usual dose 0.8–1.2 g/day in 1–2 divided doses, increased as needed up to 1.6–2 g/day in 1–2 divided doses
- Rectal: up to 1 g/day in 4 divided doses for up to 7 days (for short-term use when oral treatment not possible)
* Trigeminal neuralgia:
- Immediate-release: initial oral dose 100 mg 1–2 times per day (some patients may need higher initial dose), increase gradually according to response; usual dose 200 mg 3–4 times per day, increased as needed up to 1.6 g/day
- Modified-release: initial oral dose 100–200 mg/day in 1–2 divided doses (some patients may require higher initial dose), increase gradually according to response; usual dose 600–800 mg/day in 1–2 divided doses, increased as needed up to 1.6 g/day in 1–2 divided doses
* Prophylaxis of bipolar disorder unresponsive to lithium:
- Immediate-release: initial oral dose 400 mg/day in divided doses, increased until symptoms controlled; usual dose 400–600 mg/day; max 1.6 g/day
- Modified-release: initial oral dose 400 mg/day in 1–2 divided doses, increased until symptoms controlled; usual dose 400–600 mg/day in 1–2 divided doses; max 1.6 g/day
* Adjunct in acute alcohol withdrawal:
- Immediate-release: initial oral dose 800 mg/day in divided doses, then reduced to 200 mg/day for usual treatment duration of 7–10 days, dose to be reduced gradually over 5 days

∗Diabetic neuropathy:
• Immediate-release: initial oral dose 100 mg 1–2 times per day, increased gradually according to response; usual dose 200 mg 3–4 times per day, increased if necessary up to 1.6 g/day

Children and adolescents:

∗Unlicensed use for the prophylaxis of bipolar disorder:
• Child 1 month–11 years (initial dose either 5 mg/kg/day at night, or 2.5 mg/kg twice per day, then increased by increments of 2.5–5 mg/kg every 3–7 days as needed; maintenance 5 mg/kg 2–3 times per day, increased as needed to 20 mg/kg/day)
• Child 12–17 years (initial dose 100–200 mg 1–2 times per day, then increased to 200–400 mg 2–3 times per day, slowly increased as needed up to 1.8 g/day)

 Dosing Tips

• Higher peak levels occur with the suspension formulation than with the same dose of the tablet formulation, so suspension should generally be started at a lower dose and titrated slowly
• Take carbamazepine with food to avoid gastrointestinal effects
∗Slower dose titration may delay onset of therapeutic action, but enhance tolerability to sedating side effects
• Modified-release formulations can significantly reduce sedation and other CNS side effects
• Levels vary through the day and it is important to sample trough serum levels usually before the first dose of the day
• Should titrate slowly in the presence of other sedating agents, such as other anticonvulsants, in order to best tolerate additive sedative side effects
∗Can sometimes minimise the impact of carbamazepine upon the bone marrow by dosing slowly and monitoring closely when initiating treatment; initial trend to leucopenia/neutropenia may reverse with continued conservative dosing over time and allow subsequent dosage increases with careful monitoring
∗Carbamazepine often requires a dosage adjustment upward with time, as the drug induces its own metabolism, thus lowering its own plasma levels over the first several weeks to months of treatment

• Do not chew carbamazepine modified-release tablets as this will alter the controlled-release properties
• Plasma level of higher than 7 mg/L may be required in affective illness; levels higher than 12 mg/L are associated with higher side-effect burden

Overdose

• Can be fatal (lowest known fatal dose in adults is 3.2 g, in adolescents is 4 g, and in children is 1.6 g); nausea, vomiting, involuntary movements, irregular heartbeat, urinary retention, trouble breathing, sedation, coma
• Give repeated doses of activated charcoal by mouth

Long-Term Use

• May lower sex drive
• Monitoring of liver, kidney, thyroid functions, blood counts and sodium is advised

Habit Forming

• No

How to Stop

• Taper; may need to adjust dosage of concurrent medications as carbamazepine is being discontinued
∗Rapid discontinuation may increase the risk of relapse in bipolar disorder
• Epilepsy patients may have a seizure upon withdrawal, especially if withdrawal is abrupt
• Discontinuation symptoms uncommon

Pharmacokinetics

• Metabolised in the liver, primarily by CYP450 3A4
• Renally excreted
• Initial half-life 36 hours after a single dose; half-life 16–24 hours with repeated doses
• Active metabolite is carbamazepine-10,11 epoxide
∗Is not only a substrate for CYP450 3A4, but also an inducer of CYP450 3A4
∗Thus, carbamazepine induces its own metabolism, often requiring an upward dosage adjustment
• Is also an inducer of CYP450 2C9 and weakly of CYP450 1A2 and 2C19
• Food does not affect absorption

Drug Interactions

- Carbamazepine reduces plasma levels of most antidepressants, most antipsychotics, benzodiazepines, some cholinesterase inhibitors, methadone, thyroxine, theophylline, oestrogens and other steroids may also be reduced resulting in treatment failure
- Patients requiring contraception will need to be on higher doses of oestrogen or use non-hormonal methods
- Drugs that inhibit CYP450 3A4 will increase carbamazepine plasma levels and may precipitate toxicity, e.g. cimetidine, diltiazem, verapamil, erythromycin, some SSRIs including fluoxetine
- Enzyme-inducing antiepileptic drugs (carbamazepine itself as well as phenobarbital, phenytoin, and primidone) may increase the clearance of carbamazepine and lower its plasma levels
- Pharmacodynamic interactions also occur. Anticonvulsant activity of carbamazepine is reduced by drugs that lower the seizure threshold (e.g. antipsychotics and antidepressants). Potential for carbamazepine to cause neutropenia may be increased by drugs that have potential to depress the bone marrow (e.g. clozapine), risk of hyponatraemia may be increased by other drugs that have potential to deplete sodium (e.g. diuretics). Rarely, neurotoxicity has been reported when carbamazepine is combined with lithium
- Because carbamazepine is structurally similar to TCAs, in theory it should not be given within 14 days of discontinuing MAOI
- Combined use of carbamazepine and lithium may increase risk of neurotoxic effects
- Depressive effects are increased by other CNS depressants (alcohol, MAOIs, other anticonvulsants, etc.)
- Combined use of carbamazepine suspension with liquid formulations of chlorpromazine has been shown to result in excretion of an orange rubbery precipitate; because of this, combined use of carbamazepine suspension with any liquid medicine is not recommended

 Other Warnings/Precautions

*Patients should be monitored carefully for signs of unusual bleeding or bruising, mouth sores, infections, fever, or sore throat, as the risk of aplastic anaemia and agranulocytosis with carbamazepine use is 5–8 times greater than in the general population (risk in the untreated general population is 6 patients per 1 million per year for agranulocytosis and 2 patients per 1 million per year for aplastic anaemia)
- Leucopenia that is severe, progressive, or associated with clinical symptoms requires withdrawal (if necessary under cover of a suitable alternative)
- Use with caution in patients with a history of haematological reactions to other medications
- Use with caution in patients with cardiac disease
- Caution with skin reactions
- Because carbamazepine has a tricyclic chemical structure, use with caution with MAOIs, including 14 days after MAOIs are stopped (for the expert)
- May exacerbate angle-closure glaucoma
- Because carbamazepine can lower plasma levels of hormonal contraceptives, it may also reduce their effectiveness
- May need to restrict fluid intake, because of risk of developing syndrome of inappropriate antidiuretic hormone secretion, hyponatraemia and its complications
- Use with caution in patients with mixed seizure disorders that include atypical absence seizures, because carbamazepine has been associated with increased frequency of generalised convulsions in such patients
- May exacerbate absence and myoclonic seizures
- Warn patients and their caregivers about the possibility of activation of suicidal ideation and advise them to report such side effects immediately
- Carbamazepine is associated with antiepileptic hypersensitivity syndrome.
- Cross-sensitivity reported with oxcarbazepine and with phenytoin
- Consider vitamin D supplementation in immobilised patients or those with inadequate sun exposure or dietary calcium intake

Do Not Use

- If patient has history of bone marrow suppression
- If patient has phaeochromocytoma
- If patient has AV conduction abnormalities (unless paced)
- If patient tests positive for the HLA-B*1502 allele (individuals with the HLA-B*1502 allele are at increased risk of developing Stevens-Johnson syndrome and toxic epidermal necrolysis)
- Suspension: in patients with hereditary problems with fructose intolerance
- If there is a proven allergy to any tricyclic compound
- If there is a proven allergy to carbamazepine

SPECIAL POPULATIONS

Renal Impairment

- Carbamazepine is renally excreted, use with caution in renal impairment

Hepatic Impairment

- Drug should be used with caution
- Rare cases of hepatic failure have occurred
- Carbamazepine should be withdrawn immediately in cases of aggravated liver dysfunction or acute liver disease

Cardiac Impairment

- Drug should be used with caution

Elderly

- Some patients may tolerate lower doses better
- Elderly patients may be more susceptible to adverse effects

Children and Adolescents

- Approved use for epilepsy; therapeutic range of total carbamazepine in plasma is considered the same for children and adults
- Not licensed for use in trigeminal neuralgia or prophylaxis of bipolar disorder

Pregnancy

- *Available data suggest an increased risk of congenital malformations, the absolute risk is estimated to between 3.8 and 6.2%
- *Risk of major congenital malformations is dose dependent
- *Exposure in pregnancy is associated with malformations of the urinary tract and respiratory system, neural tube defects, and other specific malformations
- *Available data does not suggest an increased risk of neurodevelopmental delay but limited data means this cannot be excluded
- *Limited data on perinatal death, low weight for gestational age, preterm delivery and intensive care requirements mean risks are uncertain
- Use in women of childbearing potential requires weighing potential benefits to the mother against the risks to the foetus
- *For bipolar patients, carbamazepine should generally be discontinued before anticipated pregnancies
- *If drug is continued, perform tests to detect birth defects
- *If drug is continued, start on folate 5 mg/day early in pregnancy to reduce risk of neural tube defects
- Use of anticonvulsants in combination may cause a higher prevalence of teratogenic effects than anticonvulsant monotherapy
- Taper drug if discontinuing
- Seizures, even mild seizures, may cause harm to the embryo/foetus
- Recurrent bipolar illness during pregnancy can be quite disruptive
- For bipolar patients, given the risk of relapse in the postpartum period, some form of mood stabiliser treatment may need to be restarted immediately after delivery if patient is unmedicated during pregnancy
- *Antipsychotics may be preferable to carbamazepine if treatment of bipolar disorder is required during pregnancy
- Bipolar symptoms may recur or worsen during pregnancy and some form of treatment may be necessary

Breastfeeding

- Significant amount found in mother's breast milk
- Some cases of neonatal seizures, respiratory depression, vomiting and diarrhoea have been reported in infants whose mothers received carbamazepine during pregnancy

- If drug is continued while breastfeeding, infant should be monitored for possible adverse effects, including haematological effects
- If infant shows signs of irritability or sedation, drug may need to be discontinued
* Bipolar disorder may recur during the postpartum period, particularly if there is a history of prior postpartum episodes of either depression or psychosis
- Relapse rates may be lower in women who receive prophylactic treatment for postpartum episodes of bipolar disorder
- For bipolar patients, considered first-line choice for use during breastfeeding
- Antipsychotics may be preferable in some circumstances during the postpartum period when breastfeeding

THE ART OF PSYCHOPHARMACOLOGY

Potential Advantages
- Treatment-resistant bipolar and psychotic disorders

Potential Disadvantages
- Patients who do not wish to or cannot comply with blood testing and close monitoring
- Patients who cannot tolerate sedation
- Pregnant patients

Primary Target Symptoms
- Seizures
- Unstable mood, especially mania
- Pain

Pearls
- Carbamazepine was the first anticonvulsant widely used for the treatment of bipolar disorder, but has not been shown to be as effective as lithium in prophylaxis
* A modified-release formulation has better evidence of efficacy and improved tolerability in bipolar disorder than does immediate-release carbamazepine
- Dosage frequency as well as sedation, diplopia, confusion, and ataxia may be reduced with modified-release carbamazepine
- Risk of serious side effects is greatest in the first few months of treatment
- Common side effects such as sedation often abate after a few months
* May be effective in patients who fail to respond to lithium or other mood stabilisers
- May be effective for the depressed phase of bipolar disorder and for maintenance in bipolar disorder
- Interactions with concomitant medications including the oral contraceptive can make this treatment difficult to manage

Suggested Reading

Lambru G, Zakrzewska J, Matharu M. Trigeminal neuralgia: a practical guide. Pract Neurol 2021;21(5):392–402.

Leucht S, McGrath J, White P, et al. Carbamazepine for schizophrenia and schizoaffective psychoses. Cochrane Database Syst Rev 2002;(3):CD001258.

Marson AG, Williamson PR, Hutton JL, et al. Carbamazepine versus valproate monotherapy for epilepsy. Cochrane Database Syst Rev 2000;(3):CD001030.

Smith LA, Cornelius V, Warnock A, et al. Pharmacological interventions for acute bipolar mania: a systematic review of randomized placebo-controlled trials. Bipolar Disord 2007;9(6):551–60.

Weisler RH, Kalali AH, Ketter TA. A multicenter, randomized, double-blind, placebo-controlled trial of extended-release carbamazepine capsules as monotherapy for bipolar disorder patients with manic or mixed episodes. J Clin Psychiatry 2004;65:478–84.

Cariprazine

THERAPEUTICS

Brands
• Reagila

Generic?
No, not in UK

Class
• Neuroscience-based nomenclature: pharmacology domain – dopamine, serotonin; mode of action – partial agonist and antagonist
• Dopamine partial agonist (dopamine stabiliser, atypical antipsychotic, third-generation antipsychotic; sometimes included as a second-generation antipsychotic; also a mood stabiliser)

Commonly Prescribed for
(bold for BNF indication)
• **Schizophrenia**
• Acute mania/mixed mania
• Other psychotic disorders
• Bipolar maintenance
• Bipolar depression
• Treatment-resistant depression
• Behavioural disturbances in dementia
• Behavioural disturbances in children and adolescents
• Disorders associated with problems with impulse control

 ### How the Drug Works
∗ Partial agonism at dopamine 2 receptors
• Theoretically reduces dopamine output when dopamine concentrations are high, thus improving positive symptoms and mediating antipsychotic actions
• Theoretically increases dopamine output when dopamine concentrations are low, thus improving cognitive, negative, and mood symptoms
• Preferentially binds to dopamine 3 over dopamine 2 receptors at low doses; the clinical significance is unknown but could theoretically contribute to cariprazine's efficacy for negative symptoms. D3 partial agonism could theoretically be useful for treating cognition, mood, emotions, and reward/substance use
• Cariprazine also has high affinity for serotonin 1A (partial agonist) and serotonin 2B (antagonist) receptors

• Cariprazine has moderate affinity for serotonin 2A receptors (antagonist)

How Long Until It Works
• Psychotic and manic symptoms can improve within 1 week, but it may take several weeks for full effect on behaviour as well as on cognition
• Classically recommended to wait at least 4–6 weeks to determine efficacy of drug, but in practice some patients require up to 16–20 weeks to show a good response, especially on cognitive improvement and functional outcome

If It Works
• Most often reduces positive symptoms in schizophrenia but does not eliminate them
• Can improve negative symptoms, as well as aggressive, cognitive, and affective symptoms in schizophrenia
• Most patients with schizophrenia do not have a total remission of symptoms but rather a reduction of symptoms by about a third
• Perhaps 5–15% of patients with schizophrenia can experience an overall improvement of >50–60%, especially when receiving stable treatment for > 1 year
• Such patients are considered super-responders or "awakeners" since they may be well enough to work, live independently, and sustain long-term relationships
• Continue treatment until reaching a plateau of improvement
• After reaching a satisfactory plateau, continue treatment for at least 1 year after first episode of psychosis, but it may be preferable to continue treatment indefinitely to avoid subsequent episodes
• After any subsequent episodes of psychosis, treatment may need to be indefinite
• May reduce and eliminate acute manic symptoms

If It Doesn't Work
• If dose is optimised, consider watchful waiting
• If this fails, consider increasing the antipsychotic dose according to tolerability and plasma levels (limited supporting evidence)
• Try one of the other atypical antipsychotics (risperidone or olanzapine should be considered first before considering other agents such as quetiapine, amisulpride or lurasidone)

- If two or more antipsychotic monotherapies do not work, consider clozapine
- Some patients may require treatment with a conventional antipsychotic
- If no first-line atypical antipsychotic is effective, consider time-limited augmentation strategies
- Consider non-concordance and switch to another antipsychotic with fewer side effects or to a depot antipsychotic
- Consider initiating rehabilitation and psychotherapy such as cognitive remediation
- Consider presence of concomitant drug abuse

⚖ Best Augmenting Combos for Partial Response or Treatment Resistance

- Valproic acid (Depakote or Epilim)
- Other mood-stabilising anticonvulsants (carbamazepine, oxcarbazepine, lamotrigine)
- Lithium
- Benzodiazepines

Tests

Before starting an atypical antipsychotic

* Measure weight, BMI, and waist circumference
- Get baseline personal and family history of diabetes, obesity, dyslipidaemia, hypertension, and cardiovascular disease
* Check pulse and blood pressure, fasting plasma glucose or glycosylated haemoglobin (HbA1c), fasting lipid profile, and prolactin levels
- Full blood count (FBC), urea and electrolytes (including creatinine and eGFR), liver function tests (LFTs)
- Assessment of nutritional status, diet, and level of physical activity
- Determine if the patient:
  - is overweight (BMI 25.0–29.9)
  - is obese (BMI ≥30)
  - has pre-diabetes – fasting plasma glucose: 5.5 mmol/L to 6.9 mmol/L or HbA1c: 42 to 47 mmol/mol (6.0 to 6.4%)
  - has diabetes – fasting plasma glucose: >7.0 mmol/L or HbA1c: ≥48 mmol/L (≥6.5%)
  - has hypertension (BP >140/90 mm Hg)

- has dyslipidaemia (increased total cholesterol, LDL cholesterol, and triglycerides; decreased HDL cholesterol)
- Treat or refer such patients for treatment, including nutrition and weight management, physical activity counselling, smoking cessation, and medical management
- Baseline ECG for: inpatients; those with a personal history or risk factor for cardiac disease

Monitoring after starting an atypical antipsychotic

- FBC annually to detect chronic bone marrow suppression, stop treatment if neutrophils fall below 1.5×10^9/L and refer to specialist care if neutrophils fall below 0.5×10^9/L
- Urea and electrolytes (including creatinine and eGFR) annually
- LFTs annually
- Prolactin levels at 6 months and then annually (cariprazine is not likely to affect prolactin levels)
* Weight/BMI/waist circumference, weekly for the first 6 weeks, then at 12 weeks, at 1 year, and then annually
* Pulse and blood pressure at 12 weeks, 1 year, and then annually
* Fasting blood glucose, HbA1c, and blood lipids at 12 weeks, at 1 year, and then annually
* For patients with type 2 diabetes, measure HbA1c at 3–6 month intervals until stable, then every 6 months
* Even in patients without known diabetes, be vigilant for the rare but life-threatening onset of diabetic ketoacidosis, which always requires immediate treatment, by monitoring for the rapid onset of polyuria, polydipsia, weight loss, nausea, vomiting, dehydration, rapid respiration, weakness and clouding of sensorium, even coma
- If HbA1c remains ≥48 mmol/mol (6.5%) then drug therapy should be offered, e.g. metformin
- Treat or refer for treatment or consider switching to another atypical antipsychotic for patients who become overweight, obese, pre-diabetic, diabetic, hypertensive, or dyslipidaemic while receiving an atypical antipsychotic (these problems are relatively less likely with cariprazine)

SIDE EFFECTS

How Drug Causes Side Effects

- Partial agonist actions at dopamine 2 receptors in the striatum can cause motor side effects, such as akathisia
- Partial agonist actions at dopamine 2 receptors can also cause nausea, occasional vomiting, and activating side effects
* Mechanism of any possible weight gain or increased incidence of diabetes or dyslipidaemia is unknown

Notable Side Effects

* Akathisia, extrapyramidal symptoms, restlessness
* Gastrointestinal distress
- Sedation
- Theoretical risk of tardive dyskinesia

Common or very common

- Blood disorders: leucopenia, neutropenia
- CNS: agitation, dizziness, drowsiness, insomnia, movement disorders, parkinsonism, seizure, tremor
- CVS: arrhythmias, hypotension (dose-related), postural hypotension (dose-related), QT interval prolongation
- Endocrine: amenorrhoea, galactorrhoea, gynaecomastia, hyperglycaemia, hyperprolactinaemia
- GIT: constipation, dry mouth, vomiting, weight increased
- Other: erectile dysfunction, fatigue, muscle rigidity, rash, urinary retention

Uncommon

- Agranulocytosis, confusion, embolism and thrombosis, neuroleptic malignant syndrome (discontinue – potentially fatal)

Frequency not known

- Neonatal withdrawal syndrome, sudden death

 Life-Threatening or Dangerous Side Effects

- Hyperglycaemia, in some cases extreme and associated with ketoacidosis or hyperosmolar coma or death, has been reported in patients taking atypical antipsychotics
- Increased risk of death and cerebrovascular events in elderly patients with dementia-related psychosis
- Neuroleptic malignant syndrome (uncommon)
- Seizures

Weight Gain

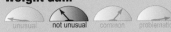

- Occurs in significant minority

Sedation

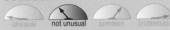

- Occurs in significant minority

What To Do About Side Effects

- Wait
- Wait
- Wait
- Low-dose benzodiazepine or beta blocker may reduce akathisia
- Weight loss, exercise programmes, and medical management for high BMIs, diabetes, and dyslipidaemia
- Switch to another antipsychotic (atypical) – quetiapine or clozapine are best in cases of tardive dyskinesia

Best Augmenting Agents for Side Effects

- Dystonia: antimuscarinic drugs (e.g. procyclidine) as oral or IM depending on the severity; botulinum toxin if antimuscarinics not effective
- Parkinsonism: antimuscarinic drugs (e.g. procyclidine)
- Akathisia: beta blocker propranolol (30–80 mg/day) or low-dose benzodiazepine (e.g. 0.5–3.0 mg/day of clonazepam) may help; other agents that may be tried include the 5HT2 antagonists such as cyproheptadine (16 mg/day) or mirtazapine (15 mg at night – caution in bipolar disorder); clonidine (0.2–0.8 mg/day) may be tried if the above ineffective
- Tardive dyskinesia: stop any antimuscarinic, consider tetrabenazine

DOSING AND USE

Usual Dosage Range

- Schizophrenia: 1.5–6 mg/day

Dosage Forms

- Capsule 1.5 mg, 3 mg, 4.5 mg, 6 mg

How to Dose

* Schizophrenia in adults:
- 1.5 mg/day, increased by increments of 1.5 mg as needed; max 6 mg/day

Dosing Tips

- Because of its long half-life, and the especially long half-life of one of its active metabolites, monitor for adverse effects and response for several weeks after starting cariprazine and with each dosage change; also washout of active drug will take several weeks
- Because of its long half-life, missing a few doses may not be as detrimental compared to other antipsychotics
- Can be taken with or without food

Overdose

- Limited experience

Long-Term Use

- Not extensively studied, but long-term maintenance treatment is often necessary for schizophrenia and bipolar mania
- Should periodically re-evaluate long-term usefulness in individual patients, but treatment may need to continue for many years in patients with schizophrenia

Habit Forming

- No

How to Stop

- Down-titration may be prudent, especially when simultaneously beginning a new antipsychotic while switching (i.e. cross-titration)
- The method for stopping cariprazine can vary depending on which agent is being switched to; see switching guidelines of individual agents for how to stop cariprazine
- However, the long half-lives of cariprazine and its two active metabolites suggest that it may be possible to stop cariprazine abruptly
- The plasma concentration of total cariprazine declines gradually following dose discontinuation. The plasma concentration of total cariprazine reduces by 50% in about 1 week and > 90% in about 3 weeks
- Rapid discontinuation could theoretically lead to rebound psychosis and worsening of symptoms, but less likely with cariprazine due to its long half-life

Pharmacokinetics

- Mainly metabolised by CYP450 3A4 into two long-lasting metabolites – desmethyl cariprazine (DCAR) and didesmethyl cariprazine (DDCAR)

- The mean terminal half-life of cariprazine is 1 to 3 days
- The mean terminal half-life of the metabolite DCAR is 1 to 3 days and of the metabolite DDCAR is 13 to 19 days
- The effective half-life is more relevant than the terminal half-life
- The effective (functional) half-life is about 2 days for cariprazine and DCAR, 8 days for DDCAR and about 1 week for total cariprazine
- Food does not affect absorption

 Drug Interactions

- Initiating a strong CYP450 3A4 inhibitor in patients on a stable dose of cariprazine: reduce the current dose of cariprazine by half (for patients taking 4.5 mg/day reduce either to 1.5 mg/day or 3 mg/day; for patients taking 1.5 mg/day reduce to 1.5 mg every other day)
- Initiating cariprazine in patients taking a strong CYP450 3A4 inhibitor: administer 1.5 mg on day 1, do not dose on day 2, administer 1.5 on day 3 and day 4; max dose 3 mg/day
- Concomitant use of cariprazine and CYP450 3A4 inducer not recommended
- May increase effects of antihypertensive agents
- May antagonise levodopa, dopamine agonists

 Other Warnings/Precautions

- All antipsychotics should be used with caution in patients with angle-closure glaucoma, blood disorders, cardiovascular disease, depression, diabetes, epilepsy and susceptibility to seizures, history of jaundice, myasthenia gravis, Parkinson's disease, photosensitivity, prostatic hypertrophy, severe respiratory disorders
- Use with caution in patients with conditions that predispose to hypotension (dehydration, overheating)
- Dysphagia has been associated with antipsychotic use, and cariprazine should be used cautiously in patients at risk for aspiration pneumonia

Do Not Use

- If there is a proven allergy to cariprazine

SPECIAL POPULATIONS

Renal Impairment
- Mild to moderate impairment: no dose adjustment necessary
- Avoid in severe impairment

Hepatic Impairment
- Mild to moderate impairment: no dose adjustment necessary
- Avoid in severe impairment

Cardiac Impairment
- Use in patients with cardiac impairment has not been studied, so use with caution

Elderly
- Dose adjustment generally not necessary, but some elderly patients may tolerate lower doses better
- Although atypical antipsychotics are commonly used for behavioural disturbances in dementia, no agent has been approved for treatment of elderly patients with dementia-related psychosis
- Elderly patients with dementia-related psychosis treated with atypical antipsychotics are at an increased risk of death compared to placebo, and also have an increased risk of cerebrovascular events

Children and Adolescents
- Not licensed for use in children and adolescents
- Safety and efficacy have not been established

Pregnancy
- Cariprazine should be avoided in pregnancy
- Controlled studies have not been conducted in pregnant women
- In rats, administration of cariprazine during organogenesis caused malformations, lower pup survival, and developmental delays at exposures less than the human exposure at maximum recommended human dose (6 mg/day); cariprazine was not teratogenic in rabbits at doses up to 4.6 times the maximum recommended human dose
- There is a risk of abnormal muscle movements and withdrawal symptoms in newborns whose mothers took an antipsychotic during the third trimester;

symptoms may include agitation, abnormally increased or decreased muscle tone, tremor, sleepiness, severe difficulty breathing, and difficulty feeding
- Psychotic symptoms may worsen during pregnancy and some form of treatment may be necessary
- Olanzapine and clozapine have been associated with maternal hyperglycaemia which may lead to developmental toxicity; risk may also apply for other atypical antipsychotics

Breastfeeding
- Unknown if cariprazine is secreted in human breast milk, but all psychotropics assumed to be secreted in breast milk
- No evidence of safety
- Haloperidol is considered to be the preferred first-generation antipsychotic, and quetiapine the preferred second-generation antipsychotic
- Infants of women who choose to breastfeed should be monitored for possible adverse effects

THE ART OF PSYCHOPHARMACOLOGY

Potential Advantages
- For patients who do not tolerate aripiprazole
- Possibly negative symptoms in schizophrenia

Potential Disadvantages
- Expensive

Primary Target Symptoms
- Positive symptoms of psychosis
- Negative symptoms of psychosis
- Cognitive symptoms
- Unstable mood and depression
- Symptoms of acute mania/mixed mania
- Aggressive symptoms
- Bipolar depression
- Mixtures of manic and depressive symptoms in bipolar disorder

Pearls
- Cariprazine is metabolised by CYP450 3A4 into two long-lasting metabolites – desmethyl cariprazine (DCAR) and didesmethyl cariprazine (DDCAR); it is therefore possible that adverse events could appear several weeks after initiation

of cariprazine due to accumulation of cariprazine and major metabolites over time
- It is also possible that cariprazine or its very long-lasting active metabolites could be developed as an 'oral depot', namely a very long-lasting oral formulation for weekly or even monthly oral administration
- Based on short-term clinical trials, cariprazine appears to have a favourable metabolic profile, with changes in triglycerides, fasting glucose, and cholesterol similar to placebo; however, it may cause a small amount of dose-dependent weight gain
- Increasing evidence suggests efficacy for cariprazine in the treatment of bipolar depression and as an adjunct for treatment-resistant unipolar depression
- D3-preferring (over D2) actions represent a novel pharmacologic profile among antipsychotics, especially at lower doses; clinical advantages of this profile remain to be determined but animal models suggest that targeting D3 receptors may have advantages for mood, negative symptoms, and substance abuse
- All antipsychotics bind to the D3 receptor in vitro, but only cariprazine has affinity for the D3 receptor greater than dopamine itself, so it is the only antipsychotic with functional D3 partial agonism in vivo in the living human brain

THE ART OF SWITCHING

 Switching from Oral Antipsychotics to Cariprazine

- It is advisable to begin cariprazine at an intermediate dose and build the dose up rapidly over 3–7 days
- Asenapine, quetiapine or olanzapine should be tapered off slowly over a period of 3–4 weeks, to allow patients to readapt to the withdrawal of blocking cholinergic, histaminergic, and alpha 1 receptors
- Clozapine should always be tapered off slowly, over a period of 4 weeks or more
- *Benzodiazepine or anticholinergic medication can be administered during cross-titration to help alleviate side effects such as insomnia, agitation, and/or psychosis

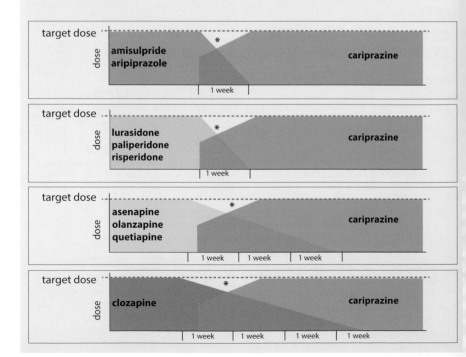

Suggested Reading

Choi YK, Adham N, Kiss B, et al. Long-term effects of cariprazine exposure on dopamine receptor subtypes. CNS Spectr 2014;19(3):268–77.

Citrome L. Cariprazine in schizophrenia: clinical efficacy, tolerability and place in therapy. Adv Ther 2013;30(2):114–26.

Earley WR, Burgess MV, Khan B, et al. Efficacy and safety of cariprazine in bipolar I depression: a double-blind, placebo-controlled phase 3 study. Bipolar Disord 2020;22(4):372–84.

Pillinger T, McCutcheon RA, Vano L, et al. Comparative effects of 18 antipsychotics on metabolic function in patients with schizophrenia, predictors of metabolic dysregulation, and association with psychopathology: a systematic review and network meta-analysis. Lancet Psychiatry 2020;7(1):64–77.

Schneider-Thoma J, Chalkou K, Dorries C, et al. Comparative efficacy and tolerability of 32 oral and long-acting injectable antipsychotics for the maintenance treatment of adults with schizophrenia: a systematic review and network meta-analysis. Lancet 2022;399(10327):824–36.

Stahl SM. Drugs for psychosis and mood: unique actions at D3, D2, and D1 dopamine receptor subtypes. CNS Spectr 2017;22(5):375–84.

Vieta E, Durgam S, Lu K, et al. Effect of cariprazine across the symptoms of mania in bipolar I disorder: analyses of pooled data from phase II/III trials. Eur Neuropsychopharmacol 2015;25(11):1882–91.

Vieta E, Earley WR, Burgess MV, et al. Long-term safety and tolerability of cariprazine as adjunctive therapy in major depressive disorder. Int Clin Psychopharmacol 2019;34(2):76–83.

Chlordiazepoxide hydrochloride

Brands
• Librium

Generic?
Yes

Class
• Neuroscience-based nomenclature: pharmacology domain – GABA; mode of action – positive allosteric modulator (PAM)
• Benzodiazepine (anxiolytic)

Commonly Prescribed for
(bold for BNF indication)
• **Short-term use in anxiety**
• **Treatment of alcohol withdrawal in moderate-severe dependence**
• Catatonia

How the Drug Works
• Binds to benzodiazepine receptors at the GABA-A ligand-gated chloride channel complex
• Enhances the inhibitory effects of GABA
• Boosts chloride conductance through GABA-regulated channels
• Inhibits neuronal activity, presumably in amygdala-centred fear circuits, to provide therapeutic benefits in anxiety disorders

How Long Until It Works
• Some immediate relief with first dosing is common; can take several weeks with daily dosing for maximal therapeutic benefit

If It Works
• For short-term symptoms of anxiety – after a few weeks, discontinue use or use on an "as-needed" basis
• For chronic anxiety disorders, the goal of treatment is complete remission of symptoms as well as prevention of future relapses
• For chronic anxiety disorders, treatment most often reduces or even eliminates symptoms, but is not a cure since symptoms can recur after medicine stopped
• For long-term symptoms of anxiety, consider switching to an SSRI or SNRI for long-term maintenance
• If long-term maintenance with a benzodiazepine is necessary, continue treatment for 6 months after symptoms resolve, and then taper dose slowly
• If symptoms re-emerge, consider treatment with an SSRI or SNRI, or consider restarting the benzodiazepine; sometimes benzodiazepines have to be used in combination with SSRIs or SNRIs for best results

If It Doesn't Work
• Consider switching to another agent or adding an appropriate augmenting agent
• Consider psychotherapy, especially cognitive behavioural psychotherapy
• Consider presence of concomitant substance abuse
• Consider presence of chlordiazepoxide abuse
• Consider another diagnosis such as a co-morbid medical condition

Best Augmenting Combos for Partial Response or Treatment Resistance
• Benzodiazepines are frequently used as augmenting agents for antipsychotics and mood stabilisers in the treatment of psychotic and bipolar disorders
• Benzodiazepines are frequently used as augmenting agents for SSRIs and SNRIs in the treatment of anxiety disorders
• Not generally rational to combine with other benzodiazepines
• Caution if using as an anxiolytic concomitantly with other sedative hypnotics for sleep

Tests
• In patients with seizure disorders, concomitant medical illness, and/or those with multiple concomitant long-term medications, periodic liver tests and blood counts may be prudent

How Drug Causes Side Effects
• Same mechanism for side effects as for therapeutic effects – namely due to excessive actions at benzodiazepine receptors
• Long-term adaptations in benzodiazepine receptors may explain the development of dependence, tolerance, and withdrawal

- Side effects are generally immediate, but immediate side effects often disappear in time

Notable Side Effects

* Sedation, fatigue, depression
* Dizziness, ataxia, slurred speech, weakness
* Forgetfulness, confusion
* Hyper excitability, nervousness
- Rare hallucinations, mania
- Rare hypotension
- Hypersalivation, dry mouth

Common or very common

- Movement disorders

Rare or very rare

- Blood disorders: agranulocytosis, bone marrow disorders, leucopenia, thrombocytopenia
- Other: abdominal distress, erectile dysfunction, menstrual disorder, skin eruption

Frequency not known

- CNS/PNS: abnormal gait, decreased level of consciousness, memory loss, suicide attempt
- Other: altered saliva, increased appetite, increased risk of fall

 Life-Threatening or Dangerous Side Effects

- Respiratory depression, especially when taken with CNS depressants in overdose
- Rare hepatic dysfunction, renal dysfunction, blood dyscrasias

Weight Gain

unusual | not unusual | common | problematic

- Reported but not expected

Sedation

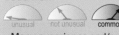
unusual | not unusual | common | problematic

- Many experience and/or can be significant in amount
- Especially at initiation of treatment or when dose increases
- Tolerance often develops over time

What to Do About Side Effects

- Wait
- Wait
- Wait
- Lower the dose
- Take largest dose at bedtime to avoid sedative effects during the day
- Switch to another agent
- Administer flumazenil if side effects are severe or life-threatening

Best Augmenting Agents for Side Effects

- Many side effects cannot be improved with an augmenting agent

DOSING AND USE

Usual Dosage Range

- Short-term use in anxiety: 10–100 mg/day in divided doses (adult); 5–50 mg/day in divided doses (elderly/debilitated)
- Treatment of alcohol withdrawal: moderate dependence (10–30 mg 4 times per day); severe dependence (10–50 mg 4 times per day)

Dosage Forms

- Capsule 5 mg, 10 mg

How to Dose

* Short-term use in anxiety (adult):
- 10 mg 3 times per day, increased as needed to 60–100 mg/day in divided doses
* Short-term use in anxiety (elderly/debilitated):
- 5 mg 3 times per day, increased as needed to 30–50 mg/day in divided doses
* Treatment of alcohol withdrawal in moderate dependence:
- 10–30 mg 4 times per day, dose to be gradually reduced over 5–7 days (consult local titration regime protocol)
* Treatment of alcohol withdrawal in severe dependence (adult):
- 10–50 mg 4 times per day and 10–40 mg as needed for the first 2 days, dose to be gradually reduced over 7–10 days; max 250 mg/day (consult local titration regime protocol)

 Dosing Tips

- Use lowest possible effective dose for the shortest possible period of time (a benzodiazepine-sparing strategy)

- Assess need for continued treatment regularly
- Risk of dependence may increase with dose and duration of treatment
- For inter-dose symptoms of anxiety, can either increase dose or maintain same total daily dose, but divide into more frequent doses
- Can also use an as-needed occasional "top up" dose for inter-dose anxiety
- Because anxiety disorders can require higher doses, the risk of dependence may be greater in these patients
- Some severely ill patients may require doses higher than the generally recommended maximum dose
- Frequency of dosing in practice is often greater than predicted from half-life, as duration of biological activity is often shorter than pharmacokinetic terminal half-life
- Chlordiazepoxide 25 mg = diazepam 10 mg

Overdose

- Fatalities can occur, hypotension, tiredness, ataxia, confusion, coma

Long-Term Use

- Evidence of efficacy up to 16 weeks
- Risk of dependence, particularly for treatment periods longer than 12 weeks and especially in patients with past or current polysubstance abuse

Habit Forming

- Chlordiazepoxide is a Class C/Schedule 4 drug
- Patients may develop dependence and/or tolerance with long-term use

How to Stop

- Patients with history of seizure may seize upon withdrawal, especially if withdrawal is abrupt
- Taper by 10 mg every 3 days to reduce chances of withdrawal effects
- For difficult to taper cases, consider reducing dose much more slowly after reaching 20 mg/day, perhaps by as little as 5 mg per week or less
- For other patients with severe problems discontinuing a benzodiazepine, dosing may need to be tapered over many months (i.e. reduce dose by 1% every 3 days by crushing tablet and suspending or

dissolving in 100 mL of fruit juice and then disposing of 1 mL while drinking the rest; 3–7 days later, dispose of 2 mL, and so on). This is both a form of very slow biological tapering and a form of behavioural desensitisation
- Be sure to differentiate re-emergence of symptoms requiring reinstitution of treatment from withdrawal symptoms
- Benzodiazepine-dependent anxiety patients are not addicted to their medications; when benzodiazepine-dependent patients stop their medication, disease symptoms can re-emerge, disease symptoms can worsen (rebound), and/or withdrawal symptoms can emerge

Pharmacokinetics

- Half-life 5–30 hours; steady state levels are usually reached within 3 days
- Pharmacologically active metabolites of chlordiazepoxide include desmethylchlordiazepoxide, demoxepam, desmethyldiazepam and oxazepam
- Active metabolite desmethyldiazepam has a half-life of 36–200 hours
- The active metabolite desmethylchlordiazepoxide has an accumulation half-life of 10–18 hours and demoxepam has an accumulation half-life of about 21–78 hours
- Steady state levels of these active metabolites are reached after 10–15 days with metabolite concentrations which are similar to those of the parent drug
- Excretion via kidneys

 Drug Interactions

- Increased depressive effects when taken with other CNS depressants (see Warnings below)

 Other Warnings/Precautions

- Warnings regarding the increased risk of CNS-depressant effects (especially alcohol) when benzodiazepines and opioid medications are used together, including specifically the risk of slowed or difficulty breathing and death
- If alternatives to the combined use of benzodiazepines and opioids are not available, clinicians should limit the dosage

and duration of each drug to the minimum possible while still achieving therapeutic efficacy
- Patients and their caregivers should be warned to seek medical attention if unusual dizziness, light-headedness, sedation, slowed or difficulty breathing, or unresponsiveness occur
- Dosage changes should be made in collaboration with prescriber
- History of drug or alcohol abuse often creates greater risk for dependency
- Some depressed patients may experience a worsening of suicidal ideation
- Some patients may exhibit abnormal thinking or behavioural changes similar to those caused by other CNS depressants (i.e. either depressant actions or disinhibiting actions)
- Avoid prolonged use and abrupt cessation
- Use lower doses in debilitated patients and the elderly
- Use with caution in patients with myasthenia gravis; respiratory disease
- Use with caution in patients with personality disorder (dependent/avoidant or anankastic types) as may increase risk of dependence
- Use with caution in patients with a history of alcohol or drug dependence/abuse
- Benzodiazepines may cause a range of paradoxical effects including aggression, antisocial behaviours, anxiety, overexcitement, perceptual abnormalities and talkativeness. Adjustment of dose may reduce impulses
- Use with caution as chlordiazepoxide can cause muscle weakness and organic brain changes

Do Not Use
- If patient has acute pulmonary insufficiency, respiratory depression, significant neuromuscular respiratory weakness, sleep apnoea syndrome or unstable myasthenia gravis
- Alone in chronic psychosis in adults
- On its own to try to treat depression, anxiety associated with depression, obsessional states or phobic states
- If patient has angle-closure glaucoma
- If there is a proven allergy to chlordiazepoxide or any benzodiazepine

Renal Impairment
- Increased risk of cerebral sensitivity to benzodiazepines
- Start with small doses in severe impairment
- Chlordiazepoxide has a long-acting active metabolite that could accumulate
- eGFR <10 mL/minute/1.73 m^2 then reduce dose by 50%
- Monitor for sedation

Hepatic Impairment
- Can precipitate coma
- If treatment is necessary, benzodiazepines with shorter half-life (such as temazepam or oxazepam) are safer
- Avoid in severe impairment

Cardiac Impairment
- Benzodiazepines have been used to treat anxiety associated with acute myocardial infarction

Elderly
- Short-term use in anxiety, 5 mg 3 times per day, increased if necessary to 30–50 mg/day in divided doses
- Cautious prescribing for the elderly due to its long elimination half-life and the risks of accumulation

 Children and Adolescents
- Not recommended in children
- Long-term effects of chlordiazepoxide in children/adolescents are unknown

 Pregnancy
- Manufacturer recommends a long wait period after completion of treatment before attempting pregnancy. This recommendation is only based on animal and in vitro studies in which not all of the assays indicated mutagenic effects. Currently there is no evidence that chlordiazepoxide use in humans in the preconception period is linked with mutagenic effects that impact foetal development
- Possible increased risk of birth defects when benzodiazepines taken during pregnancy

- Because of the potential risks, chlordiazepoxide is not generally recommended during pregnancy, especially during the first trimester
- Drug should be tapered if discontinued
- Infants whose mothers received a benzodiazepine late in pregnancy may experience withdrawal effects
- Neonatal flaccidity has been reported in infants whose mothers took a benzodiazepine during pregnancy
- Seizures, even mild seizures, may cause harm to the embryo/foetus

Breastfeeding

- Some drug is found in mother's breast milk
- Long half-life of chlordiazepoxide and active metabolites may lead to accumulation in breastfed infants
- Use of short-acting agents, e.g. oxazepam or lorazepam, preferred
- Effects of benzodiazepines on infant have been observed and include feeding difficulties, sedation, and weight loss
- Caution should be taken with the use of benzodiazepines in breastfeeding mothers, seek to use low doses for short periods to reduce infant exposure

THE ART OF PSYCHOPHARMACOLOGY

Potential Advantages

- Rapid onset of action

Potential Disadvantages

- Euphoria may lead to abuse
- Abuse especially risky in past or present substance abusers

Primary Target Symptoms

- Panic attacks
- Anxiety

Pearls

- It was the first benzodiazepine to be synthesised
- Chlordiazepoxide has a medium to long half-life (5–30 hours) but its active metabolite desmethyldiazepam has a very long half-life (36–200 hours)
- Can be a useful adjunct to SSRIs and SNRIs in the treatment of numerous anxiety disorders, but not used as frequently as some other benzodiazepines
- Not effective for treating psychosis as a monotherapy, but can be used as an adjunct to antipsychotics
- Not effective for treating bipolar disorder as a monotherapy, but can be used as an adjunct to mood stabilisers and antipsychotics
- Can both cause depression and help in the treatment of depression in different patients
- When using to treat insomnia, remember that insomnia may be a symptom of some other primary disorder itself, and thus warrant evaluation for co-morbid psychiatric and/or medical conditions
- *Remains a viable treatment option for alcohol withdrawal
- Though not systematically studied, benzodiazepines have been used effectively to treat catatonia and are the initial recommended treatment

 Suggested Reading

Baskin SI, Esdale A. Is chlordiazepoxide the rational choice among benzodiazepines? Pharmacotherapy 1982;2:110–19.

Erstad BL, Cotugno CL. Management of alcohol withdrawal. Am J Health Syst Pharm 1995;52:697–709.

Fraser AD. Use and abuse of the benzodiazepines. Ther Drug Monit 1998;20:481–9.

Liu GG, Christensen DB. The continuing challenge of inappropriate prescribing in the elderly: an update of the evidence. J Am Pharm Assoc (Wash) 2002;42(6):847–57.

Murray JB. Effects of valium and librium on human psychomotor and cognitive functions. Genet Psychol Monogr 1984;109(2D Half):167–97.

Pang D, Duffield P, Day E. A view from the acute hospital: managing patients with alcohol problems. Br J Hosp Med (Lond) 2019;80(9):500–6.

Chlorpromazine hydrochloride

Brands
- Largactil

Generic?
Yes

Class
- Neuroscience-based nomenclature: pharmacology domain – dopamine, serotonin; mode of action – antagonist
- Conventional antipsychotic (neuroleptic, phenothiazine, dopamine 2 antagonist, antiemetic); dopamine and serotonin receptor antagonist (DS-RAn)

Commonly Prescribed for
(bold for BNF indication)
- **Schizophrenia and other psychoses**
- **Mania**
- **Short-term adjunctive management of severe anxiety**
- **Psychomotor agitation, excitement, and violent or dangerously impulsive behaviour**
- **Intractable hiccup**
- **Relief of acute symptoms of psychoses (under expert supervision)**
- **Nausea and vomiting of terminal illness (where other drugs failed or not available)**

 How the Drug Works
- Blocks dopamine 2 receptors, reducing positive symptoms of psychosis and improving other behaviours
- Combination of dopamine D2, histamine H1, and cholinergic M1 blockade in the vomiting centre may reduce nausea and vomiting

How Long Until It Works
- Psychotic and manic symptoms can improve within 1 week, but may take several weeks for full effect on behaviour as well as on cognition and affective stabilisation
- Actions on nausea and vomiting are immediate

If It Works
- Most often reduces positive symptoms in schizophrenia but doesn't eliminate them
- Most patients with schizophrenia do not have a total remission of symptoms but rather a reduction of symptoms by about a third
- Continue treatment in schizophrenia until reaching a plateau of improvement
- After reaching a satisfactory plateau, continue treatment for at least a year after the first episode of psychosis
- For second and subsequent episodes of psychosis in schizophrenia, treatment may need to be indefinite
- Reduces symptoms of acute psychotic mania but not proven as a mood stabiliser or as an effective maintenance treatment in bipolar disorder
- After reducing acute psychotic symptoms in mania, switch to a mood stabiliser and/ or an atypical antipsychotic for mood stabilisation and maintenance

If It Doesn't Work
- Consider trying one of the first-line atypical antipsychotics (risperidone, olanzapine, quetiapine, aripiprazole, paliperidone, amisulpride)
- Consider trying another conventional antipsychotic
- If two or more antipsychotic monotherapies do not work, consider clozapine

 Best Augmenting Combos for Partial Response or Treatment Resistance
- Augmentation of conventional antipsychotics has not been systemically studied
- Addition of a mood-stabilising anticonvulsant such as valproate, carbamazepine, or lamotrigine may be helpful in both schizophrenia and bipolar mania
- Augmentation with lithium in bipolar mania may be helpful
- Addition of a benzodiazepine, especially short-term for agitation

Tests
Baseline
- *Measure weight, BMI, and waist circumference
- Get baseline personal and family history of diabetes, obesity, dyslipidaemia, hypertension, and cardiovascular disease
- Check for personal history of drug-induced leucopenia/neutropenia
- *Check pulse and blood pressure, fasting plasma glucose or glycosylated

haemoglobin (HbA1c), fasting lipid profile, and prolactin levels
- Full blood count (FBC)
- Assessment of nutritional status, diet, and level of physical activity
- Determine if the patient:
  - is overweight (BMI 25.0–29.9)
  - is obese (BMI ≥30)
  - has pre-diabetes – fasting plasma glucose: 5.5 mmol/L to 6.9 mmol/L or HbA1c: 42 to 47 mmol/mol (6.0 to 6.4%)
  - has diabetes – fasting plasma glucose: >7.0 mmol/L or HbA1c: ≥48 mmol/L (≥6.5%)
  - has hypertension (BP >140/90 mm Hg)
  - has dyslipidaemia (increased total cholesterol, LDL cholesterol, and triglycerides; decreased HDL cholesterol)
- Treat or refer such patients for treatment, including nutrition and weight management, physical activity counselling, smoking cessation, and medical management
- Baseline ECG for: inpatients; those with a personal history or risk factor for cardiac disease

Monitoring
- Monitor weight and BMI during treatment
- Consider monitoring fasting triglycerides monthly for several months in patients at high risk for metabolic complications and when initiating or switching antipsychotics
- While giving a drug to a patient who has gained >5% of initial weight, consider evaluating for the presence of pre-diabetes, diabetes, or dyslipidaemia, or consider switching to a different antipsychotic
- Patients with low white blood cell count (WBC) or history of drug-induced leucopenia/neutropenia should have full blood count (FBC) monitored frequently during the first few months and chlorpromazine should be discontinued at the first sign of decline of WBC in the absence of other causative factors
- Monitor prolactin levels and for signs and symptoms of hyperprolactinaemia

SIDE EFFECTS

How Drug Causes Side Effects
- By blocking dopamine 2 receptors in the striatum, it can cause motor side effects
- By blocking dopamine 2 receptors in the pituitary, it can cause elevations in prolactin
- By blocking dopamine 2 receptors excessively in the mesocortical and mesolimbic dopamine pathways, especially at high doses, it can cause worsening of negative and cognitive symptoms (neuroleptic-induced deficit syndrome)
- Anticholinergic actions may cause sedation, blurred vision, constipation and dry mouth
- Antihistaminergic actions may cause sedation and weight gain
- By blocking alpha 1 adrenergic receptors, it can cause dizziness, sedation, and hypotension
- Mechanism of weight gain and any possible increased incidence of diabetes or dyslipidaemia with conventional antipsychotics is unknown

Notable Side Effects
＊Neuroleptic-induced deficit syndrome
＊Akathisia
＊Priapism
＊Extrapyramidal side effects, parkinsonism, tardive dyskinesia
＊Galactorrhoea, amenorrhoea
- Dizziness, sedation, impaired memory
- Dry mouth, constipation, urinary retention, blurred vision
- Decreased sweating
- Sexual dysfunction
- Hypotension, tachycardia, syncope
- Weight gain

Common or very common
- Altered mood, anxiety, impaired glucose tolerance, increased muscle tone

Frequency not known
- CNS/PNS: trismus
- CVS: atrioventricular block, cardiac arrest
- Endocrine/metabolic: hyperglycaemia, hypertriglyceridaemia
- GIT: gastrointestinal disorders, hepatic disorders
- Other: accommodation disorder, angioedema, eye deposit, eye disorders, hyponatraemia, photosensitivity, respiratory disorders, sexual dysfunction, SIADH, skin reactions, systemic lupus erythematosus (SLE), temperature dysregulation
- IM use: muscle rigidity, nasal congestion

 Life-Threatening or Dangerous Side Effects
- Rare neuroleptic malignant syndrome
- Rare agranulocytosis
- Rare seizures

- Increased risk of death and cerebrovascular events

Weight Gain

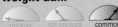

- Weight gain is a common side effect

Sedation

- Drowsiness may affect performance of skilled tasks (e.g. driving or operating machinery), especially at the start of treatment; effects of alcohol are also enhanced

What To Do About Side Effects

- Wait
- Wait
- Wait
- Reduce the dose
- Low-dose benzodiazepine or beta blocker may reduce akathisia
- Take more of the dose at bedtime to help reduce daytime sedation
- Weight loss, exercise programmes, and medical management for high BMIs, diabetes, and dyslipidaemia
- Switch to another antipsychotic (atypical) – quetiapine or clozapine are best in cases of tardive dyskinesia

Best Augmenting Agents for Side Effects

- Dystonia: antimuscarinic drugs (e.g. procyclidine) as oral or IM depending on the severity; botulinum toxin if antimuscarinics not effective
- Parkinsonism: antimuscarinic drugs (e.g. procyclidine)
- Akathisia: beta blocker propranolol (30–80 mg/day) or low-dose benzodiazepine (e.g. 0.5–3.0 mg/day of clonazepam) may help; other agents that may be tried include the 5HT2 antagonists such as cyproheptadine (16 mg/day) or mirtazapine (15 mg at night – caution in bipolar disorder); clonidine (0.2–0.8 mg/day) may be tried if the above ineffective
- Tardive dyskinesia: stop any antimuscarinic, consider tetrabenazine

DOSING AND USE

Usual Dosage Range

- 200–1000 mg/day

Dosage Forms

- Tablet 25 mg, 50 mg, 100 mg
- Oral solution 25 mg/5 mL, 100 mg/5 mL
- Solution for injection 50 mg/2 mL, 25 mg/1 mL
- Suppository (unlicensed use)

How to Dose

Adults:

＊Psychosis:
- Initial dose either 25 mg 3 times per day or 75 mg at night, adjusted according to response. Maintenance 75–300 mg/day, increased as needed up to 1 g/day. Take a third-half adult dose in elderly and debilitated patients

＊Relief of acute symptoms of psychosis (under expert supervision) by deep IM injection:
- 25–50 mg every 6–8 hours

＊Intractable hiccup:
- 25–50 mg 3–4 times per day

＊Nausea and vomiting in palliative care (where other drugs failed or not available):
- 10–25 mg every 4–6 hours (adults)

Children and adolescents:

＊Childhood schizophrenia and other psychoses – under expert supervision:
- Child 1–5 years (500 mcg/kg every 4–6 hours, adjusted according to response; max 40 mg/day)
- Child 6–11 years (10 mg 3 times per day, adjusted according to response; max 75 mg/day)
- Child 12–17 years (initial dose 25 mg 3 times per day or 75 mg at night, adjusted according to response; maintenance 75–300 mg/day, increased as needed up to 1 g/day)

＊Relief of acute symptoms of psychoses – under expert supervision:
- Child 1–5 years (500 mcg/kg IM every 6–8 hours; max 40 mg/day)
- Child 6–11 years (500 mcg/kg IM every 6–8 hours; max 75 mg/day)
- Child 12–17 years (25–50 mg IM every 6–8 hours)

Dosing Tips

- Dose adjustment may be necessary if smoking started or stopped during treatment
- For equivalent therapeutic effect 100 mg chlorpromazine base given rectally as suppository = 20–25 mg chlorpromazine hydrochloride by IM injection = 40–50 mg of chlorpromazine base of hydrochloride given by mouth
- Rectal route is not licensed

Overdose

- Extrapyramidal symptoms, sedation, hypotension, coma, respiratory depression, tachycardia, arrhythmia, pulmonary oedema, QT prolongations, seizures, dystonia, neuroleptic malignant syndrome
- Phenothiazines cause less depression of consciousness and respiration than other sedatives
- Hypotension, hypothermia, sinus tachycardia, and arrhythmias may complicate poisoning

Long-Term Use

- Some side effects may be irreversible (e.g. tardive dyskinesia)

Habit Forming

- No

How to Stop

- Slow down-titration of oral formulation (over 6–8 weeks), especially when simultaneously beginning a new antipsychotic while switching (i.e. cross-titration)
- Rapid oral discontinuation may lead to rebound psychosis and worsening of symptoms
- If anti-Parkinson agents are being used, they should be continued for a few weeks after chlorpromazine is discontinued

Pharmacokinetics

- Half-life is about 23–37 hours

 Drug Interactions

- May decrease the effects of levodopa, dopamine agonists
- May increase the effects of antihypertensive drugs except for guanethidene, whose antihypertensive actions chlorpromazine may antagonise
- Additive effects may occur if used with CNS depressants
- Some pressor agents (e.g. adrenaline) may interact with chlorpromazine to lower blood pressure
- Alcohol and diuretics may increase the risk of hypotension
- Reduces the effects of anticoagulants
- May reduce phenytoin metabolism and increase phenytoin levels
- Plasma levels of chlorpromazine and propranolol may increase if used concomitantly
- Some patients taking a neuroleptic and lithium have developed encephalopathic syndrome similar to neuroleptic malignant syndrome

 Other Warnings/Precautions

- All antipsychotics should be used with caution in patients with angle-closure glaucoma, blood disorders, cardiovascular disease, depression, diabetes, epilepsy and susceptibility to seizures, history of jaundice, myasthenia gravis, Parkinson's disease, photosensitivity, prostatic hypertrophy, severe respiratory disorders
- Skin photosensitivity may occur at higher doses. Advise to avoid undue exposure to sunlight and use sun screen if necessary
- If signs of neuroleptic malignant syndrome develop, treatment should be immediately discontinued
- Use cautiously in patients with alcohol withdrawal or convulsive disorders because of possible lowering of seizure threshold
- Avoid extreme heat exposure
- Antiemetic effect of chlorpromazine may mask signs of other disorders or overdose; suppression of cough reflex may cause asphyxia
- Use only with caution, if at all, in Lewy body disease

Do Not Use

- If there is CNS depression
- If the patient is in a comatose state
- If the patient has hypothyroidism
- If the patient has phaeochromocytoma
- If there is a proven allergy to chlorpromazine
- If there is a known sensitivity to any phenothiazine

SPECIAL POPULATIONS

Renal Impairment
- Use with caution (risk of accumulation)
- Start with small doses in renal failure due to increased cerebral sensitivity

Hepatic Impairment
- Use with caution
- Monitor closely in severe hepatic impairment due to risk of accumulation

Cardiac Impairment
- Cardiovascular toxicity can occur, especially postural hypotension

Elderly
- Use a third or half dose in the elderly or debilitated patients
- Patients should be monitored closely
- Often do not tolerate sedating actions of chlorpromazine
- Although conventional antipsychotics are commonly used for behavioural disturbances in dementia, no agent has been approved for treatment of elderly patients with dementia-related psychosis
- Elderly patients with dementia-related psychosis treated with antipsychotics are at an increased risk of death compared to placebo, and have an increased risk of cerebrovascular events

Children and Adolescents
- Indicated for use under expert supervision for childhood schizophrenia and other psychoses, as well as for the relief of the acute symptoms of psychoses
- Indicated for use in children for nausea and vomiting of terminal illness where other drugs have failed or are not available

Pregnancy
- Controlled studies have not been conducted in pregnant women
- There is a risk of abnormal muscle movements and withdrawal symptoms in newborns whose mothers took an antipsychotic during the third trimester; symptoms may include agitation, abnormally increased or decreased muscle tone, tremor, sleepiness, severe difficulty breathing, and difficulty feeding
- Reports of extrapyramidal symptoms, jaundice, hyperreflexia, hyporeflexia in infants whose mothers took a phenothiazine during pregnancy
- Psychotic symptoms may worsen during pregnancy and some form of treatment may be necessary
- Use in pregnancy may be justified if the benefit of continued treatment exceeds any associated risk
- Effects of hyperprolactinaemia on the foetus are unknown
- Switching antipsychotics may increase the risk of relapse

Breastfeeding
- Some drug is found in mother's breast milk
- Long half-life may lead to accumulation in breastfed infants
- Haloperidol is considered to be the preferred first-generation antipsychotic, and quetiapine the preferred second-generation antipsychotic
- Effects on infant have been observed (dystonia, tardive dyskinesia, sedation)
- Infants of women who choose to breastfeed should be monitored for possible adverse effects

THE ART OF PSYCHOPHARMACOLOGY

Potential Advantages
- Intramuscular formulation for emergency use
- Patients who require sedation for behavioural control

Potential Disadvantages
- Patients with tardive dyskinesia
- Children
- Elderly
- Patients who wish to avoid sedation

Primary Target Symptoms
- Positive symptoms of psychosis
- Motor and autonomic hyperactivity
- Violent or aggressive behaviour

Chlorpromazine hydrochloride (Continued)

Pearls

- Chlorpromazine is one of the earliest classical conventional antipsychotics
- Chlorpromazine has a broad spectrum of efficacy, but risk of tardive dyskinesia and the availability of alternative treatments make its use limited
- Chlorpromazine is a low-potency phenothiazine
- Sedative actions of low-potency phenothiazines are an important aspect of their therapeutic actions in some patients and side-effect profile in others
- Low-potency phenothiazines like chlorpromazine have a greater risk of cardiovascular side effects
- Patients have a very similar antipsychotic response when treated with any of the conventional antipsychotics, which is different from atypical antipsychotics where antipsychotic responses of individual patients can occasionally vary greatly from one atypical to another
- Patients with inadequate responses to atypical antipsychotics may benefit from a trial of augmentation with a conventional antipsychotic such as chlorpromazine or from switching to a conventional antipsychotic such as chlorpromazine
- However, long-term polypharmacy with a combination of a conventional antipsychotic such as chlorpromazine with an atypical antipsychotic may combine their side effects without clearly augmenting the efficacy of either
- For treatment-resistant patients, especially those with impulsivity, aggression, violence, and self-harm, long-term polypharmacy with 2 atypical antipsychotics and 1 conventional antipsychotic may be useful or even necessary while closely monitoring
- In such cases, it may be beneficial to combine 1 depot antipsychotic with 1 oral antipsychotic

 ## Suggested Reading

Adams CE, Awad G, Rathbone J, et al. Chlorpromazine versus placebo for schizophrenia. Cochrane Database Syst Rev 2007;18(2):CD000284.

Agid O, Kapur S, Arenovich T, et al. Delayed-onset hypothesis of antipsychotic action: a hypothesis tested and rejected. Arch Gen Psychiatry 2003;60(12):1228–35.

Ahmed U, Jones H, Adams CE. Chlorpromazine for psychosis induced aggression or agitation. Cochrane Database Syst Rev 2010;14(4):CD007445.

Almerie MQ, Alkhateeb H, Essali A, et al. Cessation of medication for people with schizophrenia already stable on chlorpromazine. Cochrane Database Syst Rev 2007;24(1):CD006329.

Huhn M, Nikolakopoulou A, Schneider-Thoma J, et al. Comparative efficacy and tolerability of 32 oral antipsychotics for the acute treatment of adults with multi-episode schizophrenia: a systematic review and network meta-analysis. Lancet 2019;394(10202):939–51.

Leucht C, Kitzmantel M, Chua L, et al. Haloperidol versus chlorpromazine for schizophrenia. Cochrane Database Syst Rev 2008;23(1):CD004278.

Liu X, De Haan S. Chlorpromazine dose for people with schizophrenia. Cochrane Database Syst Rev 2009;15(2):CD007778.

Samara MT, Cao H, Helfer B, et al. Chlorpromazine versus every other antipsychotic for schizophrenia: a systematic review and meta-analysis challenging the dogma of equal efficacy of antipsychotic drugs. Eur Neuropsychopharmacol 2014;24(7):1046–55.

Citalopram

Brands
- Cipramil

Generic?
Yes

Class
- Neuroscience-based nomenclature: pharmacology domain – serotonin; mode of action – reuptake inhibitor
- SSRI (selective serotonin reuptake inhibitor); antidepressant

Commonly Prescribed for
(bold for BNF indication)
- **Depressive illness**
- **Panic disorder**
- Premenstrual dysphoric disorder (PMDD)
- Obsessive-compulsive disorder (OCD)
- Generalised anxiety disorder (GAD)
- Social anxiety disorder (social phobia)

How the Drug Works
- Blocks reuptake of serotonin by its transporter at the synaptic cleft
- Increases levels of available serotonin at the synapse, augmenting serotonin neurotransmission
- Desensitises the serotonin receptors, in particular serotonin 1A autoreceptors
- Mild antagonist action at histamine H1 receptors
- Minimal effects on neuronal reuptake of noradrenaline or dopamine
- Citalopram's R-enantiomer may reduce the serotonin-enhancing action of the S-enantiomer

How Long Until It Works
- Onset of therapeutic actions with some antidepressants can be seen within 1–2 weeks, but often delayed 2–4 weeks
- Initially review at 1–2 weeks to assess for effectiveness, adherence and side effects including suicidality
- If it is not working within 3–4 weeks for depression, it may require a dosage increase

If It Works
- The goal of treatment is complete remission of current symptoms as well as prevention of future relapses

- Treatment most often reduces or even eliminates symptoms, but is not a cure since symptoms can recur after medicine is stopped
- Continue treatment until all symptoms are gone (remission), especially in depression and whenever possible in anxiety disorders
- Once symptoms are gone, continue treating for at least 6–9 months for the first episode of depression or >12 months if relapse indicators present
- If >5 episodes and/or 2 episodes in the last few years then need to continue for at least 2 years or indefinitely
- Use in anxiety disorders may also need to be indefinite

If It Doesn't Work
- Important to recognise non-response to treatment early on (3–4 weeks)
- Many patients have only a partial response where some symptoms are improved but others persist
- Other patients may be non-responders, sometimes called treatment-resistant or treatment-refractory
- Some patients who have an initial response may relapse even though they continue treatment
- Consider increasing dose, switching to another agent or adding an appropriate augmenting agent
- Lithium may be added for suicidal patients or those at high risk of relapse
- Consider psychotherapy
- Consider ECT
- Consider evaluation for another diagnosis or for a co-morbid condition (e.g. medical illness, substance abuse, etc.)
- Some patients may experience a switch into mania and so would require antidepressant discontinuation and initiation of a mood stabiliser

Best Augmenting Combos for Partial Response or Treatment Resistance
- Mood stabilisers or atypical antipsychotics for bipolar depression
- Atypical antipsychotics for psychotic depression
- Atypical antipsychotics as first-line augmenting agents (quetiapine MR 300 mg/

Citalopram (Continued)

day or aripiprazole at 2.5–10 mg/day) for treatment-resistant depression
- Atypical antipsychotics as second-line augmenting agents (risperidone 0.5–2 mg/day or olanzapine 2.5–10 mg/day) for treatment-resistant depression
- Mirtazapine at 30–45 mg/day as another second-line augmenting agent (a dual serotonin and noradrenaline combination, but observe for switch into mania, increase in suicidal ideation or rare risk of non-fatal serotonin syndrome)
- Although T3 (20–50 mcg/day) is another second-line augmenting agent the evidence suggests that it works best with tricyclic antidepressants
- Other augmenting agents but with less evidence include bupropion (up to 400 mg/day), buspirone (up to 60 mg/day) and lamotrigine (up to 400 mg/day)
- Benzodiazepines if agitation present
- Hypnotics or trazodone for insomnia (but there is a rare risk of non-fatal serotonin syndrome with trazodone)
- Augmenting agents reserved for specialist use include: modafinil for sleepiness, fatigue and lack of concentration; stimulants, oestrogens, testosterone
- Lithium is particularly useful for suicidal patients and those at high risk of relapse including with factors such as severe depression, psychomotor retardation, repeated episodes (>3), significant weight loss, or a family history of major depression (aim for lithium plasma levels 0.6–1.0 mmol/L)
- For severely ill patients other combinations may be tried especially in specialist centres
- Augmenting agents that may be tried include omega-3, SAM-e, L-methylfolate
- Additional non-pharmacological treatments such as exercise, mindfulness, CBT, and IPT can also be helpful
- If present after treatment response (4–8 weeks) or remission (6–12 weeks), the most common residual symptoms of depression include cognitive impairments, reduced energy and problems with sleep

Tests
- ECG monitoring for those at risk of cardiac disease due to risk of QT prolongation

SIDE EFFECTS

How Drug Causes Side Effects
- Theoretically due to increases in serotonin concentrations at serotonin receptors in parts of the brain and body other than those that cause therapeutic actions (e.g. unwanted actions of serotonin in sleep centres causing insomnia, unwanted actions of serotonin in the gut causing diarrhoea, etc.)
- Increasing serotonin can cause diminished dopamine release and might contribute to emotional flattening, cognitive slowing, and apathy in some patients
- Most side effects are immediate but often go away with time, in contrast to most therapeutic effects which are delayed and are enhanced over time
- *Citalopram's antihistaminergic actions may contribute to fatigue and sedation in some people

Notable Side Effects
- CNS: headache, drowsiness, dizziness, memory loss, sleep disorders, tinnitus, altered taste, tremor, visual impairment
- CVS: arrhythmias, palpitations
- GIT: abnormal appetite, constipation, diarrhoea, dry mouth, GI upset, nausea (dose-related), vomiting
- Sexual dysfunction (dose-dependent; men: delayed ejaculation, erectile dysfunction; men and women: decreased libido, anorgasmia)
- Rare SIADH (syndrome of inappropriate antidiuretic hormone secretion)
- Rare hyponatraemia (mostly in elderly patients, reversible)
- Mood elevation in diagnosed or undiagnosed bipolar disorder
- Sweating (dose-dependent)
- Bruising and rare bleeding

Common or very common
- CNS: angle-closure glaucoma, apathy, headache (migraine)
- GIT: flatulence, increased saliva
- Resp: rhinitis

Uncommon
- Oedema

Rare or very rare
- Cough, seizure

Frequency not known
- Hypokalaemia

Life-Threatening or Dangerous Side Effects

- Seizures
- Rare induction of mania
- Serotonin syndrome
- QT prolongation
- Increased bleeding risk, particularly of the upper gastrointestinal tract when in combination with aspirin and NSAIDs
- Rare increase in suicidal ideation and behaviours in adolescents and young adults (up to age 25), hence patients should be warned of this potential adverse event

Weight Gain

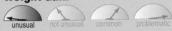

- Weight gain has been reported but is unexpected

Sedation

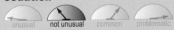

- Non-sedating generally, but can cause sedation in a significant minority

What To Do About Side Effects

- Manage side effects that are likely to be transient (e.g. nausea) by explanation, reassurance, and if necessary, dose reduction and re-titration
- Give patients simple strategies for managing mild side effects (e.g. dry mouth)
- For persistent or distressing side effects, several options exist:
  - Dose reduction and titration if possible
  - Switch drug to one with a lesser tendency to cause that side effect
  - Non-drug management of the side effect, e.g. diet and exercise for weight gain
  - Symptomatic treatment with a second drug (see below)

Best Augmenting Agents for Side Effects

- Many side effects are dose-dependent (i.e. they increase as dose increases, or they re-emerge until tolerance redevelops)
- Many side effects are time-dependent (i.e. they start immediately upon dosing and upon each dose increase, but go away with time)

- Often best to try another antidepressant monotherapy prior to resorting to augmentation strategies to treat side effects
- Trazodone, mirtazapine or hypnotic for insomnia
- Mirtazapine for agitation, and gastrointestinal side effects
- Bupropion for emotional flattening, cognitive slowing, or apathy
- For sexual dysfunction: can augment with bupropion for women, sildenafil for men; or otherwise switch to another antidepressant
- Benzodiazepines for jitteriness and anxiety, especially at initiation of treatment and especially for anxious patients
- Increased activation or agitation may represent the induction of a bipolar state, especially a mixed dysphoric bipolar condition sometimes associated with suicidal ideation, and require the addition of lithium, a mood stabiliser or an atypical antipsychotic, and/or discontinuation of the SSRI

DOSING AND USE

Usual Dosage Range

- Depression:
- 20–40 mg/day (tablet); 16–32 mg/day (oral drops)
- Panic disorder: 10–40 mg/day (tablet); 8–32 mg/day (oral drops)

Dosage Forms

- Oral drops 40 mg/mL
- Tablet 10 mg, 20 mg, 40 mg
- Intravenous 40 mg/ml (has been used as a research tool as well as used in hospital patients with severe depression; also shows better efficacy and faster response when compared with oral doses in the treatment of OCD)

How to Dose

∗Depression:
- Tablet: 20 mg/day, increased by increments of 20 mg/day at intervals of 3–4 weeks as needed; max 40 mg/day. Elderly: 10–20 mg/day; max 20 mg/day
- Oral drops: 16 mg/day, increased by increments of 16 mg/day at intervals of 3–4 weeks as needed; max 32 mg/day. Elderly: 8–16 mg/day; max 16 mg/day
∗Panic disorder:
- Tablet: 10 mg/day, increased gradually by increments of 10 mg/day as needed; usual

dose 20–30 mg/day; max 40 mg/day. Elderly: 10 mg/day, increased gradually by increments of 10 mg/ day as needed; max 20 mg/day
• Oral drops: 8 mg/day, increased gradually by increments of 8 mg as needed; usual dose 16–24 mg/day; max 32 mg/day. Elderly: 8 mg/day, increased gradually by increments of 8 mg as needed; max 16 mg/day

Dosing Tips

• Four oral drops (8 mg) is equivalent in therapeutic effect to 10 mg tablet
• No clear evidence of increased risk of arrhythmia at licensed dose
• Give once daily, at the time of day that is best tolerated by the patient

Overdose

• Rare fatalities have been reported with citalopram overdose, both alone and in combination with other drugs
• Symptoms include: nausea, vomiting, agitation, tremor, nystagmus, drowsiness, sinus tachycardia and convulsions
• Rarer, more dangerous symptoms include: serotonin syndrome, neuromuscular hyperactivity, autonomic instability, rhabdomyolysis, renal failure and coagulopathies

Long-Term Use

• Safe

Habit Forming

• No

How to Stop

• If taking SSRIs for more than 6–8 weeks, it is not recommended to stop them suddenly due to the risk of withdrawal effects (dizziness, nausea, stomach cramps, sweating, tingling, dysaesthesias)
• Taper dose gradually over 4 weeks, or longer if withdrawal symptoms emerge
• Inform all patients of the risk of withdrawal symptoms
• If withdrawal symptoms emerge, raise dose to stop symptoms and then restart withdrawal much more slowly

Pharmacokinetics

• Parent drug half-life about 36 hours
• Weak inhibitor of CYP450 2D6
• Metabolised by CYP450 3A4 and 2C19

Drug Interactions

• Tramadol increases the risk of seizures in patients taking an antidepressant
• Can increase TCA levels; use with caution with TCAs or when switching from a TCA to citalopram
• Can cause a fatal "serotonin syndrome" when combined with MAOIs, so do not use with MAOIs or for at least 14 days after MAOIs are stopped
• Do not start an MAOI for at least 5 half-lives (5 to 7 days for most drugs) after discontinuing citalopram
• Could theoretically cause weakness, hyperreflexia, and incoordination when combined with sumatriptan or possibly other triptans, requiring careful monitoring of patient
• Increased risk of bleeding when used in combination with NSAIDs, aspirin, alteplase, anti-platelets, and anticoagulants
• NSAIDs may impair effectiveness of SSRIs
• Increased risk of hyponatraemia when citalopram is used in combination with other agents that cause hyponatraemia, e.g. thiazides
• Avoid using in combination with other drugs that prolong the QT interval, e.g. amiodarone, amisulpride, haloperidol, pimozide
• Caution when administering citalopram in combination with cimetidine (potent CYP450 2D6, 3A4 and 1A2 inhibitor) as cimetidine can raise citalopram plasma levels

Other Warnings/Precautions

• Use with caution in patients with cardiac disease or a susceptibility to QT-interval prolongation
• Use with caution in patients with diabetes
• Use with caution in patients with susceptibility to angle-closure glaucoma
• Use with caution in patients receiving ECT or with a history of seizures
• Use with caution in patients with a history of bleeding disorders
• Use with caution in patients with bipolar disorder unless treated with concomitant mood-stabilising agent
• When treating children, carefully weigh the risks and benefits of pharmacological treatment against the risks and benefits

of nontreatment with antidepressants and make sure to document this in patient notes
- Warn patients and their caregivers about the possibility of activating side effects and advise them to report such symptoms immediately
- Monitor patients for activation of suicidal ideation, especially children and adolescents

Do Not Use
- If patient has poorly controlled epilepsy
- If patient enters a manic phase
- If patient has QT prolongation
- If patient is already taking an MAOI (risk of serotonin syndrome)
- If patient is taking pimozide
- If there is a proven allergy to escitalopram or citalopram

SPECIAL POPULATIONS

Renal Impairment
- Dosage adjustment is not necessary in cases of mild or moderate renal impairment
- Use with caution in severe renal impairment
- Renal failure has been reported with citalopram overdose

Hepatic Impairment
- SSRIs are hepatically metabolised and accumulate on chronic dosing
- For tablets: initial dose of 10 mg/day for mild to moderate impairment, dose can be increased to 20 mg/day
- For oral solution: initial dose of 8 mg/day for the first 2 weeks in mild-moderate impairment, dose may be increased up to a max of 16 mg/day
- Use with extra caution and careful dose titration in severe impairment

Cardiac Impairment
- Contraindicated in QT prolongation
- May cause abnormal changes in electrical activity of the heart at doses greater than 40 mg/day; use with caution post myocardial infarction (MI) but there is some evidence of safety

Elderly
- Dose reduction advised (see above 'How to Dose')

- Risk of SIADH and hyponatraemia is higher in elderly
- May cause osteopenia, increases clinical risk if the patient should have a fall
- Reduction in the risk of suicide with antidepressants compared with placebo in those aged 65 and over

Children and Adolescents
- Not licensed for use in children, but is prescribed in clinical practice for children 12–17 years
- Weigh up risks and benefits of treatment and non-treatment and document this decision in the notes
- For mild to moderate depression psychotherapy (individual or systemic) should be the first-line treatment. For moderate to severe depression, pharmacological treatment may be offered when the young person is unresponsive after 4–6 sessions of psychological therapy. Combined initial therapy (fluoxetine and psychological therapy) may be considered
- For anxiety disorders evidence-based psychological treatments should be offered as first-line treatment including psychoeducation and skills training for parents, particularly of young children, to promote and reinforce the child's exposure to feared or avoided social situations and development of skills
- For OCD, children and young people, should be offered CBT (including exposure response prevention – ERP) that involves the family or carers and is adapted to suit the developmental age of the child as the treatment of choice
- For both severe depression and anxiety disorders, pharmacological interventions may have to commence prior to psychological treatments to enable the child/young person to engage in psychological therapy
- Where a child or young person presents with self-harm and suicidal thoughts the immediate risk management may take first priority as suicidal thoughts might increase in the initial stages of treatment
- All children and young people presenting with depression/anxiety should be supported with sleep management, anxiety management, exercise and activation schedules, and healthy diet

Citalopram (Continued)

Practical notes:
- A risk management plan should be discussed prior to start of medication because of the possible increase in suicidal ideation and behaviours in adolescents and young adults
- Monitor patients face-to-face regularly, and weekly during the first 2–3 weeks of treatment or after an increase in dose
- Monitor for activation of suicidal ideation at the beginning of treatment
- Use with caution, observing for activation of known or unknown bipolar disorder and/or suicidal ideation, and inform parents or guardians of this risk so they can help observe child or adolescent patients

If it does not work:
- Review child's/young person's profile, consider new/changing contributing individual or systemic factors such as peer or family conflict. Consider physical health problems
- Consider non-concordance, especially in adolescents. In all children consider non-concordance by parent or child, address underlying reasons for non-concordance
- Consider dose adjustment before switching or augmentation. Be vigilant of polypharmacy especially in complex and highly vulnerable children/adolescents
- For all SSRIs there is a 2–3x higher incidence of behavioural activation and vomiting in children when compared to adolescents; for adolescents there is a higher incidence than in adults
- Children taking SSRIs may have slower growth; long-term effects are unknown
- Major depression: oral tablets initially 10 mg/day, increased if required to 20 mg/day, dose to be increased over 2–4 weeks; oral drops initially 8 mg/day, increased if necessary to 16 mg/day, dose to be increased over 2–4 weeks
- Effective dose range: tablets 10–40 mg/day; oral drops 8–32 mg/day (note QT effects)
- Adolescents often receive adult dose, but doses slightly lower for children
- Re-evaluate the need for continued treatment regularly

Pregnancy
- Not generally recommended for use during pregnancy, especially during first trimester
- Nonetheless, continuous treatment during pregnancy may be necessary and has not been proven to be harmful to the foetus
- Must weigh the risk of treatment (first trimester foetal development, third trimester newborn delivery) to the child against the risk of no treatment (recurrence of depression, maternal health, infant bonding) to the mother and child
- For many patients, this may mean continuing treatment during pregnancy
- Exposure to SSRIs in pregnancy has been associated with cardiac malformations, however recent studies have suggested that these findings may be due to other patient factors
- Exposure to SSRIs in pregnancy has been associated with an increased risk of spontaneous abortion, low birth weight and preterm delivery. Data is conflicting and the effects of depression cannot be ruled out from some studies
- SSRI use beyond the 20th week of pregnancy may be associated with increased risk of persistent pulmonary hypertension (PPHN) in newborns. Whilst the risk of PPHN remains low it presents potentially serious complications
- SSRI/SNRI antidepressant use in the month before delivery may result in a small increased risk of postpartum haemorrhage
- Neonates exposed to SSRIs or SNRIs late in the third trimester have developed complications requiring prolonged hospitalisation, respiratory support, and tube feeding; reported symptoms are consistent with either a direct toxic effect of SSRIs and SNRIs or, possibly, a drug discontinuation syndrome, and include respiratory distress, cyanosis, apnoea, seizures, temperature instability, feeding difficulty, vomiting, hypoglycaemia, hypotonia, hypertonia, hyperreflexia, tremor, jitteriness, irritability, and constant crying

Breastfeeding
- Small to moderate amounts found in mother's breast milk
- Small amounts may be present in nursing children whose mothers are taking citalopram
- If child becomes irritable or sedated, breastfeeding or drug may need to be discontinued

- Immediate postpartum period is a high-risk time for depression, especially in women who have had prior depressive episodes, so drug may need to be reinstituted late in the third trimester or shortly after childbirth to prevent a recurrence during the postpartum period
- Must weigh benefits of breastfeeding with risks and benefits of antidepressant treatment versus non-treatment to both the infant and the mother
- For many patients, this may mean continuing treatment during breastfeeding
- Other SSRIs (e.g. sertraline or paroxetine) may be preferable for breastfeeding mothers

THE ART OF PSYCHOPHARMACOLOGY

Potential Advantages

- Elderly patients
- Patients who are excessively sedated or activated by other SSRIs
- Patients taking concomitant medications (few drug interactions)

Potential Disadvantages

- May require dose titration to achieve optimal therapeutic effect
- Potential sedative effect
- In children: those that already exhibit psychomotor agitation, anger, irritability, or who do not have a psychiatric diagnosis

Primary Target Symptoms

- Depressed mood
- Panic attacks
- Anxiety
- Obsessive-compulsive disorder
- Sleep disturbance, both insomnia and hypersomnia

 Pearls

- May be better tolerated than some other antidepressants except for escitalopram
- May have less sexual dysfunction than some other SSRIs
- May be especially well tolerated in the elderly, however non-response might suggest underlying cognitive impairment
- Can cause affective "numbing"
- In PMDD treatment restricted to the luteal phase may be more effective than continuous treatment
- SSRIs may be less effective in women >50 years of age, especially if not on oestrogens
- SSRIs may be useful for hot flushes in perimenopausal women
- Better tolerated by adolescents than by children

THE ART OF SWITCHING

 **Switching**

- Generally, when changing from one agent to another abrupt withdrawal should be avoided
- Cross-tapering is preferred, in which the dose of the drug being changed is slowly lowered while the new drug is introduced
- The speed of cross-tapering is best decided based on patient tolerability
- However, when switching between SSRIs, cross-tapering may not be required as the two agents have similar effects, so abrupt cessation of the first SSRI and commencement of the second SSRI may be possible
- Caution is advised when switching strategies involve combining serotonin-enhancing drugs

 Suggested Reading

Apler A. Citalopram for major depressive disorder in adults: a systematic review and meta-analysis of published placebo-controlled trials. BMJ Open 2011;1:e000106.

Cipriani A, Furukawa TA, Salanti G, et al. Comparative efficacy and acceptability of 21 antidepressant drugs for the acute treatment of adults with major depressive disorder: a systematic review and network meta-analysis. Lancet 2018;391(10128):1357–66.

Citalopram (Continued)

Cipriani A, Purgato M, Furukawa TA, et al. Citalopram versus other anti-depressive agents for depression. Cochrane Database Syst Rev 2012;7(7):CD006534.

Cleare A, Pariante CM, Young AH, et al. Evidence-based guidelines for treating depressive disorders with antidepressants: a revision of the 2008 British Association for Psychopharmacology guidelines. J Psychopharmacol 2015;29(5):459–525.

Montgomery SA, Pedersen V, Tanghoj P, et al. The optimal dosing regimen for citalopram–a meta-analysis of nine placebo-controlled studies. Int Clin Psychopharmacol 1994;9 Suppl 1:35–40.

Sangkuhl K, Klein TE, Altman RB. PharmGKB summary: citalopram pharmacokinetics pathway. Pharmacogenet Genomics 2011;21(11):769–72.

Clomipramine hydrochloride

Brands
• Non-proprietary

Generic?
Yes

Class
• Neuroscience-based nomenclature: pharmacology domain – serotonin, norepinephrine; mode of action – reuptake inhibitor
• Tricyclic antidepressant (TCA)
• Parent drug is a potent serotonin reuptake inhibitor
• Active metabolite is a potent noradrenaline reuptake inhibitor

Commonly Prescribed for
(bold for BNF indication)
• **Depressive illness**
• **Phobic and obsessional states**
• **Adjunctive treatment of cataplexy associated with narcolepsy**
• Obsessive-compulsive disorder
• Severe and treatment-resistant depression
• Anxiety
• Insomnia
• Neuropathic pain/chronic pain

 ## How the Drug Works
• Boosts neurotransmitters serotonin and noradrenaline
• Blocks serotonin reuptake pump (serotonin transporter), presumably increasing serotonergic neurotransmission
• Blocks noradrenaline reuptake pump (noradrenaline transporter), presumably increasing noradrenergic neurotransmission
• Presumably desensitises both serotonin 1A receptors and beta adrenergic receptors
• Since dopamine is inactivated by noradrenaline reuptake in frontal cortex, which largely lacks dopamine transporters, trimipramine can increase dopamine neurotransmission in this part of the brain

How Long Until It Works
• May have immediate effects in treating insomnia or anxiety
• Onset of therapeutic actions with some antidepressants can be seen within 1–2 weeks, but often delayed up to 2–4 weeks

• If it is not working within 3–4 weeks for depression, it may require a dosage increase or it may not work at all
• By contrast, for generalised anxiety, onset of response and increases in remission rates may still occur after 8 weeks, and for up to 6 months after initiating dosing
• For OCD if no improvement within about 10–12 weeks, then treatment may need to be reconsidered
• May continue to work for many years to prevent relapse of symptoms

If It Works
• The goal of treatment is complete remission of current symptoms as well as prevention of future relapses
• Treatment most often reduces or even eliminates symptoms, but is not a cure since symptoms can recur after medicine is stopped
• Continue treatment until all symptoms are gone (remission), especially in depression and whenever possible in anxiety disorders
• Once symptoms are gone, continue treating for at least 6–9 months for the first episode of depression or >12 months if relapse indicators present
• If >5 episodes and/or 2 episodes in the last few years then need to continue for at least 2 years or indefinitely
• The goal of treatment in chronic neuropathic pain is to reduce symptoms as much as possible, especially in combination with other treatments
• Treatment of chronic neuropathic pain may reduce symptoms, but rarely eliminates them completely, and is not a cure since symptoms can recur after medicine has been stopped
• Use in anxiety disorders and chronic pain may also need to be indefinite, but long-term treatment is not well studied in these conditions

If It Doesn't Work
• Important to recognise non-response to treatment early on (3–4 weeks)
• Many patients have only a partial response where some symptoms are improved but others persist (especially insomnia, fatigue, and problems concentrating)
• Other patients may be non-responders, sometimes called treatment-resistant or treatment-refractory

Clomipramine hydrochloride (Continued)

- Some patients who have an initial response may relapse even though they continue treatment
- Consider increasing dose, switching to another agent or adding an appropriate augmenting agent
- Lithium may be added for suicidal patients or those at high risk of relapse
- Consider psychotherapy
- Consider ECT
- Consider evaluation for another diagnosis or for a co-morbid condition (e.g. medical illness, substance abuse, etc.)
- Some patients may experience a switch into mania and so would require antidepressant discontinuation and initiation of a mood stabiliser

⚖ Best Augmenting Combos for Partial Response or Treatment Resistance

In OCD:
- Clomipramine is a good option in treatment-resistant cases
- Consider cautious addition of an antipsychotic (risperidone, quetiapine, olanzapine, aripiprazole or haloperidol) as augmenting agent
- Alternative augmenting agents may include ondansetron, granisetron, topiramate, lamotrigine
- Combine an SSRI or clomipramine with an evidence-based psychological treatment

In depression:
- Mood stabilisers or atypical antipsychotics for bipolar depression
- Atypical antipsychotics for psychotic depression
- Atypical antipsychotics as first-line augmenting agents (quetiapine MR 300 mg per day or aripiprazole at 2.5–10 mg per day) for treatment-resistant depression
- Atypical antipsychotics as second-line augmenting agents (risperidone 0.5–2 mg per day or olanzapine 2.5–10 mg per day) for treatment-resistant depression
- Mirtazapine at 30–45 mg per day as another second-line augmenting agent (a dual serotonin and noradrenaline combination, but observe for switch into mania, increase in suicidal ideation or serotonin syndrome)
- T3 (20–50 mcg per day) is another second-line augmenting agent that works best with tricyclic antidepressants

- Other augmenting agents but with less evidence include bupropion (up to 400 mg per day), buspirone (up to 60 mg per day) and lamotrigine (up to 400 mg per day)
- Benzodiazepines if agitation present
- Hypnotics or trazodone for insomnia (but beware of serotonin syndrome with trazodone)
- Augmenting agents reserved for specialist use include: modafinil for sleepiness, fatigue and lack of concentration; stimulants, oestrogens, testosterone
- Lithium is particularly useful for suicidal patients and those at high risk of relapse including with factors such as severe depression, psychomotor retardation, repeated episodes (>3), significant weight loss, or a family history of major depression (aim for lithium plasma levels 0.6–1.0 mmol/L)
- For elderly patients lithium is a very effective augmenting agent
- For severely ill patients other combinations may be tried especially in specialist centres
- Augmenting agents that may be tried include omega-3, SAM-e, L-methylfolate
- Additional non-pharmacological treatments such as exercise, mindfulness, CBT, and IPT can also be helpful
- If present after treatment response (4–8 weeks) or remission (6–12 weeks), the most common residual symptoms of depression include cognitive impairments, reduced energy and problems with sleep
- For chronic pain: gabapentin, other anticonvulsants, or opiates if done by experts while monitoring carefully in difficult cases

Tests

- Baseline ECG is useful for patients over age 50
- ECGs may be useful for selected patients (e.g. those with personal or family history of QTc prolongation; cardiac arrhythmia; recent myocardial infarction; decompensated heart failure; or taking agents that prolong QTc interval such as pimozide, thioridazine, selected antiarrhythmics, moxifloxacin etc.)
- *Since tricyclic and tetracyclic antidepressants are frequently associated with weight gain, before starting treatment, weigh all patients and determine if the patient is already overweight (BMI 25.0–29.9) or obese (BMI ≥30)

- Before giving a drug that can cause weight gain to an overweight or obese patient, consider determining whether the patient already has:
  - Pre-diabetes – fasting plasma glucose: 5.5 mmol/L to 6.9 mmol/L or HbA1c: 42 to 47 mmol/mol (6.0 to 6.4%)
  - Diabetes – fasting plasma glucose: >7.0 mmol/L or HbA1c: ≥48 mmol/L (≥6.5%)
  - Hypertension (BP >140/90 mm Hg)
  - Dyslipidaemia (increased total cholesterol, LDL cholesterol, and triglycerides; decreased HDL cholesterol)
- Treat or refer such patients for treatment, including nutrition and weight management, physical activity counselling, smoking cessation, and medical management
* Monitor weight and BMI during treatment
* While giving a drug to a patient who has gained >5% of initial weight, consider evaluating for the presence of pre-diabetes, diabetes, dyslipidaemia, or consider switching to a different antidepressant
- Patients at risk for electrolyte disturbances (e.g. patients aged >60, patients on diuretic therapy) should have baseline and periodic serum potassium and magnesium measurements

SIDE EFFECTS
How Drug Causes Side Effects
- Anticholinergic activity may explain sedative effects, dry mouth, constipation, and blurred vision
- Sedative effects and weight gain may be due to antihistaminergic properties
- Blockade of alpha adrenergic 1 receptors may explain dizziness, sedation, and hypotension
- Cardiac arrhythmias and seizures, especially in overdose, may be caused by blockade of ion channels

Notable Side Effects
- Blurred vision, constipation, urinary retention, dry mouth, increased appetite, nausea, diarrhoea, heartburn, unusual taste in mouth, weight gain
- Fatigue, weakness, dizziness, sedation, headache, anxiety, restlessness
- Sexual dysfunction, sweating

Common or very common
- CNS/PNS: aggression, altered mood, anxiety, confusion, delirium, depersonalisation, depression exacerbated, dizziness, drowsiness, hallucination, headache, impaired concentration, memory loss, movement disorders, paraesthesia, sleep disorders, speech disorder, tinnitus, tremor, vision disorders
- CVS: arrhythmias, hypotension, palpitations
- GIT: altered taste, constipation, diarrhoea, dry mouth, gastrointestinal disorder, increased weight, nausea, vomiting
- Other: breast enlargement, fatigue, galactorrhoea, hot flush, hyperhidrosis, increased muscle tone, muscle weakness, mydriasis, photosensitivity, sexual dysfunction, skin reactions, urinary disorders, yawning

Uncommon
- Psychosis, seizure

Rare or very rare
- Blood disorders: agranulocytosis, eosinophilia, leucopenia, thrombocytopenia
- CVS: cardiac conduction disorders, QT interval prolongation
- GIT: hepatic disorders
- Other: alopecia, glaucoma, hyperpyrexia, neuroleptic malignant syndrome, oedema, respiratory disorders, vaginal haemorrhage

Frequency not known
- Rhabdomyolysis, serotonin syndrome, suicidal behaviours, withdrawal syndrome

Life-Threatening or Dangerous Side Effects
- Paralytic ileus, hyperthermia (TCAs + anticholinergic agents)
- Lowered seizure threshold and rare seizures
- Orthostatic hypotension, sudden death, arrhythmias, tachycardia
- QTc prolongation
- Hepatic failure, extrapyramidal symptoms
- Increased intraocular pressure
- Rare induction of mania and paranoid delusions
- Rare increase in suicidal ideation and behaviours in adolescents and young adults (up to age 25), hence patients should be warned of this potential adverse event

Clomipramine hydrochloride (Continued)

Weight Gain

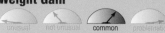

- Many experience and/or can be significant in amount
- Can increase appetite and carbohydrate craving

Sedation

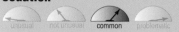

- Many experience and/or can be significant in amount
- Tolerance to sedative effects may develop with long-term use

What to Do About Side Effects

- Wait
- Wait
- Wait
- The risk of side effects is reduced by titrating slowly to the minimum effective dose (every 2–3 days)
- Consider using a lower starting dose in elderly patients
- Manage side effects that are likely to be transient (e.g. drowsiness) by explanation, reassurance and, if necessary, dose reduction and re-titration
- Giving patients simple strategies for managing mild side effects (e.g. dry mouth) may be useful
- For persistent, severe or distressing side effects the options are:
  - Dose reduction and re-titration if possible
  - Switching to an antidepressant with a lower propensity to cause that side effect
  - Non-drug management of the side effect (e.g. diet and exercise for weight gain)

Best Augmenting Agents for Side Effects

- Many side effects cannot be improved with an augmenting agent

---

DOSING AND USE

Usual Dosage Range

- Depressive illness: 30–250 mg/day (adult); 30–75 mg/day (elderly)
- Phobic and obsessional states: 100–250 mg/day (adult); 100–250 mg/day (elderly)
- Adjunctive treatment of cataplexy associated with narcolepsy: 10–75 mg/day (adult)

Dosage Forms

- Capsule 10 mg, 25 mg, 50 mg

How to Dose

*Depressive illness:
- Adult: initial dose 10 mg/day, increased gradually as needed to 30–150 mg/day in divided doses or as single dose at bedtime; max 250 mg/day
- Elderly: initial dose 10 mg/day, increased carefully over 10 days to 30–75 mg/day

*Phobic and obsessional states:
- Adult: initial dose 25 mg/day, increased gradually over 2 weeks to 100–150 mg/day; max 250 mg/day
- Elderly: initial dose 10 mg/day, increased gradually over 2 weeks to 100–150 mg/day; max 250 mg/day

*Adjunctive treatment of cataplexy associated with narcolepsy:
- Adult: initial dose 10 mg/day, increased gradually according to response up to 75 mg/day

*Obsessive-compulsive disorder:
- Children/adolescents: titrate to a max of 100 mg/day or 3 mg/kg/day after 2 weeks; after which dose may be further titrated up to a max of 200 mg/day or 3 mg/kg/day

 Dosing Tips

- If given in a single dose, should generally be administered at bedtime because of its sedative properties
- If given in split doses, largest dose should generally be given at bedtime because of its sedative properties
- If patients experience nightmares, split dose and do not give large dose at bedtime
- Patients treated for chronic pain may only require lower doses
- Patients treated for OCD may often require doses at the high end of the range (e.g. 200–250 mg/day)
- Risk of seizures increases with dose
- If intolerable anxiety, insomnia, agitation, akathisia, or activation occur either upon dosing initiation or discontinuation, consider the possibility of activated bipolar disorder, and switch to a mood stabiliser or an atypical antipsychotic

Overdose

- Can be fatal; convulsions, cardiac arrhythmias, severe hypotension, CNS depression, coma, ECG changes

Long-Term Use

- Limited data, but appears to be efficacious and safe long-term

Habit Forming

- No

How to Stop

- Taper gradually to avoid withdrawal effects
- Even with gradual dose reduction some withdrawal symptoms may appear within the first 2 weeks
- A minimum tapering period of at least 4 weeks is recommended
- If withdrawal symptoms emerge during discontinuation, raise dose to stop symptoms and then restart withdrawal much more slowly (over at least 6 months)

Pharmacokinetics

- Substrate for CYP450 2D6 and 1A2
- Clomipramine is metabolised via CYP450 1A2 to an active metabolite desmethyl-clomipramine (a predominantly noradrenaline reuptake inhibitor)
- Inhibits CYP450 2D6
- Mean half-life for clomipramine of 21 hours (range 12–36 hours), and for desmethyl-clomipramine of 36 hours
- Food does not affect absorption

 Drug Interactions

- Tramadol increases the risk of seizures in patients taking TCAs
- Use of TCAs with anticholinergic drugs may result in paralytic ileus or hyperthermia
- Fluoxetine, paroxetine, bupropion, duloxetine, terbinafine and other CYP450 2D6 inhibitors may increase TCA concentrations
- Fluvoxamine, a CYP450 1A2 inhibitor, can decrease the conversion of clomipramine to desmethyl-clomipramine, and increase clomipramine plasma concentrations
- Cimetidine may increase plasma concentrations of TCAs and cause anticholinergic symptoms

- Phenothiazines or haloperidol may raise TCA blood concentrations
- May alter effects of antihypertensive drugs; may inhibit hypotensive effects of clonidine
- Use with sympathomimetic agents may increase sympathetic activity
- Methylphenidate may inhibit metabolism of TCAs
- Clomipramine can increase the effects of adrenaline/epinephrine
- Carbamazepine decreases the exposure to clomipramine
- Both clomipramine and carbamazepine can increase the risk of hyponatraemia
- Clomipramine is predicted to increase the risk of severe toxic reaction when given with MAOIs; avoid and for 14 days after stopping the MAOI
- Both clomipramine and MAOIs can increase the risk of hypotension
- Do not start an MAOI for at least 5 half-lives (5 to 7 days for most drugs) after discontinuing clomipramine
- Activation and agitation, especially following switching or adding antidepressants, may represent the induction of a bipolar state, especially a mixed dysphoric bipolar condition sometimes associated with suicidal ideation, and require the addition of lithium, a mood stabiliser or an atypical antipsychotic, and/or discontinuation of trimipramine

 Other Warnings/Precautions

- Can possibly increase QTc interval at higher doses
- Arrhythmias may occur at higher doses and are common
- Increased risk of arrhythmias in patients with hyperthyroidism or phaeochromocytoma
- Caution if patient is taking agents capable of significantly prolonging QTc interval or if there is a history of QTc prolongation
- Caution if the patient is taking drugs that inhibit TCA metabolism, including CYP450 2D6 inhibitors
- Because TCAs can prolong QTc interval, use with caution in patients who have bradycardia or who are taking drugs that can induce bradycardia (e.g. beta blockers, calcium channel blockers, clonidine, digitalis)
- Because TCAs can prolong QTc interval, use with caution in patients who have

Clomipramine hydrochloride (Continued)

hypokalaemia and/or hypomagnesaemia or who are taking drugs that can induce hypokalaemia and/or hypomagnesaemia (e.g. diuretics, stimulant laxatives, intravenous amphotericin B, glucocorticoids, tetracosactide)
- Caution if there is reduced CYP450 2D6 function, such as patients who are poor 2D6 metabolisers
- Can exacerbate chronic constipation
- Use with caution when treating patients with epilepsy
- Use with caution in patients with a history of bipolar disorder, psychosis or significant risk of suicide
- Use with caution in patients with increased intra-ocular pressure or susceptibility to angle-closure glaucoma
- Use with caution in patients with prostatic hypertrophy or urinary retention

Do Not Use
- In patients during a manic phase
- If there is a history of cardiac arrhythmia, recent acute myocardial infarction, heart block
- In patients with acute porphyrias
- If there is a proven allergy to clomipramine

Renal Impairment
- Use with caution in severe impairment and start at lower doses

Hepatic Impairment
- Use with caution
- Avoid in severe impairment (risk of hypertensive crisis)

Cardiac Impairment
- Baseline ECG is recommended
- TCAs have been reported to cause arrhythmias, prolongation of conduction time, postural hypotension, sinus tachycardia, and heart failure, especially in the diseased heart
- Myocardial infarction and stroke have been reported with TCAs
- TCAs produce QTc prolongation, which may be enhanced by the existence of bradycardia, hypokalaemia, congenital

or acquired long QTc interval, which should be evaluated prior to administering trimipramine
- Use with caution if treating concomitantly with a medication likely to produce prolonged bradycardia, hypokalaemia, heart block, or prolongation of the QTc interval
- Avoid TCAs in patients with a known history of QTc prolongation, recent acute myocardial infarction, and decompensated heart failure
- TCAs may cause a sustained increase in heart rate in patients with ischaemic heart disease and may worsen (decrease) heart rate variability, an independent risk of mortality in cardiac populations
- Since SSRIs may improve (increase) heart rate variability in patients following a myocardial infarct and may improve survival as well as mood in patients with acute angina or following a myocardial infarction, these are more appropriate agents for cardiac population than tricyclic/tetracyclic antidepressants
- *Risk/benefit ratio may not justify use of TCAs in cardiac impairment

Elderly
- Baseline ECG is recommended for patients over age 50
- May be more sensitive to anticholinergic, cardiovascular, hypotensive, and sedative effects
- Initial dose 10 mg/day
- Initial dose should be increased with caution and under close supervision
- Reduction in the risk of suicidality with antidepressants compared to placebo in adults age 65 and older

Children and Adolescents
- Not licensed and not indicated in the BNF for use in children and adolescents
- Some cases of sudden death have occurred in children taking TCAs
- Has been studied in the treatment of obsessive-compulsive disorder in children and adolescents
- May be trialled in treatment-resistant OCD, where two or more SSRIs have failed

Clomipramine hydrochloride (Continued)

Before you prescribe:
- Carefully weigh the risks and benefits of pharmacological treatment against the risks and benefits of nontreatment with antidepressants and make sure to document this in the patient's chart
- For OCD, all children and young people should be offered CBT (including exposure response prevention – ERP) that involves the family or carers and is adapted to suit the developmental age of the child as the treatment of choice
- Where a child or young person presents with self-harm and suicidal thoughts then immediate risk management may take first priority

Practical notes:
- Inform parents and child/young person that improvements may take several weeks to emerge
- The earliest effects may only be apparent to outsiders
- A risk management plan should be discussed prior to start of medication because of the possible increase in suicidal ideation and behaviours in adolescents and young adults
- Monitor patients face-to-face regularly, and weekly during the first 2–3 weeks of treatment or after increase
- Monitor for activation of suicidal ideation at the beginning of treatment
- Use with caution, observing for activation of known or unknown bipolar disorder and/or suicidal ideation, and inform parents or guardians of this risk so they can help observe child or adolescent patients
- All children and young people presenting with anxiety should be supported with sleep management, anxiety management, exercise and activation schedules, and healthy diet

If it does not work:
- Review child/young person's profile, consider differential diagnosis and co-morbidities including developmental disorders such as ASD, ADHD and ODD.
- Consider new or changing individual or systemic contributing factors such as peer or family conflict, school environment
- Consider physical health problems
- Consider non-concordance, especially in adolescents. In all children consider non-concordance by parent or child, address underlying reasons for non-concordance

- Consider dose adjustment before switching or augmentation. Be vigilant of polypharmacy especially in complex and highly vulnerable children/adolescents
- Re-evaluate the need for continued treatment regularly

Pregnancy
- No strong evidence of TCA maternal use during pregnancy being associated with an increased risk of congenital malformations
- Risk of malformations cannot be ruled out due to limited information on specific TCAs
- Poor neonatal adaptation syndrome and/or withdrawal has been reported in infants whose mothers took a TCA during pregnancy or near delivery
- Maternal use of more than one CNS-acting medication is likely to lead to more severe symptoms in the neonate
- Must weigh the risk of treatment (first trimester foetal development, third trimester newborn delivery) to the child against the risk of no treatment (recurrence of depression, maternal health, infant bonding) to the mother and child
- For many patients this may mean continuing treatment during pregnancy

Breastfeeding
- Small amounts expected in mother's breast milk
- Infant should be monitored for sedation and poor feeding
- Immediate postpartum period is a high-risk time for depression, especially in women who have had prior depressive episodes; antidepressants may need to be reinstituted late in the third trimester or shortly after childbirth to prevent a recurrence during the postpartum period
- Must weigh benefits of breastfeeding with risks and benefits of antidepressant treatment versus nontreatment to both the infant and the mother
- For many patients this may mean continuing treatment during breastfeeding
- Other antidepressants may be preferable, e.g. imipramine or nortriptyline

Clomipramine hydrochloride (Continued)

Potential Advantages
- Patients with insomnia
- Severe or treatment-resistant depression
- Patients with co-morbid OCD and depression
- Patients with cataplexy

Potential Disadvantages
- Paediatric and geriatric patients
- Patients concerned with weight gain and sedation
- Cardiac patients
- Patients with seizure disorders

Primary Target Symptoms
- Depressed mood
- Obsessive thoughts
- Compulsive behaviours

 Pearls

* Only TCAs with proven efficacy in treating obsessional states
* One of the most favoured TCAs for treating severe depression
- Clomipramine, a potent serotonin reuptake inhibitor, at steady state is metabolised extensively via CYP450 1A2 to its active metabolite desmethyl-clomipramine, a potent noradrenaline reuptake inhibitor
- Thus, at steady state, plasma drug activity is generally more noradrenergic (with higher active metabolite levels) than serotonergic (with lower parent drug levels)
- Addition of fluvoxamine (SSRI and CYP450 1A2 inhibitor) blocks this conversion and results in higher clomipramine levels than desmethyl-clomipramine levels
- For the expert only: addition of the SSRI fluvoxamine to clomipramine in treatment-resistant OCD can powerfully enhance serotonergic activity via both pharmacodynamic and pharmacokinetic mechanisms
- TCAs are often a first-line treatment option for chronic pain
- TCAs are no longer generally considered a first-line option for depression because of their side-effect profile
- TCAs continue to be useful for severe or treatment-resistant depression
- TCAs may aggravate psychotic symptoms

* Unique among TCAs, clomipramine has a potentially fatal interaction with MAOIs in addition to the danger of hypertension characteristic of all MAOI-TCA combinations
* A potentially fatal serotonin syndrome with high fever, seizures, coma, analogous to that caused by SSRIs and MAOIs, can occur with clomipramine and SSRIs, presumably due to clomipramine's potent serotonin reuptake blocking properties
- Use with alcohol can cause additive CNS-depressant effects
- Underweight patients may be more susceptible to adverse cardiovascular effects
- Patients with inadequate hydration, and patients with cardiac disease may be more susceptible to TCA-induced cardiotoxicity than healthy adults
- Patients on tricyclics should be aware that they may experience symptoms such as photosensitivity or blue-green urine
- SSRIs may be more effective than TCAs in women, and TCAs may be more effective than SSRIs in men
- Since tricyclic/tetracyclic antidepressants are substrates for CYP450 2D6, and 7% of the population (especially Whites) may have a genetic variant leading to reduced activity of 2D6, such patients may not safely tolerate normal doses of tricyclic/tetracyclic antidepressants and may require dose reduction
- Patients who seem to have extraordinarily severe side effects at normal or low doses may have this phenotypic CYP450 2D6 variant and require low doses or switching to another antidepressant not metabolised by 2D6

 **Switching**
- Consider switching to another agent or adding an appropriate augmenting agent if it doesn't work
- Consider switching to a different antidepressant if the patient has gained >5% of initial weight
- With patients with significant side effects at normal or low doses, they may have the phenotypic CYP450 2D6 variant; consider low doses or switching to another antidepressant not metabolised by 2D6

Suggested Reading

Anderson IM. Selective serotonin reuptake inhibitors versus tricyclic antidepressants: a meta-analysis of efficacy and tolerability. J Affect Disord 2000;58(1):19–36.

Anderson IM. Meta-analytical studies on new antidepressants. Br Med Bull 2001;57:161–78.

Bassetti CLA, Kallweit U, Vignatelli L, et al. European guideline and expert statements on the management of narcolepsy in adults and children. Eur J Neurol 2021;28(9):2815–30.

Cipriani A, Furukawa TA, Salanti G, et al. Comparative efficacy and acceptability of 21 antidepressant drugs for the acute treatment of adults with major depressive disorder: a systematic review and network meta-analysis. Lancet 2018;391(10128):1357–66.

Cox BJ, Swinson RP, Morrison B, et al. Clomipramine, fluoxetine, and behavior therapy in the treatment of obsessive-compulsive disorder: a meta-analysis. J Behav Ther Exp Psychiatry 1993;24(2):149–53.

Feinberg M. Clomipramine for obsessive-compulsive disorder. Am Fam Physician 1991;43(5):1735–8.

Clonazepam

Brands
• Non-proprietary

Generic?
Yes

Class
• Neuroscience-based nomenclature: pharmacology domain – GABA; mode of action – positive allosteric modulator (PAM)
• Benzodiazepine (anxiolytic, anticonvulsant)

Commonly Prescribed for
(bold for BNF indication)
• **All forms of epilepsy**
• **Myoclonus**
• **Panic disorders (with or without agoraphobia) resistant to antidepressant therapy**
• Other anxiety disorders
• Acute mania (adjunctive)
• Acute psychosis (adjunctive)
• Insomnia
• Catatonia

 ## How the Drug Works
• Binds to benzodiazepine receptors at the GABA-A ligand-gated chloride channel complex
• Enhances the inhibitory effects of GABA
• Boosts chloride conductance through GABA-regulated channels
• Inhibits neuronal activity presumably in amygdala-centred fear circuits to provide therapeutic benefits in anxiety disorders
• Inhibitory actions in cerebral cortex may provide therapeutic benefits in seizure disorders

How Long Until It Works
• Some immediate relief with first dosing is common; can take several weeks for maximal therapeutic benefit with daily dosing

If It Works
• For short-term symptoms of anxiety – after a few weeks, discontinue use or use on an "as-needed" basis
• For chronic anxiety disorders, the goal of treatment is complete remission of symptoms as well as prevention of future relapses
• For chronic anxiety disorders, treatment most often reduces or even eliminates symptoms, but is not a cure since symptoms can recur after medicine stopped
• For long-term symptoms of anxiety, consider switching to an SSRI or SNRI for long-term maintenance
• If long-term maintenance with a benzodiazepine is necessary, continue treatment for 6 months after symptoms resolve, and then taper dose slowly
• If symptoms re-emerge, consider treatment with an SSRI or SNRI, or consider restarting the benzodiazepine; sometimes benzodiazepines have to be used in combination with SSRIs or SNRIs for best results

If It Doesn't Work
• Consider switching to another agent or adding an appropriate augmenting agent
• Consider psychotherapy, especially cognitive behavioural psychotherapy
• Consider presence of concomitant substance abuse
• Consider presence of clonazepam abuse
• Consider another diagnosis such as a co-morbid medical condition

Best Augmenting Combos for Partial Response or Treatment Resistance
• Benzodiazepines are frequently used as augmenting agents for antipsychotics and mood stabilisers in the treatment of psychotic and bipolar disorders
• Benzodiazepines are frequently used as augmenting agents for SSRIs and SNRIs in the treatment of anxiety disorders
• Not generally rational to combine with other benzodiazepines
• Caution if using as an anxiolytic concomitantly with other sedative hypnotics for sleep

Tests
• In patients with seizure disorders, concomitant medical illness, and/or those with multiple concomitant long-term medications, periodic liver tests and blood counts may be prudent

SIDE EFFECTS

How Drug Causes Side Effects
- Same mechanism for side effects as for therapeutic effects – namely due to excessive actions at benzodiazepine receptors
- Long-term adaptations in benzodiazepine receptors may explain the development of dependence, tolerance, and withdrawal
- Side effects are generally immediate, but immediate side effects often disappear in time

Notable Side Effects
* Sedation, fatigue, depression
* Dizziness, ataxia, slurred speech, weakness
* Forgetfulness, confusion
* Hyperexcitability, nervousness
- Rare hallucinations, mania
- Rare hypotension
- Hypersalivation, dry mouth

Frequency not known
- CNS/PNS: abnormal coordination, impaired concentration, nystagmus, seizures, speech impairment, suicidal behaviours
- GIT: drooling and increased salivation (in children)
- Resp: increased bronchial secretion (in children)
- Other: alopecia, decreased muscle tone, incomplete precocious puberty (in children), increased risk of falls and fractures (in adults), sexual dysfunction, skin reactions

 Life-Threatening or Dangerous Side Effects
- Respiratory depression, especially when taken with CNS depressants in overdose
- Rare hepatic dysfunction, renal dysfunction, blood dyscrasias

Weight Gain

unusual   not unusual   common   problematic
- Reported but not expected

Sedation

unusual   not unusual   common   problematic
- Many experience and/or can be significant in amount

- Especially at initiation of treatment or when dose increases
- Tolerance often develops over time

What to Do About Side Effects
- Wait
- Wait
- Wait
- Lower the dose
- Take largest dose at bedtime to avoid sedative effects during the day
- Switch to another agent
- Administer flumazenil if side effects are severe or life-threatening

Best Augmenting Agents for Side Effects
- Many side effects cannot be improved with an augmenting agent

DOSING AND USE

Usual Dosage Range
- All forms of epilepsy, myoclonus (adults): 1–8 mg/day
- All forms of epilepsy (children): 0.25–8 mg/day depending on age
- Panic disorders (with or without agoraphobia) resistant to antidepressant therapy (adult): 1–2 mg/day

Dosage Forms
- Tablet 0.5 mg, 2 mg
- Oral solution 0.5 mg/5 mL, 2 mg/5 mL

How to Dose
Adult:
* All forms of epilepsy, myoclonus (adult):
- Initial dose 1 mg/day for 4 nights, increased over 2–4 weeks, usual dose 4–8 mg at night, adjusted according to response; may be given in 3–4 divided doses
* All forms of epilepsy (elderly):
- Initial dose 0.5 mg/day for 4 nights, increased over 2–4 weeks, usual dose 4–8 mg at night, adjusted according to response; may be given in 3–4 divided doses
* Panic disorders (with or without agoraphobia) resistant to antidepressant therapy:
- 1–2 mg/day

Children and adolescents:
* All forms of epilepsy:
- Child 1–11 months: initial dose 0.25 mg/day for 4 nights, increased over 2–4 weeks,

usual dose 0.5–1 mg at night; may be given in 3 divided doses
- Child 1–4 years: initial dose 0.25 mg/day for 4 nights, increased over 2–4 weeks, usual dose 1–3 mg at night; may be given in 3 divided doses
- Child 5–11 years: initial dose 0.5 mg/day for 4 nights, increased over 2–4 weeks, usual dose 3–6 mg at night; may be given in 3 divided doses
- Child 12–17 years: initial dose 1 mg/day for 4 nights, dose increased over 2–4 weeks, usual dose 4–8 mg at night; may be given in 3–4 divided doses

 Dosing Tips

- For anxiety disorders, use lowest possible effective dose for the shortest possible period of time (a benzodiazepine-sparing strategy)
- Assess need for continuous treatment regularly
- Risk of dependence may increase with dose and duration of treatment
- For inter-dose symptoms of anxiety, can either increase dose or maintain same daily dose but divide into more frequent doses
- Can also use an as-needed occasional "top-up" dose for inter-dose anxiety
- Because seizure disorder can require doses much higher than 2 mg/day, the risk of dependence may be greater in these patients
- Because panic disorder can require doses somewhat higher than 2 mg/day, the risk of dependence may be greater in these patients than in anxiety patients maintained at lower doses
- Some severely ill seizure patients may require more than 20 mg/day
- Some severely ill panic patients may require 4 mg/day or more
- Frequency of dosing in practice is often greater than predicted from half-life, as duration of biological activity is often shorter than pharmacokinetic terminal half-life
- *Clonazepam is generally dosed half the dosage of alprazolam
- Escalation of dose may be necessary if tolerance develops in seizure disorders
- Escalation of dose usually not necessary in anxiety disorders, as tolerance to clonazepam does not generally develop in the treatment of anxiety disorders
- Clonazepam 1–2 mg = diazepam 10 mg

Overdose
- Rarely fatal in monotherapy; sedation, confusion, coma, diminished reflexes

Long-Term Use
- May lose efficacy for seizures; dose increase may restore efficacy
- Risk of dependence, particularly for treatment periods longer than 12 weeks and especially in patients with past or current polysubstance abuse

Habit Forming
- Clonazepam is a Class C/Schedule 4 drug
- Patients may develop dependence and/or tolerance with long-term use
- Around one-third of individuals treated with clonazepam for longer than 4 weeks develop a dependence on the drug and experience a withdrawal syndrome upon dose reduction. High dosage and long-term use increase the risk and severity of dependence and withdrawal symptoms

How to Stop
- Patients with history of seizure may seize upon withdrawal, especially if withdrawal is abrupt
- Taper by 0.25 mg every 3 days to reduce chances of withdrawal effects
- For difficult-to-taper cases, consider reducing dose much more slowly once reaching 1.5 mg/day, perhaps by as little as 0.125 mg per week or less
- For other patients with severe problems discontinuing a benzodiazepine, dosing may need to be tapered over many months (i.e. reduce dose by 1% every 3 days by crushing tablet and suspending or dissolving in 100 mL of fruit juice and then disposing of 1 mL while drinking the rest; 3–7 days later, dispose of 2 mL, and so on). This is both a form of very slow biological tapering and a form of behavioural desensitisation
- Be sure to differentiate re-emergence of symptoms requiring reinstitution of treatment from withdrawal symptoms
- Benzodiazepine-dependent anxiety patients are not addicted to their medications; when benzodiazepine-dependent patients stop their medication, disease symptoms can re-emerge, disease symptoms can worsen (rebound), and/or withdrawal symptoms can emerge

Pharmacokinetics

- Peak plasma concentrations are reached in most cases within 1–4 hours after an oral dose
- Long half-life compared to other benzodiazepine anxiolytics; mean elimination half-life about 30 hours (range 20–60 hours)
- Onset of action within an hour and duration of action 6–12 hours
- Substrate for CYP450 3A4
- Food does not affect absorption
- Excretion: 50–70% in urine and 10–30% in faeces

 ## Drug Interactions

- Increased depressive effects when taken with other CNS depressants (see Warnings below)
- Inhibitors of CYP450 3A4 may affect the clearance of clonazepam, but dosage adjustment usually not necessary
- Flumazenil (used to reverse the effects of benzodiazepines) may precipitate seizures and should not be used in patients treated for seizure disorders with clonazepam
- Use of clonazepam with valproate may cause absence status
- Clonazepam decreases the levels of carbamazepine. Clonazepam may affect levels of phenytoin. Clonazepam increases the levels of primidone and phenobarbital
- Azole antifungals, such as ketoconazole, may inhibit the metabolism of clonazepam

 ## Other Warnings/Precautions

- Warning regarding the increased risk of CNS-depressant effects (especially alcohol) when benzodiazepines and opioid medications are used together, including specifically the risk of slowed or difficulty breathing and death
- If alternatives to the combined use of benzodiazepines and opioids are not available, clinicians should limit the dosage and duration of each drug to the minimum possible while still achieving therapeutic efficacy
- Patients and their caregivers should be warned to seek medical attention if unusual dizziness, light-headedness, sedation, slowed or difficulty breathing, or unresponsiveness occur
- Dosage changes should be made in collaboration with prescriber
- History of drug or alcohol abuse often creates greater risk for dependency
- Some depressed patients may experience a worsening of suicidal ideation
- Some patients may exhibit abnormal thinking or behavioural changes similar to those caused by other CNS depressants (i.e. either depressant actions or disinhibiting actions)
- Avoid prolonged use and abrupt cessation
- Use lower doses in debilitated patients and the elderly
- Use with caution in patients with myasthenia gravis; respiratory disease
- Use with caution in patients with personality disorder (dependent/avoidant or anankastic types) as may increase risk of dependence
- Use with caution in patients with a history of alcohol or drug dependence/abuse
- Benzodiazepines may cause a range of paradoxical effects including aggression, antisocial behaviours, anxiety, overexcitement, perceptual abnormalities and talkativeness. Adjustment of dose may reduce impulses
- Clonazepam has been confused with clobazam; care must be taken to ensure the correct drug is prescribed and dispensed
- Clonazepam should be used with caution in patients with acute porphyrias, airway obstruction, brain damage, cerebellar or spinal ataxia

Do Not Use

- If patient has acute pulmonary insufficiency, respiratory depression, significant neuromuscular respiratory weakness, sleep apnoea syndrome or unstable myasthenia gravis
- Alone in chronic psychosis in adults
- On its own to try to treat depression, anxiety associated with depression, obsessional states or phobic states
- If patient has angle-closure glaucoma
- In a comatose patient
- If patient is currently abusing alcohol or illicit drugs
- If patient has severe liver disease
- If there is a proven allergy to clonazepam or any benzodiazepine

SPECIAL POPULATIONS

Renal Impairment
- Start with small doses in severe impairment

Hepatic Impairment
- Start with smaller initial doses or reduce dose
- Can precipitate coma
- Avoid in severe impairment
- Clonazepam may aggravate hepatic porphyria

Cardiac Impairment
- Benzodiazepines have been used to treat anxiety associated with acute myocardial infarction

Elderly
- Should receive lower doses and be monitored

Children and Adolescents
- For treating all forms of epilepsy in children and adolescents see 'How to Dose' section
- Safety and efficacy not established in panic disorder
- For anxiety, children and adolescents should generally receive lower doses (0.25–0.5 mg) and be more closely monitored
- Long-term effects of clonazepam in children/adolescents are unknown

Pregnancy
- Possible increased risk of birth defects when benzodiazepines taken during pregnancy
- Because of the potential risks, clonazepam is not generally recommended as treatment for anxiety during pregnancy, especially during the first trimester
- Drug should be tapered if discontinued
- Infants whose mothers received a benzodiazepine late in pregnancy may experience withdrawal effects
- Neonatal flaccidity has been reported in infants whose mothers took a benzodiazepine during pregnancy
- Seizures, even mild seizures, may cause harm to the embryo/foetus

Breastfeeding
- Some drug is found in mother's breast milk
- Effects of benzodiazepines on infant have been observed and include feeding difficulties, sedation, and weight loss
- Caution should be taken with the use of benzodiazepines in breastfeeding mothers, seek to use low doses for short periods to reduce infant exposure
- Use of short-acting agents, e.g. oxazepam or lorazepam, preferred

THE ART OF PSYCHOPHARMACOLOGY

Potential Advantages
- Rapid onset of action
- Less sedation than some other benzodiazepines
- Longer duration of action than some other benzodiazepines
- Well tolerated as adjunctive treatment in acute mania and for akathisia

Potential Disadvantages
- Development of tolerance may require dose increases, especially in seizure disorders
- Abuse especially risky in past or present substance abusers

Primary Target Symptoms
- Frequency and duration of seizures
- Spike and wave discharges in absence seizures (petit-mal)
- Panic attacks
- Anxiety

Pearls
- *One of the most popular benzodiazepines for anxiety, especially among psychiatrists
- Is a very useful adjunct to SSRIs and SNRIs in the treatment of numerous anxiety disorders
- Not effective for treating psychosis as a monotherapy, but can be used as an adjunct to antipsychotics
- Not effective for treating bipolar disorder as a monotherapy, but can be used as an adjunct to mood stabilisers and antipsychotics
- Generally used as second-line treatment for petit-mal seizures if succinimides are ineffective

Clonazepam (Continued)

- Can be used as an adjunct or as monotherapy for seizure disorders
- Clonazepam is the only benzodiazepine that is used as a solo maintenance treatment for seizure disorders
- *Easier to taper than some other benzodiazepines because of long half-life
- *May have less abuse potential than some other benzodiazepines
- *May cause less depression, euphoria, or dependence than some other benzodiazepines
- *Clonazepam is often considered a "longer-acting alprazolam-like anxiolytic" with improved tolerability features in terms of less euphoria, abuse, dependence, and withdrawal problems, but this has not been proven
- When using to treat insomnia, remember that insomnia may be a symptom of some other primary disorder itself, and thus warrant evaluation for co-morbid psychiatric and/or medical conditions
- Though not systematically studied, benzodiazepines have been used effectively to treat catatonia and are the initial recommended treatment
- Well tolerated as adjunctive treatment in acute mania and for akathisia

 Suggested Reading

Davidson JR, Moroz G. Pivotal studies of clonazepam in panic disorder. Psychopharmacol Bull 1998;34(2):169–74.

DeVane CL, Ware MR, Lydiard RB. Pharmacokinetics, pharmacodynamics, and treatment issues of benzodiazepines: alprazolam, adinazolam, and clonazepam. Psychopharmacol Bull 1991;27(4):463–73.

Iqbal MM, Sobhan T, Ryals T. Effects of commonly used benzodiazepines on the fetus, the neonate, and the nursing infant. Psychiatr Serv 2002;53(1):39–49.

Panayiotopoulos CP. Treatment of typical absence seizures and related epileptic syndromes. Paediatr Drugs 2001;3(5):379–403.

Riss J, Cloyd J, Gates J, et al. Benzodiazepines in epilepsy: pharmacology and pharmacokinetics. Acta Neurol Scand 2008;118(2):69–86.

Wingard L, Taipale H, Reutfors J, et al. Initiation and long-term use of benzodiazepines and Z-drugs in bipolar disorder. Bipolar Disord 2018;20(7):634–46.

Clonidine hydrochloride

Brands
• Catapres

Generic?
Yes

Class
• Neuroscience-based nomenclature: pharmacology domain – norepinephrine; mode of action – agonist
• Antihypertensive; centrally acting alpha 2 agonist hypotensive agent, nonstimulant for ADHD

Commonly Prescribed for
(bold for BNF indication)
• **Hypertension**
• **Prevention of recurrent migraine**
• **Prevention of vascular headache**
• **Menopausal symptoms, especially flushing and vasomotor conditions**
• Tourette syndrome (unlicensed use)
• Sedation (unlicensed use)
• Refractory antipsychotic-induced akathisia
• Clozapine-induced hypersalivation
• Anxiety disorders, including post-traumatic stress disorder (PTSD) and social anxiety disorder
• Attention deficit hyperactivity disorder (ADHD) – third-line agent
• Tics
• Substance withdrawal, including opiates and alcohol
• Akathisia

 ## How the Drug Works
• For hypertension, acts centrally to stimulate alpha 2 adrenergic receptors in the brain-stem, reducing sympathetic outflow from the CNS and decreasing peripheral resistance, renal vascular resistance, heart rate, and systolic and diastolic blood pressure
• For migraine and menopausal symptoms; diminishes the responsiveness of peripheral vessels to constrictor and dilator stimuli, thereby preventing vascular changes associated with migraine and flushing
• For ADHD, theoretically has central actions on postsynaptic alpha 2 receptors in the prefrontal cortex
• An imidazoline, so also interacts at imidazoline receptors

How Long Until It Works
• For ADHD, can take several weeks to see maximum therapeutic benefits
• Blood pressure may be lowered 30–60 minutes after first dose; greatest reduction seen after 2–4 hours
• May take several weeks to control blood pressure adequately
• May take 2–4 weeks until clonidine is fully effective for prevention of migraine, vascular headache or menopausal symptoms

If It Works
• The goal of treatment of ADHD is reduction of symptoms of inattentiveness, motor hyperactivity, and/or impulsiveness that disrupt social, school, and/or occupational functioning
• Continue treatment until all symptoms are under control or improvement is stable and then continue treatment indefinitely as long as improvement persists
• Re-evaluate the need for treatment periodically
• Treatment for ADHD started in childhood may need to be continued into adolescence and adulthood if ongoing benefit is observed
• For hypertension, continue treatment indefinitely and check blood pressure regularly

If It Doesn't Work
• Inform patient it may take several weeks for full effects to be seen
• Consider adjusting dose or switching to another formulation or another agent. It is important to consider if maximal dose has been achieved before deciding there has not been an effect and switching
• Consider behavioural therapy or cognitive behavioural therapy if appropriate – to address issues such as social skills with peers, problem-solving, self-control, active listening and dealing with and expressing emotions
• Consider the possibility of non-concordance and counsel patients and parents
• Consider evaluation for another diagnosis or for a co-morbid condition (e.g. bipolar disorder, substance abuse, medical illness, etc.)
• In children consider other important factors, such as ongoing conflicts, family

psychopathology, adverse environment, for which alternate interventions might be more appropriate (e.g. social care referral, trauma-informed care)

＊Some ADHD patients and some depressed patients may experience lack of consistent efficacy due to activation of latent or underlying bipolar disorder, and require either augmenting with a mood stabiliser or switching to a mood stabiliser

Best Augmenting Combos for Partial Response or Treatment Resistance

- Best to attempt another monotherapy prior to augmenting for ADHD
- Possibly combination with stimulants (with caution as benefits of combination poorly documented and there are some reports of serious adverse events)
- Combinations for ADHD should be for the expert, while monitoring the patient closely, and when other treatment options have failed
- Alternative antihypertensive for hypertension

Tests

- Blood pressure should be checked regularly during treatment

SIDE EFFECTS

How Drug Causes Side Effects

- Excessive actions on alpha 2 receptors and/or on imidazoline receptors

Notable Side Effects

＊Dry mouth
＊Dizziness, constipation, sedation

Common or very common

- CNS: depression, dizziness, fatigue, headache, sedation, sleep disorders
- GIT: constipation, dry mouth, nausea, salivary gland pain, vomiting
- Other: postural hypotension, sexual dysfunction

Uncommon

- CNS/PNS: delusions, hallucination, malaise, paraesthesia

- Other: Raynaud's phenomenon, skin reactions

Rare or very rare

- CVS: atrioventricular block
- GIT: intestinal pseudo-obstruction
- Other: alopecia, dry eye, gynaecomastia, nasal dryness

Frequency not known

- Accommodation disorders of the eye, arrhythmias, confusional state

Life-Threatening or Dangerous Side Effects

- Sinus bradycardia, atrioventricular block
- During withdrawal, hypertensive encephalopathy, cerebrovascular accidents, and death (rare)
- Intestinal pseudo-obstruction
- May exacerbate psychosis or depression

Weight Gain

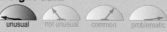

- Reported but not expected

Sedation

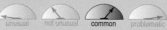

- Common or very common side effect
- Many experience and/or can be significant in amount
- Some patients may not tolerate it
- Can abate with time

What to Do About Side Effects

- Wait
- Take larger dose at bedtime to avoid daytime sedation
- Switch to another medication with better evidence of efficacy
＊For withdrawal and discontinuation reactions, may need to reinstate clonidine and taper very slowly when stabilised

Best Augmenting Agents for Side Effects

- Dose reduction or switching to another agent may be more effective since most side effects cannot be improved with an augmenting agent

DOSING AND USE

Usual Dosage Range
- ADHD/Tic: initial dose 0.5–1 mcg/kg 3 times daily, increase weekly, max 0.4 mg/day in divided doses
- Hypertension: 0.15–1.2 mg/day in divided doses
- Prevention of recurrent migraine and vascular headaches: 100 mcg–150 mcg/day in divided doses
- Menopausal symptoms: 100–150 mcg/day in divided doses
- Opioid withdrawal: 0.1 mg 3 times daily (can be higher in inpatient settings)

Dosage Forms
- Tablet 25 mcg, 100 mcg
- Oral solution 50 mcg/5 mL sugar-free solution

How to Dose
∗ Hypertension:
- Initial oral dose 50–100 mcg 3 times per day, increase dose every 2–3 days. Max dose 1.2 mg/day
∗ Prevention of recurrent migraine, vascular headache or menopausal symptoms): initial oral dose 50 mcg twice per day for 2 weeks, increased to 75 mcg twice per day as needed
∗ Clozapine-induced hypersalivation:
- oral dose 0.1 mg/day at bedtime
∗ Antipsychotic-induced akathisia:
- oral dose 0.2–0.8 mg/day
∗ ADHD:
- Start slow, go slow. Initial oral dose 0.5–1 mcg/kg 1–2 times per day. Weekly increase by 0.5–1 mcg/kg, with larger dose at bedtime (e.g. week 1: initial dose 25 mcg twice per day, week 2: 25 mcg morning, 50 mcg evening). Max dose 0.4 mg/day in divided doses
∗ Opioid withdrawal:
- Oral 0.1 mg 3 times per day; next dose should be withheld if BP falls below 90/60 mm Hg; outpatients max 3-day supply only, detoxification completed within 4–6 days for short-acting opioids

Dosing Tips
- Adverse effects are dose-related and usually transient

- The last dose of the day should occur at bedtime so that blood pressure is controlled overnight
- If clonidine is terminated abruptly, rebound hypertension may occur within 2–4 days, so taper dose in decrements of no more than 0.1 mg every 3 to 7 days when discontinuing
- Using clonidine in combination with another antihypertensive agent may attenuate the development of tolerance to clonidine's antihypertensive effects
- The likelihood of severe discontinuation reactions with CNS and cardiovascular symptoms may be greater after administration of high doses of clonidine
∗ If administered with a beta blocker, stop the beta blocker first for several days before the gradual discontinuation of clonidine in cases of planned discontinuation

Overdose
- Manifestations are due to generalised sympathetic depression
- Hypotension, hypertension, miosis, respiratory depression, seizures, bradycardia, hypothermia, coma, sedation, decreased reflexes, weakness, irritability, dysrhythmia, occasional vomiting, dry mouth
- Treatment: no specific antidote for
- clonidine overdose; activated charcoal should be administered where appropriate; supportive therapy; atropine for symptomatic bradycardia, intravenous fluids, and/or inotropic agents for hypotension; severe persistent hypertension may require correction with an alpha-adrenoreceptor- blocking drug; naloxone may be a useful adjunct for respiratory depression

Long-Term Use
- Patients may develop tolerance to the antihypertensive effects
∗ Studies have not established the utility of clonidine for long-term CNS uses
∗ Be aware that forgetting to take clonidine or running out of medication can lead to abrupt discontinuation and associated withdrawal reactions and complications

Clonidine hydrochloride (Continued)

Habit Forming
- Reports of some abuse by opiate addicts
- Reports of some abuse by non-opioid-dependent patients

How to Stop
* Discontinuation reactions are common and sometimes severe
- Sudden discontinuation can result in nervousness, agitation, headache, and tremor, with rapid rise in blood pressure
- Rare instances of hypertensive encephalopathy, cerebrovascular accident, and death have been reported after clonidine withdrawal
- Taper over 2–4 days or longer to avoid rebound effects (nervousness, increased blood pressure), especially if being used to treat hypertension
- If administered with a beta blocker, stop the beta blocker first slowly to avoid sympathetic hyperactivity before the gradual discontinuation of clonidine

Pharmacokinetics
- Dose-proportional pharmacokinetics in dose range of 75–300 mcg
- Minor first-pass effect seen
- Peak plasma concentration 1–3 hours after oral administration
- 30–40% bound to plasma proteins
- Half-life about 10–20 hours, prolonged in severe renal impairment
- Metabolised by the liver
- Main metabolite, p-hydroxy-clonidine is pharmacologically inactive
- Excreted renally, 70% excreted in urine mainly in the form of unchanged parent drug, about 20% excreted in faeces
- Crosses blood–brain barrier and placental barrier
- Antihypertensive effect reached at plasma concentrations in the range 0.2–2.0 ng/mL in patients with normal renal function. Hypotensive effect is attenuated or decreases with plasma concentrations above 2.0 ng/mL

 Drug Interactions
- The likelihood of severe discontinuation reactions with CNS and cardiovascular

symptoms may be greater when clonidine is combined with a beta blocker
- Concomitant administration of a beta-receptor blocker may cause or potentially worsen peripheral vascular disorders
- Concurrent administration of antihypertensive agents, vasodilators or diuretics may lead to increased hypotensive effect
- Increased depressive and sedative effects when taken with other CNS depressants
- Orthostatic hypotension may be provoked or aggravated by concomitant administration of tricyclic antidepressants or neuroleptics with alpha-receptor blocking action. May be necessary to adjust dosage of clonidine in patients also taking TCAs
- Corneal lesions in rats increased by use of clonidine with amitriptyline
- Use of clonidine with agents that affect sinus node function or AV nodal function (e.g. digitalis, calcium channel blockers, beta blockers) may result in bradycardia or AV block
- Medicines with alpha 2 blocking action such as mirtazapine may abolish alpha 2 receptor-mediated effects of clonidine in a dose-dependent manner
- Theoretical potentiation of the effect of tranquillisers, hypnotics and alcohol

 Other Warnings/Precautions
- There have been cases of hypertensive encephalopathy, cerebrovascular accidents, and death after abrupt discontinuation
- If used with a beta blocker, the beta blocker should be stopped several days before tapering clonidine
- Use with caution in patients with cerebrovascular disease, constipation, heart failure, history of depression, mild-moderate bradyarrhythmia, polyneuropathy, Raynaud's syndrome or other occlusive peripheral vascular disease
- Use with caution at higher than recommended doses in combination with other antihypertensive agents, as hypotensive effects may occur
- Arrhythmias have been observed in patients with pre-existing cardiac conduction abnormalities when clonidine used in high doses

Do Not Use

- If patient has severe bradyarrhythmia secondary to second- or third-degree AV block or sick sinus syndrome
- If patient has rare hereditary problems of galactose intolerance, Lapp lactase deficiency or glucose-galactose malabsorption as this medicine contains lactose
- If there is a proven allergy to clonidine

SPECIAL POPULATIONS

Renal Impairment

- Use with caution in severe impairment and possibly reduce initial dose and increase gradually
- Careful monitoring of blood pressure required

Hepatic Impairment

- Use with caution

Cardiac Impairment

- Use with caution in patients with recent myocardial infarction, severe coronary insufficiency, cerebrovascular disease

Elderly

- Elderly patients may tolerate a lower initial dose better
- Elderly patients may be more sensitive to sedative effects

Children and Adolescents

- Licensed for use for the treatment of severe hypertension for children aged 2–17
- Otherwise not licensed for use in children
- Used off-label for the treatment of ADHD or tic disorders
- Children may be more sensitive to hypertensive effects of withdrawing treatment

Before you prescribe:

- Diagnosis of ADHD should only be made by an appropriately qualified healthcare professional, e.g. specialist psychiatrist, paediatrician, and after full clinical and psychosocial assessment in different domains, full developmental and psychiatric history, observer reports across different settings and opportunity to speak to the child and carer on their own
- Children and adolescents with untreated anxiety, PTSD and mood disorders, or those who do not have a psychiatric diagnosis but social or environmental stressors, may present with anger, irritability, motor agitation, and concentration problems
- Consider undiagnosed learning disability or specific learning difficulties and sensory impairments that may potentially cause or contribute to inattention and restlessness, especially in school
- ADHD-specific advice on symptom management and environmental adaptations should be offered to all families and teachers, including reducing distractions, seating, shorter periods of focus, movement breaks and teaching assistants
- For children older than 5 years of age and young people with moderate ADHD pharmacological treatment should be considered if they continue to show significant impairment in at least one setting after symptom management and environmental adaptations have been implemented
- For severe ADHD, behavioural symptom management may not be effective until pharmacological treatment has been established

Practical notes:

ADHD

- Clonidine is a third-line treatment in children where other treatments have not been effective or who cannot tolerate stimulants or with co-morbid severely impairing tic disorder or where stimulant medication has led to sustained and impairing exacerbation of tics
- Consider a course of cognitive behavioural therapy (CBT) for young people with ADHD who have benefited from medication but whose symptoms are still causing a significant impairment in at least one domain, addressing the following areas: social skills with peers, problem-solving, self-control, active listening skills, dealing with and expressing feelings
- Medication for ADHD for a child under 5 years should only be considered on specialist advice from an ADHD service

with expertise in managing ADHD in young children (ideally a tertiary service). Use of medicines for treating ADHD is off-label in children aged less than 5 years of age
- Offer the same medication choices to people with ADHD and anxiety disorder, tic disorder or autism spectrum disorder as other people with ADHD
- Monitor behavioural response. If no change or behaviour worsens, adjust medication and/or review diagnosis, formulation and care-plan implementation

Tic disorders
- Transient tics occur in up to 20% of children. Tourette syndrome occurs in 1% of children
- Tics wax and wane over time and may be exacerbated by factors such as fatigue, inactivity, stress
- Tics are a lifelong disorder, but often get better over time. As many as 65% of young people with Tourette syndrome have only mild tics in adult life
- Co-morbid OCD, ADHD, depression, anxiety and behavioural problems should be treated first
- Most people don't require pharmacological intervention
- Psychoeducation and comprehensive behavioural interventions are recommended as first-line treatments
- It can be used as monotherapy or as adjunct

General
- Monitor patients face-to-face regularly, particularly during the first several weeks of treatment
- Children are more sensitive to side effects. Therefore: start slow and go slow with titration
- Children may be more sensitive to hypertensive effects of withdrawing treatment
- *Because children commonly have gastrointestinal illnesses that lead to vomiting, they may be more likely to abruptly discontinue clonidine and therefore be more susceptible to hypertensive episodes resulting from abrupt inability to take medication
- Children may be more likely to experience CNS depression with overdose and may even exhibit signs of toxicity with 0.1 mg of clonidine
- Sudden death in children and adolescents with serious heart problems has been reported
- Re-evaluate the need for continued treatment regularly
- Efficacy in paediatric studies for ADHD, Tourette syndrome and stuttering has not been demonstrated
- In paediatric studies, the most common side effects were drowsiness, dry mouth, headache, dizziness and insomnia

Pregnancy
- Clonidine crosses the placental barrier
- Controlled studies have not been conducted in pregnant women
- Some animal studies have shown adverse effects
- May lower foetal heart rate
- Advised to avoid oral use unless potential benefit outweighs risk
- Avoid using injection
- Use in women of childbearing potential requires weighing potential benefits to the mother against potential risks to the foetus
- *For ADHD patients, clonidine should generally be discontinued before anticipated pregnancies
- Careful monitoring of mother and child recommended
- Inadequate experience regarding long-term effects of prenatal exposure

Breastfeeding
- Significant amounts may be found in mother's breast milk
- No adverse effects have been reported in nursing infants
- Advised to avoid while breastfeeding due to presence in breast milk
- Use with caution especially in premature and newborn infants, with infant monitoring for hypotension. Consider using alternative antihypertensive
- If irritability or sedation develop in nursing infant, may need to discontinue drug or bottle feed

THE ART OF PSYCHOPHARMACOLOGY

Potential Advantages

- In children: for patients whose parents do not want them to take a stimulant or who cannot tolerate or do not respond to stimulants
- In adolescents: for patients who have a history of diverting or abusing stimulants
- Not a controlled substance

Potential Disadvantages

- Not well studied in adults with ADHD
- Withdrawal reactions
- Non-concordant patients
- Patients on concomitant CNS medications

Primary Target Symptoms

- Concentration
- Motor hyperactivity
- Oppositional and impulsive behaviour
- High blood pressure

 Pearls

In children:

- For children with co-morbid ADHD and Tourette syndrome and whose tics worsen with stimulant treatment, clonidine may improve both ADHD symptoms and tics

In adolescents:

- For adolescents with co-morbid ADHD and Tourette syndrome and whose tics worsen with stimulant treatment, clonidine may improve both ADHD symptoms and tics
- Unlike stimulants, clonidine is not a drug of abuse and has no value to friends where otherwise drug diversion of stimulants may be a problem

For all ages:

- *As monotherapy or in combination with methylphenidate for ADHD with conduct disorder or oppositional defiant disorder, may improve aggression, oppositional, and conduct disorder symptoms
- Clonidine is sometimes used in combination with stimulants to reduce side effects and enhance therapeutic effects on motor hyperactivity

- Doses of 0.1 mg in 3 divided doses have been reported to reduce stimulant-induced insomnia as well as impulsivity
- *Clonidine may also be effective for treatment of tic disorders, including Tourette syndrome
- May suppress tics especially in severe Tourette syndrome, and may be even better at reducing explosive violent behaviours in Tourette syndrome
- Sedation is often unacceptable in various patients despite improvement in CNS symptoms and leads to discontinuation of treatment, especially for ADHD and Tourette syndrome
- Considered an investigational treatment for most other CNS applications
- May block the autonomic symptoms in anxiety and panic disorders (e.g. palpitations, sweating) and improve subjective anxiety as well
- May be useful in decreasing the autonomic arousal of PTSD
- May be useful as an as-needed medication for stage fright or other predictable socially phobic situations
- May also be useful when added to SSRIs for reducing arousal and dissociative symptoms in PTSD
- May block autonomic symptoms of opioid withdrawal (e.g. palpitations, sweating) especially in inpatients, but muscle aches, irritability, and insomnia may not be well suppressed by clonidine
- May be used with naltrexone to suppress symptoms of opioid withdrawal; this requires monitoring of the patient for 8 hours on the first day due to the potential severity of naltrexone-induced withdrawal and the potential blood pressure effects of clonidine
- May be useful in decreasing the hypertension, tachycardia, and tremulousness associated with alcohol withdrawal, but not the seizures or delirium tremens in complicated alcohol withdrawal
- Clonidine may improve social relationships, affective and sensory responses in autistic disorder

Clonidine hydrochloride (Continued)

- Clonidine may reduce the incidence of menopausal flushing
- Growth hormone response to clonidine may be reduced during menses
- Clonidine stimulates growth hormone secretion (no chronic effects have been observed)
- Alcohol may reduce the effects of clonidine on growth hormone

* Guanfacine is a related centrally active alpha 2 agonist hypotensive agent that has been used for similar CNS applications
* Guanfacine may be tolerated better than clonidine in some patients (e.g. sedation) or it may work better in some patients for CNS applications than clonidine

 Suggested Reading

Besag FM, Vasey MJ, Lao KS, et al. Pharmacological treatment for Tourette syndrome in children and adults: what is the quality of the evidence? A systematic review. J Psychopharmacol 2021;35(9):1037–61.

Dunn KE, Weerts EM, Huhn AS, et al. Preliminary evidence of different and clinically meaningful opioid withdrawal phenotypes. Addict Biol 2020;25(1):e12680.

Gavras I, Manolis AJ, Gavras H. The alpha2-adrenergic receptors in hypertension and heart failure: experimental and clinical studies. J Hypertens 2001;19(12):2115–24.

Naguy A. Clonidine use in psychiatry: panacea or panache. Pharmacology 2016;98(1–2):87–92.

Schoretsanitis G, de Leon J, Eap CB, et al. Clinically significant drug-drug interactions with agents for attention-deficit/hyperactivity disorder. CNS Drugs 2019;33(12):1201–22.

Clozapine

THERAPEUTICS

Brands
- Clozaril
- Denzapine
- Zaponex

Generic?
No, not in UK

Class
- Neuroscience-based nomenclature: pharmacology domain – dopamine, serotonin, norepinephrine; mode of action – antagonist
- Atypical antipsychotic (serotonin-dopamine antagonist; second-generation antipsychotic)

Commonly Prescribed for
(bold for BNF indication)
- **Schizophrenia in patients unresponsive to, or intolerant of, conventional antipsychotic drugs**
- **Psychosis in Parkinson's disease**
- Schizoaffective disorder
- Rapid cycling bipolar disorder
- Aggression in schizophrenia
- Aggression and self-harm in emotionally unstable personality disorder
- Reduction in the risk of recurrent suicidal behaviour in schizophrenia/schizoaffective disorder

How the Drug Works
- Blocks dopamine 2 receptors, reducing positive symptoms of psychosis and stabilising affective symptoms
- Blocks serotonin 2A receptors, causing enhancement of dopamine release in certain brain regions and thus reducing motor side effects and possibly improving cognitive and affective symptoms
- Interactions at a myriad of other neurotransmitter receptors may contribute to clozapine's efficacy
- *Specifically, interactions at serotonin 2C and serotonin 1A receptors may contribute to efficacy for cognitive and affective symptoms in some patients
- Mechanism of efficacy for psychotic patients who do not respond to conventional antipsychotics is unknown

How Long Until It Works
- Likelihood of response depends on achieving trough plasma levels within a therapeutic range of 0.35–0.5 mg/L
- Median time to response after achieving therapeutic plasma levels (0.35 mg/L) is about 3 weeks
- If there is no response after 3 weeks of therapeutic plasma levels, recheck plasma levels and continue titration

If It Works
- In strictly defined refractory schizophrenia, 50–60% of patients will respond to clozapine
- The response rate to other atypical antipsychotics in the refractory patient population ranges from 0–9%
- Can improve negative symptoms, as well as aggressive, cognitive and affective symptoms in schizophrenia
- Most patients with schizophrenia do not have a total remission of symptoms but rather a reduction of symptoms by about a third
- Many patients with bipolar disorder and other disorders with psychotic, aggressive, violent, impulsive and other types of behavioural disturbances may respond to clozapine when other agents have failed
- Perhaps 5–15% of patients with schizophrenia can experience an overall improvement of greater than 50–60%, especially when receiving stable treatment for more than a year
- *Such patients are considered super-responders or "awakeners" since they may be well enough to be employed, live independently and sustain long-term relationships; super-responders are anecdotally reported more often with clozapine than with some other antipsychotics
- Treatment may not only reduce mania but also prevent recurrences of mania in bipolar disorder

If It Doesn't Work
- Obtain clozapine plasma levels and continue titration
- Levels greater than 0.7 mg/L may not be well tolerated
- No evidence to support dosing that results in plasma levels greater than 1 mg/L

- Some patients may respond better if switched to a conventional antipsychotic
- *Some patients may require augmentation with a conventional antipsychotic or with an atypical antipsychotic (e.g. amisulpride or aripiprazole)
- *Can consider augmentation with lamotrigine for negative symptoms
- Consider non-concordance and switch to another antipsychotic with fewer side effects or to an antipsychotic that can be given by depot injection
- Consider initiating rehabilitation and psychotherapy such as cognitive remediation
- Consider presence of concomitant drug abuse

 Best Augmenting Combos for Partial Response or Treatment Resistance

- Antipsychotics (for positive & negative symptoms: aripiprazole; amisulpride; for positive symptoms: risperidone; haloperidol)
- Lamotrigine potentially for negative symptoms and aggression
- Other potential augmenting agents: omega-3 fatty acids; mood stabilisers/antidepressants for affective symptoms

Tests
- A full blood count (FBC) is required before initiating clozapine
- The FBC test should include platelets, white blood cell (WBC) count and neutrophil count
- Only a green result allows for new patient initiation of clozapine:
- Green – WBC >3.5, neutrophils >2.0
- Benign ethnic neutropenia (BEN) – patients who have a low WBC because of BEN may be started on clozapine with the agreement of a haematologist

Testing for myocarditis:
- Myocarditis is rare and is most likely to occur in the first 2 months of treatment
- Baseline: consider checking troponin I/T, C-reactive protein (CRP)
- Weekly troponin I/T and CRP for the first month
- Fever is usually benign and self-limiting; suspicion of myocarditis should only be raised based on elevated troponin and other features of myocarditis

- Clozapine should be stopped if troponin ≥2x upper limits of normal or CRP >100 mg/L
- Cardiomyopathy is a late complication; consider annual ECG

Before starting an atypical antipsychotic
- *Measure weight, BMI, and waist circumference
- Get baseline personal and family history of diabetes, obesity, dyslipidaemia, hypertension, and cardiovascular disease
- *Check pulse and blood pressure, fasting plasma glucose or glycosylated haemoglobin (HbA1c), fasting lipid profile, and prolactin levels
- Full blood count (FBC), urea and electrolytes (including creatinine and eGFR), liver function tests (LFTs)
- Assessment of nutritional status, diet, and level of physical activity
- Determine if the patient:
  - is overweight (BMI 25.0–29.9)
  - is obese (BMI ≥30)
  - has pre-diabetes – fasting plasma glucose: 5.5 mmol/L to 6.9 mmol/L or HbA1c: 42 to 47 mmol/mol (6.0 to 6.4%)
  - has diabetes – fasting plasma glucose: >7.0 mmol/L or HbA1c: ≥48 mmol/L (≥6.5%)
  - has hypertension (BP >140/90 mm Hg)
  - has dyslipidaemia (increased total cholesterol, LDL cholesterol, and triglycerides; decreased HDL cholesterol)
- Treat or refer such patients for treatment, including nutrition and weight management, physical activity counselling, smoking cessation, and medical management
- Baseline ECG for: inpatients; those with a personal history or risk factor for cardiac disease

Children and adolescents:
- As for adults
- Also check history of congenital heart problems, history of dizziness when stressed or on exertion, history of long-QT syndrome, family history of long-QT syndrome, bradycardia, myocarditis, family history of cardiac myopathies, low K/low Mg/low Ca++
- Measure weight, BMI, and waist circumference plotted on a growth chart
- Pulse, BP plotted on a percentile chart
- ECG. Note for QTc interval: machine-generated may be incorrect in children as different formula needed if HR <60 or >100

Monitoring after starting an atypical antipsychotic

∗ Weight/BMI/waist circumference, weekly for the first 6 weeks, then at 12 weeks, at 1 year, and then annually
∗ Pulse and blood pressure at 12 weeks, 1 year, and then annually
∗ Fasting blood glucose, HbA1c, and blood lipids at 12 weeks, at 1 year, and then annually
∗ For patients with type 2 diabetes, measure HbA1c at 3–6 month intervals until stable, then every 6 months
∗ Even in patients without known diabetes, be vigilant for the rare but life-threatening onset of diabetic ketoacidosis, which always requires immediate treatment, by monitoring for the rapid onset of polyuria, polydipsia, weight loss, nausea, vomiting, dehydration, rapid respiration, weakness and clouding of sensorium, even coma
• If HbA1c remains ≥48 mmol/mol (6.5%) then drug therapy should be offered, e.g. metformin
• A strategy to ameliorate weight gain may include the addition of aripiprazole

Children and adolescents:
• As for adults but:
• Weight/BMI/waist circumference, weekly for the first 6 weeks, then at 12 weeks, and then every 6 months, plotted on a growth/percentile chart
• Height every 6 months, plotted on a growth chart
• Pulse and blood pressure at 12 weeks, then every 6 months plotted on a percentile chart
• ECG prior to starting and after 2 weeks after dose increase for monitoring of QTc interval. Machine-generated may be incorrect in children as different formula needed if HR <60 or >100
• Prolactin monitoring: clozapine tends not to increase prolactin above normal levels

SIDE EFFECTS

How Drug Causes Side Effects
• By blocking alpha 1 adrenergic receptors, it can cause orthostatic hypotension, tachycardia, dizziness, and sedation
• By blocking muscarinic M1 receptors, it can cause sialorrhoea, constipation, sometimes with paralytic ileus, and sedation
• By blocking histamine H1 receptors in the brain, it can cause sedation and possibly weight gain
• Mechanism of weight gain and increased risk of diabetes and dyslipidaemia with atypical antipsychotics is unknown but insulin regulation may be impaired by blocking pancreatic muscarinic M3 receptors
• By blocking dopamine 2 receptors in the striatum, it can cause motor side effects (very rare)

Notable Side Effects
• Orthostasis
• Sialorrhoea
• Constipation
• Sedation
• Tachycardia
• Weight gain
• Dyslipidaemia and hyperglycaemia
• Benign fever (about 20%)
• Rare tardive dyskinesia (note – no reports have directly implicated clozapine in the development of tardive dyskinesia)

Common or very common
• CNS: blurred vision, headache, speech impairment, visual disturbances
• CVS: hypertension, syncope
• GIT: decreased appetite, nausea, oral disorders
• Urinary disorders
• Other: abnormal sweating, eosinophilia, fever, leucocytosis, temperature dysregulation

Uncommon
• Falls

Rare or very rare
• CNS: delirium, obsessive-compulsive disorder, restlessness, sleep apnoea
• CVS: cardiac arrest, cardiac inflammation, cardiomyopathy, circulatory collapse, pericardial effusion
• Endocrine and metabolic: diabetes mellitus, dyslipidaemia, impaired glucose tolerance, ketoacidosis
• GIT: gastrointestinal disorders, hepatic disorders, intestinal obstruction (including fatal cases), pancreatitis
• Resp: respiratory disorders
• Urinary: nephritis (tubulointerstitial)
• Other: anaemia, increased risk of infection, sexual dysfunction, skin reactions, thrombocytopenia, thrombocytosis

Frequency not known
• CVS: angina pectoris, chest pain, mitral valve incompetence, myocardial infarction, palpitations

- GIT: diarrhoea, gastrointestinal discomfort
- Urinary: renal failure
- Other: angioedema, cholinergic syndrome, hypersensitivity vasculitis, muscle complaints, muscle weakness, nasal congestion, polyserositis, pseudophaeochromocytoma, rhabdomyolysis, sepsis, systemic lupus erythematosus (SLE)

Life-Threatening or Dangerous Side Effects

- Agranulocytosis (1% of patients taking clozapine)
- Severe neutropenia
- Myocarditis (first 2 months of treatment)
- Paralytic ileus or clozapine-induced gastrointestinal hypomobility
- Seizures (risk increases with dose above 600 mg/day or levels above 1.0 mg/L)
- Hyperglycaemia, in some cases extreme and associated with ketoacidosis or hyperosmolar coma or death, has been reported in patients taking atypical antipsychotics
- Pulmonary embolism (may include deep vein thrombosis or respiratory symptoms)
- Dilated cardiomyopathy
- Increased risk of death and cerebrovascular events in elderly patients with dementia-related psychosis
- Neuroleptic malignant syndrome (more likely when clozapine is used with another agent)

Weight Gain

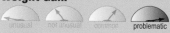

- Frequent and can be significant in amount
- May increase risk for aspiration events
- Should be managed aggressively
- More than for some other antipsychotics, but never say always as not a problem in everyone

Sedation

- Frequent and can be significant in amount
- Some patients may not tolerate it
- More than for some other antipsychotics, but never say always as not a problem in everyone
- Can wear off over time

- Can re-emerge as dose increases and then wear off again over time

What To Do About Side Effects

- Slow titration to minimise orthostasis and sedation
- Minimise use of other alpha 1 antagonists
- Take at bedtime to help reduce daytime sedation

Sialorrhoea management:
- Limited evidenced but often used clinical remedy is hyoscine hydrobromide (Kwells) 300 mcg tablets sucked or chewed up to 3 times per day or administer in the form of a patch
- Avoid use of systemic anticholinergic agents, which increase the risk of ileus (procyclidine, glycopyrronium, etc.)

Constipation management:
- Avoid bulk-forming laxatives such as ispaghula as they may worsen symptoms
- If needed, add both a stimulant (senna) and stool-softening laxative (docusate)
- Alternative and second-line agents include regular lactulose or Movicol

Weight gain and metabolic effects:
- All patients should be referred for lifestyle management and exercise; if not responding despite these measures:
- Consider adjunctive aripiprazole
- Or consider adjunctive metformin; check renal function and Vit B12 levels first; start at 500 mg for 1 week, then increase dose; may need to continue for a few months

Tachycardia:
- Limited evidence, but sometimes used is the addition of beta blocker (e.g. bisoprolol) to keep resting HR <100 bpm

Chest pain during the first 2 months:
- Obtain workup for myocarditis

Fever:
- In the absence of elevated troponin and myocarditis symptoms, fever is usually self-limited and there is no need to stop clozapine

Seizures:
- Valproate for myoclonic or generalised seizures
- Avoid phenytoin and carbamazepine because of kinetic interactions

Best Augmenting Agents for Side Effects

- Many side effects cannot be improved with an augmenting agent

DOSING AND USE

Usual Dosage Range
- Depends on plasma levels; threshold for response is trough plasma level of 0.35 mg/L; therapeutic reference range (0.35–0.50 mg/L)

Dosage Forms
- Tablet 25 mg, 50 mg, 100 mg, 200 mg
- Orodispersible tablet 12.5 mg, 25 mg, 50 mg, 100 mg, 200 mg
- Oral suspension 50 mg/mL

How to Dose
- 12.5 mg once or twice on the first day followed by 25 mg once or twice on the second day; increase by 25–50 mg/day, dose to be increased over 14–21 days. Increase to 300 mg daily in divided doses, larger dose to be given at night
- Obtain trough plasma level one week after target dose reached
- Threshold for response is 0.35 mg/L
- Levels greater than 0.7 mg/L are often not well tolerated
- No evidence to support dosing that results in plasma levels greater than 1.0 mg/L
- Doses greater than 200 mg per day may require a split dose
- The target dose will vary depending on sex and smoking status
- Please also refer to your local clozapine titration protocol
- See also The Art of Switching, after Pearls

 Dosing Tips
- Because of the monitoring schedule, prescriptions are generally given 1 week at a time for the first 18 weeks, then every 2 weeks for 18–52 weeks, and then every 4 weeks thereafter
- Plasma half-life suggests twice-daily administration, but in practice it may be given once at night
- Prior to initiating treatment with clozapine, the patient and prescriber must be registered with a manufacturer monitoring service; a Green result for a baseline WBC and neutrophil count is essential
- If treatment is discontinued for more than 2 days, reinitiate with 12.5 mg once or twice daily; if that dose is tolerated, the dose may be increased to the previously therapeutic dose more quickly than recommended for initial treatment

- Treatment breaks of over 72–96 hours will affect FBC monitoring schedules depending on which manufacturer monitoring service is being used (check with hospital pharmacy/clozapine clinic)
- If abrupt discontinuation of clozapine is necessary, the patient must be covered for cholinergic rebound; those with higher clozapine plasma levels may need extremely high doses of anticholinergic medications to prevent delirium and other rebound symptoms
- Slow off-titration is preferred if possible to avoid cholinergic rebound and rebound psychosis

Overdose
- Sometimes lethal; changes in heart rhythm, excess salivation, respiratory depression, altered state of consciousness

Long-Term Use
- Treatment to reduce risk of suicidal behaviour should be continued for at least 2 years
- Medication of choice for treatment-refractory schizophrenia

Habit Forming
- No

How to Stop
- See The Art of Switching section of individual agents for how to stop clozapine, generally over at least 4 weeks
- See Tables for guidance on stopping due to neutropenia
- *Rapid discontinuation may lead to rebound psychosis and worsening of symptoms

Pharmacokinetics
- Mean half-life about 12 hours (range 6–26 hours)
- Metabolised primarily by CYP450 1A2 and to a lesser extent by CYP450 2D6 and 3A4

 Drug Interactions
- Use clozapine plasma levels to guide treatment due to propensity for drug interactions
- In presence of a strong CYP450 1A2 inhibitor (e.g. fluvoxamine, ciprofloxacin): use 1/3 the dose of clozapine

- In the presence of a strong CYP450 1A2 inducer (e.g. cigarette smoke), clozapine plasma levels are decreased
- May need to decrease clozapine dose by up to 50% during periods of extended smoking cessation (>1 week)
- Strong CYP450 2D6 inhibitors (e.g. bupropion, duloxetine, paroxetine, fluoxetine) can raise clozapine levels; dose adjustment may be necessary
- Strong CYP450 3A4 inhibitors (e.g. ketoconazole) can raise clozapine levels; dose adjustment may be necessary
- Clozapine may enhance effects of antihypertensive drugs

 ## Other Warnings/Precautions

- All antipsychotics should be used with caution in patients with angle-closure glaucoma, blood disorders, cardiovascular disease, depression, diabetes, epilepsy and susceptibility to seizures, history of jaundice, myasthenia gravis, Parkinson's disease, photosensitivity, prostatic hypertrophy, severe respiratory disorders
- Use with caution in patients on other anticholinergic agents (procyclidine, benztropine, trihexyphenidyl, olanzapine, quetiapine, chlorpromazine, oxybutynin, and other antimuscarinics) – can worsen constipation or intestinal obstruction
- Should not be used in conjunction with agents that are known to cause neutropenia
- Myocarditis is rare but can occur in the first 2 months of treatment
- Cardiomyopathy is a late complication (consider annual ECG)
- Use with caution in patients with glaucoma

Do Not Use

- In alcoholic or toxic psychoses
- In bone-marrow disorders or patients with a history of neutropenia or agranulocytosis
- In coma or severe CNS depression
- In drug intoxication
- In patients with uncontrolled epilepsy
- In patients with a history of severe cardiac disorders (e.g. myocarditis) or circulatory collapse
- In patients with paralytic ileus
- If there is a proven allergy to clozapine

Alert ranges and monitoring for general population

Alert Colour	RED	AMBER	GREEN
Blood results	WBC <3.0 x 10^9/L or Neutrophils <1.5 x 10^9/L or Platelets <50 x 10^9/L	WBC 3.0 – <3.5 x 10^9/L or Neutrophils 1.5 – <2.0 x 10^9/L	WBC ≥ 3.5 x 10^9/L and Neutrophils ≥ 2.0 x 10^9/L and Platelets ≥ 50 x 10^9/L
Recommendation and monitoring	Immediately stop clozapine treatment, sample blood daily until haematological abnormality is resolved, monitor for infection. Do not re-expose the patient	Continue clozapine treatment, sample blood twice weekly until counts stabilise or increase	Continue clozapine treatment
The WBC and neutrophil parameters will be reduced by 0.5 x 10^9/L for patients who have been diagnosed by a consultant haematologist			

Renal Impairment
- Should be used with caution
- Avoid in severe impairment

Hepatic Impairment
- Should be used with caution

Cardiac Impairment
- Should be used with caution, particularly if patient is taking concomitant antihypertensive or alpha 1 antagonist

Elderly
- Some patients may tolerate lower doses better
- Although atypical antipsychotics are commonly used for behavioural disturbances in dementia, no agent has been approved for treatment of elderly patients with dementia-related psychosis
- Elderly patients with dementia-related psychosis treated with atypical antipsychotics are at an increased risk of death compared to placebo, and also have an increased risk of cerebrovascular events

 Children and Adolescents
- The algorithm for treatment-resistant schizophrenia is the same as for adults
- Safety and efficacy have not been established
- Preliminary research has suggested efficacy in early-onset treatment-resistant schizophrenia
- Children and adolescents taking clozapine should be monitored more often than adults

Before you prescribe:
- Do not offer antipsychotic medication when transient or attenuated psychotic symptoms or other mental state changes associated with distress, impairment, or help-seeking behaviour are not sufficient for a diagnosis of psychosis or schizophrenia. Consider individual CBT with or without family therapy and other treatments recommended for anxiety, depression, substance use, or emerging personality disorder
- For first-episode psychosis (FEP) antipsychotic medication should only be started by a specialist following a comprehensive multidisciplinary assessment and in conjunction with recommended psychological interventions (CBT, family therapy)

- As first-line treatment: allow patient to choose from aripiprazole, olanzapine or risperidone. As second-line treatment switch to alternative from list. Consider quetiapine depending on desired profile. Olanzapine should be tried before moving to clozapine. Clozapine is reserved for treatment-resistant schizophrenia
- Choice of antipsychotic medication should be an informed choice depending on individual factors and side-effect profile (metabolic, cardiovascular, extrapyramidal, hormonal, other)
- In all children and young people psychosis should be supported with sleep management, anxiety management, exercise and activation schedules, and healthy diet
- Where a child or young person presents with self-harm and suicidal thoughts the immediate risk management may take first priority
- A risk management plan is important prior to start of medication because of the possible increase in suicidal ideation and behaviours in adolescents and young adults

Practical notes:
- Carefully weigh the risks and benefits of pharmacological treatment against the risks and benefits of non-treatment and make sure to document this in the patient's chart
- Monitor weight, weekly for the first 6 weeks, then at 12 weeks, and then every 6 months (plotted on a growth chart)
- Monitor height every 6 months (plotted on a growth chart)
- Monitor waist circumference every 6 months (plotted on a percentile chart)
- Monitor pulse and blood pressure (plotted on a percentile chart) at 12 weeks and then every 6 months
- Monitor fasting blood glucose, HbA1c, blood lipid and prolactin levels at 12 weeks and then every 6 months
- Monitor for activation of suicidal ideation at the beginning of treatment. Inform parents or guardians of this risk so they can help observe child or adolescent patients
- If it does not work: review child's/young person's profile, consider new/changing contributing individual or systemic factors such as peer or family conflict. Consider drug/substance misuse. Consider dose adjustment before switching or augmentation. Be vigilant of polypharmacy especially in complex and highly vulnerable children/adolescents

Clozapine (Continued)

- Consider non-concordance by parent or child, consider non-concordance in adolescents, address underlying reasons for non-concordance
- Children are more sensitive to most side effects
  - There is an inverse relationship between age and incidence of EPS
  - Exposure to antipsychotics during childhood and young age is associated with a three-fold increase of diabetes mellitus
  - Treatment with all SGAs has been associated with changes in most lipid parameters
  - Weight gain correlates with time on treatment. Any childhood obesity is associated with obesity in adults
- May tolerate lower doses better
- Dose adjustments may be necessary in the presence of interacting drugs
- Re-evaluate the need for continued treatment regularly

Pregnancy

- Controlled studies have not been conducted in pregnant women
- There is a risk of abnormal muscle movements and withdrawal symptoms in newborns whose mothers took an antipsychotic during the third trimester; symptoms may include agitation, abnormally increased or decreased muscle tone, tremor, sleepiness, severe difficulty breathing, and difficulty feeding
- Animal studies have not shown adverse effects
- Psychotic symptoms may worsen during pregnancy and some form of treatment may be necessary
- Use in pregnancy may be justified if the benefit of continued treatment exceeds any associated risk
- Clozapine has been associated with maternal hyperglycaemia which may lead to developmental toxicity; blood glucose levels should be monitored

Breastfeeding

- Limited data suggest that clozapine may accumulate in breast milk
- Agranulocytosis and delayed speech reported in breastfed infants

- An antipsychotic that is less sedating and has a short half-life is preferred for use during breastfeeding
- Haloperidol is the preferred choice first-generation antipsychotic, and quetiapine is the preferred choice second-generation antipsychotic
- Infants of women who choose to breastfeed while on clozapine should be monitored for possible adverse effects

THE ART OF PSYCHOPHARMACOLOGY

Potential Advantages

* Treatment-resistant schizophrenia
* Violent, aggressive patients
* Patients with tardive dyskinesia
* Patients with suicidal behaviour

Potential Disadvantages

* Patients with diabetes, obesity, and/or dyslipidaemia
- Sialorrhoea, sedation, and orthostasis may be intolerable for some

Primary Target Symptoms

- Positive symptoms of psychosis
- Negative symptoms of psychosis
- Cognitive symptoms
- Affective symptoms
- Suicidal behaviour
- Violence and aggression

Pearls

* Clozapine is the gold standard treatment for refractory schizophrenia
* Clozapine is not used first-line due to side effects and monitoring burden
* However, some studies have shown that clozapine was associated with the lowest risk of mortality among the antipsychotics, causing the study authors to question if its use should continue to be restricted to resistant cases
- May reduce violence and aggression in difficult cases, including forensic cases
* Can reduce suicide in schizophrenia
- May reduce substance abuse
- May improve tardive dyskinesia
- Little or no prolactin elevation, motor side effects, or tardive dyskinesia
- Clinical improvements often continue slowly over years

- Cigarette smoke can decrease clozapine levels and patients may be at risk for relapse if they begin or increase smoking
- More weight gain than many other antipsychotics – does not mean every patient gains weight
- Patients can have much better responses to clozapine than to any other agent, but not always
- For treatment-resistant patients, especially those with impulsivity, aggression, violence, and self-harm, long-term polypharmacy with 2 atypical antipsychotics or with 1 atypical antipsychotic and 1 conventional antipsychotic may be useful or even necessary while closely monitoring
- In such cases, it may be beneficial to combine 1 depot antipsychotic with 1 oral antipsychotic
- To treat constipation and reduce risk of paralytic ileus and bowel obstruction, taper off other anticholinergic agents and consider laxatives
- Concordance with treatment and monitoring requirements may be greatly improved once response to treatment achieved

THE ART OF SWITCHING

 **Switching from Oral Antipsychotics to Clozapine**

- Clozapine should be gradually titrated (see How to Dose), ideally this should be done after other antipsychotics are withdrawn although in practice the previous antipsychotic is often cross-titrated
- Care should be taken when switching depot antipsychotics and atypical long-acting injections due to their long half-lives and the increased risk of agranulocytosis
* Benzodiazepine medication can be administered during cross-titration to help alleviate side effects such as insomnia, agitation, and/or psychosis. However, use with caution in combination with clozapine as this can increase the risk of circulatory collapse.

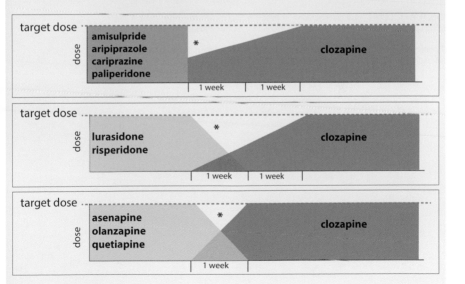

Suggested Reading

Cooper SJ, Reynolds GP, Barnes T, et al. BAP guidelines on the management of weight gain, metabolic disturbances and cardiovascular risk associated with psychosis and antipsychotic drug treatment. J Psychopharmacol 2016;30(8):717–48.

Huhn M, Nikolakopoulou A, Schneider-Thoma J, et al. Comparative efficacy and tolerability of 32 oral antipsychotics for the acute treatment of adults with multi-episode schizophrenia: a systematic review and network meta-analysis. Lancet 2019;394(10202):939–51.

Lally J, Docherty MJ, MacCabe JH. Pharmacological interventions for clozapine-induced sinus tachycardia. Cochrane Database Syst Rev 2016;(6):CD011566.

Masuda T, Misawa F, Takase M, et al. Association with hospitalization and all-cause discontinuation among patients with schizophrenia on clozapine vs other oral second-generation antipsychotics: a systematic review and meta-analysis of cohort studies. JAMA Psychiatry 2019;76(10):1052–62.

Pillinger T, McCutcheon RA, Vano L, et al. Comparative effects of 18 antipsychotics on metabolic function in patients with schizophrenia, predictors of metabolic dysregulation, and association with psychopathology: a systematic review and network meta-analysis. Lancet Psychiatry 2020;7(1):64–77.

Rajagopal S. Clozapine, agranulocytosis, and benign ethnic neutropenia. Postgrad Med J 2005;81(959):545–6.

Ronaldson KJ, Fitzgerald PD, McNeil JJ. Clozapine-induced myocarditis, a widely overlooked adverse reaction. Acta Psychiatr Scand 2015;132:231–40.

Rosenheck RA, Davis S, Covell N, et al. Does switching to a new antipsychotic improve outcomes? Data from the CATIE Trial. Schizophr Res 2009;170(1):22–9.

Schulte P. What is an adequate trial with clozapine?: therapeutic drug monitoring and time to response in treatment-refractory schizophrenia. Clin Pharmacokinet 2003;42:607–18.

Syed R, Au K, Cahill C, et al. Interventions for people with schizophrenia who have too much saliva due to clozapine treatment. Cochrane Database Syst Rev 2008;(3):CD005579.

Tiihonen J, Lonnqvist J, Wahlbeck K, et al. 11-year follow-up of mortality in patients with schizophrenia: a population-based cohort study (FIN11 study). Lancet 2009;374(9690):620–7.

Dexamfetamine sulfate

Brands
- Amfexa
- Dexedrine (imported from USA)

Generic?
Yes

Class
- Neuroscience-based nomenclature: pharmacology domain – dopamine, norepinephrine; mode of action – multimodal
- Stimulant; dopamine and noradrenaline reuptake inhibitor and releaser (DN-RIRe)

Commonly Prescribed for
- **Narcolepsy**
- **Refractory attention deficit hyperactivity disorder (initiated under specialist supervision – licensed for children aged 6 years and older; unlicensed in adults)**
- Exogenous obesity
- Treatment-resistant depression

How the Drug Works
* Increases noradrenaline and especially dopamine actions by blocking their reuptake and facilitating their release
- Enhancement of dopamine and noradrenaline actions in certain brain regions may improve attention, concentration, executive function and wakefulness (e.g. dorsolateral prefrontal cortex)
- Enhancement of dopamine actions in other brain regions (e.g. basal ganglia) may improve hyperactivity
- Enhancement of dopamine and noradrenaline in yet other brain regions (e.g. medial prefrontal cortex, hypothalamus) may improve depression, fatigue, and sleepiness

How Long Until It Works
- Some immediate effects can be seen with first dosing
- Can take several weeks to attain maximum therapeutic benefit

If It Works
- The goal of treatment of ADHD is reduction of symptoms of inattentiveness, motor hyperactivity, and/or impulsiveness that disrupt social, school, and/or occupational functioning
- Continue treatment until all symptoms are under control or improvement is stable and then continue treatment indefinitely as long as improvement persists
- Re-evaluate the need for treatment periodically
- Treatment for ADHD begun in childhood may need to be continued into adolescence and adulthood if continued benefit is documented
- For narcolepsy: used to promote wakefulness and so reduce excessive daytime sleepiness

If It Doesn't Work
ADHD:
- Inform patient it may take several weeks for full effects to be seen
- Consider adjusting dose or switching to another formulation or another agent. It is important to consider if maximal dose has been achieved before deciding there has not been an effect and switching
- Consider behavioural therapy or cognitive behavioural therapy if appropriate – to address issues such as social skills with peers, problem-solving, self-control, active listening and dealing with and expressing emotions
- Consider the possibility of non-concordance and counsel patients and parents
- Consider evaluation for another diagnosis or for a co-morbid condition (e.g. bipolar disorder, substance abuse, medical illness, etc.)
- In children consider other important factors, such as ongoing conflicts, family psychopathology, adverse environment, for which alternate interventions might be more appropriate (e.g. social care referral, trauma-informed care)
* Some ADHD patients and some depressed patients may experience lack of consistent efficacy due to activation of latent or underlying bipolar disorder, and require

either augmenting with a mood stabiliser or switching to a mood stabiliser

Narcolepsy:

- Ensure good sleep hygiene has been implemented and counselling or support has been sought
- Consider switching to an alternative stimulant such as modafinil or methylphenidate, sodium oxybate, pitolisant or antidepressants such as selective serotonin reuptake inhibitors (SSRIs), serotonin–noradrenaline reuptake inhibitors (SNRIs) or tricyclic antidepressants

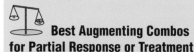

Best Augmenting Combos for Partial Response or Treatment Resistance

∗ Best to attempt other monotherapies prior to augmenting
- For the expert can combine immediate-release formulation with modified-release formulation of dexamfetamine for ADHD
- For the expert, can combine with modafinil or atomoxetine for ADHD, though there is little evidence about the efficacy or safety of this combination
- For the expert, can occasionally combine with atypical antipsychotics in highly treatment-resistant cases of ADHD

Tests

- Before treatment, assess for presence of cardiac disease (history, family history, physical exam)
- Pulse, BP, appetite, weight, height, psychiatric symptoms should be recorded at start of therapy, following every dose change and at every 6 months after that
- In children, pulse, BP, height and weight should be recorded on percentile charts; observe growth trajectory by plotting a graph
- In children, height and weight should be recorded before start of treatment, and height, weight and appetite monitored at least every 6 months during treatment
- Monitor for aggressive behaviour or hostility during initial treatment

SIDE EFFECTS

How Drug Causes Side Effects

- Increases in norepinephrine peripherally can cause autonomic side effects, including tremor, tachycardia, hypertension, and cardiac arrhythmias
- Increases in norepinephrine and dopamine centrally can cause CNS side effects such as insomnia, agitation, psychosis and substance abuse

Notable Side Effects

∗ Insomnia, headache, exacerbation of tics, nervousness, irritability, overstimulation, tremor, dizziness
∗ Anorexia, nausea, dry mouth, constipation, diarrhoea, weight loss
- Can temporarily slow normal growth in children (controversial)
- Sexual dysfunction long-term (impotence, libido changes), but can also improve sexual dysfunction short-term

Common or very common

∗ CNS/PNS: abnormal behaviour, altered mood, anxiety, depression, headache, movement disorders, sleep disorders, vertigo
∗ GIT: abdominal pain, decreased appetite, decreased weight, diarrhoea, dry mouth, nausea, poor weight gain, vomiting
∗ Other: arrhythmias, muscle cramps, palpitations

Rare or very rare

- Blood disorders: anaemia, leucopenia, thrombocytopenia
- CNS/PNS: cerebral vasculitis, cerebrovascular insufficiency, hallucination, intracranial haemorrhage, psychosis, seizure, suicidal behaviours, tic (in those at risk), vision disorders
- CVS: angina pectoris, cardiac arrest
- GIT: abnormal hepatic function, hepatic coma
- Other: fatigue, growth retardation, mydriasis, skin reactions

Frequency not known

- CNS/PNS: impaired concentration, confusion, dizziness, drug dependence, increased reflexes, obsessive-compulsive disorder, tremor
- CVS: cardiomyopathy, chest pain, circulatory collapse, myocardial infarction

- GIT: altered taste, diarrhoea, ischaemic colitis
- Other: acidosis, alopecia, hyperhidrosis, hypermetabolism, hyperpyrexia, kidney injury, neuroleptic malignant syndrome, rhabdomyolysis, sexual dysfunction, sudden death

 Life-Threatening or Dangerous Side Effects

- Psychotic episodes
- Seizures
- Palpitations, tachycardia, hypertension
- Rare activation of hypomania, mania, or suicidal ideation (controversial)
- Cardiovascular adverse effects, sudden death in patients with pre-existing cardiac abnormalities or long-QT syndrome

Weight Gain

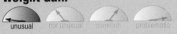
unusual | not unusual | common | problematic

- Reported but not expected
- Some patients may experience weight loss

Sedation

unusual | not unusual | common | problematic

- Reported but not expected
- Activation much more common than sedation

What To Do About Side Effects

- Wait
- Can usually be managed by symptomatic management and/or dose reduction
- If lack of appetite and weight is a clinical concern suggest taking medication with or after food and offer high calorie food or snacks early morning or late evening when stimulant effects have worn off
- If child or young person on ADHD medication shows persistent resting heart rate >120 bpm, arrhythmia, or systolic BP (measured on 2 occasions) with clinically significant increase or >95th percentile, then reduce medication dose and refer to specialist physician
- If a person taking stimulants develops tics, consider: are the tics related to the stimulant (tics naturally wax and wane)? Observe tic evolution over 3 months. Consider if the impairment associated with the tics outweighs the benefits of ADHD treatment
- If tics are stimulant related, reduce the stimulant dose, or consider changing to guanfacine (in children aged 5 years and over and young people only), atomoxetine, clonidine or stopping medication
- If a person with ADHD presents with seizures (new or worsening), review and stop any ADHD medication that could reduce the seizure threshold. Cautiously reintroduce the ADHD medication after completing necessary tests and confirming it as non-contributory towards the cause of the seizures
- If sleep becomes a problem: assess sleep at baseline. Monitor changes in sleep pattern (for example, with a sleep diary). Adjust medication accordingly. Advise on sleep hygiene as appropriate. Prescription of melatonin may be helpful to promote sleep onset where behavioural and environmental adjustments have not been effective
- Consider drug holidays to prevent growth retardation in children
- Switch to another agent, e.g. atomoxetine or guanfacine

Best Augmenting Agents for Side Effects

- Beta blockers for peripheral autonomic side effects
- Beta blockers or pregabalin for anxiety; do not prescribe benzodiazepines
- SSRIs or SNRIs for depression
- If psychosis develops, stop dexamfetamine and add antipsychotics such as olanzapine or quetiapine, consider a switch to atomoxetine
- Consider melatonin for insomnia in children
- Dose reduction or switching to another agent may be more effective

DOSING AND USE

Usual Dosage Range

Narcolepsy:
- Adult: 10–60 mg/day
- Elderly: 5–60 mg/day

ADHD:
- Adult: 10–60 mg/day
- Child (over age 6): 5–20 mg/day (some older children may require up to max of 40 mg/day)

Dosage Forms
- Tablet 5 mg, 10 mg, 20 mg
- Modified-release capsule (Dexedrine Spansules – imported from USA) 5 mg, 10 mg, 15 mg
- Oral solution 5 mg/5 mL (150 mL bottle)

How to Dose
*Narcolepsy (Adult):
- Initial dose 10 mg/day in divided doses, increased by increments of 10 mg every week, maintenance dose in 2–4 divided doses; max 60 mg/day

*Narcolepsy (Elderly):
- Initial dose 5 mg/day in divided doses, increased by increments of 5 mg every week, maintenance dose in 2–4 divided doses; max 60 mg/day

*Refractory ADHD (Child 6–17 years):
- Initial dose 2.5 mg 2–3 times per day, increased by increments of 5 mg every week as needed; usual maximum 1 mg/kg/day, up to 20 mg/day (40 mg/day in some children); maintenance dose in 2–4 divided doses

*Refractory ADHD (Adult):
- Initial dose 5 mg twice per day, increased at weekly intervals according to response, maintenance dose in 2–4 divided doses; max 60 mg/day

Dosing Tips
- Not licensed for use in adults for refractory ADHD
- Tablets can be halved
- Dose of a single capsule should not be divided, should not be chewed but should be swallowed whole
- Clinical duration of action often differs from pharmacokinetic half-life
- For use in children with ADHD aged 3–5 years is 2.5 mg/day, increased as needed by 2.5 mg/day at weekly intervals
- For use in children with ADHD aged 6 years and over, the usual starting dose is 5–10 mg/day increasing as needed by 5 mg/day at weekly intervals

*Immediate-release dexamfetamine has 3–6 hour duration of clinical action

*Modified-release dexamfetamine capsule (Dexedrine Spansule) has up to 8-hour duration of clinical action

- Elimination of lunchtime dosing may be possible in many patients with the use of the modified-release capsule

- Once-daily dosing can be an important practical element in stimulant use, eliminating the hassle and pragmatic difficulties of lunchtime dosing at school, including storage problems, potential diversion, and the need for a medical professional to supervise dosing away from home
- Avoid dosing after the morning because of the risk of insomnia

*May be possible to dose only during the school week for some ADHD patients

*May be able to give drug holidays for patients with ADHD over the summer in order to reassess therapeutic utility and effects on growth suppression as well as to assess any other side effects and the need to reinstitute stimulant treatment for the next school term

- Side effects are generally dose-related
- Taking with food may delay peak actions for 2–3 hours

Overdose
- Individual patient response may vary widely and toxic manifestations may occur with quite small overdoses
- Rarely fatal; hyperpyrexia, mydriasis, hyperreflexia, chest pain, tachycardia, cardiac arrhythmias, confusion, panic states, aggressive behaviour, hallucinations, delirium, convulsions, respiratory depression, coma, circulatory collapse
- Treatment consists of the induction of vomiting and/or gastric lavage together with supportive and symptomatic measures. Excessive stimulation or convulsions may be treated with diazepam
- Chlorpromazine antagonises the central stimulant effects of amfetamines and can be used to treat amfetamine intoxication

Long-Term Use
- Can be used long-term for ADHD when ongoing monitoring documents continued efficacy
- Dependence and/or abuse may develop
- Tolerance to therapeutic effects may develop in some patients
- Long-term stimulant use may be associated with growth suppression in children (controversial)
- Important to periodically monitor weight, blood pressure and psychiatric symptoms
- Cardiomyopathy has been reported with chronic amfetamine use

Habit Forming
- High abuse potential – dexamfetamine is a Schedule 2 drug
- Patients may develop tolerance and psychological dependence
- Decision to use dexamfetamine in children with ADHD must be based on a very thorough assessment of the severity and chronicity of the child's symptoms in relation to the child's age and potential for abuse, misuse or diversion

How to Stop
- Taper to avoid withdrawal effects
- Withdrawal following chronic therapeutic use may unmask symptoms of the underlying disorder and may require follow-up and reinstitution of treatment
- Careful supervision is required during withdrawal from abuse use since severe depression may occur
- Symptoms of withdrawal after heavy and prolonged use include dysphoric mood, fatigue, vivid and unpleasant dreams, insomnia or hypersomnia, increased appetite, psychomotor retardation or agitation, anhedonia and drug craving

Pharmacokinetics
- Half-life about 10–12 hours
- Dexamfetamine is readily absorbed from the gastrointestinal tract. It is resistant to metabolism by monoamine oxidase. It is excreted in the urine as unchanged parent drug together with some hydroxylated metabolites. Elimination is increased in acidic urine. After high doses, elimination in the urine may take several days

 Drug Interactions
- May affect blood pressure and should be used cautiously with agents used to control blood pressure
- Gastrointestinal acidifying agents (guanethidine, reserpine, glutamic acid, ascorbic acid, fruit juices, etc.) and urinary acidifying agents (ammonium chloride, sodium phosphate, etc.) lower amfetamine plasma levels, so such agents can be useful to administer after an overdose but may also lower therapeutic efficacy of amfetamines
- Gastrointestinal alkalinising agents (sodium bicarbonate, etc.) and urinary alkalinising agents (acetazolamide, some thiazides) increase amfetamine plasma levels and potentiate amfetamine's actions
- Theoretically, agents with noradrenaline reuptake blocking properties, such as venlafaxine, duloxetine, atomoxetine, and reboxetine, could add to amfetamine's CNS and cardiovascular effects
- Amfetamines may counteract the sedative effects of antihistamines
- Haloperidol, chlorpromazine, and lithium may inhibit stimulatory effects of amfetamine
- Theoretically, atypical antipsychotics should also inhibit stimulatory effects of amfetamines
- Theoretically, amfetamines could inhibit the antipsychotic actions of antipsychotics
- Theoretically, amfetamines could inhibit the mood-stabilising actions of atypical antipsychotics in some patients
- Combinations of amfetamines with mood stabilisers (lithium, anticonvulsants, atypical antipsychotics) are generally something for experts only, when monitoring patients closely and when other options fail
- Absorption of phenobarbital, phenytoin, and ethosuximide is delayed by amfetamines
- Amfetamines inhibit adrenergic blockers and enhance adrenergic effects of noradrenaline
- Amfetamines may antagonise hypotensive effects of Veratrum alkaloids and other antihypertensives
- Amfetamines can raise plasma corticosteroid levels
- MAOIs slow absorption of amfetamines and thus potentiate their actions, which can cause headache, hypertension, and rarely hypertensive crisis and malignant hyperthermia, sometimes with fatal results
- Use with MAOIs, including within 14 days of MAOI use, is not advised
- There is a risk of serotonin syndrome if dexamfetamine combined with serotonergic drugs, or other agents that increase the risk of serotonin syndrome (St John's wort, bupropion, linezolid, granisetron, ondansetron, opiates, SSRIs, SNRIs TCAs, MAOIs, lithium, or triptans)

 Other Warnings/Precautions
- Caution in patients with mild hypertension
- Caution if patient has or is susceptible to angle-closure glaucoma

Dexamfetamine sulfate (Continued)

- Children who are not growing or not gaining weight should stop treatment, at least temporarily
- May worsen motor and phonic tics
- Caution if patient has motor tics or Tourette syndrome or if there is a family history of Tourette syndrome, discontinue use if tics occur
- May worsen symptoms of thought disorder and behaviour disturbance in psychotic patients, special caution advised with bipolar disorder
- Stimulants have a high potential for abuse and must be used with caution in anyone with a current or past history of substance abuse or alcoholism or in emotionally unstable patients
- Administration of stimulants for prolonged periods of time should be avoided whenever possible or done only with close monitoring, as it may lead to marked tolerance and drug dependence, including psychological dependence with varying degrees of abnormal behaviour
- Particular attention should be paid to the possibility of subjects obtaining stimulants for non-therapeutic use or distribution to others and the drugs should in general be prescribed sparingly with documentation of appropriate use
- Usual dosing with amfetamine has been associated with sudden death in children with cardiac rhythm abnormalities, e.g. long QT
- Not a recommended treatment for depression or for normal fatigue
- Caution in patients with a history of epilepsy, may lower the seizure threshold (discontinue if seizures occur)
- Emergence or worsening of activation and agitation may represent the induction of a bipolar state, especially a mixed dysphoric bipolar condition sometimes associated with suicidal ideation, and requires the addition of a mood stabiliser and/or discontinuation of dexamfetamine

Do Not Use

- If patient has extreme anxiety/agitation or hyperexcitability
- Should generally not be administered with an MAOI, including within 14 days of MAOI use
- If patient has anorexia
- If patient has hyperthyroidism
- If patient has cerebrovascular disorder
- If patient has advanced arteriosclerosis, cardiomyopathies, cardiovascular disease, heart failure, life-threatening arrhythmias, moderate and severe hypertension, structural cardiac abnormalities
- If patient has history of alcohol or drug abuse
- If patient suffers from psychiatric disorders such as psychosis, schizophrenia, uncontrolled bipolar disorder, severe depression, borderline personality disorder
- If patient has suicidal tendencies
- Co-morbidity with psychiatric disorders is common in ADHD. If new psychiatric symptoms develop or exacerbation of psychiatric disorders occurs, continued use should only be if benefits outweigh risks
- If there is a proven allergy to any sympathomimetic agent

Renal Impairment

- Use with caution, no dose adjustment necessary

Hepatic Impairment

- Use with caution

Cardiac Impairment

- Caution in patients with mild hypertension
- Do not use if patient has advanced arteriosclerosis, cardiomyopathies, cardiovascular disease, heart failure, life-threatening arrhythmias, moderate and severe hypertension, structural cardiac abnormalities

Elderly

- Some patients may tolerate lower doses better; titrate doses up more slowly

 Children and Adolescents

Before you prescribe:
- Safety and efficacy not established in children under age 6
- Use in young children should be reserved for the expert
- Diagnosis of ADHD should only be made by an appropriately qualified healthcare professional, e.g. specialist psychiatrist, paediatrician, and after full clinical and psychosocial assessment in different domains, full developmental and psychiatric history, observer reports across different settings and opportunity to speak to the child and carer on their own

- Children and adolescents with untreated anxiety, PTSD and mood disorders, or those who do not have a psychiatric diagnosis but have social or environmental stressors, may present with anger, irritability, motor agitation, and concentration problems
- Consider undiagnosed learning disability or specific learning difficulties, and sensory impairments that may potentially cause or contribute to inattention and restlessness, especially in school
- ADHD-specific advice on symptom management and environmental adaptations should be offered to all families and teachers, including reducing distractions, seating, shorter periods of focus, movement breaks and teaching assistants
- For children aged 5 years and over and young people with moderate ADHD pharmacological treatment should be considered if they continue to show significant impairment in at least one setting after symptom management and environmental adaptations have been implemented
- For severe ADHD, behavioural symptom management may not be effective until pharmacological treatment has been established

Practical notes:
- Consider for refractory ADHD when other stimulants or second- and third-line options have not been effective. Single and divided dosing options are available. Single day dosing may improve adherence, reduce stigma, acceptability to schools
- Monitor patients face-to-face regularly, particularly during the first several weeks of treatment
- Monitor for activation of suicidal ideation at the beginning of treatment
- Consider cognitive behavioural therapy (CBT) for those whose ADHD symptoms are still causing significant difficulties in one or more domains, addressing emotion regulation, problem-solving, self-control, and social skills (including active listening skills and interactions with peers)
- Medication for ADHD for a child under 5 years should only be considered on specialist advice from an ADHD service with expertise in managing ADHD in young children (ideally a tertiary service). Use of medicines for treating ADHD is off-label in children aged <5

- Same medication choices should be offered to patients with co-morbidities (e.g. anxiety, tic disorders, or autism spectrum disorders) as to patients with ADHD alone
- Insomnia is common
- Dexamfetamine may worsen symptoms of behavioural disturbance and thought disorder in psychotic children
- Dexamfetamine has acute effects on growth hormone; long-term effects are unknown but weight and height should be monitored 6-monthly using a growth chart
- Do not use in children with structural cardiac abnormalities or other serious cardiac problems
- Sudden death in children and adolescents with serious heart problems has been reported
- American Heart Association recommends ECG prior to initiating stimulant treatment in children, although not all experts agree, and it is not usual practice in UK
- Re-evaluate the need for continued treatment regularly

Pregnancy

- Limited and confounded human data on use during pregnancy
- Possible increased risk of premature birth, low birth weight and neurodevelopmental delay in infants whose mothers take dexamfetamine during pregnancy
- Infants whose mothers take dexamfetamine during pregnancy may experience withdrawal symptoms
- In animal studies, dexamfetamine caused delayed skeletal ossification and decreased postweaning weight gain in rats; no major malformations occurred in rat or rabbit studies
- Use in women of childbearing potential requires weighing potential benefits to the mother against potential risks to the foetus
* For ADHD patients, dexamfetamine should generally be discontinued before anticipated pregnancies

Breastfeeding

- Small but significant amounts found in mother's breast milk
- Infants of women who choose to breastfeed while on lisdexamfetamine should be monitored for possible adverse effects
- If irritability, sleep disturbance, or poor weight gain develop in nursing infant, may need to discontinue drug or bottle feed

Dexamfetamine sulfate (Continued)

THE ART OF PSYCHOPHARMACOLOGY

Potential Advantages
- May work in ADHD patients unresponsive to other stimulants
- Established long-term efficacy of immediate-release and modified-release formulations

Potential Disadvantages
- Patients with current or past history of substance abuse
- Patients with current or past bipolar disorder or psychosis

Primary Target Symptoms
- Concentration, attention span
- Motor hyperactivity
- Impulsivity
- Physical and mental fatigue
- Daytime sleepiness
- Depression

 Pearls
- May be useful for the treatment of cognitive impairment, depressive symptoms, and severe fatigue in patients with HIV infection and in cancer patients
- Can be used to potentiate opioid analgesia and reduce sedation, particularly in end-of-life management

- Some patients respond to or tolerate dexamfetamine better than methylphenidate and vice versa
- *Some patients may benefit from an occasional addition of 5–10 mg of immediate-release dexamfetamine to their daily base of modified-release capsules
- *Can reverse sexual dysfunction caused by psychiatric illness and by some drugs such as SSRIs, including decreased libido, erectile dysfunction, delayed ejaculation, and anorgasmia
- Atypical antipsychotics may be useful in treating stimulant or psychotic consequences of overdose
- Taking food may delay peak actions for 2–3 hours, but this could also reduce the impact of side effects such as anxiety and agitation
- Half-life and duration of clinical action tend to be shorter in younger children
- Drug abuse may actually be lower in ADHD adolescents treated with stimulants than in ADHD adolescents who are not treated
- It is a popular drug on the black market and is used as an athletic performance and cognitive enhancer, and recreationally as an aphrodisiac and euphoriant
- Sometimes it is prescribed off-label for depression or obesity

Suggested Reading

Castells X, Blanco-Silvente L, Cunhill R. Amphetamines for attention deficit hyperactivity disorder (ADHD) in adults. Cochrane Database Syst Rev 2018;8(8):CD007813.

Cortese S. Pharmacologic treatment of attention deficit-hyperactivity disorder. N Engl J Med 2020;383(11):1050–6.

Cortese S, Newcorn JH, Coghill D. A practical, evidence-informed approach to managing stimulant-refractory attention deficit hyperactivity disorder (ADHD). CNS Drugs 2021;35(10):1035–51.

Greenhill LL, Swanson JM, Hechtman L. Trajectories of growth associated with long-term stimulant medication in the multimodal treatment study of attention-deficit/hyperactivity disorder. J Am Acad Child Adolesc Psychiatry 2020;59(8):978–89.

Heal DJ, Smith SL, Gosden J, et al. Amphetamine, past and present – a pharmacological and clinical perspective. J Psychopharmacol 2013;27(6):479–96.

Shindler J, Schacter M, Brincat, S et al. Amphetamine, mazindol, and fencamfamin in narcolepsy. Br Med J (Clin Res Ed) 1985;290(6476):1167–70.

Stevenson RD, Wolraich ML. Stimulant medication therapy in the treatment of children with attention deficit hyperactivity disorder. Pediatr Clin North Am 1989;36(5):1183–97.

Diazepam

THERAPEUTICS

Brands
- Diazemuls
- Stesolid

Generic?
Yes

Class
- Neuroscience-based nomenclature: pharmacology domain – GABA; mode of action – positive allosteric modulator (PAM)
- Benzodiazepine (anxiolytic, muscle relaxant, anticonvulsant)

Commonly Prescribed for
(bold for BNF indication)
- **Muscle spasm (of varied aetiology; acute muscle spasm; muscle spasm in cerebral spasticity or in postoperative skeletal muscle spasm)**
- **Tetanus**
- **Anxiety (severe acute anxiety; control of acute panic attacks; acute anxiety and agitation)**
- **Insomnia associated with anxiety**
- **Acute alcohol withdrawal**
- **Acute drug-induced dystonic reactions (including life-threatening reactions)**
- **Premedication**
- **Sedation (in dental procedures carried out in hospital; conscious sedation for procedures, and in conjunction with local anaesthesia; sedative cover for minor surgical and medical procedures)**
- **Status epilepticus, febrile convulsions, convulsions due to poisoning**
- **Dyspnoea associated with anxiety in palliative care**
- **Pain of muscle spasm in palliative care**
- Catatonia

How the Drug Works
- Binds to benzodiazepine receptors at the GABA-A ligand-gated chloride channel complex
- Enhances the inhibitory effects of GABA
- Boosts chloride conductance through GABA-regulated channels
- Inhibits neuronal activity presumably in amygdala-centred fear circuits to provide therapeutic benefits in anxiety disorders
- Inhibiting actions in cerebral cortex may provide therapeutic benefits in seizure disorders
- Inhibitory actions in spinal cord may provide therapeutic benefits for muscle spasms

How Long Until It Works
- Some immediate relief with first dosing is common; can take several weeks with daily dosing for maximal therapeutic benefit

If It Works
- For short-term symptoms of anxiety or muscle spasms – after a few weeks, discontinue use or use on an "as-needed" basis
- Chronic muscle spasms may require chronic diazepam treatment
- For chronic anxiety disorders, the goal of treatment is complete remission of symptoms as well as prevention of future relapses
- For chronic anxiety disorders, treatment most often reduces or even eliminates symptoms, but is not a cure since symptoms can recur after medicine stopped
- For long-term symptoms of anxiety, consider switching to an SSRI or SNRI for long-term maintenance
- Avoid long-term maintenance with a benzodiazepine
- If symptoms re-emerge after stopping a benzodiazepine, consider treatment with an SSRI or SNRI, or consider restarting the benzodiazepine; sometimes benzodiazepines have to be used in combination with SSRIs or SNRIs at the start of treatment for best results

If It Doesn't Work
- Consider switching to another agent or adding an appropriate augmenting agent
- Consider psychotherapy, especially cognitive behavioural psychotherapy
- Consider presence of concomitant substance abuse
- Consider presence of diazepam abuse
- Consider another diagnosis, such as a co-morbid medical condition

Diazepam (Continued)

Best Augmenting Combos for Partial Response or Treatment Resistance

- Benzodiazepines are frequently used as augmenting agents for antipsychotics and mood stabilisers in the treatment of psychotic and bipolar disorders
- Benzodiazepines are frequently used as augmenting agents for SSRIs and SNRIs in the treatment of anxiety disorders
- Not generally rational to combine with other benzodiazepines
- Caution if using as an anxiolytic concomitantly with other sedative hypnotics for sleep

Tests

- In patients with seizure disorders, concomitant medical illness, and/or those with multiple concomitant long-term medications, periodic liver tests and blood counts may be prudent

SIDE EFFECTS

How Drug Causes Side Effects

- Same mechanism for side effects as for therapeutic effects – namely due to excessive actions at benzodiazepine receptors
- Long-term adaptations in benzodiazepine receptors may explain the development of dependence, tolerance, and withdrawal
- Side effects are generally immediate, but immediate side effects often disappear in time

Notable Side Effects

* Sedation, fatigue, depression
* Dizziness, ataxia, slurred speech, weakness
* Forgetfulness, confusion
* Hyperexcitability, nervousness
* Pain at injection site
- Rare hallucinations, mania
- Rare hypotension
- Hypersalivation, dry mouth

Common or very common

- CNS/PNS: impaired concentration, movement disorders, muscle spasms, sensory disorder
- CVS: palpitations
- GIT: abnormal appetite, vomiting

Uncommon

- CNS: slurred speech
- GIT: constipation, diarrhoea, increased saliva
- Other: skin reactions (intravenous, oral or rectal use)

Rare or very rare

- CNS: loss of consciousness, memory loss, psychiatric disorder (IV or oral use)
- CVS: bradycardia, cardiac arrest, heart failure, syncope
- Resp: increased bronchial secretion, respiratory arrest
- Other: dry mouth, gynaecomastia, leucopenia, sexual dysfunction

Frequency not known

- Apnoea, nystagmus
- IM use (in adults): chest pain, embolism and thrombosis, fall, increased dementia risk, psychiatric disorders, soft tissue necrosis, urticaria

Life-Threatening or Dangerous Side Effects

- Respiratory depression, especially when taken with CNS depressants in overdose
- Rare hepatic dysfunction, renal dysfunction, blood dyscrasias

Weight Gain

unusual   not unusual   common   problematic

- Reported but not expected

Sedation

unusual   not unusual   common   problematic

- Many experience and/or can be significant in amount
- Especially at initiation of treatment or when dose increases
- Tolerance often develops over time

What to Do About Side Effects

- Wait
- Wait
- Wait
- Lower the dose
- Take largest dose at bedtime to avoid sedative effects during the day
- Switch to another agent
- Administer flumazenil if side effects are severe or life-threatening

Best Augmenting Agents for Side Effects
- Many side effects cannot be improved with an augmenting agent

DOSING AND USE

Usual Dosage Range
- Anxiety: oral 6–30 mg/day in divided doses (adult); oral 3–15 mg/day in divided doses (elderly)
- Insomnia associated with anxiety: oral 5–15 mg/day (at bedtime)
- Severe acute anxiety, control of acute panic attacks, acute alcohol withdrawal: IM or slow intravenous injection 10 mg, then 10 mg after at least 4 hours as needed
- Acute drug-induced dystonic reactions: intravenous injection: 5–10 mg, then 5–10 mg after at least 10 minutes as needed
- Acute anxiety and agitation: rectal 500 mcg/kg, then 500 mcg/kg after 12 hours as required (adult); 250 mcg/kg, then 250 mcg/kg after 12 hours as needed (elderly)
- Life-threatening acute drug-induced dystonic reactions: intravenous injection 100 mcg/kg, repeated as needed, to be given over 3–5 minutes (child 1 month–11 years); 5–10 mg, repeated as needed, to be given over 3–5 minutes (child 12–17 years)

Dosage Forms
- Tablet 2 mg, 5 mg, 10 mg
- Emulsion for injection 10 mg/2 mL x 10 ampoules
- Solution for injection 10 mg/2 mL x 10 ampoules
- Oral suspension 2 mg/5 mL
- Oral solution 2 mg/5 mL
- Enema 2.5 mg, 5 mg, 10 mg

How to Dose
*Anxiety:
- Oral 2 mg 3 times per day, increased as needed to 15–30 mg/day in divided doses; for debilitated patients, use elderly dose: 1 mg 3 times per day, increased as needed to 7.5–15 mg/day in divided doses
- Liquid formulation should be mixed with water, fruit juice or pudding

- Because of risk of respiratory depression, rectal diazepam treatment should not be given more than once in 5 days or more than twice during a treatment course, especially for alcohol withdrawal or status epilepticus

 Dosing Tips
* Only benzodiazepine with a formulation specifically for rectal administration
* One of the few benzodiazepines available in an oral liquid formulation
* One of the few benzodiazepines available in an injectable formulation
- Diazepam injection is intended for acute use; patients who require long-term treatment should be switched to the oral formulation
- Use lowest possible effective dose for the shortest possible period of time (a benzodiazepine-sparing strategy)
- Assess need for continued treatment regularly
- Risk of dependence may increase with dose and duration of treatment
- For inter-dose symptoms of anxiety, can either increase dose or maintain same total daily dose but divide into more frequent doses
- Can also use an as-needed occasional "top up" dose for inter-dose anxiety
- Because some anxiety disorder patients and muscle spasm patients can require doses higher than 40 mg/day or more, the risk of dependence may be greater in these patients
- Frequency of dosing in practice is often greater than predicted from half-life, as duration of biological activity is often shorter than pharmacokinetic terminal half-life

Overdose
- Fatalities can occur; hypotension, tiredness, ataxia, confusion, coma

Long-Term Use
- Some evidence of efficacy up to 16 weeks, but long-term use should be avoided
- Risk of dependence, particularly for treatment periods longer than 12 weeks and especially in patients with past or current polysubstance abuse

- Not recommended for long-term treatment of seizure disorders

Habit forming

- Diazepam is a Class C/Schedule 4 drug
- Patients may develop dependence and/or tolerance with long-term use

How to Stop

- Patients with history of seizure may seize upon withdrawal, especially if withdrawal is abrupt
- Taper by 2 mg every 3 days to reduce chances of withdrawal effects
- For difficult-to-taper cases, consider reducing dose much more slowly after reaching 20 mg/day, perhaps by as little as 0.5–1 mg every week or less
- For other patients with severe problems discontinuing a benzodiazepine, dosing may need to be tapered over many months (i.e. reduce dose by 1% every 3 days by crushing tablet and suspending or dissolving in 100 mL of fruit juice and then disposing of 1 mL while drinking the rest; 3–7 days later, dispose of 2 mL, and so on). This is both a form of very slow biological tapering and a form of behavioural desensitisation
- Be sure to differentiate re-emergence of symptoms requiring reinstitution of treatment from withdrawal symptoms
- Benzodiazepine-dependent anxiety patients and insulin-dependent diabetics are not addicted to their medications. When benzodiazepine-dependent patients stop their medication, disease symptoms can re-emerge, disease symptoms can worsen (rebound), and/or withdrawal symptoms can emerge

Pharmacokinetics

- Elimination half-life for diazepam about 50 hours (range 20–100 hours). Main active metabolite desmethyldiazepam half-life ranging from 36–200 hours
- Substrate for CYP450 2C19 and 3A4
- Food does not affect absorption
- Excretion via kidneys

 Drug Interactions

- Increased depressive side effects when taken with other CNS depressants
- Cimetidine may reduce the clearance and raise the levels of diazepam

- Flumazenil (used to reverse the effects of benzodiazepines) may precipitate seizures and should not be used in patients treated for seizure disorders with diazepam
- Fluvoxamine inhibits both CYP450 3A4 and 2C19 which leads to inhibition of the oxidative metabolism of diazepam leading to near doubling of diazepam plasma levels

 Other Warnings/Precautions

- Warning regarding the increased risk of CNS-depressant effects when benzodiazepines and opioid medications are used together, including specifically the risk of slowed or difficulty breathing and death
- If alternatives to the combined use of benzodiazepines and opioids are not available, clinicians should limit the dosage and duration of each drug to the minimum possible while still achieving therapeutic efficacy
- Patients and their caregivers should be warned to seek medical attention if unusual dizziness, light-headedness, sedation, slowed or difficulty breathing, or unresponsiveness occur
- Dosage changes should be made in collaboration with prescriber
- History of drug or alcohol abuse often creates greater risk for dependency
- Some depressed patients may experience a worsening of suicidal ideation
- Some patients may exhibit abnormal thinking or behavioural changes similar to those caused by other CNS depressants (i.e. either depressant actions or disinhibiting actions)
- Avoid prolonged use and abrupt cessation
- Use lower doses in debilitated patients and the elderly
- Use with caution in patients with myasthenia gravis; respiratory disease
- Use with caution in patients with personality disorder (dependent/avoidant or anankastic types) as may increase risk of dependence
- Use with caution in patients with a history of alcohol or drug dependence/abuse
- Benzodiazepines may cause a range of paradoxical effects including aggression, antisocial behaviours, anxiety, overexcitement, perceptual abnormalities and talkativeness. Adjustment of dose may reduce impulses
- Use with caution as diazepam can cause muscle weakness and organic brain changes

- With parenteral administration close observation is required until full recovery achieved from sedation
- With intravenous use: high risk of venous thrombophlebitis with intravenous use (reduced by using an emulsion formulation). When given intravenously, facilities for reversing respiratory depression with mechanical ventilation must be immediately available

Do Not Use

- If patient has acute pulmonary insufficiency, respiratory depression, significant neuromuscular respiratory weakness, sleep apnoea syndrome or unstable myasthenia gravis
- In patients with CNS depression, compromised airway or hyperkinesis
- Alone in chronic psychosis in adults
- On its own to try to treat depression, anxiety associated with depression, obsessional states or phobic states
- If patient has angle-closure glaucoma
- Injections containing benzyl alcohol in neonates
- If there is a proven allergy to diazepam or any benzodiazepine

Renal Impairment

- Increased cerebral sensitivity to benzodiazepines
- Start with small doses in severe impairment

Hepatic Impairment

- Can precipitate coma
- If treatment is necessary, benzodiazepines with shorter half-life are safer, such as temazepam or oxazepam
- Avoid in severe impairment

Cardiac Impairment

- Benzodiazepines have been used to treat anxiety associated with acute myocardial infarction
- Diazepam may be used as an adjunct during cardiovascular emergencies

Elderly

- Anxiety: oral 3–15 mg/day in divided doses

Children and Adolescents

- Safety and efficacy data limited
- Indications in children include: tetanus; muscle spasm in cerebral spasticity or in postoperative skeletal muscle spasm; seizures (status epilepticus, febrile convulsions, convulsions due to poisoning); life-threatening acute drug-induced dystonic reactions
- Long-term effects of diazepam in children/ adolescents are unknown
- Should generally receive lower doses and be more closely monitored
- Hallucinations in children 6–17 have been reported

Pregnancy

- Possible increased risk of birth defects when benzodiazepines taken during pregnancy
- Because of the potential risks, diazepam is not generally recommended as treatment for anxiety during pregnancy, especially during the first trimester
- Drug should be tapered if discontinued
- Infants whose mothers received a benzodiazepine late in pregnancy may experience withdrawal effects
- Neonatal flaccidity has been reported in infants whose mothers took a benzodiazepine during pregnancy
- Seizures, even mild seizures, may cause harm to the embryo/foetus
- Women who have seizures in the second half of pregnancy should be assessed for eclampsia before any change is made to antiepileptic treatment. Status epilepticus should be treated according to the standard protocol

Breastfeeding

- Some drug is found in mother's breast milk
- Effects of benzodiazepines on infant have been observed and include feeding difficulties, sedation, and weight loss
- Caution should be taken with the use of benzodiazepines in breastfeeding mothers; seek to use low doses for short periods to reduce infant exposure
- Diazepam may accumulate in the breastfed infant
- Use of short-acting agents, e.g. oxazepam or lorazepam, preferred

Diazepam (Continued)

THE ART OF PSYCHOPHARMACOLOGY

Potential Advantages
- Rapid onset of action
- Availability of oral liquid, rectal, and injectable dosage formulations

Potential Disadvantages
- Euphoria may lead to abuse
- Abuse especially risky in past or present substance abusers
- Can be sedating at doses necessary to treat moderately severe anxiety disorders

Primary Target Symptoms
- Panic attacks
- Anxiety
- Incidence of seizures (adjunct)
- Muscle spasms

 Pearls

- NICE Guidelines recommend medication for insomnia only as a second-line treatment after non-pharmacological treatment options have been tried (e.g. cognitive behavioural therapy for insomnia)
- Can be a useful adjunct to SSRIs and SNRIs in the treatment of numerous anxiety disorders, but not used as frequently as other benzodiazepines for this purpose
- Not effective for treating psychosis as a monotherapy, but can be used as an adjunct to antipsychotics
- Not effective for treating bipolar disorder as a monotherapy, but can be used as an adjunct to mood stabilisers and antipsychotics

*Diazepam is often the first-choice benzodiazepine to treat status epilepticus, and is administered either intravenously or rectally
- Because diazepam suppresses stage 4 sleep, it may prevent night terrors in adults
- May both cause depression and treat depression in different patients
- Was once one of the most commonly prescribed drugs in the world and the most commonly prescribed benzodiazepine
*Remains a popular benzodiazepine for treating muscle spasms
- A commonly used benzodiazepine to treat sleep disorders
*Remains a popular benzodiazepine to treat acute alcohol withdrawal
- Not especially useful as an oral anticonvulsant
*Multiple dosage formulations (oral tablet, oral liquid, rectal gel, injectable) allow more flexibility of administration compared to most other benzodiazepines
- When using to treat insomnia, remember that insomnia may be a symptom of some other primary disorder itself, and thus warrants evaluation for co-morbid psychiatric and/or medical conditions
- Though not systematically studied, benzodiazepines have been used effectively to treat catatonia and are the initial recommended treatment
- Diazepam is a long-acting benzodiazepine without a sharp peak of effects and so with some reduction in the risk of abuse in comparison to some other benzodiazepines

 Suggested Reading

Ashton H. Guidelines for the rational use of benzodiazepines. When and what to use. Drugs 1994;48(1):25–40.

De Negri M, Baglietto MG. Treatment of status epilepticus in children. Paediatr Drugs 2001;3(6):411–20.

Mandelli M, Tognoni G, Garattini S. Clinical pharmacokinetics of diazepam. Clin Pharmacokinet 1978;3(1):72–91.

Rey E, Treluyer JM, Pons G. Pharmacokinetic optimization of benzodiazepine therapy for acute seizures. Focus on delivery routes. Clin Pharmacokinet 1999;36(6):409–24.

Soyka M. Treatment of benzodiazepine dependence. N Engl J Med 2017;376(12):1147–57.

Disulfiram

Brands
- Antabuse
- Esperal

Generic?
Yes

Class
- Neuroscience-based nomenclature: pharmacology domain – alcohol; mode of action – enzyme inhibitor
- Alcohol dependence treatment; enzyme inhibitor (mainly liver)

Commonly Prescribed for
(bold for BNF indication)
- **Adjunct in treatment of alcohol dependence (under expert supervision)**

 ## How the Drug Works
- Irreversibly inhibits aldehyde dehydrogenase, the enzyme involved in second-stage metabolism of alcohol
- Alcohol is metabolised to acetaldehyde, which in turn is metabolised by aldehyde dehydrogenase; thus, disulfiram blocks this second-stage metabolism
- If alcohol is consumed by a patient taking disulfiram, toxic levels of acetaldehyde build up, causing prominent unpleasant physical symptoms (similar effects to that of a hangover and felt immediately following alcohol consumption)
- The knowledge of this potential aversive experience deters patients from consuming alcohol
- If alcohol is consumed then the aversive experience can lead to negative conditioning, in which patients abstain from alcohol in order to avoid the unpleasant effects
- Disulfiram can thus be used post-detox to support abstinence

How Long Until It Works
- Disulfiram's effects are immediate; patients should not take disulfiram until at least 24 hours after stopping drinking

If It Works
- Increases abstinence from alcohol

If It Doesn't Work
- Patients who drink alcohol while taking disulfiram experience adverse effects, including alcohol toxicity
- Evaluate for and address contributing factors
- Consider switching to another agent

 ## Best Augmenting Combos for Partial Response or Treatment Resistance
- Augmentation with behavioural, educational, and/or supportive therapy in groups or as an individual including couple/family therapy or community reinforcement approaches is probably key to successful treatment
- Witnessing (supervision) either by a professional or carer optimises concordance and contributes to effectiveness

Tests
- Baseline and follow-up liver function tests every 2 weeks for the first 2 months, then monthly for the following 4 months, and then every 6 months

How Drug Causes Side Effects
- One of disulfiram's metabolites is carbon disulfide, which may be excreted through the lungs; this could account for the side effect of metallic taste
- When alcohol is consumed by a patient taking disulfiram, levels of acetaldehyde build up, causing side effects of alcohol toxicity

Notable Side Effects
- Metallic taste, dermatitis, sedation
- If alcohol is consumed: dyspnoea, flushing, headache, hyperventilation, hypotension, nausea, sweating, tachycardia, vomiting

Frequency not known
- CNS: depression, drowsiness, encephalopathy, mania, nerve disorders, paranoia, psychosis
- GIT: hepatocellular injury, nausea, vomiting

- Other: allergic dermatitis, decreased libido, fatigue, halitosis

 Life-Threatening or Dangerous Side Effects

- Hepatotoxicity (this can be rapid and unpredictable, therefore advise patients that if they feel unwell or develop a fever or jaundice that they should stop taking disulfiram and seek urgent medical attention)
- If alcohol is consumed: myocardial infarction, congestive heart failure, respiratory depression, other signs of alcohol and acetaldehyde toxicity such as arrhythmias, hypotension, collapse

Weight Gain

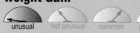

- Reported but not expected

Sedation

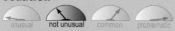

- Occurs in significant minority

What to Do About Side Effects

- Wait
- Reduce dose
- Take at night to reduce sedation

Best Augmenting Agents for Side Effects

- Dose reduction or switching to another agent may be more effective since most side effects cannot be improved with an augmenting agent

DOSING AND USE

Usual Dosage Range

- 200–500 mg/day; 1-year duration

Dosage Forms

- Tablet 200 mg, 250 mg, 500 mg

How to Dose

- The patient should not take disulfiram until at least 24 hours after drinking
- Initial dose 200 mg/day for 1–2 weeks increased as needed
- Usually dosed in the morning, but can be dosed at night if sedation is a problem
- Maintenance dose usually 250 mg/day; max dose 500 mg/day

 Dosing Tips

- Patients and carers should be fully informed about the disulfiram–alcohol reactions
- Reactions may occur following exposure to small amounts found in perfume, aerosol sprays, cough medicines or low alcohol and "non-alcohol" beers and wines
- Symptoms may be severe and life-threatening: can include nausea, flushing, palpitations, arrhythmias, hypotension, respiratory depression and coma
- Should also be counselled on signs of hepatotoxicity
- Patients should discontinue treatment and seek immediate medical attention if they feel unwell or have symptoms such as fever or jaundice
- Patients should carry an emergency card stating that they are taking disulfiram
- Probably safe to restart at previous dose after a period of non-adherence

Overdose

- Disulfiram alone has low toxicity
- Most patients develop symptoms within the first 12 hours, but for some the clinical presentation may be delayed for days after an overdose, with slow recovery and long-term effects
- Symptoms include nausea, vomiting, abdominal pain, diarrhoea, drowsiness, delirium, hallucinations, lethargy, tachycardia, tachypnoea, hyperthermia and hypotension
- Hypotonia may be prominent, especially in children, and tendon reflexes may be reduced
- Hyperglycaemia, leucocytosis, ketosis and methaemoglobinaemia reported
- Severe cases may lead to cardiovascular collapse, coma and convulsions
- Rare complications include sensorimotor neuropathy, EEG abnormalities, encephalopathy, psychosis and catatonia, which may appear several days after overdose. Dysarthria, myoclonus, ataxia, dystonia and akinesia may also occur. Movement disorders may be related to direct toxic effects on the basal ganglia

Long-Term Use

- Maintenance treatment should be continued until the patient is recovered
- Monitor at least every 2 weeks for the first 2 months, then each month for the following 4 months, and at least every 6 months thereafter

Habit Forming

- No

How to Stop

- Taper not necessary
- A disulfiram–alcohol reaction may occur for up to 2 weeks after disulfiram is stopped

Pharmacokinetics

- Half-life of parent drug 60–120 hours
- Half-life of metabolites 13.9 hours (diethyldithiocarbamate) and 8.9 hours (carbon disulfide)
- Disulfiram is an inhibitor of CYP450 2E1
- Excretion is primarily via kidneys

 Drug Interactions

- Disulfiram may increase blood levels of phenytoin; baseline and follow-up levels of phenytoin should be taken
- Disulfiram may prolong prothrombin time, requiring dose adjustment of oral anticoagulants
- Use with isoniazid may lead to unsteady gait or change in mental status
- Disulfiram may reduce caffeine clearance via CYP450 1A2 inhibltion

 Other Warnings/Precautions

- Not recommended for patients above the age of 60
- Take extreme caution if using in patients with hypothyroidism, epilepsy, diabetes, respiratory disease or cerebral damage
- Patients taking disulfiram should not be exposed to ethylene dibromide or its vapours, as this has resulted in a higher incidence of tumours in rats

Do Not Use

- If the patient is in a state of alcohol intoxication
- Without the patient's full knowledge
- For at least 24 hours after the patient last drank

- If patient is taking metronidazole, fosamprenavir, ritonavir or sertraline
- If patient has psychosis, severe personality disorder or is a suicide risk
- If patient has history of cardiac failure, coronary artery disease, hypertension or history of cerebrovascular accident
- In acute porphyrias, renal or hepatic failure including cirrhosis or portal hypertension
- If there is a proven allergy to disulfiram
- If there is a proven allergy to thiuram derivatives

Renal Impairment

- Not recommended for patients with chronic renal failure

Hepatic Impairment

- Not recommended

Cardiac Impairment

- Contraindicated

Elderly

- Not generally recommended for patients older than 60 years of age
- Some patients may tolerate lower doses better

 Children and Adolescents

- Safety and efficacy have not been established

 Pregnancy

- Very limited data on disulfiram use in pregnancy
- Data confounded by possible underreporting of alcohol and substance misuse
- Some animal studies have shown adverse effects
- Pregnant women needing to stop drinking may consider behavioural therapy before pharmacotherapy
- Not generally recommended for use during pregnancy, especially during first trimester

Breastfeeding

- Disulfiram is expected to be secreted in human breast milk

Disulfiram (Continued)

- Risk of breastfeeding by an alcohol-dependent mother should be assessed
- Disulfiram is contraindicated in breastfeeding mothers due to the risk of the infant being exposed to alcohol, either from the breast milk or from another source
- Acamprosate and naltrexone may be considered as alternative treatment options

THE ART OF PSYCHOPHARMACOLOGY

Potential Advantages

- Individuals who are motivated to abstain from alcohol and those who want a psychological barrier to drinking alcohol

Potential Disadvantages

- Adherence rates can be low

Primary Target Symptoms

- Alcohol dependence

 Pearls

- Disulfiram is recommended as a second-line option for moderate-to-severe alcohol dependence for patients who are not suitable for acamprosate or naltrexone or have specified a preference for disulfiram and aim to stay abstinent from alcohol
- Some evidence of efficacy in co-morbid alcohol use disorder and PTSD
- Preliminary evidence of efficacy for use in cocaine dependence, both alone and co-morbid with alcohol use disorder, partly acting by inhibiting dopamine metabolism (increasing dopamine levels and reducing norepinephrine levels)
- Disulfiram has been studied as a possible treatment for other conditions such as cancer, parasitic infections and latent HIV infection

Suggested Reading

Barth KS, Malcolm RJ. Disulfiram: an old therapeutic with new applications. CNS Neurol Disord Drug Targets 2010;9(1):5–12.

Jiao Y, Hannafon BN, Ding WQ. Disulfiram's anticancer activity: evidence and mechanisms. Anticancer Agents Med Chem 2016;16(11):1378–84.

Jorgensen CH, Pedersen B, Tonnesen H. The efficacy of disulfiram for the treatment of alcohol use disorder. Alcohol Clin Exp Res 2011;35(10):1749–58.

Lee SA, Elliott JH, McMahon J, et al. Population pharmacokinetics and pharmacodynamics of disulfiram on inducing latent HIV-1 transcription in a phase IIb trial. Clin Pharmacol Ther 2019;105(3):692–702.

Pani PP, Troqu E, Vacca R, et al. Disulfiram for the treatment of cocaine dependence. Cochrane Database Syst Rev 2010;20(1):CD007024.

Shirley D-A, Sharma I, Warren CA, et al. Drug repurposing of the alcohol abuse medication disulfiram as an anti-parasitic agent. Front Cell Infect Microbiol 2021;11:633194.

Donepezil hydrochloride

Brands
• Aricept
• Aricept Evess

Generic?
Yes

Class
• Neuroscience-based nomenclature: pharmacology domain – acetylcholine; mode of action – enzyme inhibitor
• Cholinesterase inhibitor (selective acetylcholinesterase inhibitor); cognitive enhancer

Commonly Prescribed for
(bold for BNF indication)
• **Mild-moderate dementia in Alzheimer's disease**
• Mild-moderate dementia in Parkinson's disease
• Dementia with Lewy bodies
• Alzheimer's disease of atypical or mixed type (when vascular dementia and Alzheimer's disease are co-morbid)

How the Drug Works
• Reversibly but non-competitively inhibits centrally active acetylcholinesterase (AChE), making more acetylcholine available
• Increased availability of acetylcholine compensates in part for degenerating cholinergic neurons in neocortex which regulate memory
• Does not inhibit butyrylcholinesterase and does not act as a nicotine modulator

How Long Until It Works
• May take up to 6 weeks before any improvement in baseline memory or behaviour is evident
• May take months before any stabilisation in degenerative course is evident
• In moderate or severe Alzheimer's disease continued treatment with donepezil is associated with significant functional benefits over 12 months

If It Works
• May improve symptoms of disease, or slow progression, but does not reverse the degenerative process

If It Doesn't Work
• Consider adjusting dose, switching to a different cholinesterase inhibitor or consider adding memantine in moderate or severe Alzheimer's disease
• Reconsider diagnosis and rule out other conditions such as depression or a dementia other than Alzheimer's disease

Best Augmenting Combos for Partial Response or Treatment Resistance
• Augmenting agents may help with managing non-cognitive symptoms
✳Memantine for moderate to severe Alzheimer's disease
✳Atypical antipsychotics should only be used for severe aggression or psychosis when this is causing significant distress
• Careful consideration needs to be undertaken for co-morbid conditions and the benefits and risks of treatment in view of the increased risk of stroke and death with antipsychotic drugs in dementia
✳Antidepressants if concomitant depression, apathy, or lack of interest, however efficacy may be limited
• Not rational to combine with another cholinesterase inhibitor

Tests
• None for healthy individuals

How Drug Causes Side Effects
• Peripheral inhibition of acetylcholinesterase can cause gastrointestinal side effects
• Central inhibition of acetylcholinesterase may contribute to nausea, vomiting, weight loss, and sleep disturbances

Notable Side Effects
✳Gastrointestinal side effects including nausea, diarrhoea, vomiting, reduced appetite and weight loss, increased gastric secretion
• Insomnia, dizziness
• Muscle cramps, fatigue, depression, abnormal dreams

Donepezil hydrochloride (Continued)

Common or very common

- CNS: aggression, agitation, dizziness, hallucination, headache, sleep disorders
- GIT: decreased appetite, diarrhoea, gastrointestinal disorders, nausea, vomiting
- Other: common cold, fatigue, injury, muscle cramps, pain, skin reactions, syncope, urinary incontinence

Uncommon

- Bradycardia, gastrointestinal haemorrhage, increased saliva, seizure

Rare or very rare

- Cardiac conduction disorders, extrapyramidal symptoms, hepatic disorders, neuroleptic malignant syndrome, rhabdomyolysis

 Life-Threatening or Dangerous Side Effects

- Seizures
- Syncope
- Neuroleptic malignant syndrome

Weight Gain

- Reported but not expected
- Some patients may experience weight loss

Sedation

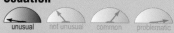

- Reported but not expected

What to Do About Side Effects

- Wait
- Side effects such as nausea improve with time
- Take in daytime to reduce insomnia or take with food to reduce nausea
- Use slower dose titration
- Consider lowering dose, switching to a different agent or adding an appropriate augmenting agent

Best Augmenting Agents for Side Effects

- Many side effects cannot be improved with an augmenting agent

---

DOSING AND USE

Usual Dosage Range

- 5–10 mg at night

Dosage Forms

- Tablet 5 mg, 10 mg
- Orodispersible tablet 5 mg, 10 mg
- Oral solution 1 mg/mL (150 mL)

How to Dose

- Initial dose 5 mg/day at bedtime; may increase to 10 mg/day after 4 weeks

 Dosing Tips

- Side effects occur more frequently at higher doses
- Slower titration (e.g. 6 weeks to 10 mg/day) may reduce the risk of side effects
- Food does not affect the absorption of donepezil
- Probably best to utilise highest tolerated dose within the usual dosage range
- In those patients showing intolerance to a cholinesterase inhibitor, switching to another agent should be done only after complete resolution of side effects following discontinuation of the first agent (for donepezil allow a 2-week washout period which equates to 5x half-life of the drug)
- If there is a lack of efficacy switching can be done more quickly
- Switching to another cholinesterase inhibitor is not recommended in patients who are no longer receiving beneficial effects from the drug several years later

Overdose

- Can be lethal; nausea, vomiting, excess salivation, sweating, hypotension, bradycardia, collapse, convulsions, muscle weakness (weakness of respiratory muscles can lead to death)

Long-Term Use

- Drug may lose effectiveness in slowing degenerative course of Alzheimer's disease after 6 months
- Can be effective in some patients for several years and stopping medication is then not recommended if the disease becomes severe and the medication is well tolerated

Habit Forming

- No

How to Stop

- Taper recommended (reduce dose to 5 mg/day for a month and monitor before completely stopping the drug)
- Discontinuation may lead to notable deterioration in memory and behaviour, which may not be restored when drug is restarted or another cholinesterase inhibitor is initiated

Pharmacokinetics

- Metabolised by CYP450 2D6 and 3A4
- Elimination half-life about 70 hours

 Drug Interactions

- Donepezil may increase the effects of anaesthetics and should be discontinued prior to surgery
- Inhibitors of CYP450 2D6 and 3A4 may inhibit donepezil metabolism and increase its plasma levels
- Inducers of CYP450 2D6 and 3A4 may increase clearance of donepezil and decrease its plasma levels
- Donepezil may interact with anticholinergic agents and the combination may decrease the efficacy of both
- May have synergistic effect if administered with cholinomimetics (e.g. bethanechol)
- Bradycardia may occur if combined with beta blockers
- Theoretically, could reduce the efficacy of levodopa in Parkinson's disease
- Not rational to combine with another cholinesterase inhibitor

 Other Warnings/Precautions

- May exacerbate asthma or chronic obstructive pulmonary disease
- Increased gastric acid secretion may increase the risk of ulcers
- Caution when using in patients with sick sinus syndrome or supraventricular conduction abnormalities
- Bradycardia or heart block may occur in patients with or without cardiac impairment

Do Not Use

- If there is a proven allergy to donepezil

Renal Impairment

- Limited data available but dose adjustment is most likely unnecessary

Hepatic Impairment

- Caution in hepatic impairment

Cardiac Impairment

- Use with caution due to effects on heart rate (e.g. bradycardia) especially in patients with "sick sinus syndrome" or other supraventricular cardiac disturbances, such as sinoatrial or atrioventricular block
- Use with caution in patients taking medications that reduce heart rate (e.g. digoxin or beta blockers)
- Syncopal episodes have been reported with the use of donepezil

Elderly

- Some patients may tolerate lower doses better
- Use of cholinesterase inhibitors may be associated with increased rates of syncope, bradycardia, pacemaker insertion, and hip fracture in older adults with dementia

 Children and Adolescents

- Safety and efficacy have not been established

 Pregnancy

- Controlled studies have not been conducted in pregnant women
- Not recommended for use in pregnant women or women of childbearing potential

Breastfeeding

- Unknown if donepezil is secreted in human breast milk, but all psychotropics assumed to be secreted in breast milk
- *Recommended either to discontinue drug or bottle feed
- Donepezil is not recommended for use in nursing women

Donepezil hydrochloride (Continued)

Potential Advantages

- Once a day dosing
- May work in some patients who do not respond to other cholinesterase inhibitors
- May work in some patients who do not tolerate other cholinesterase inhibitors

Potential Disadvantages

- Patients with insomnia

Primary Target Symptoms

- Memory loss in Alzheimer's disease
- Behavioural symptoms in Alzheimer's disease
- Memory loss in dementia in Parkinson's disease

Pearls

- Dramatic reversal of symptoms of Alzheimer's disease is not generally seen with cholinesterase inhibitors
- Can lead to unnecessary therapeutic nihilism among prescribers and lack of an appropriate trial of a cholinesterase inhibitor
- Perhaps only 50% of Alzheimer's patients are diagnosed, and only 50% of those diagnosed are treated, and only 50% of those treated are given a cholinesterase inhibitor, and then only for 200 days in a disease that lasts 7–10 years
- Must evaluate lack of efficacy and loss of efficacy over months not weeks
- The benefits of donepezil treatment on cognitive function, activities of daily living and behaviour have been observed in meta-analyses, but not observed on quality-of-life scores
- Cholinesterase inhibitors have at best a modest impact on non-cognitive features of dementia such as apathy, disinhibition, delusions, anxiety, lack of cooperation, pacing, but in the absence of safe and effective alternatives a trial of a cholinesterase inhibitor is appropriate
- Treat the patient but ask the caregiver about efficacy

What to expect from a cholinesterase inhibitor:

- Patients do not generally improve dramatically, although this can be observed in a significant minority of patients
- Onset of behavioural problems and nursing home placement can be delayed
- Functional outcomes including activities of daily living may be preserved
- Caregiver burden and stress can be reduced
- Delay in progression in Alzheimer's disease is not evidence of disease-modifying actions of cholinesterase inhibition
- Cholinesterase inhibitors like donepezil depend upon the presence of intact targets for acetylcholine for maximum effectiveness and thus may be most effective in the early stages of Alzheimer's disease
- Benefits of the higher dose (10 mg) are marginal so if a patient can only tolerate the lower dose of 5 mg this is also worthwhile
- The most prominent side effects of donepezil are gastrointestinal effects, which are usually mild and transient
- May cause more sleep disturbances than some other cholinesterase inhibitors
- Weight loss can be a problem in Alzheimer's disease patients with debilitation and muscle wasting
- Use with caution in underweight or frail patients
- Cognitive improvement may be linked to substantial (>65%) inhibition of acetylcholinesterase
- Donepezil has greater action on CNS acetylcholinesterase than on peripheral acetylcholinesterase
- Some Alzheimer's disease patients who fail to respond to donepezil may respond to another cholinesterase inhibitor
- Some Alzheimer's disease patients who fail to respond to another cholinesterase inhibitor may respond when switched to donepezil
- Not recommended by NICE for patients with Mild Cognitive Impairment (MCI)
- May be useful in Parkinson's disease-related dementia and for dementia with Lewy bodies (DLB, constituted by early loss of attentiveness and visual perception with possible hallucinations, Parkinson's disease-like movement problems, fluctuating cognition such as daytime drowsiness and lethargy, staring into space for long periods, episodes of disorganised speech)
- May decrease delusions, apathy, agitation, and hallucinations in dementia with Lewy bodies

Donepezil hydrochloride (Continued)

- Only consider AChE inhibitors or memantine for people with vascular dementia if they have suspected co-morbid Alzheimer's disease, Parkinson's disease dementia or dementia with Lewy bodies
- Do not offer AChE inhibitors or memantine to people with frontotemporal dementia

- Do not offer AChE inhibitors or memantine to people with cognitive impairment caused by multiple sclerosis
- May be helpful for dementia in Down's syndrome

 Suggested Reading

Birks JS, Harvey RJ. Donepezil for dementia due to Alzheimer's disease. Cochrane Database Syst Rev 2006;(1):CD001190.

Cummings JL. Use of cholinesterase inhibitors in clinical practice: evidence-based recommendations. Am J Geriatr Psychiatry 2003;11(2):131–45.

Hansen RA, Gartlehner G, Webb AP, et al. Efficacy and safety of donepezil, galantamine, and rivastigmine for the treatment of Alzheimer's disease: a systematic review and meta-analysis. Clin Interv Aging 2008;3(2):211–25.

Howard R, McShane R, Lindesay J, et al. Donepezil and memantine for moderate-to-severe Alzheimer's disease. N Engl J Med 2012;366(10):893–903.

Lee J-H, Jeong S-K, Kim BC, et al. Donepezil across the spectrum of Alzheimer's disease: dose optimization and clinical relevance. Acta Neurl Scand 2015;131(5):259–67.

Stinton C, McKeith I, Taylor J-P, et al. Pharmacological management of Lewy body dementia: a systematic review and meta-analysis. Am J Psychiatry 2015;172(8):731–42.

Dosulepin hydrochloride

Brands

• Prothiaden

Generic?

Yes

Class

• Neuroscience-based nomenclature: pharmacology domain – serotonin, norepinephrine; mode of action – reuptake inhibitor
• Tricyclic antidepressant (TCA)

Commonly Prescribed for

(bold for BNF indication)
• **Depressive illness, where sedation required (not recommended – risk of fatality in overdose; initiated by a specialist)**
• Anxiety
• Insomnia
• Neuropathic pain/chronic pain
• Treatment-resistant depression

 ## How the Drug Works

• Boosts neurotransmitters serotonin and noradrenaline
• Blocks serotonin reuptake pump (serotonin transporter), presumably increasing serotonergic neurotransmission
• Blocks noradrenaline reuptake pump (noradrenaline transporter), presumably increasing noradrenergic neurotransmission
• Inhibits presynaptic alpha 2 adrenergic receptors, thereby facilitating the release of noradrenaline
• Presumably desensitises both serotonin 1A receptors and beta-adrenergic receptors
• Since dopamine is inactivated by noradrenaline reuptake in frontal cortex, which largely lacks dopamine transporters, dosulepin can increase dopamine neurotransmission in this part of the brain
• Since the noradrenaline transporter is responsible for the re-uptake of both noradrenaline and dopamine in the prefrontal cortex, which largely lacks dopamine transporters, dosulepin can also increase prefrontal dopaminergic neurotransmission

How Long Until It Works

• May have immediate effects in treating insomnia or anxiety
• Onset of therapeutic actions with some antidepressants can be seen within 1–2 weeks, but often delayed up to 2–4 weeks
• If it is not working within 3–4 weeks for depression, it may require a dosage increase or it may not work at all
• By contrast, for generalised anxiety, onset of response and increases in remission rates may still occur after 8 weeks, and for up to 6 months after initiating dosing

If It Works

• The goal of treatment is complete remission of current symptoms as well as prevention of future relapses
• Treatment most often reduces or even eliminates symptoms, but is not a cure since symptoms can recur after medicine is stopped
• Continue treatment until all symptoms are gone (remission), especially in depression and whenever possible in anxiety disorders
• Once symptoms are gone, continue treating for at least 6–9 months for the first episode of depression or >12 months if relapse indicators present
• If >5 episodes and/or 2 episodes in the last few years then need to continue for at least 2 years or indefinitely
• The goal of treatment in chronic neuropathic pain is to reduce symptoms as much as possible, especially in combination with other treatments
• Treatment of chronic neuropathic pain may reduce symptoms, but rarely eliminates them completely, and is not a cure since symptoms can recur after medicine has been stopped
• Use in anxiety disorders and chronic pain may also need to be indefinite, but long-term treatment is not well studied in these conditions

If It Doesn't Work

• Important to recognise non-response to treatment early on (3–4 weeks)
• Many patients have only a partial response where some symptoms are improved but others persist (especially insomnia, fatigue, and problems concentrating)

Dosulepin hydrochloride (Continued)

- Other patients may be non-responders, sometimes called treatment-resistant or treatment-refractory
- Some patients who have an initial response may relapse even though they continue treatment
- Consider increasing dose, switching to another agent or adding an appropriate augmenting agent
- Lithium may be added for suicidal patients or those at high risk of relapse
- Consider psychotherapy
- Consider ECT
- Consider evaluation for another diagnosis or for a co-morbid condition (e.g. medical illness, substance abuse, etc.)
- Some patients may experience a switch into mania and so would require antidepressant discontinuation and initiation of a mood stabiliser

⚖️ Best Augmenting Combos for Partial Response or Treatment Resistance

- Mood stabilisers or atypical antipsychotics for bipolar depression
- Atypical antipsychotics for psychotic depression
- Atypical antipsychotics as first-line augmenting agents (quetiapine MR 300 mg/day or aripiprazole at 2.5–10 mg/day) for treatment-resistant depression
- Atypical antipsychotics as second-line augmenting agents (risperidone 0.5–2 mg/day or olanzapine 2.5–10 mg/day) for treatment-resistant depression
- Mirtazapine at 30–45 mg/day as another second-line augmenting agent (a dual serotonin and noradrenaline combination, but observe for switch into mania, increase in suicidal ideation or serotonin syndrome)
- T3 (20–50 mcg/day) is another second-line augmenting agent that works best with tricyclic antidepressants
- Other augmenting agents but with less evidence include bupropion (up to 400 mg/day), buspirone (up to 60 mg/day) and lamotrigine (up to 400 mg/day)
- Benzodiazepines if agitation present
- Hypnotics or trazodone for insomnia (but beware of serotonin syndrome with trazodone)

- Augmenting agents reserved for specialist use include: modafinil for sleepiness, fatigue and lack of concentration; stimulants, oestrogens, testosterone
- Lithium is particularly useful for suicidal patients and those at high risk of relapse including with factors such as severe depression, psychomotor retardation, repeated episodes (>3), significant weight loss, or a family history of major depression (aim for lithium plasma levels 0.6–1.0 mmol/L)
- For elderly patients lithium is a very effective augmenting agent
- For severely ill patients other combinations may be tried especially in specialist centres
- Augmenting agents that may be tried include omega-3, SAM-e, L-methylfolate
- Additional non-pharmacological treatments such as exercise, mindfulness, CBT, and IPT can also be helpful
- If present after treatment response (4–8 weeks) or remission (6–12 weeks), the most common residual symptoms of depression include cognitive impairments, reduced energy and problems with sleep
- For chronic pain: gabapentin, other anticonvulsants, or opiates if done by experts while monitoring carefully in difficult cases

Tests

- Baseline ECG is useful for patients over age 50
- ECGs may be useful for selected patients (e.g. those with personal or family history of QTc prolongation; cardiac arrhythmia; recent myocardial infarction; decompensated heart failure; or taking agents that prolong QTc interval such as pimozide, thioridazine, selected antiarrhythmics, moxifloxacin etc.)
- *Since tricyclic and tetracyclic antidepressants are frequently associated with weight gain, before starting treatment, weigh all patients and determine if the patient is already overweight (BMI 25.0–29.9) or obese (BMI ≥30)
- Before giving a drug that can cause weight gain to an overweight or obese patient, consider determining whether the patient already has:
  - Pre-diabetes – fasting plasma glucose: 5.5 mmol/L to 6.9 mmol/L or HbA1c: 42 to 47 mmol/mol (6.0 to 6.4%)

- Diabetes – fasting plasma glucose: >7.0 mmol/L or HbA1c: ≥48 mmol/L (≥6.5%)
- Hypertension (BP >140/90 mm Hg)
- Dyslipidaemia (increased total cholesterol, LDL cholesterol, and triglycerides; decreased HDL cholesterol)
- Treat or refer such patients for treatment, including nutrition and weight management, physical activity counselling, smoking cessation, and medical management
* Monitor weight and BMI during treatment
* While giving a drug to a patient who has gained >5% of initial weight, consider evaluating for the presence of pre-diabetes, diabetes, dyslipidaemia, or consider switching to a different antidepressant
- Patients at risk for electrolyte disturbances (e.g. patients aged >60, patients on diuretic therapy) should have baseline and periodic serum potassium and magnesium measurements

SIDE EFFECTS

How Drug Causes Side Effects
- Anticholinergic activity may explain sedative effects, dry mouth, constipation, and blurred vision
- Sedative effects and weight gain may be due to antihistaminergic properties
- Blockade of alpha adrenergic 1 receptors may explain dizziness, sedation, and hypotension
- Cardiac arrhythmias and seizures, especially in overdose, may be caused by blockade of ion channels

Notable Side Effects
- Blurred vision, constipation, urinary retention, increased appetite, dry mouth, nausea, diarrhoea, heartburn, unusual taste in mouth, weight gain
- Fatigue, weakness, dizziness, sedation, headache, anxiety, nervousness, restlessness
- Sexual dysfunction, sweating

Frequency not known
- Blood disorders: agranulocytosis, eosinophilia, leucopenia, thrombocytopenia
- CNS/PNS: altered mood, confusion, dizziness, drowsiness, movement disorders, nervousness, paranoid delusions, psychosis, seizures, speech disorder, suicidal behaviours, tremor
- CVS: arrhythmias, cardiac conduction disorder, hypertension, hypotension
- Endocrine: endocrine disorder, galactorrhoea, gynaecomastia
- GIT: abnormal appetite, constipation, dry mouth, epigastric discomfort, hepatic disorders, nausea, vomiting, weight changes
- Other: accommodation disorder, alveolitis, anticholinergic syndrome, asthenia, bone marrow depression, hyperhidrosis, hyponatraemia, photosensitivity, risk of fractures, sexual dysfunction, SIADH, skin reactions, testicular hypertrophy, urinary hesitation, withdrawal syndrome

Life-Threatening or Dangerous Side Effects
- Paralytic ileus, hyperthermia (TCAs + anticholinergic agents)
- Lowered seizure threshold and rare seizures (dose-related)
- Orthostatic hypotension, sudden death, arrhythmias, tachycardia
- QTc prolongation
- Hepatic failure, extrapyramidal symptoms
- Increased intraocular pressure
- Rare induction of mania and paranoid delusions
- Rare increase in suicidal ideation and behaviours in adolescents and young adults (up to age 25), hence patients should be warned of this potential adverse event

Weight Gain

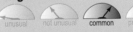

- Many experience and/or can be significant in amount
- Can increase appetite and carbohydrate craving

Sedation

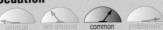

- Many experience and/or can be significant in amount
- Tolerance to sedative effects may develop with long-term use

What To Do About Side Effects
- Wait
- Wait
- Wait

Dosulepin hydrochloride (Continued)

- The risk of side effects is reduced by titrating slowly to the minimum effective dose (every 2–3 days)
- Consider using a lower starting dose in elderly patients
- Manage side effects that are likely to be transient (e.g. drowsiness) by explanation, reassurance and, if necessary, dose reduction and re-titration
- Giving patients simple strategies for managing mild side effects (e.g. dry mouth) may be useful
- For persistent, severe or distressing side effects the options are:
  - Dose reduction and re-titration if possible
  - Switching to an antidepressant with a lower propensity to cause that side effect
  - Non-drug management of the side effect (e.g. diet and exercise for weight gain)

Best Augmenting Agents for Side Effects

- Many side effects cannot be improved with an augmenting agent

DOSING AND USE

Usual Dosage Range

- 75–150 mg/day

Dosage Forms

- Capsule 25 mg
- Tablet 75 mg

How to Dose

- Adult: initial dose 75 mg/day either in divided doses or once daily at bedtime, increased gradually as needed to 150 mg/day; up to 225 mg/day in some circumstances, e.g. inpatient setting
- Elderly: initial dose 50–75 mg/day either in divided doses or once daily at bedtime, increased gradually as needed to 75–150 mg/day; up to 225 mg/day in some circumstances, e.g. inpatient setting

 Dosing Tips

- If given in a single dose, should generally be administered at bedtime because of its sedative properties
- If given in split doses, largest dose should generally be given at bedtime because of its sedative properties
- If patients experience nightmares, split dose and do not give large dose at bedtime

- Patients treated for chronic pain may only require lower doses
- If intolerable anxiety, insomnia, agitation, akathisia, or activation occur either upon dosing initiation or discontinuation, consider the possibility of activated bipolar disorder, and switch to a mood stabiliser or an atypical antipsychotic

Overdose

- Can be fatal; convulsions, cardiac arrhythmias, severe hypotension, CNS depression, coma, ECG changes
- The relative toxicity of dosulepin is 2.7 times that of amitriptyline

Long-Term Use

- Safe

Habit Forming

- No

How to Stop

- Taper gradually to avoid withdrawal effects
- Even with gradual dose reduction some withdrawal symptoms may appear within the first 2 weeks
- It is best to reduce the dose gradually over 4 weeks or longer if withdrawal symptoms emerge
- If severe withdrawal symptoms emerge during discontinuation, raise dose to stop symptoms and then restart withdrawal much more slowly (over at least 6 months in patients on long-term maintenance treatment)

Pharmacokinetics

- Substrate for CYP450 2D6 and 3A4
- Half-life of parent drug is about 14–40 hours
- Half-life of active metabolite desmethy-dosulepin is 22–60 hours

 Drug Interactions

- Tramadol increases the risk of seizures in patients taking TCAs
- Use of TCAs with anticholinergic drugs may result in paralytic ileus or hyperthermia
- Fluoxetine, paroxetine, bupropion, duloxetine, terbinafine and other CYP450 2D6 inhibitors may increase TCA concentrations
- Cimetidine may increase plasma concentrations of TCAs and cause anticholinergic symptoms

- Phenothiazines or haloperidol may raise TCA blood concentrations
- May alter effects of antihypertensive drugs; may inhibit hypotensive effects of clonidine
- Use with sympathomimetic agents may increase sympathetic activity
- Methylphenidate may inhibit metabolism of TCAs
- Dosulepin can increase the effects of adrenaline/epinephrine
- Strong CYP450 3A4 inducers (e.g. carbamazepine, phenobarbital) can reduce dosulepin plasma levels; dose adjustment may be necessary
- Both dosulepin and carbamazepine can increase the risk of hyponatraemia
- The risk of hyponatraemia is increased in patients taking diuretics, trimethoprim, bupropion, NSAIDs and SSRIs
- Dosulepin is predicted to increase the risk of severe toxic reaction when given with MAOIs; avoid and for 14 days after stopping the MAOI
- Both dosulepin and MAOIs can increase the risk of hypotension
- Do not start an MAOI for at least 5 half-lives (5 to 7 days for most drugs) after discontinuing dosulepin
- Dosulepin may increase the risk of neurotoxicity when given with lithium
- Alcohol and other sedative medications (e.g. promethazine) may compound the sedative properties of dosulepin (beware respiratory depression)
- Activation and agitation, especially following switching or adding antidepressants, may represent the induction of a bipolar state, especially a mixed dysphoric bipolar condition sometimes associated with suicidal ideation, and require the addition of lithium, a mood stabiliser or an atypical antipsychotic, and/or discontinuation of dosulepin

 Other Warnings/Precautions

- Can possibly increase QTc interval at higher doses
- Arrhythmias may occur at higher doses, but are rare
- Increased risk of arrhythmias in patients with hyperthyroidism or phaeochromocytoma

- Caution if patient is taking agents capable of significantly prolonging QTc interval or if there is a history of QTc prolongation
- Caution if the patient is taking drugs that inhibit TCA metabolism, including CYP450 2D6 inhibitors
- Because TCAs can prolong QTc interval, use with caution in patients who have bradycardia or who are taking drugs that can induce bradycardia (e.g. beta blockers, calcium channel blockers, clonidine, digitalis)
- Because TCAs can prolong QTc interval, use with caution in patients who have hypokalaemia and/or hypomagnesaemia or who are taking drugs that can induce hypokalaemia and/or hypomagnesaemia (e.g. diuretics, stimulant laxatives, intravenous amphotericin B, glucocorticoids, tetracosactide)
- Caution if there is reduced CYP450 2D6 function, such as patients who are poor 2D6 metabolisers
- Epidemiological data show that TCAs are associated with an increased risk of fracture which may be secondary to their sedative or hypotensive effect
- Can exacerbate chronic constipation
- Use caution when treating patients with epilepsy
- Use with caution in patients with diabetes
- Use with caution in patients with increased intra-ocular pressure or susceptibility to angle-closure glaucoma
- Use with caution in patients with prostatic hypertrophy or urinary retention
- Use with caution in patients with a history of bipolar disorder, psychosis or significant risk of suicide
- Limited quantities of dosulepin should be prescribed at any one time due to the considerable risk in overdose
- Consider a maximum prescription equivalent to 2 weeks' supply of 75 mg daily in patients with increased risk factors for suicide

Do Not Use

- In patients during a manic phase
- If there is a history of cardiac arrhythmia, recent acute myocardial infarction, heart block
- In patients with acute porphyrias
- If there is a proven allergy to dosulepin

Dosulepin hydrochloride (Continued)

Renal Impairment
- Use with caution
- The majority of active metabolites are renally excreted and may accumulate in renal failure; adjust dose if eGFR <20 mL/minute/1.73 m^2, start with a small dose and titrate to response (monitor for adverse effects)

Hepatic Impairment
- Use with caution in mild-moderate impairment; avoid in severe impairment

Cardiac Impairment
- Baseline ECG is recommended
- TCAs have been reported to cause arrhythmias, prolongation of conduction time, orthostatic hypotension, sinus tachycardia, and heart failure, especially in the diseased heart
- Myocardial infarction and stroke have been reported with TCAs
- An increased incidence of myocardial infarction and stroke has been reported with TCAs
- TCAs produce QTc prolongation, which may be enhanced by the existence of bradycardia, hypokalaemia, congenital or acquired long QTc interval, which should be evaluated prior to administering dosulepin
- Use with caution if treating concomitantly with a medication likely to produce prolonged bradycardia, hypokalaemia, slowing of intracardiac conduction, or prolongation of the QTc interval
- Avoid TCAs in patients with a known history of QTc prolongation, recent acute myocardial infarction, and decompensated heart failure
- TCAs may cause a sustained increase in heart rate in patients with ischaemic heart disease and may worsen (decrease) heart rate variability, an independent risk of mortality in cardiac populations
- Since SSRIs may improve (increase) heart rate variability in patients following a myocardial infarct and may improve survival as well as mood in patients with acute angina or following a myocardial infarction, these are more appropriate agents for cardiac population than tricyclic/tetracyclic antidepressants
- *Risk/benefit ratio may not justify use of TCAs in cardiac impairment

Elderly
- Baseline ECG is recommended for patients over age 50
- May be more sensitive to anticholinergic, cardiovascular, hypotensive, and sedative effects (beware falls)
- Consider a starting dose of 50–75 mg/day
- Reduction in the risk of suicidality with antidepressants compared to placebo in adults age 65 and older
- Therapeutic response can be delayed; the elderly may take longer to respond to antidepressants than younger adults

 Children and Adolescents
- Not recommended for use in children under age 18
- TCAs are more cardiotoxic in young people than in adults
- TCAs are not effective in prepubertal children, and may have moderate efficacy in adolescents and young adults
- Dosulepin has previously been used to treat enuresis or hyperactive/impulsive behaviours
- Some cases of sudden death have occurred in children taking TCAs

 Pregnancy
- No strong evidence of TCA maternal use during pregnancy being associated with an increased risk of congenital malformations
- Risk of malformations cannot be ruled out due to limited information on specific TCAs
- Poor neonatal adaptation syndrome and/or withdrawal have been reported in infants whose mothers took a TCA during pregnancy or near delivery
- Maternal use of more than one CNS-acting medication is likely to lead to more severe symptoms in the neonate
- Must weigh the risk of treatment (first trimester foetal development, third trimester newborn delivery) to the child against the risk of no treatment (recurrence of depression, maternal health, infant bonding) to the mother and child
- For many patients this may mean continuing treatment during pregnancy

Breastfeeding

- Small amounts found in mother's breast milk
- Infant should be monitored for sedation and poor feeding
- Immediate postpartum period is a high-risk time for depression, especially in women who have had prior depressive episodes, antidepressants may need to be reinstituted late in the third trimester or shortly after childbirth to prevent a recurrence during the postpartum period
- Must weigh benefits of breastfeeding with risks and benefits of antidepressant treatment versus nontreatment to both the infant and the mother
- For many patients this may mean continuing treatment during breastfeeding
- Other antidepressants may be preferable, e.g. imipramine or nortriptyline

THE ART OF PSYCHOPHARMACOLOGY

Potential Advantages

- Patients with insomnia
- Severe or treatment-resistant depression
- Anxious depression

Potential Disadvantages

- Paediatric and geriatric patients
- Patients concerned with weight gain
- Cardiac patients
- Risk of fatality in overdose

Primary Target Symptoms

- Depressed mood
- Chronic pain

Pearls

- Close structural similarity to amitriptyline
- TCAs are often a first-line treatment option for chronic pain
- TCAs are no longer generally considered a first-line option for depression because of their side-effect profile
- TCAs continue to be useful for severe or treatment-resistant depression
- TCAs may aggravate psychotic symptoms
- Use with alcohol can cause additive CNS-depressant effects

- Underweight patients may be more susceptible to adverse cardiovascular effects
- Patients with inadequate hydration and patients with cardiac disease may be more susceptible to TCA-induced cardiotoxicity than healthy adults
- Patients on tricyclics should be aware that they may experience symptoms such as photosensitivity or blue-green urine
- SSRIs may be more effective than TCAs in women, and TCAs may be more effective than SSRIs in men
- Dosulepin, alone of the TCAs, may be better tolerated than SSRIs; however, young women may tolerate TCAs less well than men
- Since tricyclic/tetracyclic antidepressants are substrates for CYP450 2D6, and 7% of the population (especially Whites) may have a genetic variant leading to reduced activity of 2D6, such patients may not safely tolerate normal doses of tricyclic/tetracyclic antidepressants and may require dose reduction
- Patients who seem to have extraordinarily severe side effects at normal or low doses may have this phenotypic CYP450 2D6 variant and require low doses or switching to another antidepressant not metabolised by 2D6
- In overdose patients may present with Brugada-like changes on ECG

THE ART OF SWITCHING

 Switching

- Dosulepin should be gradually titrated, ideally after the previous antidepressant has been withdrawn
- Additional care should be taken when switching from bupropion, duloxetine, paroxetine, and fluoxetine as these are all potent CYP450 2D6 inhibitors, and may increase plasma levels of dosulepin
- In treating unipolar depression, the effective dose of dosulepin 150 mg/day is approximately equivalent to fluoxetine 40 mg/day
- When switching from dosulepin, consider that the half-life of active metabolites is 22–60 hours, but may be longer in patients with renal impairment

Dosulepin hydrochloride (Continued)

 Suggested Reading

Anderson IM. Selective serotonin reuptake inhibitors versus tricyclic antidepressants: a meta-analysis of efficacy and tolerability. J Affect Disord 2000;58(1):19–36.

Anderson IM. Meta-analytical studies on new antidepressants. Br Med Bull 2001;57:161–78.

Cleare A, Pariante CM, Young AH, et al. Evidence-based guidelines for treating depressive disorders with antidepressants: a revision of the 2008 British Association for Psychopharmacology guidelines. J Psychopharmacol 2015;29(5):459–525.

Donovan S, Dearden L, Richardson L. The tolerability of dothiepin: a review of clinical studies between 1963 and 1990 in over 13,000 depressed patients. Prog Neuropsychopharmacol Biol Psychiatry 1994;18(7):1143–62.

Lancaster SG, Gonzalez JP. Dothiepin. A review of its pharmacodynamic and pharmacokinetic properties, and therapeutic efficacy in depressive illness. Drugs 1989;38(1):123–47.

Doxepin

THERAPEUTICS

Brands
• Xepin

Generic?
Yes

Class
• Neuroscience-based nomenclature: low-dose doxepin: pharmacology domain – histamine; mode of action – receptor antagonist; upper-dose doxepin: pharmacology domain – norepinephrine, serotonin; mode of action – multimodal
• Tricyclic antidepressant (TCA)
• Serotonin and noradrenaline reuptake inhibitor
• Antihistamine

Commonly Prescribed for
(bold for BNF indication)
• **Depressive illness (particularly where sedation is required)**
• **Pruritus in eczema**
✽ Pruritus/itching (topical)
• Dermatitis, atopic (topical)
• Lichen simplex chronicus (topical)
• Anxiety
• Insomnia
• Neuropathic pain/chronic pain

How the Drug Works
At antidepressant doses:
• Boosts neurotransmitters serotonin and noradrenaline
• Blocks serotonin reuptake pump (serotonin transporter), presumably increasing serotonergic neurotransmission
• Blocks noradrenaline reuptake pump (noradrenaline transporter), presumably increasing noradrenergic neurotransmission
• Presumably desensitises both serotonin 1A receptors and beta adrenergic receptors
• Since dopamine is inactivated by noradrenaline reuptake in frontal cortex, which largely lacks dopamine transporters, doxepin can thus increase dopamine neurotransmission in this part of the brain
• May be effective in treating skin conditions because of its strong antihistamine properties

• Selectively and potently blocks histamine 1 receptors, presumably decreasing wakefulness and thus promoting sleep

How Long Until It Works
• May have immediate effects in treating insomnia or anxiety
• Onset of therapeutic actions with some antidepressants can be seen within 1–2 weeks, but often delayed 2–4 weeks
• If it is not working within 3–4 weeks for depression, it may require a dosage increase or it may not work at all
• By contrast, for generalised anxiety, onset of response and increases in remission rates may still occur after 8 weeks, and for up to 6 months after initiating dosing
• May continue to work for many years to prevent relapse of symptoms

If It Works
• The goal of treatment is complete remission of current symptoms as well as prevention of future relapses
• Treatment most often reduces or even eliminates symptoms, but is not a cure since symptoms can recur after medicine is stopped
• Continue treatment until all symptoms are gone (remission), especially in depression and whenever possible in anxiety disorders
• Once symptoms are gone, continue treating for at least 6–9 months for the first episode of depression or >12 months if relapse indicators present
• If >5 episodes and/or 2 episodes in the last few years then need to continue for at least 2 years or indefinitely
• The goal of treatment of insomnia is to improve quality of sleep, including effects on total wake time and number of night time awakenings
• The goal of treatment of chronic neuropathic pain is to reduce symptoms as much as possible, especially in combination with other treatments
• Treatment of chronic neuropathic pain may reduce symptoms, but rarely eliminates them completely, and is not a cure since symptoms can recur after medicine is stopped
• Use in anxiety disorders, chronic pain, and skin conditions may also need to be indefinite, but long-term treatment is not well studied in these conditions

If It Doesn't Work

- Important to recognise non-response to treatment early on (3–4 weeks)
- Many patients have only a partial response where some symptoms are improved but others persist (especially insomnia, fatigue, and problems concentrating)
- Other patients may be non-responders, sometimes called treatment-resistant or treatment-refractory
- Some patients who have an initial response may relapse even though they continue treatment
- Consider increasing dose, switching to another agent or adding an appropriate augmenting agent
- Lithium may be added for suicidal patients or those at high risk of relapse
- Consider psychotherapy
- Consider ECT
- Consider evaluation for another diagnosis or for a co-morbid condition (e.g. medical illness, substance abuse, etc.)
- Some patients may experience a switch into mania and so would require antidepressant discontinuation and initiation of a mood stabiliser

⚖ Best Augmenting Combos for Partial Response or Treatment Resistance

- Mood stabilisers or atypical antipsychotics for bipolar depression
- Atypical antipsychotics for psychotic depression
- Atypical antipsychotics as first-line augmenting agents (quetiapine MR 300 mg/day or aripiprazole at 2.5–10 mg/day) for treatment-resistant depression
- Atypical antipsychotics as second-line augmenting agents (risperidone 0.5–2 mg/day or olanzapine 2.5–10 mg/day) for treatment-resistant depression
- Mirtazapine at 30–45 mg/day as another second-line augmenting agent (a dual serotonin and noradrenaline combination, but observe for switch into mania, increase in suicidal ideation or serotonin syndrome)
- Although T3 (20–50 mcg/day) is another second-line augmenting agent the evidence suggests that it works best with tricyclic antidepressants

- Other augmenting agents but with less evidence include bupropion (up to 400 mg/day), buspirone (up to 60 mg/day) and lamotrigine (up to 400 mg/day)
- Benzodiazepines if agitation present
- Hypnotics or trazodone for insomnia (but beware of serotonin syndrome with trazodone)
- Augmenting agents reserved for specialist use include: modafinil for sleepiness, fatigue and lack of concentration; stimulants, oestrogens, testosterone
- Lithium is particularly useful for suicidal patients and those at high risk of relapse including with factors such as severe depression, psychomotor retardation, repeated episodes (>3), significant weight loss, or a family history of major depression (aim for lithium plasma levels 0.6–1.0 mmol/L)
- For elderly patients lithium is a very effective augmenting agent
- For severely ill patients other combinations may be tried especially in specialist centres
- Augmenting agents that may be tried include omega-3, SAM-e, L-methylfolate
- Additional non-pharmacological treatments such as exercise, mindfulness, CBT, and IPT can also be helpful
- If present after treatment response (4–8 weeks) or remission (6–12 weeks), the most common residual symptoms of depression include cognitive impairments, reduced energy and problems with sleep
- Gabapentin, tiagabine, other anticonvulsants, even opiates if done by experts while monitoring carefully in difficult cases (for chronic pain)

Tests

- Baseline ECG is useful for patients over age 50
- ECGs may be useful for selected patients (e.g. those with personal or family history of QTc prolongation; cardiac arrhythmia; recent myocardial infarction; decompensated heart failure; or taking agents that prolong QTc interval such as pimozide, thioridazine, selected antiarrhythmics, moxifloxacin etc.)
- ∗Since tricyclic and tetracyclic antidepressants are frequently associated with weight gain, before starting treatment, weigh all patients and determine if the patient is already overweight (BMI 25.0–29.9) or obese (BMI ≥30)
- Before giving a drug that can cause weight gain to an overweight or obese patient,

---

consider determining whether the patient already has:

- Pre-diabetes – fasting plasma glucose: 5.5 mmol/L to 6.9 mmol/L or HbA1c: 42 to 47 mmol/mol (6.0 to 6.4%)
- Diabetes – fasting plasma glucose: >7.0 mmol/L or HbA1c: ≥48 mmol/L (≥6.5%)
- Hypertension (BP >140/90 mm Hg)
- Dyslipidaemia (increased total cholesterol, LDL cholesterol, and triglycerides; decreased HDL cholesterol)
- Treat or refer such patients for treatment, including nutrition and weight management, physical activity counselling, smoking cessation, and medical management

* Monitor weight and BMI during treatment
* While giving a drug to a patient who has gained >5% of initial weight, consider evaluating for the presence of pre-diabetes, diabetes, dyslipidaemia, or consider switching to a different antidepressant

- Patients at risk for electrolyte disturbances (e.g. patients aged >60, patients on diuretic therapy) should have baseline and periodic serum potassium and magnesium measurements

SIDE EFFECTS

How Drug Causes Side Effects

- At antidepressant doses, anticholinergic activity may explain sedative effects, dry mouth, constipation, and blurred vision
- Sedative effects and weight gain may be due to antihistamine properties
- At antidepressant doses, blockade of alpha adrenergic 1 receptors may explain dizziness, sedation, and hypotension
- Cardiac arrhythmias and seizures, especially in overdose, may be caused by blockade of ion channels

Notable Side Effects

- Anticholinergic: dry mouth, blurred vision, constipation, urinary retention
- Nausea, diarrhoea, heartburn, unusual taste in mouth, increased appetite, weight gain
- Fatigue, weakness, dizziness, sedation, headache, anxiety, nervousness, restlessness
- Sexual dysfunction, sweating

Frequency not known

With oral use:
- Blood disorders: agranulocytosis, eosinophilia, haemolytic anaemia, leucopenia, thrombocytopenia

- CNS/PNS: abnormal sensation, agitation, confusion, hallucination, mania, movement disorders, paranoid delusions, psychosis, seizure, sleep disorders, tinnitus, tremor
- CVS: cardiovascular effects, postural hypotension, tachycardia
- Endocrine: galactorrhoea, gynaecomastia
- GIT: decreased appetite, jaundice, oral ulceration, weight increased
- Other: alopecia, anticholinergic syndrome, asthenia, asthma exacerbated, bone marrow depression, breast enlargement, chills, face oedema, flushing, hyperhidrosis, hyperpyrexia, increased risk of fracture, photosensitivity, sexual dysfunction, SIADH, testicular swelling

With topical use:
- Dry eye, fever, paraesthesia

 ### Life-Threatening or Dangerous Side Effects

- Paralytic ileus, hyperthermia (TCAs + anticholinergic agents)
- Lowered seizure threshold and rare seizures
- Orthostatic hypotension, sudden death, arrhythmias, tachycardia
- QTc prolongation
- Hepatic failure, extrapyramidal symptoms
- Increased intraocular pressure
- Rare induction of mania and paranoid delusions
- Rare increase in suicidal ideation and behaviours in adolescents and young adults (up to age 25), hence patients should be warned of this potential adverse event

Weight Gain

- Many experience and/or can be significant in amount (antidepressant doses)
- Can increase appetite and carbohydrate craving
- Weight gain is unusual at hypnotic doses

Sedation

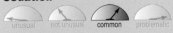

- Many experience and/or can be significant in amount
- Tolerance to sedative effect may develop with long-term use
- Sedation is not unusual at hypnotic doses

What to Do About Side Effects

- Wait
- Wait
- Wait
- The risk of side effects is reduced by titrating slowly to the minimum effective dose (every 2–3 days)
- Consider using a lower starting dose in elderly patients
- Manage side effects that are likely to be transient (e.g. drowsiness) by explanation, reassurance and, if necessary, dose reduction and re-titration
- Giving patients simple strategies for managing mild side effects (e.g. dry mouth) may be useful
- For persistent, severe or distressing side effects the options are:
- Dose reduction and re-titration if possible
- Switching to an antidepressant with a lower propensity to cause that side effect
- Non-drug management of the side effect (e.g. diet and exercise for weight gain)
- Switch to another hypnotic

Best Augmenting Agents for Side Effects

- Many side effects cannot be improved with an augmenting agent

DOSING AND USE

Usual Dosage Range

- Depressive illness: 25 mg/day once daily to 300 mg/day in divided doses

Dosage Forms

- Capsule 25 mg, 50 mg
- Topical 5% cream, 30 g unit

How to Dose

*Depressive illness:
- Adult; child 12–17 years: initial dose 75 mg/day at bedtime or in divided doses; increase gradually; maintenance dose 25–300 mg/day; max dose 300 mg/day; doses above 100 mg should be given in 3 divided doses
- Elderly: start at smaller doses and titrate up very gradually
*Pruritus in eczema:
- Topical – for children over 12 years and adults: apply up to 3 g 3–4 times per day to cover <10% of body surface area; max 12 g/day

Dosing Tips

- If given in a single antidepressant dose, should generally be administered at bedtime because of its sedative properties
- If given in split antidepressant doses, largest dose should generally be given at bedtime because of its sedative properties
- If patients experience nightmares, split antidepressant dose and do not give large dose at bedtime
- Patients treated for chronic pain may only require lower doses
*Topical administration is absorbed systematically and can cause the same systematic side effects as oral administration
- If intolerable anxiety, insomnia, agitation, akathisia, or activation occur either upon dosing initiation or discontinuation, consider the possibility of activated bipolar disorder, and switch to a mood stabiliser or an atypical antipsychotic

Overdose

- Can be fatal; convulsions, CNS depression, coma of varying degree, severe hypotension, hypothermia, hyperreflexia, cardiac conduction defects and arrhythmias, ECG changes. Dilated pupils and urinary retention also occur

Long-Term Use

- Safe

Habit Forming

- No

How to Stop

- Taper gradually to avoid withdrawal effects
- Even with gradual dose reduction some withdrawal symptoms may appear within the first 2 weeks
- It is best to reduce the dose gradually over 4 weeks or longer if withdrawal symptoms emerge
- If severe withdrawal symptoms emerge during discontinuation, raise dose to stop symptoms and then restart withdrawal much more slowly (over at least 6 months in patients on long-term maintenance treatment)

Pharmacokinetics

- Substrate for CYP450 2D6
- Half-life about 8–24 hours

 Drug Interactions

- Tramadol increases the risk of seizures in patients taking TCAs
- Use of TCAs with anticholinergic drugs may result in paralytic ileus or hyperthermia
- Fluoxetine, paroxetine, bupropion, duloxetine, and other CYP450 2D6 inhibitors may increase TCA concentrations
- Cimetidine may increase plasma concentrations of TCAs and cause anticholinergic symptoms
- Dronedarone is predicted to increase exposure to doxepin
- Phenothiazines or haloperidol may raise TCA blood concentrations
- May alter effects of antihypertensive drugs; may inhibit hypotensive effects of clonidine
- Use with sympathomimetic agents may increase sympathetic activity
- Methylphenidate may inhibit metabolism of TCAs
- Anecdotal evidence to suggest increased risk of neurotoxicity when given with lithium
- Predicted to increase risk of severe toxic reaction when given with monoamine oxidase inhibitors, such as isocarboxazid, tranylcypromine and moclobemide
- Most drug interactions may be less likely at low doses (1–6 mg/day – not used in UK) due to the lack of effects on receptors other than the histamine 1 receptors
- Activation and agitation, especially following switching or adding antidepressants, may represent the induction of a bipolar state, especially a mixed dysphoric bipolar condition sometimes associated with suicidal ideation, and require the addition of lithium, a mood stabiliser or an atypical antipsychotic, and/or discontinuation of doxepin

 Other Warnings/Precautions

- Add or initiate other antidepressants with caution for up to 2 weeks after discontinuing doxepin
- Generally, do not use with MAOIs, including 14 days after MAOIs are stopped; do not start an MAOI for at least 5 half-lives (5 to 7 days for most drugs) after discontinuing doxepin, but see Pearls
- Use with caution in patients with epilepsy, diabetes, and chronic constipation
- Use with caution in patients with prostatic hypertrophy, urinary retention, susceptibility to angle-closure glaucoma, and increased intraocular pressure
- Use with caution in patients with cardiovascular disease, heart block, in the immediate recovery period from myocardial infarction, hyperthyroidism, and phaeochromocytoma
- TCAs can increase QTc interval, especially at toxic doses, which can be attained not only by overdose but also by combining with drugs that inhibit TCA metabolism via CYP450 2D6, potentially causing torsade de pointes-type arrhythmia or sudden death
- Because TCAs can prolong QTc interval, use with caution in patients with arrhythmias or bradycardia or who are taking drugs that can induce bradycardia (e.g. beta blockers, calcium channel blockers, clonidine, digitalis)
- Because TCAs can prolong QTc interval, use with caution in patients who have hypokalaemia and/or hypomagnesaemia or who are taking drugs that can induce hypokalaemia and/or hypomagnesaemia (e.g. diuretics, stimulant laxatives, intravenous amphotericin B, glucocorticoids, tetracosactide)
- Use with caution in patients with a history of bipolar disorder or psychosis and patients with a significant risk of suicide
- When treating children, carefully weigh the risks and benefits of pharmacological treatment against the risks and benefits of nontreatment with antidepressants and make sure to document this in the patient's chart
- Warn patients and their caregivers about the possibility of activating side effects and advise them to report such symptoms immediately
- Monitor patients for activation of suicidal ideation, especially children and adolescents

Do Not Use

- If patient is taking agents capable of significantly prolonging QTc interval (e.g. pimozide, thioridazine, selected antiarrhythmics, moxifloxacin)

- If there is severe heart disease including a known history of QT prolongation
- If patient has acute porphyria
- In patients during a manic phase
- If patient is taking drugs that inhibit TCA metabolism, including CYP450 2D6 inhibitors, except by an expert
- If there is reduced CYP450 2D6 function, such as patients who are poor 2D6 metabolisers, except by an expert and at low doses
- If patient has angle-closure glaucoma or severe urinary retention
- If there is a proven allergy to doxepin

SPECIAL POPULATIONS

Renal Impairment

- Use with caution, reduce dose in severe impairment

Hepatic Impairment

- Use with caution – may need lower than usual adult dose
- Sedative effects are increased in hepatic impairment
- Avoid in severe liver disease

Cardiac Impairment

- Baseline ECG is recommended
- TCAs have been reported to cause arrhythmias, prolongation of conduction time, orthostatic hypotension, sinus tachycardia, and heart failure, especially in the diseased heart
- Myocardial infarction and stroke have been reported with TCAs
- TCAs produce QTc prolongation, which may be enhanced by the existence of bradycardia, hypokalaemia, congenital or acquired long QTc interval, which should be evaluated prior to administering doxepin
- Use with caution if treating concomitantly with a medication likely to produce prolonged bradycardia, hypokalaemia, slowing of intracardiac conduction, or prolongation of the QTc interval
- Avoid TCAs in patients with a known history of QTc prolongation, recent acute myocardial infarction, and decompensated heart failure
- TCAs may cause a sustained increase in heart rate in patients with ischaemic heart disease and may worsen (decrease) heart rate variability, an independent risk of mortality in cardiac populations
- Since SSRIs may improve (increase) heart rate variability in patients following a myocardial infarct and may improve survival as well as mood in patients with acute angina or following a myocardial infarction, these are more appropriate agents for cardiac population than tricyclic/ tetracyclic antidepressants
- *Risk/benefit ratio may not justify use of TCAs in cardiac impairment

Elderly

- Baseline ECG required
- May be more sensitive to anticholinergic, cardiovascular, hypotensive, and sedative effects
- Dose selection should be cautious, starting at the low end of the dosing range
- Reduction in the risk of suicidality with antidepressants compared to placebo in adults age 65 and older

 Children and Adolescents

- Indicated for use in depressive illness particularly where sedation is required (child 12–17 years)
- Topical doxepin indicated for pruritus in eczema

 Pregnancy

- No strong evidence of TCA maternal use during pregnancy being associated with an increased risk of congenital malformations
- Risk of malformations cannot be ruled out due to limited information on specific TCAs
- Poor neonatal adaptation syndrome and/or withdrawal has been reported in infants whose mothers took a TCA during pregnancy or near delivery
- Maternal use of more than one CNS-acting medication is likely to lead to more severe symptoms in the neonate
- Must weigh the risk of treatment (first trimester foetal development, third trimester newborn delivery) to the child against the risk of no treatment (recurrence of depression, maternal health, infant bonding) to the mother and child

- For many patients this may mean continuing treatment during pregnancy

Breastfeeding

- Small amounts found in mother's breast milk
- Significant drug levels have been detected in some nursing infants
∗Recommended either to discontinue drug or bottle feed
- Immediate postpartum period is a high-risk time for depression, especially in women who have had prior depressive episodes, so drug may need to be reinstituted late in the third trimester or shortly after childbirth to prevent a recurrence during the postpartum period
- Must weigh benefits of breastfeeding with risks and benefits of antidepressant treatment versus nontreatment to both the infant and the mother
- For many patients this may mean continuing treatment during breastfeeding
- Other antidepressants may be preferable, e.g. imipramine or nortriptyline

THE ART OF PSYCHOPHARMACOLOGY

Potential Advantages

- Patients with insomnia
- Severe or treatment-resistant depression
- Patients with neurodermatitis and itching

Potential Disadvantages

- Elderly patients
- Patients concerned with weight gain
- Cardiac patients

Primary Target Symptoms

- Depressed mood
- Anxiety
- Disturbed sleep, energy
- Somatic symptoms
- Itching skin

 Pearls

∗Only TCA available in topical formulation
∗Topical administration may reduce symptoms in patients with various neurodermatitis syndromes, especially itching
- Can be lethal in overdose, therefore requires careful consideration and risk assessment before prescribing for patients with suicidal ideation
- At low doses (3–6 mg/day as used in some countries outside UK), there is no tolerance to hypnotic actions
- At low doses, there is little or no weight gain
- At low doses doxepin is selective for the histamine 1 receptor and thus can improve sleep without causing side effects associated with other neurotransmitter systems
- In particular, low-dose doxepin does not appear to cause anticholinergic symptoms, memory impairment, or weight gain, nor is there evidence of tolerance, rebound insomnia, or withdrawal effects
- TCAs are often a first-line treatment option for chronic pain
- TCAs are no longer generally considered a first-line option for depression because of their side-effect profile
- TCAs continue to be useful for severe or treatment-resistant depression
- TCAs may aggravate psychotic symptoms
- Alcohol should be avoided because of additive CNS effects
- Underweight patients may be more susceptible to adverse cardiovascular effects
- Children, patients with inadequate hydration, and patients with cardiac disease may be more susceptible to TCA-induced cardiotoxicity than healthy adults
- For the expert only: although generally prohibited, a heroic but potentially dangerous treatment for severely treatment-resistant patients is to give a tricyclic/tetracyclic antidepressant other than clomipramine simultaneously with an MAOI for patients who fail to respond to numerous other antidepressants
- If this option is elected, start the MAOI with the tricyclic/tetracyclic antidepressant simultaneously at low doses after appropriate drug washout, then alternately increase doses of these agents every few days to a week as tolerated
- Although very strict dietary and concomitant drug restrictions must be observed to prevent hypertensive crises and serotonin syndrome, the most common side effects of MAOI/tricyclic or tetracyclic combinations may be weight gain and orthostatic hypotension

- Patients on TCAs should be aware that they may experience symptoms such as photosensitivity or blue-green urine
- SSRIs may be more effective than TCAs in women, and TCAs may be more effective than SSRIs in men
- Since tricyclic/tetracyclic antidepressants are substrates for CYP450 2D6, and 7% of the population (especially Whites) may have a genetic variant leading to reduced activity of 2D6, such patients may not safely tolerate normal doses of tricyclic/tetracyclic antidepressants and may require dose reduction

- Phenotypic testing may be necessary to detect this genetic variant prior to dosing with a tricyclic/tetracyclic antidepressant, especially in vulnerable populations such as children, elderly, cardiac populations, and those on concomitant medications
- Patients who seem to have extraordinarily severe side effects at normal or low doses may have this phenotypic CYP450 2D6 variant and require low doses or switching to another antidepressant not metabolised by 2D6

 ## Suggested Reading

Anderson IM. Selective serotonin reuptake inhibitors versus tricyclic antidepressants: a meta-analysis of efficacy and tolerability. J Affect Disord 2000;58(1):19–36.

Anderson IM. Meta-analytical studies on new antidepressants. Br Med Bull 2001;57:161–78.

Godfrey RG. A guide to the understanding and use of tricyclic antidepressants in the overall management of fibromyalgia and other chronic pain syndromes. Arch Intern Med 1996;156(10):1047–52.

Roth T, Rogowski R, Hull S, et al. Efficacy and safety of doxepin 1 mg, 3 mg, and 6 mg in adults with primary insomnia. Sleep 2007;30(11):1555–61.

Singh H, Becker PM. Novel therapeutic usage of low-dose doxepin hydrochloride. Expert Opin Investig Drugs 2007;16(8):1295–305.

Stahl SM. Selective histamine H1 antagonism: novel hypnotic and pharmacologic actions challenge classical notions of antihistamines. CNS Spectr 2008;13(12):1027–38.

Duloxetine

THERAPEUTICS

Brands
- Yentreve
- Cymbalta
- Depalta
- Duciltia

Generic?
Yes

Class
- Neuroscience-based nomenclature: pharmacology domain – norepinephrine, serotonin; mode of action – reuptake inhibitor
- Second-generation SNRI (dual serotonin and norepinephrine reuptake inhibitor)
- Main action as an antidepressant, but has additional indications

Commonly Prescribed for
(bold for BNF indication)
- **Major depressive disorder**
- **Generalised anxiety disorder**
- **Diabetic neuropathy**
- **Moderate-severe stress urinary incontinence**

 How the Drug Works
- Increases the transmission of serotonin, noradrenaline and dopamine by blocking the reuptake of these neurotransmitters at the synaptic cleft (only weak inhibition of dopamine reuptake)
- Presumed to desensitise the serotonin 1A autoreceptors and beta-adrenergic receptors at the cleft
- Usually noradrenaline reuptake at the synapses in the frontal cortex inactivates dopamine and thus SNRIs relieve dopamine from this inactivating effect

How Long Until It Works
- Initially review at 1–2 weeks to assess for effectiveness, adherence and side effects including suicidality
- Therapeutic effects should be evident within 2–4 weeks
- Can improve neuropathic pain within 1 week, but its onset may be longer
- If it is not working within 3–4 weeks for depression, it may require a dosage increase or it may not work at all

- By contrast, for generalised anxiety, onset of response and increases in remission rates may still occur after 8 weeks, and for up to 6 months after initiating dosing
- May continue to work for many years to prevent relapse of symptoms

If It Works
- The goal of treatment is complete remission of current symptoms as well as prevention of future relapses
- Treatment most often reduces or even eliminates symptoms, but is not a cure since symptoms can recur after medicine is stopped
- Continue treatment until all symptoms are gone (remission), especially in depression and whenever possible in anxiety disorders
- Once symptoms are gone, continue treating for at least 6–9 months for the first episode of depression or >12 months if relapse indicators present
- If >5 episodes and/or 2 episodes in the last few years then need to continue for at least 2 years or indefinitely
- Use in anxiety disorders may also need to be indefinite

If It Doesn't Work
- Important to recognise non-response to treatment early on (3–4 weeks)
- Many patients have only a partial response where some symptoms are improved but others persist
- Other patients may be non-responders, sometimes called treatment-resistant or treatment-refractory
- Consider increasing dose, switching to another agent or adding an appropriate augmenting agent
- Lithium may be added for suicidal patients or those at high risk of relapse
- Consider psychotherapy
- Consider ECT
- Check adherence or consider evaluation for another diagnosis or for a co-morbid condition (e.g. medical illness, substance abuse, etc.)
- Some patients may experience a switch into mania and so would require antidepressant discontinuation and initiation of a mood stabiliser

Duloxetine (Continued)

⚖ Best Augmenting Combos for Partial Response or Treatment Resistance

- Mood stabilisers or atypical antipsychotics for bipolar depression
- Atypical antipsychotics for psychotic depression
- Atypical antipsychotics as first-line augmenting agents (quetiapine MR 300 mg/day or aripiprazole at 2.5–10 mg/day) for treatment-resistant depression
- Atypical antipsychotics as second-line augmenting agents (risperidone 0.5–2 mg/day or olanzapine 2.5–10 mg/day) for treatment-resistant depression
- Mirtazapine at 30–45 mg/day as another second-line augmenting agent (a dual serotonin and noradrenaline combination, but observe for switch into mania, increase in suicidal ideation or rare risk of non-fatal serotonin syndrome)
- Although T3 (20–50 mcg/day) is another second-line augmenting agent the evidence suggests that it works best with tricyclic antidepressants
- The combination of buproprion (up to 400 mg/day) and duloxetine has been shown to be effective in patients who had not responded to either drug as monotherapy
- Other augmenting agents but with less evidence include buspirone (up to 60 mg/day) and lamotrigine (up to 400 mg/day)
- Benzodiazepines if agitation present
- Hypnotics or trazodone for insomnia (but there is a rare risk of non-fatal serotonin syndrome with trazodone)
- Augmenting agents reserved for specialist use include: modafinil for sleepiness, fatigue and lack of concentration; stimulants, oestrogens, testosterone
- Lithium is particularly useful for suicidal patients and those at high risk of relapse including with factors such as severe depression, psychomotor retardation, repeated episodes (>3), significant weight loss, or a family history of major depression (aim for lithium plasma levels 0.6–1.0 mmol/L)
- For elderly patients lithium is a very effective augmenting agent
- For severely ill patients other combinations may be tried especially in specialist centres
- Augmenting agents that may be tried include omega-3, SAM-e, L-methylfolate
- Additional non-pharmacological treatments such as exercise, mindfulness, CBT, and IPT can also be helpful
- If present after treatment response (4–8 weeks) or remission (6–12 weeks), the most common residual symptoms of depression include cognitive impairments, reduced energy and problems with sleep
- In treatment of anxiety, consider gabapentin or pregabalin as augmentation therapy
- In treatment of neuropathic pain, other available agents include gabapentin and pregabalin, although expert supervision is required

Tests

- Blood pressure should be checked prior to initiation of therapy and at regular intervals throughout the treatment course

SIDE EFFECTS

How Drug Causes Side Effects

- Side effects potentially caused by the increase in serotonergic and noradrenergic transmission at unintended locations within the body, e.g. increased serotonin levels in the sleep centre causing insomnia, or increased acetylcholine release causing decreased appetite
- Most side effects are apparent immediately but last only temporarily

Notable Side Effects

- Nausea, diarrhoea, decreased appetite, dry mouth, constipation (dose-dependent)
- Insomnia, sedation, dizziness
- Sexual dysfunction (men: abnormal ejaculation/orgasm, impotence, decreased libido; women: abnormal orgasm)
- Sweating
- Increase in blood pressure (up to 2 mm Hg)
- Urinary retention

Common or very common

- CNS/PNS: anxiety, drowsiness, fall, headache, paraesthesia, sleep disorders, tinnitus, tremor, vision disorders
- CVS: palpitations
- GIT: constipation, decreased appetite, diarrhoea, dry mouth, gastrointestinal discomfort, gastrointestinal disorders, nausea, vomiting, weight changes

- Other: fatigue, flushing, muscle complaints, pain, sexual dysfunction, skin reactions, sweat changes, urinary disorders, yawning

Uncommon

- CNS/PNS: abnormal behaviour, abnormal gait, altered temperature sensation, apathy, disorientation, feeling abnormal, impaired concentration, movement disorders, peripheral coldness, suicidal behaviours, vertigo
- CVS: arrhythmias, postural hypotension, syncope
- GIT: altered taste, burping, dysphagia, hepatic disorders, thirst
- Other: chills, ear pain, haemorrhage, hyperglycaemia, increased risk of infection, malaise, menstrual disorder, mydriasis, photosensitivity reaction, testicular pain, throat tightness

Rare or very rare

- CNS/PNS: hallucination, mania, seizure
- CVS: hypertensive crisis
- GIT: oral disorders
- Other: abnormal urine odour, angioedema, cutaneous vasculitis, dehydration, galactorrhoea, glaucoma, hyperprolactinaemia, hyponatraemia, hypothyroidism, menopausal symptoms, serotonin syndrome, SIADH, Stevens-Johnson syndrome

Life-Threatening or Dangerous Side Effects

- Hypertensive crisis
- Risk of seizure induction
- Rare induction of mania
- Rare increase in suicidal ideation and behaviours in adolescents and young adults (up to age 25), hence patients should be warned of this potential adverse event

Weight Gain

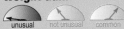

- Uncommon

Sedation

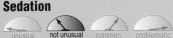

- Occurs in significant minority

What To Do About Side Effects

- Manage side effects that are likely to be transient (e.g. nausea) by explanation, reassurance, and if necessary, dose reduction and re-titration
- Rule out other possible causes for the symptoms
- Give patients simple strategies for managing mild side effects (e.g. dry mouth)
- For persistent or distressing side effects, several options exist
- Dose reduction and titration if possible
- Switch drug to one with a lesser tendency to cause that side effect
- Non-drug management of the side effect
- Symptomatic treatment with a second drug (see below)

Best Augmenting Agents for Side Effects

- Many side effects are dose-dependent (i.e. they increase as dose increases, or they re-emerge until tolerance redevelops)
- Many side effects are time-dependent (i.e. they start immediately upon dosing and upon each dose increase, but go away with time)
- Often best to try another antidepressant monotherapy prior to resorting to augmentation strategies to treat side effects
- Trazodone or a hypnotic for insomnia
- For sexual dysfunction: can augment with bupropion for women, sildenafil for men; or otherwise switch to another antidepressant
- Urinary retention can be treated with an alpha 1 blocker, e.g. tamsulosin
- Mirtazapine for insomnia, agitation, and gastrointestinal side effects
- Benzodiazepines for jitteriness and anxiety, especially at initiation of treatment and especially for anxious patients
- Increased activation or agitation may represent the induction of a bipolar state, especially a mixed dysphoric bipolar condition sometimes associated with suicidal ideation, and requires the addition of lithium, a mood stabiliser or an atypical antipsychotic, and/or discontinuation of duloxetine

DOSING AND USE

Usual Dosage Range

- Major depressive disorder: 60 mg/day
- Generalised anxiety disorder: 30–120 mg/day
- Diabetic neuropathy: 60–120 mg/day in 1–2 divided doses
- Stress urinary incontinence in females: 20–40 mg twice per day

Dosage Forms

- Capsule (gastro-resistant) 20 mg, 30 mg, 40 mg, 60 mg

How to Dose

* Major depressive disorder:
- 60 mg/day
* Generalised anxiety disorder:
- Initial dose 30 mg/day, increased to 60 mg/day (max 120 mg/day)
* Diabetic neuropathy:
- 60 mg/day, max dose 120 mg/day in divided doses. Review at least every 3 months
* Stress urinary incontinence in females:
- Initial dose 20 mg twice per day for 2 weeks; can increase further to 40 mg twice per day. Review after 2–4 weeks

Dosing Tips

- There is insufficient data to support use of duloxetine doses greater than 60 mg in depression
- If using daily doses of 120 mg, divide the daily dose and only prescribe on expert advice

Overdose

- Toxicity is low in overdose
- Signs of overdose may include drowsiness, bradycardia, hypotension
- Rare fatalities have been reported, including serotonin syndrome and coma induction

Long-Term Use

- Regular monitoring of blood pressure required

Habit Forming

- No

How to Stop

- If taking duloxetine for more than 6-8 weeks, it is not recommended to stop it suddenly due to the risk of withdrawal effects (nausea, vomiting, headache, anxiety, sleep disturbance, tremor, dizziness and paraesthesia)
- Taper dose gradually over 4 weeks, or longer if withdrawal symptoms emerge
- Inform all patients of the risk of withdrawal symptoms
- If withdrawal symptoms emerge, raise dose to stop symptoms and then restart withdrawal much more slowly

Pharmacokinetics

- Elimination half-life of about 8–17 hours
- Duloxetine inhibits CYP450 2D6
- CYP450 1A2 inhibition increases duloxetine exposure to a degree that is clinically relevant
- Several factors affect the pharmacokinetics of the drug, including sex, age and smoking status, but only hepatic impairment and severe renal failure warrant dose reductions or warnings
- Smoking is associated with a 30% decrease in duloxetine concentration
- Absorption may be impaired and clearance increased by up to one-third for an evening dose compared to a morning dose
- No relationship between ingestion of food and absorption

Drug Interactions

- Tramadol increases the risk of seizures in patients taking an antidepressant
- Can cause a fatal "serotonin syndrome" when combined with MAOIs, so do not use with MAOI or for at least 14 days after MAOIs are stopped
- Do not start an MAOI for at least 5 half-lives (5 to 7 days for most drugs) after discontinuing duloxetine
- Possible increased risk of bleeding, especially when combined with anticoagulants (e.g. warfarin, NSAIDs)
- Inhibition of CYP450 1A2 may increase plasma clozapine levels
- Inhibition of CYP450 2D6 can render tamoxifen (prodrug) ineffective, resulting in treatment failure and potentially increased mortality
- Can increase TCA levels – if switching between duloxetine and a TCA, a slow cross-taper is advised, with a low dose of TCA to start
- Risk of serotonin syndrome if used in conjunction with other serotonin transmission enhancing agents

Other Warnings/Precautions

- Duloxetine can increase systolic blood pressure, so monitoring of blood pressure is recommended
- Warn patients and their family about the risks of treatment, inform them of side effects and encourage early reporting

- Caution in patients with bleeding disorders, the elderly, history of mania or history of seizures
- Caution in patients with cardiac disease and hypertension
- Caution in patients with raised intra-ocular pressure or susceptibility to angle-closure glaucoma
- When treating children, carefully weigh the risks and benefits of pharmacological treatment against the risks and benefits of nontreatment with antidepressants and make sure to document this in patient notes
- Warn patients and their caregivers about the possibility of activating side effects and advise them to report such symptoms immediately
- Monitor patients for activation of suicidal ideation, especially children and adolescents

Do Not Use
- If patient has uncontrolled angle-closure glaucoma
- In uncontrolled hypertension
- If patient is taking an MAOI
- If there is a proven allergy to duloxetine

SPECIAL POPULATIONS

Renal Impairment
- No dose adjustment needed in moderate impairment
- Start with very low dose in severe impairment; avoid in chronic kidney disease as it can accumulate

Hepatic Impairment
- Avoid in hepatic impairment
- Clearance of duloxetine is markedly decreased even in minimal hepatic impairment
- There have been reports of deranged liver enzymes with duloxetine use, alongside reports of hepatic or cholestatic injury, although these are very rare

Cardiac Impairment
- Caution is advised in individuals with cardiac disease
- Use cautiously in hypertension, as its use can cause elevation of systolic blood pressure
- Caution should also be taken in those having recently suffered a myocardial infarction

- There is limited clinical evidence of its use in cardiac impairment, and therefore its use is not recommended

Elderly
- Caution in the elderly population
- Trials have shown its use to be safe in the elderly for treatment of depression, with most commonly reported side effects including dry mouth, constipation and nausea
- SNRIs may be particularly useful for elderly suffering with pain alongside depression
- The elderly may require a lower starting dose – start at 30 mg/day, with potential to increase to 120 mg/day in divided doses as needed
- Risk of hyponatraemia, raised systolic blood pressure and bleeding (gastrointestinal or haemorrhagic strokes)

 ### Children and Adolescents
- Not licensed for use in children in UK
- Duloxetine has been approved in USA for use in treatment of paediatric generalised anxiety disorder, often employed third-line after a trial of 2 different SSRIs proves ineffective

 ### Pregnancy
- Controlled studies have not been conducted in pregnant women
- Not generally recommended for use during pregnancy, especially during first trimester
- Nonetheless, continuous treatment during pregnancy may be necessary and has not been proven to be harmful to the foetus
- Must weigh the risk of treatment (first trimester foetal development, third trimester newborn delivery) to the child against the risk of no treatment (recurrence of depression, maternal health, infant bonding) to the mother and child
- For many patients this may mean continuing treatment during pregnancy
- Although there is no data to substantiate, there is a theoretical risk that as with SSRIs when used beyond the 20th week of pregnancy there is increased risk of persistent pulmonary hypertension (PPHN) in newborns

Duloxetine (Continued)

- SSRI/SNRI antidepressant use in the month before delivery may result in a small increased risk of postpartum haemorrhage
- Neonates exposed to SSRIs or SNRIs late in the third trimester have developed complications requiring prolonged hospitalisation, respiratory support, and tube feeding; reported symptoms are consistent with either a direct toxic effect of SSRIs and SNRIs or, possibly, a drug discontinuation syndrome, and include respiratory distress, cyanosis, apnoea, seizures, temperature instability, feeding difficulty, vomiting, hypoglycaemia, hypotonia, hypertonia, hyperreflexia, tremor, jitteriness, irritability, and constant crying

Breastfeeding

- Small amounts found in mother's breast milk
- If child becomes irritable or sedated, breastfeeding or drug may need to be discontinued
- Immediate postpartum period is a high-risk time for depression, especially in women who have had prior depressive episodes, so drug may need to be reinstituted late in the third trimester or shortly after childbirth to prevent a recurrence during the postpartum period
- Must weigh benefits of breastfeeding with risks and benefits of antidepressant treatment versus nontreatment to both the infant and the mother
- For many patients, this may mean continuing treatment during breastfeeding
- Other antidepressants may be preferable, e.g. paroxetine, sertraline, imipramine, or nortriptyline

THE ART OF PSYCHOPHARMACOLOGY
Potential Advantages
- Those with physical symptoms of depression
- Those with atypical depression
- Those with co-morbid anxiety

- Those with depression may experience higher remission rates with SNRIs versus SSRIs
- Those who do not respond or remit on treatment with SSRIs

Potential Disadvantages
- Those with urology disorders, e.g. enlarged prostate
- Those who are sensitive to nausea

Primary Target Symptoms
- Depressed mood
- Sleep disturbance
- Anxiety
- Physical symptoms
- Pain

 Pearls
- Useful for the painful symptoms of depression
- Powerful pro-noradrenaline actions may occur at dose >60 mg/day
- SNRIs may lead to higher remission rates than SSRIs
- Caution when switching with another pro-noradrenaline agent (e.g. atomoxetine, reboxetine, other SNRI, nortriptyline)
- Caution when switching with a CYP450 2D6 substrate (e.g. atomoxetine, nortriptyline)

THE ART OF SWITCHING
 Switching
- When changing from one agent to another, sudden discontinuation is not recommended unless switching between agents with similar action, e.g. duloxetine and other SSRIs and SNRIs
- Cross-tapering is preferred, in which the dose of duloxetine is gradually reduced, usually weekly, as the other agent is slowly introduced
- The speed of cross-tapering will be determined by the patient and any adverse effects or lack of tolerability
- Rare risk of non-fatal serotonin syndrome if two agents that act to potentiate serotonin transmission are co-administered

Suggested Reading

Abdey NA, Gerhart K. Duloxetine withdrawal syndrome in a newborn. Clin Pediatr (Phila) 2013;52(10):976–7.

Cipriani A, Furukawa TA, Salanti G, et al. Comparative efficacy and acceptability of 21 antidepressant drugs for the acute treatment of adults with major depressive disorder: a systematic review and network meta-analysis. Lancet 2018;391(10128):1357–66.

Cleare A, Pariante CM, Young AH, et al. Evidence-based guidelines for treating depressive disorders with antidepressants: a revision of the 2008 British Association for Psychopharmacology guidelines. J Psychopharmacol 2015;29(5);459–525.

Hoog SL, Cheng Y, Elpers J, et al. Duloxetine and pregnancy outcomes: safety surveillance findings. Int J Med Sci 2013;10(4):413–19.

Knadler MP, Lobo E, Chappell J, et al. Duloxetine: clinical pharmacokinetics and drug interactions. Clin Pharmacokinet 2011;50(5):281–94.

Nagler EV, Webster AC, Vanholder R, et al. Antidepressants for depression in stage 3–5 chronic kidney disease: a systematic review of pharmacokinetics, efficacy and safety with recommendations by European Renal Best Practice (ERBP). Nephrol Dial Transplant 2012;27(10):3736–45.

Oakes TM, Katona C, Liu P, et al. Safety and tolerability of duloxetine in elderly patients with major depressive disorder: a pooled analysis of two placebo-controlled studies. Int Clin Psychopharmacol 2013;28(1):1–11.

Papakostas GI, Worthington 3rd JJ, Iosifescu DV, et al. The combination of duloxetine and bupropion for treatment-resistant major depressive disorder. Depress Anxiety 2006;23(3):178–81.

Wernicke J, Acharya N, Strombom I, et al. Hepatic effects of duloxetine-II: spontaneous reports and epidemiology of hepatic events. Curr Drug Saf 2008;3(2):143–53.

Escitalopram

Brands
- Cipralex

Generic?
Yes

Class
- Neuroscience-based nomenclature: pharmacology domain – serotonin; mode of action – reuptake inhibitor
- SSRI (selective serotonin reuptake inhibitor); often classified as an antidepressant, but it is not just an antidepressant

Commonly Prescribed for
(bold for BNF indication)
- **Depressive illness**
- **Generalised anxiety disorder (GAD)**
- **Panic disorder**
- **Obsessive-compulsive disorder (OCD)**
- **Social anxiety disorder (social phobia)**
- Post-traumatic stress disorder (PTSD)
- Premenstrual dysphoric disorder

 How the Drug Works
- Boosts neurotransmitter serotonin
- Blocks serotonin reuptake pump (serotonin transporter)
- Desensitises serotonin receptors, especially serotonin 1A autoreceptors
- Presumably increases serotonergic neurotransmission

How Long Until It Works
- Onset of therapeutic actions with some antidepressants can be seen within 1–2 weeks, but often delayed 2–4 weeks
- If it is not working within 3–4 weeks for depression, it may require a dosage increase or it may not work at all
- By contrast, for generalised anxiety, onset of response and increases in remission rates may still occur after 8 weeks, and for up to 6 months after initiating dosing
- For OCD if no improvement within about 10–12 weeks, then treatment may need to be reconsidered
- May continue to work for many years to prevent relapse of symptoms

If It Works
- The goal of treatment is complete remission of current symptoms as well as prevention of future relapses
- Treatment most often reduces or even eliminates symptoms, but is not a cure since symptoms can recur after medicine is stopped
- Continue treatment until all symptoms are gone (remission), especially in depression and whenever possible in anxiety disorders (e.g. OCD, PTSD)
- Once symptoms are gone, continue treating for at least 6–9 months for the first episode of depression or >12 months if relapse indicators present
- If >5 episodes and/or 2 episodes in the last few years then need to continue for at least 2 years or indefinitely
- For OCD continue treatment for at least 12 months for patients that have responded to treatment
- Use in anxiety disorders may need to be indefinite

If It Doesn't Work
- Important to recognise non-response to treatment in depression early on (3–4 weeks)
- Many patients have only a partial response where some symptoms are improved but others persist (especially insomnia, fatigue, and problems concentrating in depression)
- Other patients may be non-responders, sometimes called treatment-resistant or treatment-refractory
- Some patients who have an initial response may relapse even though they continue treatment
- Consider increasing dose, switching to another agent, or adding an appropriate augmenting agent
- Lithium may be added for suicidal patients or those at high risk of relapse in depression
- Consider psychotherapy
- Consider ECT in depression
- Consider evaluation for another diagnosis or for a co-morbid condition (e.g. medical illness, substance abuse, etc.)
- Some patients may experience a switch into mania and so would require antidepressant discontinuation and initiation of a mood stabiliser

Best Augmenting Combos for Partial Response or Treatment Resistance

In OCD:
- Consider cautious addition of an antipsychotic (risperidone, quetiapine, olanzapine, aripiprazole or haloperidol) as augmenting agent
- Alternative augmenting agents may include ondansetron, granisetron, topiramate, lamotrigine
- A switch to clomipramine may be a better option in treatment-resistant cases
- Combine an SSRI or clomipramine with an evidence-based psychological treatment

In depression:
- Mood stabilisers or atypical antipsychotics for bipolar depression
- Atypical antipsychotics for psychotic depression
- Atypical antipsychotics as first-line augmenting agents (quetiapine MR 300 mg/day or aripiprazole at 2.5–10 mg/day) for treatment-resistant depression
- Atypical antipsychotics as second-line augmenting agents (risperidone 0.5–2 mg/day or olanzapine 2.5–10 mg/day) for treatment-resistant depression
- Mirtazapine at 30–45 mg/day as another second-line augmenting agent (a dual serotonin and noradrenaline combination, but observe for switch into mania, increase in suicidal ideation or rare risk of non-fatal serotonin syndrome)
- Although T3 (20–50 mcg/day) is another second-line augmenting agent the evidence suggests that it works best with tricyclic antidepressants
- Other augmenting agents but with less evidence include bupropion (up to 400 mg/day), buspirone (up to 60 mg/day) and lamotrigine (up to 400 mg/day)
- Benzodiazepines may be considered if agitation or anxiety present with appropriate warnings about dependence issues
- Hypnotics or trazodone for insomnia (but there is a rare risk of non-fatal serotonin syndrome with trazodone)
- Augmenting agents reserved for specialist use include: modafinil for sleepiness, fatigue and lack of concentration; stimulants, oestrogens, testosterone
- Lithium is particularly useful for suicidal patients and those at high risk of relapse including with factors such as severe depression, psychomotor retardation, repeated episodes (>3), significant weight loss, or a family history of major depression (aim for lithium plasma levels 0.6–1.0 mmol/L)
- For elderly patients lithium is a very effective augmenting agent
- For severely ill patients other combinations may be tried especially in specialist centres
- Augmenting agents that may be tried include omega-3, SAM-e, L-methylfolate
- Additional non-pharmacological treatments such as exercise, mindfulness, CBT, and IPT can also be helpful
- If present after treatment response (4–8 weeks) or remission (6–12 weeks), the most common residual symptoms of depression include cognitive impairments, reduced energy and problems with sleep
- If all else fails for anxiety disorders, consider pregabalin or gabapentin

Tests
- ECG monitoring for those at risk of cardiac disease due to risk of QT prolongation

SIDE EFFECTS
How Drug Causes Side Effects
- Theoretically due to increases in serotonin concentrations at serotonin receptors in parts of the brain and body other than those that cause therapeutic actions (e.g. unwanted actions of serotonin in sleep centres causing insomnia, unwanted actions of serotonin in the gut causing diarrhoea, etc.)
- Increasing serotonin can cause diminished dopamine release and might contribute to emotional flattening, cognitive slowing and apathy in some patients
- Most side effects are immediate but often go away with time, in contrast to most therapeutic effects which are delayed and are enhanced over time
- *As escitalopram has no known important secondary pharmacologic properties, its side effects are presumably all mediated by its serotonin reuptake blockade

Notable Side Effects
- CNS: headache, drowsiness, dizziness, memory loss, sleep disorders, tinnitus, altered taste, tremor, visual impairment
- CVS: arrhythmias, palpitations

- GIT: abnormal appetite, constipation, diarrhoea, dry mouth, GI upset, nausea (dose-related), vomiting
- Sexual dysfunction (dose-dependent; men: delayed ejaculation, erectile dysfunction; men and women: decreased libido, anorgasmia)
- Rare SIADH (syndrome of inappropriate antidiuretic hormone secretion)
- Rare hyponatraemia (mostly in elderly patients, reversible)
- Mood elevation in diagnosed or undiagnosed bipolar disorder
- Sweating (dose-dependent)
- Bruising and rare bleeding

Common or very common
- Sinusitis

Uncommon
- Oedema

 Life-Threatening or Dangerous Side Effects
- Rare seizures
- Rare induction of mania
- Rare increase in suicidal ideation and behaviours in adolescents and young adults (up to age 25), hence patients should be warned of this potential adverse event

Weight Gain

unusual / not unusual / common / problematic

- Reported but not expected

Sedation

unusual / not unusual / common / problematic

- Reported but not expected

What to Do About Side Effects
- Manage side effects that are likely to be transient (e.g. nausea) by explanation, reassurance, and if necessary, dose reduction and re-titration
- Give patients simple strategies for managing mild side effects (e.g. dry mouth)
- For persistent or distressing side effects, several options exist:
  - Dose reduction and titration if possible
  - Switch drug to one with a lesser tendency to cause that side effect
  - Non-drug management of the side effect, e.g. diet and exercise for weight gain

- Symptomatic treatment with a second drug (see below)

Best Augmenting Agents for Side Effects
- Many side effects are dose-dependent (i.e. they increase as dose increases, or they re-emerge until tolerance redevelops)
- Many side effects are time-dependent (i.e. they start immediately upon dosing and upon each dose increase, but go away with time)
- Often best to try another antidepressant monotherapy prior to resorting to augmentation strategies to treat side effects
- Trazodone, mirtazapine or hypnotic for insomnia
- Mirtazapine for agitation, and gastrointestinal side effects
- Bupropion for emotional flattening, cognitive slowing, or apathy
- For sexual dysfunction: can augment with bupropion for women, sildenafil for men; or otherwise switch to another antidepressant
- Benzodiazepines for jitteriness and anxiety, especially at initiation of treatment and especially for anxious patients
- Increased activation or agitation may represent the induction of a bipolar state, especially a mixed dysphoric bipolar condition sometimes associated with suicidal ideation, and requires the addition of lithium, a mood stabiliser or an atypical antipsychotic, and/or discontinuation of the SSRI

DOSING AND USE

Usual Dosage Range
- Depressive illness, GAD, OCD: 10–20 mg/day
- Panic disorder, social anxiety disorder: 5–20 mg/day
- Elderly for depressive illness, GAD, OCD and panic disorder: 5–10 mg/day

Dosage Forms
- Tablet 5 mg, 10 mg, 20 mg
- Oral drops 20 mg/mL

How to Dose
* Depressive illness, GAD, OCD:
- Initial dose 10 mg/day; increased to 20 mg/day as needed
* Panic disorder:
- Initial dose 5 mg/day for 1 week, increased to 10 mg/day, max 20 mg/day
* Social anxiety disorder:
- 10 mg/day for 2–4 weeks, adjust to 5–20 mg/day

Dosing Tips

- Given once daily, usually in the morning to avoid insomnia
- *10 mg of escitalopram may be comparable in efficacy to 40 mg of citalopram with fewer side effects
- Thus, give an adequate trial of 10 mg prior to giving 20 mg
- Some patients require dosing with 30 or 40 mg (unlicensed)
- If intolerable anxiety, insomnia, agitation, akathisia, or activation occur either upon dosing initiation or discontinuation, consider the possibility of activated bipolar disorder and switch to a mood stabiliser or an atypical antipsychotic

Overdose

- Few reports of escitalopram overdose, but probably similar to citalopram overdose
- Rare fatalities have been reported in citalopram overdose, both in combination with other drugs and alone
- Symptoms associated with citalopram overdose include vomiting, sedation, heart rhythm disturbances, dizziness, sweating, nausea, tremor, and rarely amnesia, confusion, coma, convulsions
- Severe overdose can result in serotonin syndrome – symptoms and signs include: neuromuscular hyperactivity, autonomic instability, hyperthermia, rhabdomyolysis, renal failure and coagulopathies

Long-Term Use

- Safe

Habit Forming

- No

How to Stop

- If taking SSRIs for more than 6–8 weeks, it is not recommended to stop them suddenly due to the risk of withdrawal effects (dizziness, nausea, stomach cramps, sweating, tingling, dysaesthesias)
- Taper dose gradually over 4 weeks, or longer if withdrawal symptoms emerge
- Inform all patients of the risk of withdrawal symptoms
- If withdrawal symptoms emerge, raise dose to stop symptoms and then restart withdrawal much more slowly

Pharmacokinetics

- Mean elimination half-life about 30 hours
- Steady-state plasma concentrations achieved within 1 week
- No significant actions on CYP450 enzymes

 Drug Interactions

- Tramadol increases the risk of seizures in patients taking an antidepressant
- Can increase TCA levels; use with caution with TCAs or when switching from a TCA to escitalopram
- Can cause a fatal "serotonin syndrome" when combined with MAOIs, so do not use with MAOIs or for at least 14 days after MAOIs are stopped
- Do not start an MAOI for at least 5 half-lives (5 to 7 days for most drugs) after discontinuing escitalopram
- Could theoretically cause weakness, hyperreflexia, and incoordination when combined with sumatriptan or possibly other triptans, requiring careful monitoring of patient
- Increased risk of bleeding when used in combination with NSAIDs, aspirin, alteplase, anti-platelets, and anticoagulants
- NSAIDs may impair effectiveness of SSRIs
- Increased risk of hyponatraemia when escitalopram is used in combination with other agents that cause hyponatraemia, e.g. thiazides
- Avoid using in combination with other drugs that prolong the QT interval, e.g. amiodarone, amisulpride, haloperidol, pimozide
- Caution when administering escitalopram in combination with cimetidine (potent CYP450 2D6, 3A4 and 1A2 inhibitor) as cimetidine can raise escitalopram plasma levels

 Other Warnings/Precautions

- Drug causes a dose-dependent prolongation of QT interval
- Use with caution in patients with diabetes
- Use with caution in patients with susceptibility to angle-closure glaucoma
- Use with caution in patients receiving ECT or with a history of seizures
- Use with caution in patients with a history of bleeding disorders
- Use with caution in patients with bipolar disorder unless treated with concomitant mood-stabilising agent

- When treating children, carefully weigh the risks and benefits of pharmacological treatment against the risks and benefits of nontreatment with antidepressants and make sure to document this in patient notes
- Warn patients and their caregivers about the possibility of activating side effects and advise them to report such symptoms immediately
- Monitor patients for activation of suicidal ideation, especially children and adolescents

Do Not Use

- If patient has poorly controlled epilepsy
- If patient enters a manic phase
- If patient has QT prolongation
- If patient is already taking an MAOI (risk of serotonin syndrome)
- If patient is taking pimozide
- If there is a proven allergy to escitalopram or citalopram

SPECIAL POPULATIONS

Renal Impairment

- No dose adjustment for mild to moderate impairment
- Use cautiously in patients with severe impairment

Hepatic Impairment

- Recommended dose in mild-moderate impairment 5 mg/day for 2 weeks then increased up to 10 mg/day according to response
- Dose should be titrated cautiously in severe impairment

Cardiac Impairment

- Risk of QT prolongation with citalopram and escitalopram
- Contraindicated in QT prolongation
- Treating depression with SSRIs in patients with acute angina or following myocardial infarction may reduce cardiac events and improve survival as well as mood

Elderly

- Depressive illness, GAD, OCD, panic disorder: recommended dose 5 mg/day, max dose 10 mg/day
- Risk of SIADH with SSRIs is higher in the elderly
- Reduction in the risk of suicidality with antidepressants compared to placebo in adults age 65 and older

- May cause osteopenia, increases clinical risk if the patient should have a fall

 ### Children and Adolescents

- Escitalopram is not licensed for use in children and adolescents
- If used this should be under child and adolescent consultant psychiatrist supervision
- For mild to moderate depression psychotherapy (individual or systemic) should be the first-line treatment. For moderate to severe depression, pharmacological treatment may be offered when the young person is unresponsive after 4–6 sessions of psychological therapy. Combined initial therapy (fluoxetine and psychological therapy) may be considered
- For anxiety disorders evidence-based psychological treatments should be offered as first-line treatment including psychoeducation and skills training for parents, particularly of young children, to promote and reinforce the child's exposure to feared or avoided social situations and development of skills
- For OCD, children and young people, should be offered CBT (including exposure response prevention – ERP) that involves the family or carers and is adapted to suit the developmental age of the child as the treatment of choice
- For both severe depression and anxiety disorders, pharmacological interventions may have to commence prior to psychological treatments to enable the child/young person to engage in psychological therapy
- Where a child or young person presents with self-harm and suicidal thoughts the immediate risk management may take first priority as suicidal thoughts might increase in the initial stages of treatment
- All children and young people presenting with depression/anxiety should be supported with sleep management, anxiety management, exercise and activation schedules, and healthy diet

Practical notes:
- A risk management plan should be discussed prior to start of medication because of the possible increase in suicidal ideation and behaviours in adolescents and young adults

- Monitor patients face-to-face regularly, and weekly during the first 2–3 weeks of treatment or after an increase in dose
- Monitor for activation of suicidal ideation at the beginning of treatment
- Use with caution, observing for activation of known or unknown bipolar disorder and/or suicidal ideation, and inform parents or guardians of this risk so they can help observe child or adolescent patients

If it does not work:
- Review child's/young person's profile, consider new/changing contributing individual or systemic factors such as peer or family conflict. Consider physical health problems
- Consider non-concordance, especially in adolescents. In all children consider non-concordance by parent or child, address underlying reasons for non-concordance
- Consider dose adjustment before switching or augmentation. Be vigilant of polypharmacy especially in complex and highly vulnerable children/adolescents
- For all SSRIs children can have a two-to three-fold higher incidence of behavioural activation and vomiting than adolescents, who also have a somewhat higher incidence than adults
- Children taking SSRIs may have slower growth; long-term effects are unknown
- Adolescents often receive adult dose, but doses slightly lower for children
- Re-evaluate the need for continued treatment regularly

Pregnancy

- Not generally recommended for use during pregnancy, especially during first trimester
- Nonetheless, continuous treatment during pregnancy may be necessary and has not been proven to be harmful to the foetus
- Must weigh the risk of treatment (first trimester foetal development, third trimester newborn delivery) to the child against the risk of no treatment (recurrence of depression, maternal health, infant bonding) to the mother and child
- For many patients, this may mean continuing treatment during pregnancy
- Exposure to SSRIs in pregnancy has been associated with cardiac malformations, however recent studies have suggested that these findings may be due to other patient factors
- Exposure to SSRIs in pregnancy has been associated with an increased risk of spontaneous abortion, low birth weight and preterm delivery. Data is conflicting and the effects of depression cannot be ruled out from some studies
- SSRI use beyond the 20th week of pregnancy may be associated with increased risk of persistent pulmonary hypertension (PPHN) in newborns. Whilst the risk of PPHN remains low it presents potentially serious complications
- SSRI/SNRI antidepressant use in the month before delivery may result in a small increased risk of postpartum haemorrhage
- Neonates exposed to SSRIs or SNRIs late in the third trimester have developed complications requiring prolonged hospitalisation, respiratory support, and tube feeding; reported symptoms are consistent with either a direct toxic effect of SSRIs and SNRIs or, possibly, a drug discontinuation syndrome, and include respiratory distress, cyanosis, apnoea, seizures, temperature instability, feeding difficulty, vomiting, hypoglycaemia, hypotonia, hypertonia, hyperreflexia, tremor, jitteriness, irritability, and constant crying

Breastfeeding

- Small amounts found in mother's breast milk
- Small amounts may be present in nursing children whose mothers are taking escitalopram
- Case report of necrotising enterocolitis in an infant exposed to escitalopram during pregnancy and breastfeeding
- If child becomes irritable or sedated, breastfeeding or drug may need to be discontinued
- Immediate postpartum period is a high-risk time for depression, especially in women who have had prior depressive episodes, so drug may need to be reinstituted late in the third trimester or shortly after childbirth to prevent a recurrence during the postpartum period
- Must weigh benefits of breastfeeding with risks and benefits of antidepressant treatment versus nontreatment to both the infant and the mother

- For many patients, this may mean continuing treatment during breastfeeding
- Other SSRIs (e.g. sertraline or paroxetine) may be preferable for breastfeeding mothers

THE ART OF PSYCHOPHARMACOLOGY

Potential Advantages

- Patients taking concomitant medications (few drug interactions and fewer even than with citalopram)
- Patients requiring faster onset of action

Potential Disadvantages

- More expensive than citalopram in markets where citalopram is generic
- Not licensed for children
- In children: those who already show psychomotor agitation, anger, irritability, or who do not have a psychiatric diagnosis

Primary Target Symptoms

- Depressed mood
- Anxiety
- Panic attacks, avoidant behaviour, re-experiencing, hyperarousal
- Sleep disturbance, both insomnia and hypersomnia

Pearls

* May be among the best-tolerated antidepressants

- May have less sexual dysfunction than some other SSRIs
- May be better tolerated than citalopram
- Can cause cognitive and affective "flattening"
  * R-citalopram may interfere with the binding of S-citalopram at the serotonin transporter
  * For this reason, S-citalopram may be more than twice as potent as R,S-citalopram (i.e. citalopram)
- Thus, 10 mg starting dose of S-citalopram may have the therapeutic efficacy of 40 mg of R,S-citalopram
- Thus, escitalopram may have faster onset and better efficacy with reduced side effects compared to R,S-citalopram
  * Escitalopram is commonly used with augmenting agents, as it is the SSRI with the least interaction at either CYP450 2D6 or 3A4, therefore causing fewer pharmacokinetically mediated drug interactions with augmenting agents than other SSRIs
- SSRIs may be less effective in women over 50, especially if they are not taking oestrogen
- SSRIs may be useful for hot flushes in perimenopausal women
- Some postmenopausal women's depression will respond better to escitalopram plus oestrogen augmentation than to escitalopram alone
- Non-response to escitalopram in elderly may require consideration of mild cognitive impairment or Alzheimer's disease

 Suggested Reading

Baldwin DS, Reines EH, Guiton C, et al. Escitalopram therapy for major depression and anxiety disorders. Ann Pharmacother 2007;41(10):1583–92.

Bareggi SR, Mundo E, Dell'Osso B, et al. The use of escitalopram beyond major depression: pharmacological aspects, efficacy and tolerability in anxiety disorders. Expert Opin Drug Metab Toxicol 2007;3(5):741–53.

Burke WJ. Escitalopram. Expert Opin Investig Drugs 2002;11(10):1477–86.

Cipriani A, Furukawa TA, Salanti G, et al. Comparative efficacy and acceptability of 21 antidepressant drugs for the acute treatment of adults with major depressive disorder: a systematic review and network meta-analysis. Lancet 2018;391(10128):1357–66.

Esketamine

Brands

- Spravato
- Vesierra

Generic?

Yes (solution for injection only)

Class

- Neuroscience-based nomenclature: pharmacology domain – glutamate; mode of action – antagonist
- Glutamate N-methyl-D-aspartate (NMDA) receptor antagonist

Commonly Prescribed for

(bold for BNF indication)

- **Major depressive disorder (specialist use only)**
- **Induction and maintenance of anaesthesia (specialist use only)**
- **Analgesic supplementation of regional and local anaesthesia (specialist use only)**
- **Analgesia in emergency medicine (specialist use only)**

 How the Drug Works

- Esketamine is a nonselective, noncompetitive open channel inhibitor of the NMDA receptor; specifically, it binds to the phencyclidine site of the NMDA receptor
- This leads to downstream glutamate release and consequent stimulation of other glutamate receptors, including AMPA receptors
- Theoretically, esketamine may have antidepressant effects because activation of AMPA receptors leads to activation of signal transduction cascades, including mTORC1, and an increase in growth factors such as BDNF that cause the expression of synaptic proteins and an increase in the density of dendritic spines

How Long Until It Works

- Antidepressant effects can occur within 24 hours

If It Works

- Can immediately alleviate depressed mood and suicidal ideation
- Use of esketamine does not preclude the need for hospitalisation if clinically warranted, even if patients experience improvement after an initial dose of esketamine

If It Doesn't Work

- Try another antidepressant or electroconvulsive therapy

 Best Augmenting Combos for Partial Response or Treatment Resistance

- Esketamine can itself act as an augmenting agent

Tests

- Assess blood pressure (BP) before dosing: if baseline BP is elevated (e.g. >140 mmHg systolic, >90 mmHg diastolic), consider the risks of short-term increases in BP and the benefit of esketamine treatment, and do not administer esketamine if an increase in BP or intracranial pressure poses a serious risk
- Given its potential to induce dissociative effects, carefully assess patients with psychosis before administering esketamine

How Drug Causes Side Effects

- Direct effect on NMDA receptors

Notable Side Effects

- Dissociation, dizziness, sedation, vertigo, anxiety, lethargy, feeling drunk, numbness, hypoaesthesia, BP increased, euphoric mood
- Nausea, vomiting
- Lower urinary tract symptoms, including polyuria

Common or very common

- General side effects: anxiety, dizziness, nausea, vomiting
- Specific side effects (intranasal use):
- CNS: abnormal sensation, altered mood, altered perception, blurred vision, dissociation, drowsiness, dysarthria, feeling abnormal, hallucinations, headache, hyperacusia, psychiatric disorders, tinnitus, tremor, vertigo
- CVS: hypertension, tachycardia
- GIT: altered taste, dry mouth, oral disorders
- Other: feeling of body temperature change, hyperhidrosis, nasal complaints, urinary disorders

Esketamine (Continued)

- Specific side effects (parenteral use):
- CNS: movement disorders, sleep disorders, vision disorders
- CVS: arrhythmias
- GIT: hypersalivation
- Resp: respiratory disorders, respiratory secretion increased

Uncommon
- Specific side effects (parenteral use): increased muscle tone, nystagmus, skin reactions

Rare or very rare
- Specific side effects (parenteral use): hypotension

Frequency not known
- Specific side effects (intranasal use): cystitis
- Specific side effects (parenteral use): disorientation, drug-induced liver injury, dysphoria, hallucination

 Life-Threatening or Dangerous Side Effects
- Sedation
- Increased BP (peak at about 40 minutes post-administration and lasts about 4 hours)
- Short-term cognitive impairment (generally resolves by 2 hours post-dose)

Weight Gain

unusual not unusual common problematic

- Reported but not expected

Sedation

unusual not unusual common problematic

- Many experience and/or can be significant in amount

What To Do About Side Effects
- Use lower dose
- For CNS side effects, if clinically appropriate, discontinuing non-essential centrally acting medications may help
- If BP remains high seek specialist advice from practitioners experienced in BP management
- Refer patients experiencing symptoms of hypertensive crisis (e.g. chest pain, shortness of breath) or hypertensive encephalopathy (e.g. sudden severe headache, visual disturbances, seizures, diminished consciousness, or focal neurological deficits) immediately for emergency care

Best Augmenting Agents for Side Effects
- Many side effects cannot be improved with an augmenting agent

Usual Dosage Range
* **Major depressive disorder:**
- Administration in conjunction with an oral antidepressant
  Adult:
- Induction phase: initial dose 56 mg on day 1, then 56–84 mg twice per week for weeks 1–4
- Maintenance phase: 56–84 mg once per week for weeks 5–8
- Maintenance phase: 56–84 mg every 1–2 weeks from week 9 onwards (use least frequent dosing to maintain remission/response)
- Periodically review continued treatment, treatment is recommended for at least 6 months after depressive symptoms improve, all dose adjustments to be made in 28 mg increments
  Elderly or adults of Japanese origin:
- Induction phase: initial dose 28 mg on day 1, then 28–84 mg twice per week for weeks 1–4
- Maintenance phase: 28–84 mg once per week for weeks 5–8
- Maintenance phase: 28–84 mg every 1–2 weeks from week 9 onwards (use least frequent dosing to maintain remission/response)
- Periodically review continued treatment, treatment is recommended for at least 6 months after depressive symptoms improve, all dose adjustments to be made in 28 mg increments

* **Induction and maintenance of anaesthesia:**
- Adult (slow IV injection): 0.5–1 mg/kg, then maintenance 0.25–0.5 mg/kg every 10–15 minutes, adjusted according to response

- Adult (IM injection): 2–4 mg/kg, then maintenance 1–2 mg/kg every 10–15 minutes, adjusted according to response
- Adult (continuous IV infusion): 0.5–3 mg/kg/hour, adjusted according to response

＊Analgesic supplementation of regional and local anaesthesia:
- Adult (continuous IV infusion): 0.125–0.25 mg/kg/hour, adjusted according to response

＊Analgesia in emergency medicine:
- Adult (IM injection): 0.25–0.5 mg/kg, adjusted according to response
- Adult (slow IV injection): 0.125–0.25 mg/kg, adjusted according to response

Dosage Forms
- Spray 28 mg/0.2 mL nasal spray unit dose (esketamine hydrochloride 140 mg/mL)
- Solution for injection 25 mg/5 mL, 250 mg/10 mL, 50 mg/2 mL

How to Dose

＊Major depressive disorder:
- Give in conjunction with an oral antidepressant
- Administered intranasally under the supervision of a healthcare provider
- Each nasal spray delivers 2 sprays containing a total of 28 mg of esketamine
- To prevent loss of medication, do not prime the device before use
- Patient should recline head at 45 degrees during administration to keep medication inside the nose
- Patient should blow nose before first device only
- Use 2 devices (for a 56 mg dose) or 3 devices (for an 84 mg dose) with a 5-minute rest period between each device
- BP must be assessed before administration; if BP is raised weigh the risks versus benefits of esketamine administration
- After dosing with esketamine BP should be reassessed at about 40 minutes and subsequently as clinically warranted
- Because of the possibility of sedation, dissociation and elevated BP, patients must be monitored by a healthcare professional until the patient is considered clinically stable and ready to leave the clinic
- Patients should be monitored for at least 2 hours at each treatment session; if BP is decreasing and patient is clinically stable

for at least 2 hours, the patient may be discharged; if not continue to monitor
- Advise the patient not to engage in potentially hazardous activities, such as driving or operating machinery until the next day after a restful sleep; patients need to arrange transportation home

 Dosing Tips
- A patient guide should be provided
- Nausea and vomiting are potential side effects, so advise patients to avoid food for 2 hours before administration and liquids for at least 30 minutes before administration
- Nasal corticosteroid or nasal decongestant should not be used within an hour prior to administration of esketamine
- If patient misses treatment sessions and there is a worsening of symptoms, consider returning to previous dosing schedule (i.e. fortnightly to weekly; weekly to bi-weekly)
- For treatment-resistant depression, evidence of therapeutic benefit should be evaluated at the end of the induction phase to determine the need for continued treatment
- For depression with suicidality, evidence of therapeutic benefit should be evaluated after 4 weeks to determine the need for continued treatment; use beyond 4 weeks has not been systematically evaluated

Overdose
- The maximum single esketamine nasal spray dose of 112 mg did not show evidence of toxicity and/or adverse clinical outcomes, but was associated with higher rates of side effects such as dizziness, feeling abnormal, hyperhidrosis, hypoaesthesia, somnolence, nausea and vomiting
- Life-threatening symptoms expected based on experience with ketamine at 25x usual anaesthetic dose: convulsions, cardiac arrhythmias, respiratory arrest. Administration of comparable supratherapeutic dose of esketamine by intranasal route not likely to be feasible

Long-Term Use
- Long-term cognitive effects of esketamine have not been evaluated beyond 1 year

- Long-term cognitive and memory impairment have been reported with repeated ketamine misuse or abuse
- Long-term use has been associated with bladder disorder

Habit Forming

- Yes
- Esketamine is a Schedule 2 controlled drug
- Only available under specialist supervision

How to Stop

- Taper not necessary

Pharmacokinetics

- Rapidly absorbed by the nasal mucosa, can be measured in plasma within 7 minutes
- Time to maximum plasma concentration (tmax) is about 20–40 minutes after the last administered nasal spray
- Mean terminal half-life following administration as nasal spray is 7–12 hours
- Metabolised primarily by CYP450 2B6 and CYP450 3A4, and to a lesser extent by CYP450 2C9 and 2C19
- No significant actions on CYP450 enzymes, although esketamine has modest induction effects on CYP450 2B6 and 3A4 in human hepatocytes

 Drug Interactions

- Little potential to affect metabolism of drugs cleared by CYP450 enzymes
- Use with caution with other drugs that block NMDA receptors (e.g. amantadine, memantine)
- Esketamine may increase the effects of other sedatives, including benzodiazepines, barbiturates, opioids, anaesthetics, and alcohol
- Concomitant use with stimulants or monoamine oxidase inhibitors (MAOIs) may increase BP
- Esketamine may increase the risk of seizures when given with aminophylline or theophylline
- Esketamine may increase the risk of elevated BP when given with ergometrine

 Other Warnings/Precautions

- Esketamine can raise BP; patients with cardiovascular (clinically unstable or significant) and cerebrovascular conditions and risk factors may be at an increased risk of adverse effects
- Use with caution in patients with hypertension, raised intracranial pressure, thyroid dysfunction, respiratory conditions (clinically unstable or significant)
- BP should be monitored post-administration of esketamine, and prompt medical care should be sought if BP remains high; refer patients with symptoms of hypertensive crisis or hypertensive encephalopathy for immediate emergency care
- In patients with a history of hypertensive encephalopathy, more intensive monitoring, including more frequent BP and symptom assessment, is warranted because these patients are at higher risk for developing encephalopathy even with small increases in BP
- For patients with cardiovascular or respiratory conditions esketamine should be administered by appropriately trained staff and with resuscitation facilities available
- Because of the risks of delayed or prolonged sedation and dissociation, patients must be monitored at each treatment session, followed by an assessment to determine when the patient is clinically stable and ready to leave the clinic
- Because of the risk of dissociation, carefully assess patients with psychosis before administering esketamine and only initiate treatment if the potential benefits outweigh the risks
- Monitor patients for activation of suicidal ideation
- Esketamine may impair attention, judgement, thinking, reaction speed, and motor skills
- Esketamine may impair ability to drive and operate machinery
- Patients and carers should be counselled on effects on driving and performance of skilled tasks – risk of anxiety, dissociation, dizziness, perceptual disturbances, sedation, somnolence, vertigo
- Whenever possible, warn patients and carers about the possibility of activating side effects, and advise them to report such symptoms immediately
- Monitor patients for activation of suicidal ideation especially in younger adults

- When prescribing for depression caution must be used in patients with active/previous history of mania, bipolar disorder or psychosis

Do Not Use
- If patient has acute porphyria
- If patient has aneurysmal vascular disease
- If patient has an intracerebral haemorrhage
- In a patient with a recent cardiovascular event (e.g. within 6 weeks of a myocardial infarction)
- If there is a proven allergy to esketamine or ketamine

SPECIAL POPULATIONS

Renal Impairment
- No dose adjustment necessary

Hepatic Impairment
- Caution in moderate impairment when using maximum dose (84 mg)
- Avoid in severe impairment

Cardiac Impairment
- Patients with cardiovascular and cerebrovascular conditions and risk factors may be at an increased risk of associated adverse events
- Contraindicated if patient has aneurysmal vascular disease (including thoracic and abdominal aorta, intracranial and peripheral arterial vessels)

Elderly
- Safety profile equivalent to that in adults
- Elderly may have a greater risk of falling once mobilised, therefore they need to be carefully monitored
- In clinical trials pharmacokinetic parameters such as maximum serum concentration (Cmax) and area under the curve (AUC) were higher in elderly subjects
- Thus, best to initiate with a lower dose
- However, in the maintenance phase can use up to the maximum adult dose

Children and Adolescents
- Not approved for a paediatric population
- Safety and efficacy have not been established

Pregnancy
- Not recommended during pregnancy and in women of childbearing potential not on contraception
- There are limited data on use of esketamine in pregnant women
- Animal studies have shown that ketamine (racemic mixture of arketamine and esketamine) induces neurotoxicity in the developing foetus. A similar risk with esketamine cannot be ruled out
- If a woman becomes pregnant while being treated with esketamine, treatment should be discontinued, and the patient should be counselled about potential risk to the foetus and clinical/therapeutic options as soon as possible

Breastfeeding
- Esketamine is present in human milk
- Risk to the breastfeeding infant cannot be excluded
- A decision must be made whether to stop breastfeeding or to discontinue esketamine treatment when trying to balance the benefits of breastfeeding versus the benefit of treatment for the woman

THE ART OF PSYCHOPHARMACOLOGY
Potential Advantages
- Moderate-severe treatment-resistant depression
- Reducing suicidal ideation
- More rapid response than other treatments for depression

Potential Disadvantages
- For use under specialist supervision only
- Must be administered in the presence of a healthcare professional
- Requires post-administration monitoring until patient is clinically stable and ready to leave the clinic

Primary Target Symptoms
- Treatment-resistant depression

Esketamine (Continued)

Pearls

- Esketamine is the 'S' enantiomer of ketamine
- Several studies suggest a rapid reduction in depressive symptoms in depressed patients with active suicidal ideation and intent
- Studies of esketamine or IV ketamine administered during psychotherapy sessions suggest potential improvement of substance and alcohol abuse

 Suggested Reading

Canuso CM, Singh JB, Fedgchin M, et al. Efficacy and safety of intranasal esketamine for the rapid reduction of symptoms of depression and suicidality in patients at imminent risk for suicide: results of a double-blind, randomized, placebo-controlled study. Am J Psychiatry 2018;175(7):620–30.

Daly EJ, Trivedi MH, Janik A, et al. Efficacy of esketamine nasal spray plus oral antidepressant treatment for relapse prevention in patients with treatment-resistant depression: a randomized clinical trial. JAMA Psychiatry 2019;76(9):893–903.

Fedgchin M, Trivedi M, Daly EJ, et al. Efficacy and safety of fixed-dose esketamine nasal spray combined with a new oral antidepressant in treatment-resistant depression: results of a randomized, double-blind, active-controlled study (TRANSFORM-1). Int J Neuropsychopharmacol 2019;22(10):616–30.

Fu DJ, Ionescu DF, Li X, et al. Esketamine nasal spray for rapid reduction of major depressive disorder symptoms in patients who have active suicidal ideation with intent: double-blind, randomized study (ASPIRE I). J Clin Psychiatry 2020;81(3):19m13191.

Ionescu DF, Fu DJ, Qiu X, et al. Esketamine nasal spray for rapid reduction of depressive symptoms in patients with major depressive disorder who have active suicide ideation with intent: results of a phase 3, double-blind, randomized study (ASPIRE II). Int J Neuropsychopharmacol 2021;24(1):22–31.

Ochs-Ross R, Daly EJ, Zhang Y, et al. Efficacy and safety of esketamine nasal spray plus an oral antidepressant in elderly patients with treatment-resistant depression – TRANSFORM-3. Am J Geriatr Psychiatry 2020;28(2):121–41.

Popova V, Daly EJ, Trivedi M, et al. Efficacy and safety of flexibly dosed esketamine nasal spray combined with a newly initiated oral antidepressant in treatment-resistant depression: a randomized double-blind active-controlled study. Am J Psychiatry 2019;176(6):428–38.

Flumazenil

Brands
• Non-proprietary

Generic?
Yes

Class
• Neuroscience-based nomenclature: pharmacology domain – GABA; mode of action – antagonist
• Benzodiazepine receptor antagonist

Commonly Prescribed for
(bold for BNF indication)
• **Reversal of sedative effects of benzodiazepines (in anaesthesia and clinical procedures; in intensive care including if drowsiness recurs after injection)**
• Management of benzodiazepine overdose
• Reversal of conscious sedation induced with benzodiazepines (paediatric patients)

 ## How the Drug Works
• Blocks benzodiazepine receptors at GABA-A ligand-gated chloride channel complex, preventing benzodiazepines from binding there

How Long Until It Works
• Onset of action 1–2 minutes; peak effect 6–10 minutes

If It Works
• Reverses sedation and psychomotor retardation rapidly but may not restore memory completely
• Patients treated for benzodiazepine overdose may experience CNS excitation
• Patients who receive flumazenil to reverse benzodiazepine effects should be monitored for up to 2 hours for re-sedation, respiratory depression or other lingering benzodiazepine effects

If It Doesn't Work
• Sedation is most likely not due to a benzodiazepine and treatment with flumazenil should be discontinued and other causes of sedation investigated

 ## Best Augmenting Combos for Partial Response or Treatment Resistance
• None – flumazenil is used as a monotherapy antidote to reverse the actions of benzodiazepines

Tests
• None for healthy individuals

How Drug Causes Side Effects
• Blocks benzodiazepine receptors at GABA-A ligand-gated chloride channel complex, preventing benzodiazepines from binding there

Notable Side Effects
• May precipitate benzodiazepine withdrawal in patients dependent upon or tolerant to benzodiazepines
• Dizziness, injection site pain, sweating, headache, blurred vision

Common or very common
• CNS/PNS: anxiety, diplopia, headache, insomnia, paraesthesia, speech disorder, tremor, vertigo
• Other: dry mouth, eye disorders, flushing, hiccups, hyperhidrosis, hyperventilation, hypotension, nausea, palpitations, vomiting

Uncommon
• CNS/PNS: abnormal hearing, seizures
• CVS: arrhythmias, chest pain
• Resp: cough, dyspnoea, nasal congestion
• Other: chills

Frequency not known
• Withdrawal syndrome

 ## Life-Threatening or Dangerous Side Effects
• Seizures (more common in patients with epilepsy)
• Cardiac arrhythmias

Weight Gain

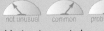

unusual — not unusual — common — problematic

• Reported but not expected

Flumazenil (Continued)

Sedation

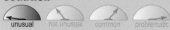

unusual not unusual common problematic

- Reported but not expected
- Patients may experience re-sedation if the effects of flumazenil wear off before the effects of the benzodiazepine

What To Do About Side Effects

- Monitor patient
- Restrict ambulation because of dizziness, blurred vision and possibility of re-sedation

Best Augmenting Agents for Side Effects

- None – augmenting agents are not appropriate to treat side effects associated with flumazenil use

DOSING AND USE

Usual Dosage Range

- Reversal of sedative effects of benzodiazepines in anaesthesia and clinical procedures: 0.2–1.0 mg
- Reversal of sedative effects of benzodiazepines in intensive care: 0.3–2.0 mg
- Reversal of sedative effects of benzodiazepines in intensive care (if drowsiness recurs after injection): 100–400 mcg/hour, adjusted according to response (intravenous infusion) or 300 mcg, adjusted according to response (intravenous injection)

Dosage Forms

- Solution for injection 500 mcg/5 mL
- Solution for injection/infusion 0.1 mg/mL; 100 mcg/mL

How to Dose

*Reversal of sedative effects of benzodiazepines in anaesthesia and clinical procedures:
- 200 mcg administered over 15 seconds, then 100 mcg every 1 minute as needed; usual dose 300–600 mcg; max 1 mg per course

*Reversal of sedative effects of benzodiazepines in intensive care:
- 300 mcg dose administered over 15 seconds, then 100 mcg every 1 minute as needed; max 2 mg per course

*Reversal of sedative effects of benzodiazepines in intensive care (if drowsiness recurs after injection):

- Initial dose by IV infusion 100–400 mcg/hour, adjusted according to response, alternatively (by IV injection) 300 mcg, adjusted according to response

Dosing Tips

- May need to administer follow-up doses to reverse actions of benzodiazepines that have a longer half-life than flumazenil (i.e. longer than 1 hour)

Overdose

- Anxiety, agitation, increased muscle tone, hyperaesthesia, convulsions

Long-Term Use

- Not a long-term treatment

Habit Forming

- No

How to Stop

- Not applicable

Pharmacokinetics

- Terminal half-life 41–79 minutes

Drug Interactions

- Food increases its clearance

Other Warnings/Precautions

- Flumazenil should only be administered by, or under the direct supervision of, personnel experienced in its use
- Use with caution in patients with benzodiazepine dependence (may precipitate withdrawal symptoms)
- Flumazenil may induce seizures, particularly in patients tolerant to or dependent on benzodiazepines, or who have overdosed on cyclic antidepressants, received recent/repeated doses of parenteral benzodiazepines or have jerking or convulsion during overdose
- Use with caution in patients with head injury
- Patients with a history of panic disorder have a risk of recurrence
- Use with caution in cases of mixed overdose, because toxic effects of other drugs used in overdose (e.g. convulsions) may appear when the effects of the benzodiazepine are reversed

Do Not Use

- Should not be used until after neuromuscular blockers have been reversed
- Should not be used if benzodiazepine was prescribed to control a life-threatening condition (e.g. status epilepticus, raised intracranial pressure)
- Should not be used in patients with epilepsy who have been receiving long-term benzodiazepines
- Avoid rapid injection following major surgery, in high-risk or anxious patients
- If patient exhibits signs of serious cyclic antidepressant overdose
- If there is a proven allergy to flumazenil or benzodiazepines

SPECIAL POPULATIONS

Renal Impairment

- Dose adjustment may not be necessary

Hepatic Impairment

- Cautious dose titration advised due to risk of increased half-life in hepatic impairment

Cardiac Impairment

- Dose adjustment may not be necessary

Elderly

- Dose adjustment may not be necessary

Children and Adolescents

- More variable pharmacokinetics
- Unlicensed use
- Used for: reversal of sedative effects of benzodiazepines by intravenous injection in neonates and children; reversal of sedative effects of benzodiazepines (if drowsiness recurs after injection) by intravenous infusion in neonates and children; reversal of sedative effects of benzodiazepines in intensive care by intravenous injection in children

Pregnancy

- Very few reports of use in pregnancy
- Controlled studies have not been conducted in pregnant women
- The indication for flumazenil means that the benefit to the mother is likely to outweigh any potential risk to the foetus

Breastfeeding

- Unknown if flumazenil is secreted in human breast milk, but all psychotropics assumed to be secreted in breast milk
- If treatment with flumazenil is necessary, it should be administered with caution
- Short half-life means rapidly eliminated, consideration may be given to interrupting breastfeeding for 24 hours to minimise risk to infant

THE ART OF PSYCHOPHARMACOLOGY

Potential Advantages

- To reverse a low dose of a short-acting benzodiazepine

Potential Disadvantages

- May be too short-acting

Primary Target Symptoms

- Effects of benzodiazepine
- Sedative effects
- Recall and psychomotor impairments
- Ventilatory depression

Pearls

- Can precipitate benzodiazepine withdrawal seizures
- * Can wear off before the benzodiazepine it is reversing
- * Can precipitate anxiety or panic in conscious patients with anxiety disorders

Flumazenil (Continued)

 ## Suggested Reading

Malizia AL, Nutt DJ. The effects of flumazenil in neuropsychiatric disorders. Clin Neuropharmacol 1995;18(3):215–32.

McCloy RF. Reversal of conscious sedation by flumazenil: current status and future prospects. Acta Anaesthesiol Scand Suppl 1995;108:35–42.

Weinbroum AA, Flaishon R, Sorkine P, et al. A risk-benefit assessment of flumazenil in the management of benzodiazepine overdose. Drug Saf 1997;17(3):181–96.

Whitwam JG. Flumazenil and midazolam in anaesthesia. Acta Anaesthesiol Scand Suppl 1995;108:15–22.

Whitwam JG, Amrein R. Pharmacology of flumazenil. Acta Anaesthesiol Scand Suppl 1995;108:3–14.

Fluoxetine

THERAPEUTICS

Brands
- Olena
- Prozep

Generic?
Yes

Class
- Neuroscience-based nomenclature: pharmacology domain – serotonin; mode of action – reuptake inhibitor
- SSRI (selective serotonin reuptake inhibitor); often classified as an antidepressant, but it is not just an antidepressant

Commonly Prescribed for
(bold for BNF indication)
- **Major depression**
- **Bulimia nervosa**
- **Obsessive-compulsive disorder (OCD)**
- **Menopausal symptoms, particularly hot flushes, in women with breast cancer, except those on tamoxifen**
- Premenstrual dysphoric disorder (PMDD)
- Panic disorder
- Bipolar depression [in combination with olanzapine]
- Treatment-resistant depression [in combination with olanzapine]
- Social anxiety disorder (social phobia)
- Post-traumatic stress disorder (PTSD)

 ### How the Drug Works
- Boosts neurotransmitter serotonin
- Blocks serotonin reuptake pump (serotonin transporter)
- Desensitises serotonin receptors, especially serotonin 1A receptors
- Presumably increases serotonergic neurotransmission
- *Fluoxetine also has antagonist properties at serotonin 2C receptors, which could increase norepinephrine and dopamine neurotransmission

How Long Until It Works
- *Some patients may experience increased energy or activation early after initiation of treatment
- Onset of therapeutic actions with some antidepressants can be seen within 1–2 weeks, but often delayed 2–4 weeks
- If it is not working within 3–4 weeks for depression, it may require a dosage increase or it may not work at all
- For OCD if no improvement within about 10–12 weeks, then treatment may need to be reconsidered
- May continue to work for many years to prevent relapse of symptoms

If It Works
- The goal of treatment is complete remission of current symptoms as well as prevention of future relapses
- Treatment most often reduces or even eliminates symptoms, but is not a cure since symptoms can recur after medicine is stopped
- Continue treatment until all symptoms are gone (remission), especially in depression and whenever possible in anxiety disorders
- Once symptoms are gone, continue treating for at least 6–9 months for the first episode of depression or >12 months if relapse indicators present
- If >5 episodes and/or 2 episodes in the last few years then need to continue for at least 2 years or indefinitely
- For OCD continue treatment for at least 12 months for patients that have responded to treatment
- For anxiety disorders and bulimia, treatment may need to be indefinite

If It Doesn't Work
- Important to recognise non-response to treatment early on (3–4 weeks)
- Many patients have only a partial response where some symptoms are improved but others persist (especially insomnia, fatigue, and problems concentrating)
- Other patients may be non-responders, sometimes called treatment-resistant or treatment-refractory
- Some patients who have an initial response may relapse even though they continue treatment
- Consider increasing dose, switching to another agent, or adding an appropriate augmenting agent
- Lithium may be added for suicidal patients or those at high risk of relapse
- Consider psychotherapy

Fluoxetine (Continued)

- Consider ECT
- Consider evaluation for another diagnosis or for a co-morbid condition (e.g. medical illness, substance abuse, etc.)
- Some patients may experience a switch into mania and so would require antidepressant discontinuation and initiation of a mood stabiliser

Best Augmenting Combos for Partial Response or Treatment Resistance

In OCD:
- Consider cautious addition of an antipsychotic (risperidone, quetiapine, olanzapine, aripiprazole or haloperidol) as augmenting agent
- Alternative augmenting agents may include ondansetron, granisetron, topiramate, lamotrigine
- A switch to clomipramine may be a better option in treatment-resistant cases
- Combine an SSRI or clomipramine with an evidence-based psychological treatment

In depression:
- *Fluoxetine has been specifically studied in combination with olanzapine (olanzapine-fluoxetine combination) with excellent results for bipolar depression, treatment-resistant unipolar depression, and psychotic depression (combination of fluoxetine and olanzapine is superior to SSRI alone, but not to monotherapy with another class of antidepressant, such as TCAs or SNRIs)
- Mood stabilisers or atypical antipsychotics for bipolar depression
- Atypical antipsychotics for psychotic depression
- Atypical antipsychotics as first-line augmenting agents (quetiapine MR 300 mg/day or aripiprazole at 2.5–10 mg/day) for treatment-resistant depression
- Atypical antipsychotics as second-line augmenting agents (risperidone 0.5–2 mg/day or olanzapine 2.5–10 mg/day) for treatment-resistant depression
- Mirtazapine at 30–45 mg/day as another second-line augmenting agent (a dual serotonin and noradrenaline combination, but observe for switch into mania, increase in suicidal ideation or rare risk of non-fatal serotonin syndrome)
- Although T3 (20–50 mcg/day) is another second-line augmenting agent the evidence suggests that it works best with tricyclic antidepressants
- Other augmenting agents but with less evidence include bupropion (up to 400 mg/day), buspirone (up to 60 mg/day) and lamotrigine (up to 400 mg/day)
- Benzodiazepines if agitation present
- Hypnotics or trazodone for insomnia (but there is a rare risk of non-fatal serotonin syndrome with trazodone)
- Augmenting agents reserved for specialist use include: modafinil for sleepiness, fatigue and lack of concentration; stimulants, oestrogens, testosterone
- Lithium is particularly useful for suicidal patients and those at high risk of relapse including with factors such as severe depression, psychomotor retardation, repeated episodes (>3), significant weight loss, or a family history of major depression (aim for lithium plasma levels 0.6–1.0 mmol/L)
- For elderly patients lithium is a very effective augmenting agent
- For severely ill patients other combinations may be tried especially in specialist centres
- Augmenting agents that may be tried include omega-3, SAM-e, L-methylfolate
- Additional non-pharmacological treatments such as exercise, mindfulness, CBT, and IPT can also be helpful
- If present after treatment response (4–8 weeks) or remission (6–12 weeks), the most common residual symptoms of depression include cognitive impairments, reduced energy and problems with sleep

Tests
- None for healthy individuals

How Drug Causes Side Effects
- Theoretically due to increases in serotonin concentrations at serotonin receptors in parts of the brain and body other than those that cause therapeutic actions (e.g. unwanted actions of serotonin in sleep centres causing insomnia, unwanted actions of serotonin in the gut causing diarrhoea, etc.)
- Increasing serotonin can cause diminished dopamine release and might contribute to emotional flattening, cognitive slowing, and apathy in some patients

- Most side effects are immediate but often go away with time, in contrast to most therapeutic effects which are delayed and are enhanced over time
* Fluoxetine's unique serotonin 2C antagonist properties could contribute to agitation, anxiety, and undesirable activation, especially early in dosing

Notable Side Effects

- CNS: insomnia but also sedation, agitation, tremors, headache, dizziness
- GIT: decreased appetite, nausea, diarrhoea, constipation, dry mouth
- Sexual dysfunction (men: delayed ejaculation, erectile dysfunction; men and women: decreased sexual desire, anorgasmia)
- SIADH (syndrome of inappropriate antidiuretic hormone secretion)
- Mood elevation in diagnosed or undiagnosed bipolar disorder
- Sweating (dose-dependent)
- Bruising and rare bleeding

Common or very common
- CNS: blurred vision, feeling abnormal
- Other: chills, postmenopausal haemorrhage, uterine disorder, vasodilation

Uncommon
- CNS: abnormal thinking, altered mood, self-injurious behaviour
- Other: altered temperature sensation, cold sweat, dysphagia, dyspnoea, hypotension, muscle twitching

Rare or very rare
- Blood disorders: leucopenia, neutropenia
- CNS: speech disorder
- Other: buccoglossal syndrome, oesophageal pain, pharyngitis, respiratory disorders, serum sickness, vasculitis

Frequency not known
- Bone fracture

 Life-Threatening or Dangerous Side Effects

- Rare seizures
- Rare induction of mania
- Rare increase in suicidal ideation and behaviours in adolescents and young adults (up to age 25), hence patients should be warned of this potential adverse event

Weight Gain

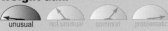

- Reported but not expected
- Possible weight loss, especially short-term

Sedation

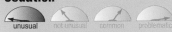

- Reported but not expected

What to Do About Side Effects

- Wait
- Wait
- Wait
- If fluoxetine is activating, take in the morning to help reduce insomnia
- Reduce dose to 10 mg, and either stay at this dose if tolerated and effective, or consider increasing again to 20 mg or more if tolerated but not effective at 10 mg
- In a few weeks, switch or add other drugs

Best Augmenting Agents for Side Effects

- Many side effects are dose-dependent (i.e. they increase as dose increases, or they re-emerge until tolerance redevelops)
- Many side effects are time-dependent (i.e. they start immediately upon dosing and upon each dose increase, but go away with time)
- Often best to try another antidepressant monotherapy prior to resorting to augmentation strategies to treat side effects
- Trazodone, mirtazapine or hypnotic for insomnia
- Mirtazapine for agitation, and gastrointestinal side effects
- Bupropion for emotional flattening, cognitive slowing, or apathy
- For sexual dysfunction: can augment with bupropion for women, sildenafil for men; or otherwise switch to another antidepressant
- Benzodiazepines for jitteriness and anxiety, especially at initiation of treatment and especially for anxious patients
- Increased activation or agitation may represent the induction of a bipolar state, especially a mixed dysphoric bipolar condition sometimes associated with suicidal ideation, and requires the addition of lithium, a mood stabiliser or an atypical antipsychotic, and/or discontinuation of the SSRI

Fluoxetine (Continued)

DOSING AND USE

Usual Dosage Range
- Depression and anxiety disorders: 20–60 mg/day
- Bulimia nervosa: 60 mg/day

Dosage Forms
- Capsule 10 mg, 20 mg, 30 mg, 40 mg, 60 mg
- Tablet 10 mg
- Dispersible tablet 20 mg
- Oral solution 20 mg/5 mL (70 mL bottle)

How to Dose
∗Depression and OCD:
- Adults and elderly: initial dose 20 mg/day in morning, wait 3–4 weeks to assess benefits before increasing dose; max dose 60 mg/day for adults, usually 40 mg/day for elderly
- Children between 8 and 17 years for depression: initial dose 10 mg/day, increased to 20 mg/day after 1–2 weeks as needed

∗Bulimia nervosa:
- Initial dose 60 mg/day in morning for adults, usually 40 mg/day for elderly; can be given in divided doses
- Some patients require lower starting dose and slower titration

∗Menopausal symptoms, particularly hot flushes, in women with breast cancer (except those taking tamoxifen):
- 20 mg/day

Dosing Tips
- Give once daily, often in the mornings, but at any time of day tolerated
- Occasional patients are dosed above 80 mg (unlicensed)
- Liquid formulation easiest for doses below 10 mg when used for cases that are very intolerant to fluoxetine or for very slow up- and down-titration needs
∗For some patients, weekly dosing with the weekly formulation may enhance concordance
- The more anxious and agitated the patient, the lower the starting dose, the slower the titration, and the more likely the need for a concomitant agent such as trazodone or a benzodiazepine
- If intolerable anxiety, insomnia, agitation, akathisia, or activation occur either upon dosing initiation or discontinuation, consider the possibility of activated bipolar disorder and switch to a mood stabiliser or an atypical antipsychotic

Overdose
- Rarely lethal in monotherapy overdose; respiratory depression especially with alcohol, ataxia, sedation, possible seizures
- Rarely, severe poisoning may result in serotonin syndrome, with marked neuropsychiatric effects, neuromuscular hyperactivity, and autonomic instability; hyperthermia, rhabdomyolysis, renal failure, and coagulopathies may develop

Long-Term Use
- Safe

Habit Forming
- No

How to Stop
- Taper rarely necessary since fluoxetine tapers itself after immediate discontinuation, due to the long half-life of fluoxetine and its active metabolites

Pharmacokinetics
- Active metabolite (norfluoxetine) has 4–16 days half-life
- Parent drug has 4–6 days half-life
- Inhibits CYP450 2D6
- Inhibits CYP450 3A4
- The long half-life of fluoxetine and its active metabolites means that dose changes will not be fully reflected in plasma levels for several weeks, lengthening titration to final dose and extending withdrawal from treatment

Drug Interactions
- Tramadol increases the risk of seizures in patients taking an antidepressant
- Can increase TCA levels; use with caution with TCAs or when switching from a TCA to fluoxetine
- Can cause a fatal "serotonin syndrome" when combined with MAOIs, so do not use with MAOIs or for at least 14 days after MAOIs are stopped
- Do not start an MAOI for at least 5 weeks after discontinuing fluoxetine

- Can rarely cause weakness, hyperreflexia, and incoordination when combined with sumatriptan, or possibly with other triptans, requiring careful monitoring of patient
- Increased risk of bleeding when used in combination with NSAIDs, aspirin, alteplase, anti-platelets, and anticoagulants
- NSAIDs may impair effectiveness of SSRIs
- Increased risk of hyponatraemia when fluoxetine is used in combination with other agents that cause hyponatraemia, e.g. thiazides
- Via CYP450 2D6 inhibition, could theoretically interfere with the therapeutic actions of codeine and tamoxifen, and increase the plasma levels of some beta blockers and of atomoxetine
- Via CYP450 3A4 inhibition, fluoxetine could theoretically increase the concentrations of pimozide, and cause QTc prolongation and dangerous cardiac arrhythmias

 Other Warnings/Precautions

＊Add or initiate other antidepressants with caution for up to 5 weeks after discontinuing fluoxetine
- Use with caution in patients with diabetes
- Use with caution in patients with susceptiblity to angle-closure glaucoma
- Use with caution in patients receiving ECT or with a history of seizures
- Use with caution in patients with a history of bleeding disorders
- Use with caution in patients with bipolar disorder unless treated with concomitant mood-stabilising agent
- When treating children, carefully weigh the risks and benefits of pharmacological treatment against the risks and benefits of nontreatment with antidepressants and make sure to document this in patient notes
- Warn patients and their caregivers about the possibility of activating side effects and advise them to report such symptoms immediately
- Monitor patients for activation of suicidal ideation, especially children and adolescents

Do Not Use
- If patient has poorly controlled epilepsy
- If patient enters a manic phase
- If patient is already taking an MAOI (risk of serotonin syndrome)
- If patient is taking pimozide or tamoxifen
- If there is a proven allergy to fluoxetine

Renal Impairment
- No dose adjustment required in moderate-severe impairment; caution in renal failure, start with low dose and adjust according to response
- Not removed by haemodialysis

Hepatic Impairment
- Lower dose or give less frequently, perhaps by half

Cardiac Impairment
- Preliminary research suggests that fluoxetine is safe in these patients – no evidence of QT prolongation
- Treating depression with SSRIs in patients with acute angina or following myocardial infarction may reduce cardiac events and improve survival as well as mood

Elderly
- Some patients may tolerate lower doses better
- Risk of SIADH with SSRIs is higher in the elderly
- Reduction in the risk of suicidality with antidepressants compared to placebo in adults age 65 and older

 Children and Adolescents

Before you prescribe:
- Carefully weigh the risks and benefits of pharmacological treatment against the risks and benefits of nontreatment with antidepressants and make sure to document this in the patient's chart
- For mild to moderate depression psychotherapy (individual or systemic) should be the first-line treatment. For moderate to severe depression, pharmacological treatment may be offered when the young person is unresponsive after 4–6 sessions of psychological therapy. Combined initial therapy (fluoxetine and psychological therapy) may be considered
- For anxiety disorders evidence-based psychological treatments should be

offered as first-line treatment including psychoeducation and skills training for parents, particularly of young children, to promote and reinforce the child's exposure to feared or avoided social situations and development of skills

- For OCD, children and young people, should be offered CBT (including ERP) that involves the family or carers and is adapted to suit the developmental age of the child as the treatment of choice
- For both severe depression and anxiety disorders, pharmacological interventions may have to commence prior to psychological treatments to enable the child/young person to engage in psychological therapy
- Where a child or young person presents with self-harm and suicidal thoughts the immediate risk management may take first priority as suicidal thoughts might increase in the initial stage of treatment
- All children and young people presenting with depression/anxiety should be supported with sleep management, anxiety management, exercise and activation schedules, and healthy diet

Practical notes:
- A risk management plan should be discussed prior to start of medication because of the possible increase in suicidal ideation and behaviours in adolescents and young adults
- Monitor patients face-to-face regularly, and weekly during the first 2–3 weeks of treatment or after increase
- Monitor for activation of suicidal ideation at the beginning of treatment
- Use with caution, observing for activation of known or unknown bipolar disorder and/ or suicidal ideation, and inform parents or guardians of this risk so they can help observe child or adolescent patients

If it does not work:
- Review child's/young person's profile, consider new/changing contributing individual or systemic factors such as peer or family conflict. Consider physical health problems
- Consider non-concordance, especially in adolescents. In all children consider non-concordance by parent or child, address underlying reasons for non-concordance
- Consider dose adjustment before switching or augmentation. Be vigilant of polypharmacy especially in complex and highly vulnerable children/adolescents

- For all SSRIs children can have a two-to three-fold higher incidence of behavioural activation and vomiting than adolescents, who also have a somewhat higher incidence than adults
- Recommended max dose for depression is 20 mg/day
- Adolescents often receive adult dose, but doses slightly lower for children
- Children taking fluoxetine may have slower growth; long-term effects are unknown
- Re-evaluate the need for continued treatment regularly

Pregnancy

- Not generally recommended for use during pregnancy, especially during first trimester
- Nonetheless, continuous treatment during pregnancy may be necessary and has not been proven to be harmful to the foetus
- Must weigh the risk of treatment (first trimester foetal development, third trimester newborn delivery) to the child against the risk of no treatment (recurrence of depression, maternal health, infant bonding) to the mother and child
- For many patients, this may mean continuing treatment during pregnancy
- Exposure to SSRIs in pregnancy has been associated with cardiac malformations, however recent studies have suggested that these findings may be due to other patient factors
- Exposure to SSRIs in pregnancy has been associated with an increased risk of spontaneous abortion, low birth weight and preterm delivery. Data is conflicting and the effects of depression cannot be ruled out from some studies
- SSRI use beyond the 20th week of pregnancy may be associated with increased risk of persistent pulmonary hypertension (PPHN) in newborns. Whilst the risk of PPHN remains low it presents potentially serious complications
- SSRI/SNRI antidepressant use in the month before delivery may result in a small increased risk of postpartum haemorrhage
- Neonates exposed to SSRIs or SNRIs late in the third trimester have developed complications requiring prolonged hospitalisation, respiratory support, and tube feeding; reported symptoms are

consistent with either a direct toxic effect of SSRIs and SNRIs or, possibly, a drug discontinuation syndrome, and include respiratory distress, cyanosis, apnoea, seizures, temperature instability, feeding difficulty, vomiting, hypoglycaemia, hypotonia, hypertonia, hyperreflexia, tremor, jitteriness, irritability, and constant crying

Breastfeeding

- Moderate to significant amounts of drug are found in mother's breast milk
- Small amounts may be present in nursing children whose mothers are on fluoxetine
- Case reports of possible side effects in the infant include: colic, decreased sleep, vomiting, hyperactivity, and serotonin syndrome
- If child becomes irritable or sedated, breastfeeding or drug may need to be discontinued
- Immediate postpartum period is a high-risk time for depression, especially in women who have had prior depressive episodes, so drug may need to be reinstituted late in the third trimester or shortly after childbirth to prevent a recurrence during the postpartum period
- Must weigh benefits of breastfeeding with risks and benefits of antidepressant treatment versus nontreatment to both the infant and the mother
- For many patients this may mean continuing treatment during breastfeeding
- Other SSRIs (e.g. sertraline or paroxetine) may be preferable for breastfeeding mothers

THE ART OF PSYCHOPHARMACOLOGY

Potential Advantages

- Patients with atypical depression (hypersomnia, increased appetite)
- Patients with fatigue and low energy
- Patients with co-morbid eating and affective disorders
- Children with depression
- Off-label – also prescribed for OCD or anxiety in children and adolescents

Potential Disadvantages

- Patients with anorexia
- Initiating treatment in anxious, agitated patients
- Initiating treatment in severe insomnia
- In children – those that already show psychomotor agitation, anger,

irritability, or who do not have a psychiatric diagnosis

Primary Target Symptoms

- Depressed mood
- Energy, motivation, and interest
- Anxiety (eventually, but can actually increase anxiety, especially short-term)
- Sleep disturbance, both insomnia and hypersomnia (eventually, but may actually cause insomnia, especially short-term)

 Pearls

- * May be a first-line choice for atypical depression (e.g. hypersomnia, hyperphagia, low energy, mood reactivity)
- Consider avoiding in agitated insomnia
- Can cause cognitive and affective "flattening"
- Not as well tolerated as some other SSRIs for panic disorder and other anxiety disorders, especially when dosing is initiated, unless given with co-therapies such as benzodiazepines or trazodone
- Long half-life; even longer lasting active metabolite, therefore not associated with withdrawal symptoms and can be stopped abruptly
- Concordance in adolescence can be even more challenging than in adults. Omissions are less problematic for fluoxetine than in other SSRIs due to long half-life
- Low risk in overdose, therefore relatively safe where there is a risk of impulsive overdose, e.g. in adolescents
- Can be used to switch patients from other SSRIs before discontinuing, or to relieve withdrawal symptoms caused by abrupt cessation of other SSRIs
- * Actions at serotonin 2C receptors may explain its activating properties
- * Actions at serotonin 2C receptors may explain in part fluoxetine's efficacy in combination with olanzapine for bipolar depression and treatment-resistant depression, since both agents have this property
- For sexual dysfunction, can augment with bupropion or sildenafil or switch to a non-SSRI such as mirtazapine
- Mood disorders can be associated with eating disorders (especially in adolescent females) and be treated successfully with fluoxetine

Fluoxetine (Continued)

- SSRIs may be less effective in women over 50, especially if they are not taking oestrogen
- SSRIs may be useful for hot flushes in perimenopausal women
- Some postmenopausal depression will respond better to fluoxetine plus oestrogen augmentation than to fluoxetine alone

- Non-response to fluoxetine in elderly may require consideration of mild cognitive impairment or Alzheimer's disease
- SSRIs may not cause as many patients to attain remission of depression as some other classes of antidepressants (e.g. SNRIs)

 ## Suggested Reading

Anderson IM. Selective serotonin reuptake inhibitors versus tricyclic antidepressants: a meta-analysis of efficacy and tolerability. J Affect Disord 2000;58(1):19–36.

Beasley Jr CM, Ball SG, Nilsson ME, et al. Fluoxetine and adult suicidality revisited: an updated meta-analysis using expanded data sources from placebo-controlled trials. J Clin Psychopharmacol 2007;27(6):682–6.

Cipriani A, Furukawa TA, Salanti G, et al. Comparative efficacy and acceptability of 21 antidepressant drugs for the acute treatment of adults with major depressive disorder: a systematic review and network meta-analysis. Lancet 2018;391(10128):1357–66.

Hagan KE, Walsh TB. State of the art: the therapeutic approaches to bulimia nervosa. Clin Ther 2021;43(1):40–9.

March JS, Silva S, Petrycki S, et al. The treatment for adolescents with depression study (TADS): long-term effectiveness and safety outcomes. Arch Gen Psychiatry 2007;64(10):1132–43.

Wagstaff AJ, Goa KL. Once-weekly fluoxetine. Drugs 2001;61(15):2221–8;discussion 2229–30.

Flupentixol

Brands
- Fluanxol
- Depixol
- Depixol Low Volume
- Psytixol

Generic?
No, not in UK

Class
- Neuroscience-based nomenclature: pharmacology domain, serotonin – dopamine; mode of action – antagonist
- Conventional antipsychotic (neuroleptic, thioxanthene, dopamine 2 antagonist)

Commonly Prescribed for
(bold for BNF indication)
- **Schizophrenia and other psychoses, particularly with apathy and withdrawal but not mania or psychomotor hyperactivity**
- **Depressive illness**
- **Flupentixol decanoate for maintenance in schizophrenia and other psychoses**

 ## How the Drug Works
- Blocks dopamine 2 receptors, reducing positive symptoms of psychosis

How Long Until It Works
- With oral formulation, psychotic symptoms can improve within 1 week, but it may take several weeks for full effect on behaviour
- With injection, psychotic symptoms can improve within a few days, but it may take 1–2 weeks for notable improvement
- For the injection the time to peak is 7 days with a plasma half-life of 8–17 days, and time to steady state of 9 weeks

If It Works
- Most often reduces positive symptoms in schizophrenia, but does not eliminate them
- Most patients with schizophrenia do not have a total remission of symptoms but rather a reduction of symptoms by about a third
- Continue treatment in schizophrenia until reaching a plateau of improvement
- After reaching a satisfactory plateau, continue treatment for at least a year after first episode of psychosis in schizophrenia
- For second and subsequent episodes of psychosis in schizophrenia, treatment may need to be indefinite
- Depression: flupentixol has a mood-elevating effect and is well tolerated

If It Doesn't Work
- Consider trying one of the first-line atypical antipsychotics (risperidone, olanzapine, quetiapine, aripiprazole, paliperidone, amisulpride)
- Consider trying another conventional antipsychotic
- If 2 or more antipsychotic monotherapies do not work, consider clozapine

 ## Best Augmenting Combos for Partial Response or Treatment Resistance
- Augmentation of conventional antipsychotics has not been systematically studied
- Addition of a mood-stabilising anticonvulsant such as valproate, carbamazepine, or lamotrigine may be helpful in schizophrenia
- Addition of a benzodiazepine, especially short-term for agitation

Tests
Baseline
- *Measure weight, BMI, and waist circumference
- Get baseline personal and family history of diabetes, obesity, dyslipidaemia, hypertension, and cardiovascular disease
- Check for personal history of drug-induced leucopenia/neutropenia
- *Check pulse and blood pressure, fasting plasma glucose or glycosylated haemoglobin (HbA1c), fasting lipid profile, and prolactin levels
- Full blood count (FBC)
- Assessment of nutritional status, diet, and level of physical activity
- Determine if the patient:
  - is overweight (BMI 25.0–29.9)
  - is obese (BMI ≥30)
  - has pre-diabetes – fasting plasma glucose: 5.5 mmol/L to 6.9 mmol/L or HbA1c: 42 to 47 mmol/mol (6.0 to 6.4%)
  - has diabetes – fasting plasma glucose: >7.0 mmol/L or HbA1c: ≥48 mmol/L (≥6.5%)

- has hypertension (BP >140/90 mm Hg)
- has dyslipidaemia (increased total cholesterol, LDL cholesterol, and triglycerides; decreased HDL cholesterol)
- Treat or refer such patients for treatment, including nutrition and weight management, physical activity counselling, smoking cessation, and medical management
- Baseline ECG for: inpatients; those with a personal history or risk factor for cardiac disease

Monitoring

- Monitor weight and BMI during treatment
- Consider monitoring fasting triglycerides monthly for several months in patients at high risk for metabolic complications and when initiating or switching antipsychotics
- While giving a drug to a patient who has gained >5% of initial weight, consider evaluating for the presence of pre-diabetes, diabetes, or dyslipidaemia, or consider switching to a different antipsychotic
- Patients with low white blood cell count (WBC) or history of drug-induced leucopenia/neutropenia should have full blood count (FBC) monitored frequently during the first few months and flupentixol should be discontinued at the first sign of decline of WBC in the absence of other causative factors
- Monitor prolactin levels and for signs and symptoms of hyperprolactinaemia

SIDE EFFECTS

How Drug Causes Side Effects

- By blocking dopamine 2 receptors in the striatum, it can cause motor side effects
- By blocking dopamine 2 receptors in the pituitary, it can cause elevations in prolactin
- By blocking dopamine 2 receptors excessively in the mesocortical and mesolimbic dopamine pathways, especially at high doses, it can cause worsening of negative and cognitive symptoms (neuroleptic-induced deficit syndrome)
- Anticholinergic actions may cause sedation, blurred vision, constipation, dry mouth
- Antihistaminergic actions may cause sedation, weight gain
- By blocking alpha 1 adrenergic receptors, it can cause dizziness, sedation, and hypotension

- Mechanism of weight gain and any possible increased incidence of diabetes or dyslipidaemia with conventional antipsychotics is unknown

Notable Side Effects

*Neuroleptic-induced deficit syndrome
*Extrapyramidal symptoms (more common at start of treatment), parkinsonism
*Insomnia, restlessness, agitation, sedation
*Tardive dyskinesia (risk increases with duration of treatment and with dose)
*Galactorrhoea, amenorrhoea
- Tachycardia
- Hypomania
- Rare eosinophilia

Common or very common

- CNS/PNS: depression, headache, impaired concentration, nervousness, vision disorders
- GIT: abnormal appetite, diarrhoea, gastrointestinal discomfort, hypersalivation
- Other: asthenia, dyspnoea, hyperhidrosis, muscle complaints, palpitations, sexual dysfunction, skin reactions, urinary disorder

Uncommon

- CNS: confusion, oculogyric crisis, speech disorder
- GIT: flatulence, nausea
- Other: hot flush, photosensitivity

Rare or very rare

- Impaired glucose tolerance and hyperglycaemia, jaundice, thrombocytopenia

Frequency not known

- Suicidal tendencies

 Life-Threatening or Dangerous Side Effects

- Torsades de pointes
- Rare neuroleptic malignant syndrome
- Rare seizures
- Rare jaundice, leucopenia
- Increased risk of death and cerebrovascular events in elderly patients with dementia-related psychosis

Weight Gain

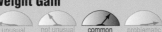

- Many experience and/or can be significant in amount

Sedation

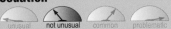

unusual   not unusual   common   problematic

- Occurs in significant minority

What To Do About Side Effects

- Wait
- Wait
- Wait
- Reduce the dose
- Low-dose benzodiazepine or beta blocker may reduce akathisia
- Take more of the dose at bedtime to help reduce daytime sedation
- Weight loss, exercise programmes, and medical management for high BMIs, diabetes, and dyslipidaemia
- Switch to another antipsychotic (atypical) – quetiapine or clozapine are best in cases of tardive dyskinesia
- For depot, side effects may persist until the drug has been cleared from its depot site

Best Augmenting Agents for Side Effects

- Dystonia: antimuscarinic drugs (e.g. procyclidine) as oral or IM depending on the severity; botulinum toxin if antimuscarinics not effective
- Parkinsonism: antimuscarinic drugs (e.g. procyclidine)
- Akathisia: beta blocker propranolol (30–80 mg/day) or low-dose benzodiazepine (e.g. 0.5–3.0 mg/day of clonazepam) may help; other agents that may be tried include the 5HT2 antagonists such as cyproheptadine (16 mg/day) or mirtazapine (15 mg at night – caution in bipolar disorder); clonidine (0.2–0.8 mg/day) may be tried if the above ineffective
- Tardive dyskinesia: stop any antimuscarinic, consider tetrabenazine

DOSING AND USE

Usual Dosage Range

- Schizophrenia and other psychoses, particularly with apathy and withdrawal but not mania or psychomotor hyperactivity: 6–18 mg/day in divided doses
- Depressive illness: 1–3 mg/day
- Maintenance in schizophrenia and other psychoses: IM depot injections 20 mg every 2 weeks – 400 mg every week

Dosage Forms

- Tablet 0.5 mg, 1 mg, 3 mg
- IM solution (flupentixol decanoate) 20 mg/mL, 40 mg/2 mL, 50 mg/0.5 mL, 100 mg/mL, 200 mg/mL

How to Dose

∗Schizophrenia and other psychoses, with apathy and withdrawal not mania or psychomotor hyperactivity:
- Initial dose 3–9 mg twice per day, adjusted according to response; max 18 mg/day
- Debilitated patients and elderly: initial dose 0.75–4.5 mg twice daily, adjusted according to response

∗Depressive illness:
- Initial dose 1 mg in morning, increased as needed to 2 mg/day after 1 week, doses above 2 mg in divided doses, last dose before late afternoon; discontinue if no benefits after 1 week at max dosage; max 3 mg/day

∗Maintenance in schizophrenia and other psychoses:
- Deep IM injection – test dose 20 mg injected into upper outer buttock or lateral thigh, then 20–40 mg after at least 7 days, then 20–40 mg every 2–4 weeks, adjusted according to response, maintenance 50 mg every 4 weeks to 300 mg every 2 weeks; max 400 mg per week

Dosing Tips

- Equivalent dose (consensus) for oral flupentixol is 3 mg/day. Range of values in the literature is 2–3 mg/day
- Equivalent dose (consensus) for flupentixol depot is 10 mg/week. Range of values in the literature is 10–20 mg/week
- Licensed injection site is buttock or thigh
- Test dose of 20 mg required
- Dose range: 50 mg every 4 weeks to 400 mg per week
- Dosing interval is 2–4 weeks
- Max licensed dose is high relative to other depot injections
- When transferring from oral to depot therapy, the dose by mouth should be reduced gradually

Overdose

- Somnolence or coma, extrapyramidal symptoms, convulsions, hypotension, shock, hyper- or hypothermia. ECG changes, QT prolongation, torsade de

pointes, cardiac arrest and ventricular arrhythmias have been reported when administered in overdose together with drugs known to affect the heart
- Do not use adrenaline in the event of an overdose

Long-Term Use
- Safe

Habit Forming
- No

How to Stop
- Slow down-titration of oral formulation (over 6–8 weeks), especially when simultaneously beginning a new antipsychotic while switching (i.e. cross-titration)
- Rapid oral discontinuation may lead to rebound psychosis and worsening of symptoms
- If anti-Parkinson agents are being used, they should be continued for a few weeks after flupentixol is discontinued

Pharmacokinetics
Oral:
- Maximum plasma concentrations within 3–8 hours
- Mean plasma half-life is about 35 hours
Depot:
- After IM injection, the ester is slowly released from the oil depot and is rapidly hydrolysed to release flupentixol. Flupentixol is widely distributed in the body and extensively metabolised in the liver
- Peak circulating levels occur around 7 days after administration with a plasma half-life of 8–17 days, and time to steady state of 9 weeks

 ## Drug Interactions
- May decrease the effects of levodopa, dopamine agonists
- May increase the effects of antihypertensive drugs except for guanethidine, whose antihypertensive actions flupenthixol may antagonise
- CNS effects may be increased if used with other CNS depressants
- Combined use with adrenaline may lower blood pressure
- Ritonavir may increase plasma levels of flupentixol

- May increase carbamazepine plasma levels
- Some patients taking a neuroleptic and lithium have developed an encephalopathic syndrome similar to neuroleptic malignant syndrome
- Avoid concomitant administration of drugs that prolong QT interval

 ## Other Warnings/Precautions
- All antipsychotics should be used with caution in patients with angle-closure glaucoma, blood disorders, cardiovascular disease, depression, diabetes, epilepsy and susceptibility to seizures, history of jaundice, myasthenia gravis, Parkinson's disease, photosensitivity, prostatic hypertrophy, severe respiratory disorders
- Use with caution in cerebral arteriosclerosis, QT-interval prolongation
- Use with caution in hypothyroidism and hyperthyroidism
- Use with caution in acute porphyrias
- Use with caution in Parkinson's disease
- Use with caution in phaeochromocytoma
- Use with caution in the elderly and senile confusional state
- An alternative antipsychotic may be necessary if symptoms such as aggression or agitation appear

Do Not Use
- In children
- In overactive or excitable patients
- If there is circulatory collapse
- If there is CNS depression
- If the patient is in a comatosed state or has impaired consciousness
- If there is a proven allergy to flupentixol

Renal Impairment
- Start with small doses of antipsychotic drugs in severe renal impairment because of increased cerebral sensitivity
- Caution in renal failure

Hepatic Impairment
- Can precipitate coma
- Consider serum-flupentixol concentration monitoring in hepatic impairment
- Caution in hepatic failure

Cardiac Impairment
- Use with caution in QT interval prolongation

Elderly

- Schizophrenia and other psychoses, particularly with apathy and withdrawal but not mania or psychomotor hyperactivity: initial dose 0.75–4.5 mg twice per day, adjusted according to response
- Depressive illness: initial dose 500 mcg in the morning, then increased if necessary to 1 mg/day after 1 week, doses above 1 mg to be given in divided doses, last dose to be taken before 4 pm; discontinue if no response after 1 week at max dosage; max 1.5 mg/day
- Maintenance in schizophrenia and other psychoses: by deep IM injection – dose is initially quarter to half adult dose

 Children and Adolescents

- Contraindicated

 Pregnancy

- Controlled studies have not been conducted in pregnant women
- There is a risk of abnormal muscle movements and withdrawal symptoms in newborns whose mothers took an antipsychotic during the third trimester; symptoms may include agitation, abnormally increased or decreased muscle tone, tremor, sleepiness, severe difficulty breathing, and difficulty feeding
- Reports of extrapyramidal symptoms, jaundice, hyperreflexia, hyporeflexia in infants whose mothers took a conventional antipsychotic during pregnancy
- Psychotic symptoms may worsen during pregnancy and some form of treatment may be necessary
- Use in pregnancy may be justified if the benefit of continued treatment exceeds any associated risk
- Switching antipsychotics may increase the risk of relapse
- Antipsychotics may be preferable to anticonvulsant mood stabilisers if treatment is required for mania during pregnancy
- Effects of hyperprolactinaemia on the foetus are unknown
- Depot antipsychotics should only be used when there is a good response to the depot and a history of non-concordance with oral medication

Breastfeeding

- Small amounts in mother's breast milk
- Risk of accumulation in infant due to long half-life
- Haloperidol is considered to be the preferred first-generation antipsychotic, and quetiapine is the preferred second-generation antipsychotic
- Infants of women who choose to breastfeed should be monitored for possible adverse effects

THE ART OF PSYCHOPHARMACOLOGY

Potential Advantages
- Non-concordant patients

Potential Disadvantages
- Children
- Elderly
- Patients with tardive dyskinesia

Primary Target Symptoms
- Positive symptoms of psychosis
- Negative symptoms of psychosis
- Aggressive symptoms

 Pearls

- Flupentixol may be helpful in schizophrenia patients with negative or affective symptoms
- Due to its effects on mood flupentixol may be used in conjunction with an antidepressant in the treatment of depression
- Less sedation and orthostatic hypotension but more extrapyramidal symptoms than some other conventional antipsychotics
- Patients have very similar antipsychotic responses to any conventional antipsychotic, which is different from atypical antipsychotics where antipsychotic responses of individual patients can occasionally vary greatly from one atypical antipsychotic to another
- Patients with inadequate responses to atypical antipsychotics may benefit from a trial of augmentation with a conventional antipsychotic such as flupentixol or from

switching to a conventional antipsychotic such as flupentixol

- However, long-term polypharmacy with a combination of a conventional antipsychotic such as flupentixol with an atypical antipsychotic may combine their side effects without clearly augmenting the efficacy of either
- For treatment-resistant patients, especially those with impulsivity, aggression, violence, and self-harm, long-term polypharmacy with 2 atypical antipsychotics or with 1 atypical antipsychotic and 1 conventional antipsychotic may be useful or even necessary while closely monitoring
- In such cases, it may be beneficial to combine 1 depot antipsychotic with 1 oral antipsychotic
- Although a frequent practice by some prescribers, adding 2 conventional antipsychotics together has little rationale and may reduce tolerability without clearly enhancing efficacy

FLUPENTIXOL DECANOATE
Usual Dosage Range

- Maintenance in schizophrenia and other psychoses
- Adult: usual maintenance dose 50 mg every 4 weeks to 300 mg every 2 weeks; max 400 mg per week (max licensed dose is very high as compared to other depots)
- Elderly: dose is initially quarter to half adult dose

How to Dose

- Adult: test dose 20 mg, dose to be injected into the upper outer buttock or lateral thigh, then 20–40 mg after at least 7 days, then 20–40 mg every 2–4 weeks, adjusted according to response, usual maintenance dose 50 mg every 4 weeks to 300 mg every 2 weeks; max 400 mg per week
- Elderly: test dose 5–10 mg, dose to be injected into the upper outer buttock or lateral thigh, then 5–20 mg after at least 7 days, then 5–20 mg every 2–4 weeks, adjusted according to response, usual maintenance dose 12.5 mg every 4 weeks to 150 mg every 2 weeks; max 200 mg per week
- An interval of at least one week should be allowed before the second injection is given at a dose consistent with the patient's condition

Dosing Tips

- Depixol/Psytixol injection 20 mg/mL is not intended for use in patients requiring doses of greater than 60 mg (3 mL) of flupentixol. Injection volumes of 2–3 mL should be distributed between two injection sites
- More concentrated solutions of flupentixol decanoate (Depixol Conc Injection or Depixol Low Volume Injection) should be used if doses greater than 3 mL (60 mg) are required
- The injection volumes selected for Depixol Conc Injection or Depixol Low Volume Injection should not exceed 2 mL

FLUPENTIXOL DECANOATE	
Flupentixol Decanoate Properties	
Vehicle	Thin vegetable oil (derived from coconuts)
Duration of action	3–4 weeks
Tmax	7–10 days
T1/2 with single dosing	8 days
T1/2 with multiple dosing	17 days
Time to reach steady state	About 9 weeks
Dosing schedule (maintenance)	1–4 weeks
Injection site	Intramuscular (gluteal)
Needle gauge	21
Dosage forms	20 mg, 100 mg, 200 mg
Injection volume	20 mg/mL, 100 mg/mL, 200 mg/mL; not to exceed 2–3 mL

Flupentixol (Continued)

- Adequate control of severe psychotic symptoms may take up to 4 to 6 months at high enough dosage. Once stabilised lower maintenance doses may be considered, but must be sufficient to prevent relapse
- With depot injections, the absorption rate constant is slower than the elimination rate constant, thus resulting in "flip-flop" kinetics – i.e. time to steady state is a function of absorption rate, while concentration at steady state is a function of elimination rate
- The rate-limiting step for plasma drug levels for depot injections is not drug metabolism, but rather slow absorption from the injection site
- In general, 5 half-lives of any medication are needed to achieve 97% of steady-state levels
- The long half-life of depot antipsychotics means that one must either adequately load the dose (if possible) or provide oral supplementation
- The failure to adequately load the dose leads either to prolonged cross-titration from oral antipsychotic or to sub-therapeutic antipsychotic plasma levels for weeks or months in patients who are not receiving (or adhering to) oral supplementation
- Because plasma antipsychotic levels increase gradually over time, dose requirements may ultimately decrease from initial; if possible obtaining periodic plasma levels can be beneficial to prevent unnecessary plasma level creep
- The time to get a blood level for patients receiving depot is the morning of the day they will receive their next injection

THE ART OF SWITCHING

 Switching From Oral Antipsychotics To Flupentixol Decanoate

- Discontinuation of oral antipsychotic can begin immediately if adequate loading is pursued; however, oral coverage may still be necessary for the first week
- How to discontinue oral formulations:
  - Down-titration is not required for: amisulpride, aripiprazole, cariprazine, paliperidone
  - 1-week down-titration is required for: lurasidone, risperidone
  - 3–4-week down-titration is required for: asenapine, olanzapine, quetiapine
  - 4+-week down-titration is required for: clozapine
  - For patients taking benzodiazepine or anticholinergic medication, this can be continued during cross-titration to help alleviate side effects such as insomnia, agitation, and/or psychosis. Once the patient is stable on the depot, these can be tapered one at a time as appropriate

Suggested Reading

Bailey L, Taylor D. Estimating the optimal dose of flupentixol decanoate in the maintenance treatment of schizophrenia–a systematic review of the literature. Psychopharmacology (Berl) 2019;236(11):3081–92.

Gerlach J. Depot neuroleptics in relapse prevention: advantages and disadvantages. Int Clin Psychopharmacol 1995;(9 Suppl 5):S17–20.

Huhn M, Nikolakopoulou A, Schneider-Thoma J, et al. Comparative efficacy and tolerability of 32 oral antipsychotics for the acute treatment of adults with multi-episode schizophrenia: a systematic review and network meta-analysis. Lancet 2019;394(10202):939–51.

Mahapatra J, Quraishi SN, David A, et al. Flupenthixol decanoate (depot) for schizophrenia or other similar psychotic disorders. Cochrane Database Syst Rev 2014;2014(6):CD001470.

Pillinger T, McCutcheon RA, Vano L, et al. Comparative effects of 18 antipsychotics on metabolic function in patients with schizophrenia, predictors of metabolic dysregulation, and association with psychopathology: a systematic review and network meta-analysis. Lancet Psychiatry 2020;7(1):64–77.

Quraishi S, David A. Depot flupenthixol decanoate for schizophrenia or other similar psychotic disorders. Cochrane Database Syst Rev 2000;(2):CD001470.

Flupentixol (Continued)

Shen X, Xia J, Adams CE. Flupenthixol versus placebo for schizophrenia. Cochrane Database Syst Rev 2012;11:CD009777.

Soyka M, De Vry J. Flupenthixol as a potential pharmacotreatment of alcohol and cocaine abuse/dependence. Eur Neuropsychopharmacol 2000;10(5):325–32.

Tardy M, Dold M, Engel RR, et al. Flupenthixol versus low-potency first-generation antipsychotic drugs for schizophrenia. Cochrane Database Syst Rev 2014;(9):CD009227.

Flurazepam

THERAPEUTICS

Brands
• Dalmane

Generic?
No, not in UK

Class
• Neuroscience-based nomenclature: pharmacology domain – GABA; mode of action – positive allosteric modulator (PAM)
• Benzodiazepine (hypnotic)

Commonly Prescribed for
(bold for BNF indication)
• **Insomnia (short-term use)**
• Insomnia characterised by difficulty in falling asleep, frequent nocturnal awakenings, and/or early morning awakening
• Recurring insomnia or poor sleeping habits
• Acute or chronic medical situations requiring restful sleep
• Catatonia

How the Drug Works
• Binds to benzodiazepine receptors at the GABA-A ligand-gated chloride channel complex
• Enhances the inhibitory effects of GABA
• Boosts chloride conductance through GABA-regulated channels
• Inhibitory actions in sleep centres may provide sedative hypnotic effects

How Long Until It Works
• Generally takes effect in less than an hour

If It Works
• Improves quality of sleep
• Effects on total wake-time and number of night time awakenings may be decreased over time
• Flurazepam is a long-acting benzodiazepine and so it may be used in cases where there are difficulties in maintaining sleep

If It Doesn't Work
• If insomnia does not improve after 7–10 days, it may be a manifestation of a primary psychiatric or physical illness such as obstructive sleep apnoea or restless leg syndrome, which requires independent evaluation
• Increase the dose

• Improve sleep hygiene
• Switch to another agent

Best Augmenting Combos for Partial Response or Treatment Resistance
• Generally best to switch to another agent:
  • Alternative benzodiazepine – e.g. temazepam
  • 'Z' drugs – e.g. zopiclone
  • Agents with antihistamine actions (e.g. promethazine)

Tests
• In patients with seizure disorders, concomitant medical illness, and/or those with multiple concomitant long-term medications, periodic liver tests and blood counts may be prudent

SIDE EFFECTS

How Drug Causes Side Effects
• Same mechanism for side effects as for therapeutic effects – namely due to excessive actions at benzodiazepine receptors
• Long-term adaptations in benzodiazepine receptors may explain the development of dependence, tolerance, and withdrawal
• Side effects are generally immediate, but immediate side effects often disappear in time

Notable Side Effects
＊Sedation, fatigue, depression
＊Dizziness, ataxia, slurred speech, weakness
＊Forgetfulness, confusion
＊Hyperexcitability, nervousness
• Rare hallucinations, mania
• Rare hypotension
• Hypersalivation, dry mouth
• Rebound insomnia when withdrawing from long-term treatment

Common or very common
• Altered taste

Rare or very rare
• Abdominal discomfort, skin eruption

Frequency not known
• Blood disorders: agranulocytosis, leucopenia, pancytopenia, thrombocytopenia
• CNS/PNS: extrapyramidal symptoms, suicide attempt

Life-Threatening or Dangerous Side Effects

- Respiratory depression, especially when taken with CNS depressants in overdose
- Rare hepatic dysfunction, renal dysfunction, blood dyscrasias

Weight Gain

- Reported but not expected

Sedation

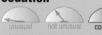

- Many experience and/or can be significant in amount

What to Do About Side Effects

- Wait
- To avoid problems with memory, only take flurazepam if planning to have a full night's sleep
- Lower the dose
- Switch to a shorter-acting sedative hypnotic
- Switch to a non-benzodiazepine hypnotic
- Administer flumazenil if side effects are severe or life-threatening

Best Augmenting Agents for Side Effects

- Many side effects cannot be improved with an augmenting agent

DOSING AND USE

Usual Dosage Range

- Insomnia (short-term use): 15–30 mg at bedtime

Dosage Forms

- Capsule 15 mg, 30 mg

How to Dose

Adult: 15–30 mg at bedtime; for debilitated patients use elderly dose
Elderly: 15 mg at bedtime

 Dosing Tips

* Because flurazepam tends to accumulate over time, perhaps not the best hypnotic for chronic nightly use
- Use lowest possible effective dose and assess need for continued treatment regularly
- Flurazepam should generally not be prescribed in quantities greater than a 2–4 week supply
- Patients with lower body weights may require lower doses
- Risk of dependence may increase with dose and duration of treatment

Overdose

- No death reported in monotherapy; sedation, slurred speech, poor coordination, confusion, coma, respiratory depression

Long-Term Use

- Not generally intended for long-term use
* Because of its relatively longer half-life, flurazepam may cause some daytime sedation and/or impaired motor/cognitive function, and may do so progressively over time
- Long-term use of flurazepam is associated with drug tolerance and dependence, rebound insomnia and CNS-related adverse effects

Habit Forming

- Flurazepam is a Class C/Schedule 4 drug
- Some patients may develop dependence and/or tolerance; risk may be greater with higher doses
- History of drug addiction may increase risk of dependence
- After discontinuation of flurazepam a rebound effect or benzodiazepine withdrawal syndrome may occur about 4 days after discontinuation of medication
- Flurazepam shares cross-tolerance with barbiturates

How to Stop

- If taken for more than a few weeks, taper to reduce chances of withdrawal effects
- Patients with seizure history may seize upon sudden withdrawal

- Rebound insomnia may occur the first 1–2 nights after stopping
- For patients with severe problems discontinuing a benzodiazepine, dosing may need to be tapered over many months (i.e. reduce dose by 1% every 3 days by crushing tablet and suspending or dissolving in 100 mL of fruit juice and then disposing of 1 mL while drinking the rest; 3–7 days later, dispose of 2 mL, and so on). This is both a form of very slow biological tapering and a form of behavioural desensitisation
- Be sure to differentiate re-emergence of symptoms requiring reinstitution of treatment from withdrawal symptoms
- Benzodiazepine-dependent anxiety patients are not addicted to their medications; when benzodiazepine-dependent patients stop their medication, disease symptoms can re-emerge, disease symptoms can worsen (rebound), and/or withdrawal symptoms can emerge

Pharmacokinetics

- Hepatic metabolism
- Two pharmacologically active major metabolites N1-hydroxyethyl-flurazepam and N1-desalkyl flurazepam
- Half-life of parent drug about 2–3 hours
- Half-life of N1-hydroxyethyl-flurazepam about 2–4 hours
- Half-life of N1-desalkyl flurazepam about 47–100 hours (elderly 71–289 hours)
- Excretion via kidneys

Drug Interactions

- Cimetidine may decrease flurazepam clearance and thus raise flurazepam levels
- Flurazepam and kava combined use may affect clearance of either drug
- Increased depressive effects when taken with other CNS depressants (see Warnings below)

Other Warnings/Precautions

- Warning regarding the increased risk of CNS-depressant effects (especially alcohol) when benzodiazepines and opioid medications are used together, including specifically the risk of slowed or difficulty breathing and death
- If alternatives to the combined use of benzodiazepines and opioids are not available, clinicians should limit the dosage and duration of each drug to the minimum possible while still achieving therapeutic efficacy
- Patients and their caregivers should be warned to seek medical attention if unusual dizziness, light-headedness, sedation, slowed or difficulty breathing, or unresponsiveness occur
- Dosage changes should be made in collaboration with prescriber
- History of drug or alcohol abuse often creates greater risk for dependency
- Some depressed patients may experience a worsening of suicidal ideation
- Some patients may exhibit abnormal thinking or behavioural changes similar to those caused by other CNS depressants (i.e. either depressant actions or disinhibiting actions)
- Avoid prolonged use and abrupt cessation
- Use lower doses in debilitated patients and the elderly
- Use with caution in patients with myasthenia gravis; respiratory disease
- Use with caution in patients with acute porphyrias; hypoalbuminaemia
- Use with caution in patients with personality disorder (dependent/avoidant or anankastic types) as may increase risk of dependence
- Use with caution in patients with a history of alcohol or drug dependence/abuse
- Benzodiazepines may cause a range of paradoxical effects including aggression, antisocial behaviours, anxiety, overexcitement, perceptual abnormalities and talkativeness. Adjustment of dose may reduce impulses
- Use with caution as flurazepam can cause muscle weakness
- Insomnia may be a symptom of a primary disorder, rather than a primary disorder itself
- Flurazepam should be administered only at bedtime

Do Not Use

- If patient has acute pulmonary insufficiency, respiratory depression, significant

neuromuscular respiratory weakness, sleep apnoea syndrome or unstable myasthenia gravis
- Alone in chronic psychosis in adults
- On its own to try to treat depression, anxiety associated with depression, obsessional states or phobic states
- If patient has angle-closure glaucoma
- If there is a proven allergy to flurazepam or any benzodiazepine

SPECIAL POPULATIONS

Renal Impairment
- Increased cerebral sensitivity to benzodiazepines
- Recommended dose of 15 mg/day
- Start with small doses in severe impairment

Hepatic Impairment
- Recommended dose of 15 mg/day in mild to moderate impairment

Cardiac Impairment
- Benzodiazepines have been used to treat anxiety associated with acute myocardial infarction

Elderly
- Recommended dose 15 mg/day at bedtime
- May be more sensitive to sedative or respiratory effects

Children and Adolescents
- Safety and efficacy have not been established
- Long-term effects of flurazepam in children/adolescents are unknown

Pregnancy
- Possible increased risk of birth defects when benzodiazepines taken during pregnancy
- Because of the potential risks, flurazepam is not generally recommended as treatment for insomnia during pregnancy, especially during the first trimester
- Drug should be tapered if discontinued

- Infants whose mothers received a benzodiazepine late in pregnancy may experience withdrawal effects
- Neonatal flaccidity has been reported in infants whose mothers took a benzodiazepine during pregnancy
- Seizures, even mild seizures, may cause harm to the embryo/foetus

Breastfeeding
- Unknown if flurazepam is secreted in human breast milk, but all psychotropics assumed to be secreted in breast milk
- Effects on infant have been observed and include feeding difficulties, sedation, and weight loss
- Caution should be taken with the use of benzodiazepines in breastfeeding mothers; seek to use low doses for short periods to reduce infant exposure
- Long half-life of active metabolites may lead to accumulation in breastfed infants
- Use of shorter-acting 'Z' drugs zopiclone or zolpidem preferred
- Mothers taking hypnotics should be warned about the risks of co-sleeping

THE ART OF PSYCHOPHARMACOLOGY

Potential Advantages
- Transient insomnia

Potential Disadvantages
- Chronic nightly insomnia

Primary Target Symptoms
- Time to sleep onset
- Total sleep time
- Night time awakenings

Pearls
- NICE Guidelines recommend medication for insomnia only as a second-line treatment after non-pharmacological treatment options have been tried (e.g. cognitive behavioural therapy for insomnia)
- *Flurazepam has a longer half-life than some other sedative hypnotics, so it may be less likely to cause rebound insomnia on discontinuation
- Flurazepam may not be as effective on the first night as it is on subsequent nights

- Was once one of the most widely used hypnotics
*Long-term accumulation of flurazepam and its active metabolites may cause insidious onset of confusion or falls, especially in the elderly
- Though not systematically studied, benzodiazepines have been used effectively to treat catatonia and are the initial recommended treatment

- Flurazepam was one of the first benzodiazepine hypnotics (sleeping pills) to be marketed
- Flurazepam shares cross-tolerance with barbiturates
- After discontinuation of flurazepam a rebound effect or benzodiazepine withdrawal syndrome may occur about 4 days after discontinuation of medication

 Suggested Reading

Greenblatt DJ. Pharmacology of benzodiazepine hypnotics. J Clin Psychiatry 1992;53(Suppl):7–13.

Hilbert JM, Battista D. Quazepam and flurazepam: differential pharmacokinetic and pharmacodynamic characteristics. J Clin Psychiatry 1991;52(Suppl):21–6.

Johnson LC, Chernik DA, Sateia MJ. Sleep, performance, and plasma levels in chronic insomniacs during 14-day use of flurazepam and midazolam: an introduction. J Clin Psychopharmacol 1990;10(4 Suppl):5S–9S.

Roth T, Roehrs TA. A review of the safety profiles of benzodiazepine hypnotics. J Clin Psychiatry 1991;52(Suppl):38–41.

Fluvoxamine maleate

Brands
• Faverin

Generic?
Yes

Class
• Neuroscience-based nomenclature: pharmacology domain – serotonin; mode of action – reuptake inhibitor
• SSRI (selective serotonin reuptake inhibitor); often classified as an antidepressant, but it is not just an antidepressant

Commonly Prescribed for
(bold for BNF indication)
• **Depressive illness**
• **Obsessive-compulsive disorder (OCD)**
• Social anxiety disorder
• Panic disorder
• Generalised anxiety disorder (GAD)
• Post-traumatic stress disorder (PTSD)

 ## How the Drug Works
• Boosts neurotransmitter serotonin
• Blocks serotonin reuptake pump (serotonin transporter)
• Desensitises serotonin receptors, especially serotonin 1A receptors
• Presumably increases serotonergic neurotransmission
∗Fluvoxamine also binds at sigma 1 receptors

How Long Until It Works
∗Some patients may experience relief of insomnia or anxiety early after initiation of treatment
• Onset of therapeutic actions with some antidepressants can be seen within 1–2 weeks, but often delayed 2–4 weeks
• If it is not working within 3–4 weeks for depression, it may require a dosage increase or it may not work at all
• By contrast, for OCD if no improvement within about 10–12 weeks, then treatment may need to be reconsidered
• May continue to work for many years to prevent relapse of symptoms

If It Works
• The goal of treatment is complete remission of current symptoms as well as prevention of future relapses
• Treatment most often reduces or even eliminates symptoms, but is not a cure since symptoms can recur after medicine is stopped
• Continue treatment until all symptoms are gone (remission), especially in depression and whenever possible in anxiety disorders (e.g. OCD)
• Once symptoms are gone, continue treating for at least 6–9 months for the first episode of depression or >12 months if relapse indicators present
• For depression if >5 episodes in a lifetime and/or 2 episodes in the last few years then need to continue for at least 2 years or indefinitely
• For OCD continue treatment for at least 12 months for patients that have responded to treatment
• Use in anxiety disorders may need to be indefinite

If It Doesn't Work
• Important to recognise non-response to treatment in depression early on (3–4 weeks)
• Many patients have only a partial response where some symptoms are improved but others persist (especially insomnia, fatigue, and problems concentrating in depression)
• Other patients may be non-responders, sometimes called treatment-resistant or treatment-refractory
• Some patients who have an initial response may relapse even though they continue treatment
• Consider increasing dose, switching to another agent, or adding an appropriate augmenting agent
• Lithium may be added for suicidal patients or those at high risk of relapse in depression
• Consider psychotherapy
• Consider ECT in depression
• Consider evaluation for another diagnosis or for a co-morbid condition (e.g. medical illness, substance abuse, etc.)
• Some patients may experience a switch into mania and so would require antidepressant

discontinuation and initiation of a mood stabiliser

 Best Augmenting Combos for Partial Response or Treatment Resistance

In OCD:

- Consider cautious addition of an antipsychotic (risperidone, quetiapine, olanzapine, aripiprazole or haloperidol) as augmenting agent
- Alternative augmenting agents may include ondansetron, granisetron, topiramate, lamotrigine
- A switch to clomipramine may be a better option in treatment-resistant cases
- Combine an SSRI or clomipramine with an evidence-based psychological treatment

In depression:

- Mood stabilisers or atypical antipsychotics for bipolar depression
- Atypical antipsychotics for psychotic depression
- Atypical antipsychotics as first-line augmenting agents (quetiapine MR 300 mg/day or aripiprazole at 2.5–10 mg/day) for treatment-resistant depression
- Atypical antipsychotics as second-line augmenting agents (risperidone 0.5–2 mg/day or olanzapine 2.5–10 mg/day) for treatment-resistant depression
- Mirtazapine at 30–45 mg/day as another second-line augmenting agent (a dual serotonin and noradrenaline combination, but observe for switch into mania, increase in suicidal ideation or rare risk of non-fatal serotonin syndrome)
- Although T3 (20–50 mcg/day) is another second-line augmenting agent the evidence suggests that it works best with tricyclic antidepressants
- Other augmenting agents but with less evidence include bupropion (up to 400 mg/day), buspirone (up to 60 mg/day) and lamotrigine (up to 400 mg/day)
- Benzodiazepines may be considered if agitation or anxiety present with appropriate warnings about dependence issues
- Hypnotics or trazodone for insomnia (but there is a rare risk of non-fatal serotonin syndrome with trazodone)
- Augmenting agents reserved for specialist use include: modafinil for sleepiness, fatigue and lack of concentration; stimulants, oestrogens, testosterone
- Lithium is particularly useful for suicidal patients and those at high risk of relapse including with factors such as severe depression, psychomotor retardation, repeated episodes (>3), significant weight loss, or a family history of major depression (aim for lithium plasma levels 0.6–1.0 mmol/L)
- For elderly patients lithium is a very effective augmenting agent
- For severely ill patients other combinations may be tried especially in specialist centres
- Augmenting agents that may be tried include omega-3, SAM-e, L-methylfolate
- Additional non-pharmacological treatments such as exercise, mindfulness, CBT, and IPT can also be helpful
- If present after treatment response (4–8 weeks) or remission (6–12 weeks), the most common residual symptoms of depression include cognitive impairments, reduced energy and problems with sleep

Tests

- None for healthy individuals

SIDE EFFECTS

How Drug Causes Side Effects

- Theoretically due to increases in serotonin concentrations at serotonin receptors in parts of the brain and body other than those that cause therapeutic actions (e.g. unwanted actions of serotonin in sleep centres causing insomnia, unwanted actions of serotonin in the gut causing diarrhoea, etc.)
- Increasing serotonin can cause diminished dopamine release and might contribute to emotional flattening, cognitive slowing, and apathy in some patients
- Most side effects are immediate but often go away with time, in contrast to most therapeutic effects which are delayed and are enhanced over time
- *Fluvoxamine's sigma 1 agonist properties may contribute to sedation and fatigue in some patients

Notable Side Effects

- CNS: insomnia but also sedation, agitation, tremors, headache, dizziness
- GIT: decreased appetite, nausea, diarrhoea, constipation, dry mouth

- Sexual dysfunction (men: delayed ejaculation, erectile dysfunction; men and women: decreased sexual desire, anorgasmia)
- SIADH (syndrome of inappropriate antidiuretic hormone secretion)
- Mood elevation in diagnosed or undiagnosed bipolar disorder
- Sweating (dose-dependent)
- Bruising and rare bleeding

Rare or very rare
- Abnormal hepatic function (discontinue)

Frequency not known
- Bone fracture, glaucoma, neonatal withdrawal syndrome, neuroleptic malignant syndrome

 Life-Threatening or Dangerous Side Effects
- Rare seizures
- Rare induction of mania
- Neuroleptic malignant syndrome
- Bone fracture
- Rare increase in suicidal ideation and behaviours in adolescents and young adults (up to age 25), hence patients should be warned of this potential adverse event

Weight Gain

unusual   not unusual   common   problematic

- Reported but not expected
- Patients may actually experience weight loss

Sedation

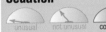
unusual   not unusual   common   problematic

- Many experience and/or can be significant in amount

What to Do About Side Effects
- Wait
- Wait
- Wait
- Nausea may be more common than for other SSRIs
- If fluvoxamine is sedating, take at night to reduce drowsiness
- Reduce dose
- In a few weeks, switch or add other drugs

Best Augmenting Agents for Side Effects
- Many side effects are dose-dependent (i.e. they increase as dose increases, or they re-emerge until tolerance redevelops)
- Many side effects are time-dependent (i.e. they start immediately upon dosing and upon each dose increase, but go away with time)
- Often best to try another antidepressant monotherapy prior to resorting to augmentation strategies to treat side effects
- Trazodone, mirtazapine or hypnotic for insomnia
- Mirtazapine for agitation and gastrointestinal side effects
- Bupropion for emotional flattening, cognitive slowing, or apathy
- For sexual dysfunction: can augment with bupropion for women, sildenafil for men; or otherwise switch to another antidepressant
- Benzodiazepines for jitteriness and anxiety, especially at initiation of treatment and especially for anxious patients
- Increased activation or agitation may represent the induction of a bipolar state, especially a mixed dysphoric bipolar condition sometimes associated with suicidal ideation, and requires the addition of lithium, a mood stabiliser or an atypical antipsychotic, and/or discontinuation of the SSRI

DOSING AND USE

Usual Dosage Range
- Depressive illness or OCD: 50–300 mg/day

Dosage Forms
- Tablet 50 mg, 100 mg

How to Dose
* Depressive illness:
- Initial dose 50–100 mg at evening, gradually increased up to 300 mg/day as needed. Doses above 150 mg/day in divided doses. Maintenance 100 mg/day
* OCD:
- Initial dose 50–100 mg at evening, gradually increased up to 300 mg/day as needed. Doses above 150 mg/day in divided doses. Maintenance 100–300 mg/day

Fluvoxamine maleate (Continued)

- If no improvement within 10 weeks, consider alternative treatment
- Children and adolescents 8–17 years:
- Initial dose 25 mg/day, increased by 25 mg every 4–7 days (max 100 mg twice per day). Doses above 50 mg in 2 divided doses

Dosing Tips

- If intolerable anxiety, insomnia, agitation, akathisia, or activation occur either upon dosing initiation or discontinuation, consider the possibility of activated bipolar disorder and switch to a mood stabiliser or an atypical antipsychotic

Overdose

- Rare fatalities have been reported, both in combination with other drugs and alone; sedation, dizziness, vomiting, diarrhoea, irregular heartbeat, seizures, coma, breathing difficulty
- Severe overdose can result in serotonin syndrome – symptoms and signs include: neuromuscular hyperactivity, autonomic instability, hyperthermia, rhabdomyolysis, renal failure and coagulopathies

Long-Term Use

- Safe

Habit Forming

- No

How to Stop

- If taking SSRIs for more than 6–8 weeks, it is not recommended to stop them suddenly due to the risk of withdrawal effects (dizziness, nausea, stomach cramps, sweating, tingling, dysaesthesias)
- Taper dose gradually over 4 weeks, or longer if withdrawal symptoms emerge
- Inform all patients of the risk of withdrawal symptoms
- If withdrawal symptoms emerge, raise dose to stop symptoms and then restart withdrawal much more slowly

Pharmacokinetics

- Parent drug has 13–22-hour half-life

- Inhibits CYP450 3A4
- Inhibits CYP450 1A2
- Inhibits CYP450 2C9/2C19

Drug Interactions

- Tramadol increases the risk of seizures in patients taking an antidepressant
- Can increase TCA levels; use with caution with TCAs or when switching from a TCA to fluvoxamine
- Can cause a fatal "serotonin syndrome" when combined with MAOIs, so do not use with MAOIs or for at least 14 days after MAOIs are stopped
- Do not start an MAOI for at least 5 half-lives (5 to 7 days for most drugs) after discontinuing fluvoxamine
- Can rarely cause weakness, hyperreflexia, and incoordination when combined with sumatriptan or possibly with other triptans, requiring careful monitoring of patient
- Increased risk of bleeding when used in combination with NSAIDs, aspirin, alteplase, anti-platelets, and anticoagulants
- NSAIDs may impair effectiveness of SSRIs
- Increased risk of hyponatraemia when fluvoxamine is used in combination with other agents that cause hyponatraemia, e.g. thiazides
- Via CYP450 1A2 inhibition, fluvoxamine may reduce clearance of theophylline and clozapine, thus raising their levels and requiring their dose to be lowered
- Fluvoxamine administered with either caffeine or theophylline can thus cause jitteriness, excessive stimulation, or rarely seizures, so concomitant use should proceed cautiously
- Metabolism of fluvoxamine may be enhanced in smokers and thus its levels lowered, requiring higher dosing
- Fluvoxamine can markedly increase the effects of melatonin and so the combination is not recommended
- Combinations of fluvoxamine with dexamfetamine/lisdexamfetamine or ondansetron or tizanidine can increase the risk of "serotonin syndrome"

- Via CYP450 3A4 inhibition, fluvoxamine may reduce clearance of carbamazepine and benzodiazepines such as alprazolam and thus require dose reductions
- Via CYP450 3A4 inhibition, fluvoxamine could theoretically increase the concentrations of pimozide, and cause QTc prolongation and dangerous cardiac arrhythmias

 Other Warnings/Precautions

- Add or initiate other antidepressants with caution for up to 2 weeks after discontinuing fluvoxamine
- May cause photosensitivity
- Use with caution in patients with diabetes
- Use with caution in patients with susceptibility to angle-closure glaucoma
- Use with caution in patients receiving ECT or with a history of seizures
- Use with caution in patients with a history of bleeding disorders
- Use with caution in patients with bipolar disorder unless treated with concomitant mood-stabilising agent
- When treating children, carefully weigh the risks and benefits of pharmacological treatment against the risks and benefits of nontreatment with antidepressants and make sure to document this in patient notes
- Warn patients and their caregivers about the possibility of activating side effects and advise them to report such symptoms immediately
- Monitor patients for activation of suicidal ideation, especially children and adolescents

Do Not Use

- If patient has poorly controlled epilepsy
- If patient enters a manic phase
- If patient is already taking an MAOI (risk of serotonin syndrome)
- If patient is taking ondansetron, pimozide, tizanidine
- If there is a proven allergy to fluvoxamine

Renal Impairment
- Start with lower initial dose

Hepatic Impairment
- Start with lower dose

Cardiac Impairment
- Preliminary research suggests that fluvoxamine is safe in these patients
- Treating depression with SSRIs in patients with acute angina or following myocardial infarction may reduce cardiac events and improve survival as well as mood

Elderly
- May require lower initial dose and slower titration
- Commonly causes sedation in the elderly, titrate dose carefully to reduce falls risk
- Reduction in the risk of suicidality with antidepressants compared to placebo in adults age 65 and older

 Children and Adolescents

- At present fluvoxamine should not be used in children and adolescents under the age of 18 for the treatment of major depressive illness
- Fluvoxamine can be used to treat OCD in those >8 years; initial dose 25 mg/day at bedtime; increase by 25 mg/day every 4–7 days; max dose 200 mg/day; doses above 50 mg/day should be divided into 2 doses with the larger dose administered at night
- Preliminary evidence suggests some efficacy for other anxiety disorders and depression in children and adolescents

Before you prescribe:
- Carefully weigh the risks and benefits of pharmacological treatment against the risks and benefits of nontreatment with antidepressants and make sure to document this in the patient's chart
- For OCD, children and young people should be offered CBT (including ERP) that involves the family or carers and is adapted to suit the developmental age of the child as the treatment of choice

Fluvoxamine maleate (Continued)

- For severe OCD pharmacological interventions may have to commence prior to psychological treatments to enable the child/young person to engage in psychological therapy
- Where a child or young person presents with self-harm and suicidal thoughts the immediate risk management may take first priority

Practical notes:

- A risk management plan is important prior to start of medication because of the possible increase in suicidal ideation and behaviours in adolescents and young adults
- Monitor patients face-to-face regularly, and weekly during the first 2–3 weeks of treatment or after increase
- Monitor for activation of suicidal ideation at the beginning of treatment
- Use with caution, observing for activation of known or unknown bipolar disorder and/ or suicidal ideation, and inform parents or guardians of this risk so they can help observe child or adolescent patients

If it does not work:

- Review child's/young person's profile, consider new/changing contributing individual or systemic factors such as peer or family conflict. Consider dose adjustment before switching or augmentation. Be vigilant of polypharmacy especially in complex and highly vulnerable children/ adolescents
- Consider non-concordance by parent or child, address underlying reasons for non-concordance
- Wait for at least 12 weeks at the maximum tolerated dose before considering alternatives
- For all SSRIs children can have a two- to threefold higher incidence of behavioural activation and vomiting than adolescents, who also have a somewhat higher incidence than adults
- Children taking fluvoxamine may have slower growth; long-term effects are unknown
- Re-evaluate the need for continued treatment regularly

Pregnancy

- Controlled studies have not been conducted in pregnant women
- Not generally recommended for use during pregnancy, especially during first trimester
- Nonetheless, continuous treatment during pregnancy may be necessary and has not been proven to be harmful to the foetus
- Must weigh the risk of treatment (first trimester foetal development, third trimester newborn delivery) to the child against the risk of no treatment (recurrence of depression, maternal health, infant bonding) to the mother and child
- For many patients, this may mean continuing treatment during pregnancy
- Exposure to SSRIs in pregnancy has been associated with cardiac malformations, however recent studies have suggested that these findings may be due to other patient factors
- Exposure to SSRIs in pregnancy has been associated with an increased risk of spontaneous abortion, low birth weight and preterm delivery. Data is conflicting and the effects of depression cannot be ruled out from some studies
- SSRI use beyond the 20th week of pregnancy may be associated with increased risk of persistent pulmonary hypertension (PPHN) in newborns. Whilst the risk of PPHN remains low it presents potentially serious complications
- SSRI/SNRI antidepressant use in the month before delivery may result in a small increased risk of postpartum haemorrhage
- Neonates exposed to SSRIs or SNRIs late in the third trimester have developed complications requiring prolonged hospitalisation, respiratory support, and tube feeding; reported symptoms are consistent with either a direct toxic effect of SSRIs and SNRIs or, possibly, a drug discontinuation syndrome, and include respiratory distress, cyanosis, apnoea, seizures, temperature instability, feeding

difficulty, vomiting, hypoglycaemia, hypotonia, hypertonia, hyperreflexia, tremor, jitteriness, irritability, and constant crying

Breastfeeding

- Small amounts found in mother's breast milk
- Small amounts may be present in nursing children whose mothers are taking fluvoxamine
- If child becomes irritable or sedated, breastfeeding or drug may need to be discontinued
- Immediate postpartum period is a high-risk time for depression, especially in women who have had prior depressive episodes, so drug may need to be reinstituted late in the third trimester or shortly after childbirth to prevent a recurrence during the postpartum period
- Must weigh benefits of breastfeeding with risks and benefits of antidepressant treatment versus nontreatment to both the infant and the mother
- For many patients, this may mean continuing treatment during breastfeeding
- Other SSRIs (e.g. sertraline or paroxetine) may be preferable for breastfeeding mothers

THE ART OF PSYCHOPHARMACOLOGY

Potential Advantages

- Patients with mixed anxiety/depression
- Generic is less expensive than brand name where available

Potential Disadvantages

- Patients with irritable bowel or multiple gastrointestinal complaints
- Can require dose titration and twice-daily dosing
- Interactions with other drugs

Primary Target Symptoms

- Depressed mood
- Anxiety

Pearls

* Often a preferred treatment of anxious depression as well as major depressive disorder co-morbid with anxiety disorders
* Interactions with several psychotropic and non-psychotropic drugs limit use of fluvoxamine
- Some withdrawal effects, especially gastrointestinal effects
- May have lower incidence of sexual dysfunction than other SSRIs
- Preliminary research suggests that fluvoxamine is efficacious in obsessive-compulsive symptoms in schizophrenia when combined with antipsychotics
- SSRIs may be useful for hot flushes in perimenopausal women
* Actions at sigma 1 receptors may explain in part fluvoxamine's sometimes rapid onset effects in anxiety disorders and insomnia
* Actions at sigma 1 receptors may explain potential advantages of fluvoxamine for psychotic depression and delusional depression
* For treatment-resistant OCD, could consider cautious combination of fluvoxamine and clomipramine by an expert
- Normally, clomipramine (CMI), a potent serotonin reuptake blocker, at steady state is metabolised extensively to its active metabolite desmethyl-clomipramine (de-CMI), a potent norepinephrine reuptake blocker
- At steady state, plasma drug activity is more noradrenergic (higher de-CMI levels) than serotonergic (lower parent CMI levels)
- Addition of fluvoxamine as a CYP450 1A2 inhibitor blocks this conversion and results in higher CMI levels than de-CMI levels
- Thus, addition of the SSRI fluvoxamine to CMI in treatment-resistant OCD can powerfully enhance serotonergic activity, not only due to the inherent serotonergic activity of fluvoxamine, but also due to a favourable pharmacokinetic interaction inhibiting CYP450 1A2 and thus converting CMI's metabolism to a more powerful serotonergic portfolio of parent drug

Fluvoxamine maleate (Continued)

 Suggested Reading

Cheer SM, Figgitt DP. Spotlight on fluvoxamine in anxiety disorders in children and adolescents. CNS Drugs 2002;16(2):139–44.

Cipriani A, Furukawa TA, Salanti G, et al. Comparative efficacy and acceptability of 21 antidepressant drugs for the acute treatment of adults with major depressive disorder: a systematic review and network meta-analysis. Lancet 2018;391(10128):1357–66.

Edinoff AN, Fort JM, Woo JJ, et al. Selective serotonin reuptake inhibitors and clozapine: clinically relevant interactions and considerations. Neurol Int 2021;13(3):445–63.

Edwards JG, Anderson I. Systematic review and guide to selection of selective serotonin reuptake inhibitors. Drugs 1999;57(4):507–33.

Figgitt DP, McClellan KJ. Fluvoxamine. An updated review of its use in the management of adults with anxiety disorders. Drugs 2000;60(4):925–54.

Omori IM, Watanabe N, Nakagawa A, et al. Fluvoxamine versus other anti-depressive agents for depression. Cochrane Database Syst Rev 2010;(3):CD006114.

Pigott TA, Seay SM. A review of the efficacy of selective serotonin reuptake inhibitors in obsessive-compulsive disorder. J Clin Psychiatry 1999;60(2):101–6.

Gabapentin

Brands
• Neurontin

Generic?
Yes

Class
• Neuroscience-based nomenclature: pharmacology domain – glutamate; mode of action – channel blocker
• Anticonvulsant, antineuralgic for chronic pain, alpha 2 delta ligand at voltage-sensitive calcium channels

Commonly Prescribed for
(Bold for BNF indication)
• **Focal seizures (adjunctive treatment of focal seizures with or without secondary generalisation; monotherapy of focal seizures with or without secondary generalisation)**
• **Peripheral neuropathic pain**
• **Menopausal symptoms, particularly hot flushes, in women with breast cancer (not licensed)**
• **Oscillopsia in multiple sclerosis (not licensed)**
• **Spasticity in multiple sclerosis (not licensed)**
• **Muscular symptoms in motor neurone disease (not licensed)**
• Anxiety (adjunctive, off-licence use)
• Bipolar disorder (adjunctive, off-licence use)

 ## How the Drug Works
• Gabapentin is a leucine analogue and is transported both into the blood from the gut, and also across the blood–brain barrier from the blood by the system L transport system
∗ Binds to the alpha 2 delta subunit of voltage-sensitive calcium channels
• This closes N and P/Q presynaptic calcium channels, diminishing excessive neuronal activity and neurotransmitter release
• Although structurally related to gamma-aminobutyric acid (GABA), it has no known direct actions on GABA or its receptors

How Long Until It Works
• Should reduce seizures by 2 weeks

• Should also reduce pain in postherpetic neuralgia by 2 weeks; some patients respond earlier
• May reduce pain in other neuropathic pain syndromes within a few weeks
• If it is not reducing pain within 6–8 weeks, it may require a dosage increase or it may not work at all
• May reduce anxiety in a variety of disorders within a few weeks
• Not yet clear if it has mood-stabilising effects in bipolar disorder or anti-neuralgic actions in chronic neuropathic pain, but some patients may respond and, if so, would be expected to show clinical effects by 2 weeks, although it may take several weeks to months to optimise

If It Works
• The goal of treatment is complete remission of symptoms (e.g. seizures)
• The goal of treatment of chronic neuropathic pain is to reduce symptoms as much as possible, especially in combination with other treatments
• Treatment of chronic neuropathic pain most often reduces but does not eliminate symptoms and is not a cure since symptoms usually recur after medicine is stopped
• Continue treatment until all symptoms are gone or until improvement is stable, and then continue treating indefinitely as long as improvement persists

If It Doesn't Work (for neuropathic pain or bipolar disorder)
∗ Many patients have only a partial response where some symptoms are improved but others persist, or continue to wax and wane without stabilisation of pain or mood
• Other patients may be non-responders, sometimes called treatment-resistant or treatment-refractory
• Consider increasing dose, switching to another agent, or adding an appropriate augmenting agent
• Consider biofeedback or hypnosis for pain
• Consider the presence of non-concordance and counsel patient
• Switch to another agent with fewer side effects
• Consider evaluation for another diagnosis or co-morbid condition (e.g. medical illness, substance abuse, etc.)

Best Augmenting Combos for Partial Response or Treatment Resistance

* *Gabapentin may act as an augmenting agent to numerous other anticonvulsants in treating epilepsy
* For postherpetic neuralgia, gabapentin can decrease concomitant opiate use
* For neuropathic pain, gabapentin can augment TCAs and SNRIs as well as tiagabine, other anticonvulsants, and even opiates if done by experts while carefully monitoring in difficult cases
* For anxiety, gabapentin may act to augment SSRIs, SNRIs, or benzodiazepines
* *For bipolar disorder, gabapentin has been tried off-label as an adjunctive agent to augment other treatments in bipolar disorder, but review of controlled studies does not suggest a role for gabapentin in monotherapy or adjunctive treatment in bipolar disorder

Tests

* None for healthy individuals
* False-positive readings with some urinary protein tests (e.g. Ames N-Multistix SG dipstick test) have been reported when gabapentin was administered with other anticonvulsants

SIDE EFFECTS

How Drug Causes Side Effects

* CNS side effects may be due to excessive blockade of voltage-sensitive calcium channels

Notable Side Effects

* *Sedation (dose-dependent), dizziness
* *Ataxia (dose-dependent), fatigue, nystagmus, tremor
* Peripheral oedema
* Blurred vision
* Vomiting, dyspepsia, diarrhoea, dry mouth, constipation, weight gain
* Additional effects in children under age 12: hostility, emotional lability, hyperkinesia, thought disorder, weight gain

Common or very common

* CNS/PNS: abnormal behaviour, abnormal gait, abnormal reflexes, abnormal sensation, abnormal thinking, anxiety, confusion, depression, dizziness, drowsiness, dysarthria, emotional lability, headache, insomnia, memory loss, movement, tremor disorders, nystagmus, vertigo, visual impairment
* CVS: hypertension, vasodilation
* GIT: abnormal appetite, constipation, diarrhoea, dry mouth, flatulence, gastrointestinal discomfort, nausea, vomiting
* Resp: cough, dyspnoea
* Other: arthralgia, asthenia, fever, increased risk of infection, malaise, muscle complaints, oedema, pain, sexual dysfunction, skin reactions, tooth disorder

Uncommon

* Cognitive impairment, dysphagia, palpitations

Rare or very rare

* Respiratory depression

Frequency not known

* Blood disorders: thrombocytopenia
* CNS: drug use disorders, hallucination, suicidal behaviours, tinnitus
* Endocrine: breast enlargement, gynaecomastia
* GIT: hepatic disorders, pancreatitis
* Other: acute kidney injury, alopecia, angioedema, hyponatraemia, rhabdomyolysis, severe cutaneous adverse reactions (SCARs), urinary incontinence, withdrawal syndrome

 Life-Threatening or Dangerous Side Effects

* Anaphylaxis and angioedema
* Sudden unexplained deaths have occurred in epilepsy (unknown if related to gabapentin use)
* Suicidal ideation and behaviour (suicidality)
* Associated with a rare risk of severe respiratory depression even without concomitant opioid medicines
* Significant dizziness or drowsiness leading to accidental physical injuries or road traffic incidents

Weight Gain

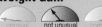

* Occurs in a significant minority

Sedation

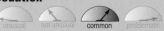

* Many experience and/or can be significant in amount

- Dose-related; can be problematic at high doses
- Can wear off with time, but might not wear off at high doses

What To Do About Side Effects

- Wait
- Take more of the dose at night to reduce daytime sedation
- Lower the dose
- Switch to another agent

Best Augmenting Agents for Side Effects

- Many side effects cannot be improved with an augmenting agent

DOSING AND USE

Usual Dosage Range

- 900–3600 mg/day in 3 divided doses (maximum per dose 1600 mg 3 times a day)

Dosage Forms

- Capsule 100 mg, 300 mg, 400 mg
- Tablet 600 mg, 800 mg
- Oral solution 50 mg/mL (150 mL bottle)

How to Dose

*Peripheral neuropathic pain:
- Initial dose 300 mg/day on day 1, then 300 mg twice per day on day 2, then 300 mg 3 times per day on day 3, then increased in steps of 300 mg every 2–3 days in 3 divided doses, adjusted according to response; max dose 3600 mg/day

*Seizures (age 18 and older):
- Initial dose 300 mg/day on day 1, then 300 mg twice per day on day 2, then 300 mg 3 times per day on day 3, then increased in steps of 300 mg every 2–3 days in 3 divided doses, adjusted according to response; usual dose 900–3600 mg/day

*Seizures (age under 18):
- See Children and Adolescents
- See also The Art of Switching, after Pearls

 Dosing Tips

- Gabapentin should not be taken until 2 hours after administration of an antacid

Overdose

- Gabapentin overdoses of less than 49 grams have not been associated with lethality
- Symptoms of the overdose may include diarrhoea, dizziness, double vision, drowsiness, lethargy, loss of consciousness, slurred speech
- Overdoses of gabapentin may result in coma particularly in combination with other CNS depressants

Long-Term Use

- Safe

Habit Forming

- Gabapentin is a Class C/Schedule 3 drug, but is exempt from safe custody requirements
- Observe patients for signs of abuse and dependence
- Withdrawal symptoms typically occur 1–2 days after abruptly stopping gabapentin

How to Stop

- Taper over a minimum of 1 week independent of the indication
- Epilepsy patients may seize upon withdrawal, especially if withdrawal is abrupt
- Rapid discontinuation may increase the risk of relapse in bipolar disorder
- Discontinuation symptoms uncommon

Pharmacokinetics

- Gabapentin is not metabolised but excreted intact renally
- Not protein bound
- Elimination half-life about 5–7 hours

 Drug Interactions

- Antacids may reduce bioavailability of gabapentin
- Antipsychotics, tricyclics and SSRIs antagonise the anticonvulsant effect of antiepileptics (convulsant threshold lowered), so either avoid concomitant administration or undertake with caution and monitoring
- Morphine increases bioavailability of gabapentin, thus gabapentin plasma levels increase over time

⚠ Other Warnings/Precautions

- Evaluate patients carefully for a history of drug abuse before prescribing pregabalin and gabapentin and observe patients

Gabapentin (Continued)

for development of signs of abuse and dependence
- Use with caution in patients with low body weight, those with diabetes mellitus and the elderly
- Patients with compromised respiratory function, respiratory or neurological disorders, renal impairment, concomitant use of CNS depressants, and elderly at higher risk of severe respiratory depression; dose adjustments may be necessary
- Depressive effects may be increased by other CNS depressants (alcohol, MAOIs, other anticonvulsants, etc.)
- Patients who require concomitant treatment with opioids should be carefully observed for signs of CNS depression, such as somnolence, sedation, and respiratory depression
- Dizziness and sedation could increase the chances of accidental injury (falls) in the elderly
- Pancreatic acinar adenocarcinomas have developed in male rats that were given gabapentin, but clinical significance is unknown
- Development of new tumours or worsening of tumours has occurred in humans taking gabapentin; it is unknown whether gabapentin affected the development or worsening of tumours
- Warn patients and their caregivers about the possibility of activation of suicidal ideation and advise them to report such side effects immediately
- Levels of acesulfame K, propylene glycol and saccharin sodium may exceed the limits of the recommended daily intake if high-dose gabapentin (oral solution – Rosemont) is given to patients (adults or adolescents) with low body weight (39–50 kg)
- Although there is no evidence of rebound seizures with gabapentin, abrupt withdrawal of anticonvulsant agents in epileptic patients may precipitate status epilepticus
- Gabapentin is not considered effective against primary generalised seizures such as absences and may aggravate these seizures in some patients, thus gabapentin should be used with caution in patients with mixed seizures including absences

Do Not Use
- If there is a proven allergy to gabapentin or pregabalin

Renal Impairment
- Gabapentin is renally excreted, so the dose may need to be lowered
- Reduce dose to 600–1800 mg daily in 3 divided doses if eGFR 50–80 mL/minute/1.73m^2
- Reduce dose to 300–900 mg daily in 3 divided doses if eGFR 30–50 mL/minute/1.73 m^2
- Reduce dose to 300 mg on alternate days (up to max 600 mg/day) in 3 divided doses if eGFR 15–30 mL/minute/1.73m^2
- Reduce dose to 300 mg on alternate days (up to max 300 mg/day) in 3 divided doses if eGFR less than 15 mL/minute/1.73m^2
- In children reduce dose if estimated glomerular filtration rate less than 80 mL/minute/1.73m^2

DOSAGE OF GABAPENTIN IN ADULTS BASED ON RENAL FUNCTION	
Creatinine Clearance (ml/min)	Total Daily Dose (mg/day)
≥ 80	900–3600
50–79	600–1800
30–49	300–900
15–29	150–600
<15	150–300

Gabapentin can be removed by haemodialysis; patients receiving haemodialysis may require supplemental doses of gabapentin. On dialysis-free days, there should be no treatment with gabapentin

Hepatic Impairment
- No available data but not metabolised by the liver, and clinical experience suggests the normal dosing

Cardiac Impairment
- No specific recommendations

Elderly
- Use with caution
- Some patients may tolerate lower doses better
- Elderly patients may be more susceptible to adverse effects, including peripheral oedema and ataxia
- Gabapentin treatment has been associated with dizziness and somnolence, which could increase the occurrence of accidental injury (fall) in the elderly population

Children and Adolescents

*Adjunct for focal seizures with or without secondary generalisation:
- Child 6–11 years: 10 mg/kg/day (max per dose 300 mg) on day 1, 10 mg/kg twice per day on day 2, 10 mg/kg 3 times per day on day 3; usual dose 25–35 mg/kg/day in 3 divided doses. Some children may tolerate a slower titration better (up to weekly). Max dose 70 mg/kg/day
- Child 12–17 years: initial dose 300 mg/day on day 1, 300 mg twice per day on day 2, 300 mg 3 times per day on day 3. Alternatively, initial dose 300 mg 3 times per day on day 1, increased by increments of 300 mg every 2–3 days in 3 divided doses, adjusted according to response

*Monotherapy for focal seizures with or without secondary generalisation:
- Child 12–17 years: initial dose 300 mg/day on day 1, 300 mg twice per day on day 2, 300 mg 3 times per day on day 3. Alternatively, initial dose 300 mg 3 times per day on day 1, increased by increments of 300 mg every 2–3 days in 3 divided doses, adjusted according to response; usual dose 900 mg–3600 mg/day in 3 divided doses (max 1600 mg 3 times per day), some children may tolerate a slower titration better (up to weekly)

Pregnancy

- Limited human data
- Use in women of childbearing potential requires weighing potential benefits to the mother against the risks to the foetus
- Taper drug if discontinuing
- Seizures, even mild seizures, may cause harm to the embryo/foetus
*Lack of convincing efficacy for treatment of bipolar disorder or psychosis suggests risk/benefit ratio is in favour of discontinuing gabapentin during pregnancy for these indications
*For bipolar patients, gabapentin should generally be discontinued before anticipated pregnancies
*For bipolar patients, given the risk of relapse in the postpartum period, mood-stabiliser treatment, especially with agents with better evidence of efficacy than gabapentin, should generally be restarted immediately after delivery if patient is unmedicated during pregnancy
*Atypical antipsychotics may be preferable to gabapentin if treatment of bipolar disorder is required during pregnancy
- Bipolar symptoms may recur or worsen during pregnancy and some form of treatment may be necessary

Breastfeeding

- Small amounts found in mother's breast milk
- If drug is continued while breastfeeding, infant should be monitored for possible adverse effects
- If infant becomes irritable or sedated, breastfeeding or drug may need to be discontinued
*Bipolar disorder may recur during the postpartum period, particularly if there is a history of prior postpartum episodes of either depression or psychosis
*Relapse rates may be lower in women who receive prophylactic treatment for postpartum episodes of bipolar disorder
- Atypical antipsychotics may be safer and more effective than gabapentin during the postpartum period when treating a nursing mother with bipolar disorder

THE ART OF PSYCHOPHARMACOLOGY

Potential Advantages
- Chronic neuropathic pain
- Has relatively mild side-effect profile
- Has few pharmacokinetic drug interactions

Potential Disadvantages
- Controlled drug
- Usually requires 3 times a day dosing
- Poor documentation of efficacy for many off-label uses, especially bipolar disorder

Primary Target Symptoms
- Seizures
- Pain
- Anxiety

Pearls
- Gabapentin is generally well tolerated, but significant side effects such as drowsiness and dizziness may occur especially in the elderly
- There is concern about the addictive potential of gabapentin, as well as harms when used together with opioids

Gabapentin (Continued)

- Gabapentin is a Class C/Schedule 3 drug, but is exempt from safe custody requirements
- Well studied in epilepsy and postherpetic neuralgia
- *Most use is off-label
- *Off-label use for first-line treatment of neuropathic pain may be justified
- *Off-label use for second-line treatment of anxiety may be justified (doses of more than 600 mg/day required; greater efficacy seen at doses above 900 mg/day)
- * For bipolar disorder, gabapentin has been tried off-label as an adjunctive agent to augment other treatments in bipolar disorder, but review of controlled studies does not suggest a role for gabapentin in monotherapy or adjunctive treatment in bipolar disorder
- *However, no clinical trials have been conducted to study the efficacy of gabapentin in the treatment of anxiety in bipolar disorder
- *Other anticonvulsants such as lamotrigine may be used in bipolar depression
- *Off-label use as an adjunct for schizophrenia may not be justified
- May be useful for some patients in alcohol withdrawal
- *One of the few agents that enhances slow-wave delta sleep, which may be helpful in chronic neuropathic pain syndromes

- *May be a useful adjunct for fibromyalgia
- Drug absorption and clinical efficacy may not necessarily be proportionately increased at high doses, and thus response to high doses may not be consistent
- In the 1990s there was a controversial promotion of off-label prescription for unapproved uses which led to large payouts to settle lawsuits
- In 2020, it was the tenth most commonly prescribed medication in USA, with more than 49 million prescriptions

THE ART OF SWITCHING

 Switching

- When substituting gabapentin with an alternative medication, the dose should be tapered gradually over a minimum of a week to minimise the risk of increased seizure frequency where it is being used for patients with seizure disorders
- The clinical importance of a slow withdrawal in patients in whom gabapentin is being used for neuropathic pain or anxiety is unknown
- Recommendations about switching to gabapentin following pregabalin treatment or vice versa cannot be made due to lack of detailed data

 ## Suggested Reading

Gomes FA, Cerqueira RO, Lee Y, et al. What not to use in bipolar disorders: a systematic review of non-recommended treatments in clinical practice guidelines. J Affect Disord 2022;298(Pt A):565–76.

Henney JE. Safeguarding patient welfare: who's in charge?. Ann Intern Med 2006;145(4):305–7.

MacDonald KJ, Young LT. Newer antiepileptic drugs in bipolar disorder. CNS Drugs 2002;16(8):549–62.

Marson AG, KadirZA, Hutton JL, et al. Gabapentin for drug-resistant partial epilepsy. Cochrane Database Syst Rev 2000;(3):CD001415.

Patorno E, Bohn RL, Wahl PM, et al. Anticonvulsant medications and the risk of suicide, attempted suicide, or violent death. JAMA 2010;303(14):1401–9.

Stahl SM. Anticonvulsants and the relief of chronic pain: pregabalin and gabapentin as alpha(2) delta ligands at voltage-gated calcium channels. J Clin Psychiatry 2004;65(5):596–7.

Stahl SM. Anticonvulsants as anxiolytics, part 2: pregabalin and gabapentin as alpha(2)delta ligands at voltage-gated calcium channels. J Clin Psychiatry 2004;65(4):460–1.

Wiffen PJ, Derry S, Bell RF, et al. Gabapentin for chronic neuropathic pain in adults. Cochrane Database Syst Rev 2017;6(6):CD007938.

Galantamine

Brands
• Reminyl
• Luventa
see index for additional brand names

Generic?
Yes

Class
• Neuroscience-based nomenclature: pharmacology domain – acetylcholine; mode of action – multimodal
• Cholinesterase inhibitor (acetylcholinesterase inhibitor); allosteric nicotinic cholinergic modulator; cognitive enhancer

Commonly Prescribed for
(bold for BNF indication)
• **Mild-moderate dementia in Alzheimer's disease**
• Parkinson's disease dementia – mild to moderate (NICE indication)
• Dementia with Lewy bodies
• Alzheimer's disease of atypical or mixed type

 How the Drug Works
∗ Reversibly and competitively inhibits centrally active acetylcholinesterase (AChE), making more acetylcholine available
• Helps to compensate for the degeneration of memory-regulating cholinergic neurons in the neocortex by increasing the availability of acetylcholine
∗ Modulates nicotinic receptors, which enhances actions of acetylcholine
• Nicotinic modulation may also enhance the actions of other neurotransmitters by increasing the release of dopamine, norepinephrine (noradrenaline), serotonin, GABA, and glutamate
• Does not inhibit butyrylcholinesterase
• May release growth factors or interfere with amyloid deposition

How Long Until It Works
• May take up to 6 weeks before any improvement in baseline memory or behaviour is evident
• May take months before any stabilisation in degenerative course is evident

If It Works
• May improve symptoms and slow progression of disease, but does not reverse the degenerative process

If It Doesn't Work
• Consider adjusting dose, switching to a different cholinesterase inhibitor or adding an appropriate augmenting agent
• Reconsider diagnosis and rule out other conditions such as depression or a dementia other than Alzheimer's disease

 Best Augmenting Combos for Partial Response or Treatment Resistance
• Augmenting agents may help with managing non-cognitive symptoms
∗ Memantine for moderate to severe Alzheimer's disease
∗ Atypical antipsychotics should only be used for severe aggression or psychosis when this is causing significant distress
• Careful consideration needs to be undertaken for co-morbid conditions and the benefits and risks of treatment in view of the increased risk of stroke and death with antipsychotic drugs in dementia
∗ Antidepressants if concomitant depression, apathy, or lack of interest, however efficacy may be limited
• Not rational to combine with another cholinesterase inhibitor

Tests
• None for healthy individuals

How Drug Causes Side Effects
• Peripheral inhibition of acetylcholinesterase can cause gastrointestinal side effects
• Central inhibition of acetylcholinesterase may contribute to nausea, vomiting, weight loss, and sleep disturbances

Notable Side Effects
∗ GIT: abdominal pain, anorexia, diarrhoea, dyspepsia, nausea, vomiting, weight loss
• Headache, dizziness
• Fatigue, depression

Common or very common
• CNS/PNS: depression, dizziness, drowsiness, hallucinations, headache, tremor

- CVS: arrhythmias, hypertension, syncope
- GIT: decreased appetite, diarrhoea, gastrointestinal discomfort, nausea, vomiting, weight decreased
- Other: asthenia, fall, malaise, muscle spasms, skin reactions

Uncommon
- CNS/PNS: blurred vision, hypersomnia, muscle weakness, paraesthesia, seizure, tinnitus
- CVS: atrioventricular block, hypotension, palpitations
- GIT: altered taste
- Other: dehydration, flushing, hyperhidrosis

Rare or very rare
- Hepatitis, severe cutaneous adverse reactions (SCARs)

 Life-Threatening or Dangerous Side Effects

- Patients should be warned of the signs of serious skin reactions, and should stop taking galantamine immediately and seek medical advice if symptoms occur
- Seizures (uncommon)
- Syncope

Weight Gain

unusual   not unusual   common   problematic

- Reported but not expected
- Some patients may experience weight loss

Sedation

unusual   not unusual   common   problematic

- Reported but not expected

What to Do About Side Effects
- Wait
- Side effects such as nausea improve with time
- Take in daytime to reduce insomnia or take with food to reduce nausea
- Use slower dose titration
- Consider lowering dose, switching to a different agent or adding an appropriate augmenting agent

Best Augmenting Agents for Side Effects
- Many side effects cannot be improved with an augmenting agent

DOSING AND USE

Usual Dosage Range
- Mild-moderately severe dementia in Alzheimer's disease: 8–16 mg/day (immediate-release); 8–24 mg/day (modified-release)

Dosage Forms
- Tablet 8 mg, 12 mg
- Modified-release capsule 8 mg, 16 mg, 24 mg
- Oral solution 4 mg/mL, 20 mg/5 mL (100 mL bottle)

How to Dose
- Immediate-release: initial dose 4 mg twice per day; after 4 weeks may increase dose to 8 mg twice per day; after 4 more weeks may increase to 12 mg twice per day; maintenance (8–12 mg twice per day)
- Modified-release: initial dose 8 mg/day; after 4 weeks may increase dose to 16 mg/day; after 4 more weeks may increase to 24 mg/day; maintenance (16–24 mg/day)

 Dosing Tips

- Gastrointestinal side effects may be reduced if drug is administered with food
- Gastrointestinal side effects may also be reduced if dose is titrated slowly
- Probably best to utilise highest tolerated dose within the usual dosing range
- *When switching to another cholinesterase inhibitor, if done for intolerance, this should be done only after complete resolution of side effects following discontinuation of the initial agent
- In the case of lack of efficacy, switching can be done overnight with a quicker titration scheme thereafter

Overdose
- Can be lethal: nausea, vomiting, excess salivation, sweating, hypotension, bradycardia, collapse, convulsions, muscle weakness (weakness of respiratory muscles can lead to death)

Long-Term Use
- Drug may lose effectiveness in slowing degenerative course of Alzheimer's disease after 6 months
- Can be effective in some patients for several years and stopping medication is

not recommended if the disease becomes severe and the medication is well tolerated

Habit Forming
• No

How to Stop
• Taper not mandatory but recommended to reduce dose for a month and monitor before completely stopping the drug
• Discontinuation may lead to notable deterioration in memory and behaviour, which may not be restored when drug is restarted or another cholinesterase inhibitor is initiated

Pharmacokinetics
• Terminal elimination half-life about 8–10 hours
• Metabolised by CYP450 2D6 and 3A4

Drug Interactions
• Galantamine may increase the effects of anaesthetics and should be discontinued prior to surgery
• Inhibitors of CYP450 2D6 and CYP450 3A4 may inhibit galantamine metabolism and raise galantamine plasma levels
• Galantamine may interact with anticholinergic agents and the combination may decrease the efficacy of both
• Cimetidine may increase bioavailability of galantamine
• May have synergistic effect if administered with cholinomimetics (e.g. bethanechol)
• Bradycardia may occur if combined with other bradycardic medications such as beta blockers or digoxin
• Use caution when prescribing with drugs that lengthen QT interval; require ECG if co-prescribing
• Theoretically, could reduce the efficacy of levodopa in Parkinson's disease
• Not rational to combine with another cholinesterase inhibitor

Other Warnings/Precautions
• May exacerbate asthma or other pulmonary disease
• Increased gastric acid secretion may increase the risk of ulcers
• Bradycardia or heart block may occur in patients with or without cardiac impairment

• Use with caution in cardiac disease, congestive heart failure, sick sinus syndrome, supraventricular conduction abnormalities, unstable angina
• Use with caution if patient has electrolyte disturbances or history of seizures

Do Not Use
• If patient has gastrointestinal obstruction or is recovering from gastrointestinal surgery
• If patient has urinary outflow obstruction or is recovering from bladder surgery
• If there is a proven allergy to galantamine

SPECIAL POPULATIONS

Renal Impairment
• Use with caution and start with lower doses; avoid in end-stage renal disease

Hepatic Impairment
• Dose adjustments are advised in moderate impairment
• For immediate-release preparations dose at 4 mg/day for 7 days, then 4 mg twice per day for at least 4 weeks, before titrating to max dose of 8 mg twice per day
• For modified-release preparations dose at 8 mg alternate days for 7 days, then 8 mg/day for at least 4 weeks, before titrating to max dose of 16 mg/day
• Not recommended for use in patients with severe hepatic impairment

Cardiac Impairment
• Use with caution due to effects on heart rate (e.g. bradycardia) especially in patients with "sick sinus syndrome" or other supraventricular cardiac disturbances, such as sinoatrial or atrioventricular block
• Use with caution in cardiac disease, congestive heart failure, unstable angina
• Use with caution in patients taking medications that reduce heart rate (e.g. digoxin or beta blockers)
• Syncopal episodes have been reported with the use of galantamine
• Use caution when prescribing with drugs that lengthen QT interval; require ECG if co-prescribing

Elderly
• Clearance is reduced in elderly patients
• Use of cholinesterase inhibitors may be associated with increased rates of syncope,

Galantamine (Continued)

bradycardia, pacemaker insertion, and hip fracture in older adults with dementia

Children and Adolescents
- Safety and efficacy have not been established

Pregnancy
- Controlled studies have not been conducted in pregnant women
- Animal studies do not show adverse effects
* Not recommended for use in pregnant women or in women of childbearing potential

Breastfeeding
- Unknown if galantamine is secreted in human breast milk, but all psychotropics assumed to be secreted in breast milk
* Recommended either to discontinue drug or bottle feed
- Galantamine is not recommended for use in nursing women

THE ART OF PSYCHOPHARMACOLOGY
Potential Advantages
- Theoretically, nicotinic modulation may provide added therapeutic benefits for memory and behaviour in some Alzheimer's dementia patients
- Theoretically, nicotinic modulation may also provide efficacy for cognitive disorders other than Alzheimer's disease

Potential Disadvantages
- Patients who have difficulty taking medication twice daily; consider once-daily modified-release preparations

Primary Target Symptoms
- Memory loss in Alzheimer's disease
- Behavioural symptoms in Alzheimer's disease

Pearls
- Dramatic reversal of symptoms of Alzheimer's disease is not generally seen with cholinesterase inhibitors

- Can lead to therapeutic nihilism among prescribers and lack of an appropriate trial of a cholinesterase inhibitor
- Perhaps only 50% of Alzheimer's dementia patients are diagnosed, and only 50% of those diagnosed are treated, and only 50% of those treated are given a cholinesterase inhibitor, and then only for 200 days in a disease that lasts 7–10 years
- Must evaluate lack of efficacy and loss of efficacy over months, not weeks
- Treat the patient but ask the caregiver about efficacy
- What you see may depend upon how early you treat
- Cholinesterase inhibitors have at best a modest impact on non-cognitive features of dementia such as apathy, disinhibition, delusions, anxiety, lack of cooperation, pacing; however, in the absence of safe and effective alternatives a trial of a cholinesterase inhibitor is appropriate
- The first symptoms of Alzheimer's disease are generally mood changes; thus, Alzheimer's disease may initially be misdiagnosed as depression

What to expect from a cholinesterase inhibitor:
- Patients do not generally improve dramatically although this can be observed in a significant minority of patients
- Onset of behavioural problems and nursing home placement can be delayed
- Functional outcomes, including activities of daily living, can be preserved
- Caregiver burden and stress can be reduced
- Delay in progression in Alzheimer's disease is not evidence of disease-modifying actions of cholinesterase inhibition
- Cholinesterase inhibitors like galantamine depend upon the presence of intact targets for acetylcholine for maximum effectiveness and thus may be most effective in the early stages of Alzheimer's disease
- The most prominent side effects of galantamine are gastrointestinal effects, which are usually mild and transient
- For patients with intolerable side effects, generally allow a washout period with resolution of side effects prior to switching to another cholinesterase inhibitor
- Weight loss can be a problem in Alzheimer's dementia patients with debilitation and muscle wasting

- Women over 85, particularly with low body weights, may experience more adverse effects
- Use with caution in underweight or frail patients
- Cognitive improvement may be linked to substantial (>65%) inhibition of acetylcholinesterase
* Galantamine is a natural product present in daffodils and snowdrops
- Modified-release formulation allows for once-daily dosing
* Actions at nicotinic receptors enhance not only the release of acetylcholine but also that of other neurotransmitters, which may boost attention and improve behaviours caused by deficiencies in those neurotransmitters in Alzheimer's disease
- Some Alzheimer's dementia patients who fail to respond to another cholinesterase inhibitor may respond when switched to galantamine and vice versa

- To prevent potential clinical deterioration, generally switch from long-term treatment with one cholinesterase inhibitor to another without a washout period
* Galantamine may slow the progression of mild cognitive impairment to Alzheimer's dementia
- Consider galantamine for people with mild to moderate dementia with Lewy bodies if donepezil and rivastigmine are not tolerated
- Only consider AChE inhibitors or memantine for people with vascular dementia if they have suspected co-morbid Alzheimer's disease, Parkinson's disease dementia or dementia with Lewy bodies
- Do not offer AChE inhibitors or memantine to people with frontotemporal dementia
- Do not offer AChE inhibitors or memantine to people with cognitive impairment caused by multiple sclerosis
- May be helpful for dementia in Down's syndrome

Suggested Reading

Campbell NL, Perkins AJ, Gao S, et al. Adherence and tolerability of Alzheimer's disease medications: a pragmatic randomized trial. J Am Geriatr Soc 2017;65(7):1497–504.

Haake A, Nguyen K, Friedman L, et al. An update on the utility and safety of cholinesterase inhibitors for the treatment of Alzheimer's disease. Expert Opin Drug Saf 2020;19(2):147–57.

Hershey LA, Coleman-Jackson R. Pharmacological management of dementia with Lewy bodies. Drugs Aging 2019;36(4):309–19.

Li D-D, Zhang Y-H, Zhang W, et al. Meta-analysis of randomized controlled trials on the efficacy and safety of donepezil, galantamine, rivastigmine, and memantine for the treatment of Alzheimer's disease. Front Neurosci 2019;13:472.

Loy C, Schneider L. Galantamine for Alzheimer's disease and mild cognitive impairment. Cochrane Database Syst Rev 2006;(1):CD001747.

O'Brien JT, Holmes C, Jones M, et al. Clinical practice with anti-dementia drugs: a revised (third) consensus statement from the British Association for Psychopharmacology. J Psychopharmacol 2017;31(2):147–68.

Stahl SM. Cholinesterase inhibitors for Alzheimer's disease. Hosp Pract (1995) 1998;33(11):131–6.

Stahl SM. The new cholinesterase inhibitors for Alzheimer's disease, part 1: their similarities are different. J Clin Psychiatry 2000;61(10):710–1.

Stahl SM. The new cholinesterase inhibitors for Alzheimer's disease, part 2: illustrating their mechanisms of action. J Clin Psychiatry 2000;61(11):813–14.

Guanfacine

Brands
• Intuniv

Generic?
No, not in UK

Class
• Neuroscience-based nomenclature: pharmacology domain – norepinephrine; mode action – agonist
• Centrally acting alpha 2A agonist; antihypertensive; nonstimulant for ADHD

Commonly Prescribed for
(bold for BNF indication)
• **Attention deficit hyperactivity disorder (ADHD) in children aged 6–17 (Intuniv, monotherapy)**
• Oppositional defiant disorder
• Conduct disorder
• Pervasive developmental disorders
• Motor tics
• Tourette syndrome

 ## How the Drug Works
• For ADHD, theoretically has central actions on postsynaptic alpha 2A receptors in the prefrontal cortex
• Guanfacine is 15–20 times more selective for alpha 2A receptors than for alpha 2B or alpha 2C receptors
• The prefrontal cortex is thought to be responsible for modulation of working memory, attention, impulse, control, and planning

How Long Until It Works
• For ADHD, can take several weeks to see maximum therapeutic benefits

If It Works
• The goal of treatment of ADHD is reduction of symptoms of inattentiveness, motor hyperactivity, and/or impulsiveness that disrupt social, school, and/or occupational functioning
• Continue treatment until all symptoms are under control or improvement is stable and then continue treatment indefinitely as long as improvement persists
• Re-evaluate the need for treatment periodically

• Treatment for ADHD begun in childhood may need to be continued into adolescence and adulthood if continued benefit is documented

If It Doesn't Work
• Inform patient it may take several weeks for full effects to be seen
• Consider adjusting dose or switching to another formulation or another agent. It is important to consider if maximal dose has been achieved before deciding there has not been an effect and switching
• Consider behavioural therapy or cognitive behavioural therapy if appropriate – to address issues such as social skills with peers, problem-solving, self-control, active listening and dealing with and expressing emotions
• Consider the possibility of non-concordance and counsel patients and parents
• Consider evaluation for another diagnosis or for a co-morbid condition (e.g. bipolar disorder, substance abuse, medical illness, etc.)
• In children consider other important factors, such as ongoing conflicts, family psychopathology, adverse environment, for which alternate interventions might be more appropriate (e.g. social care referral, trauma-informed care)
∗ Some ADHD patients and some depressed patients may experience lack of consistent efficacy due to activation of latent or underlying bipolar disorder, and require either augmenting with a mood stabiliser or switching to a mood stabiliser

Best Augmenting Combos for Partial Response or Treatment Resistance
• Best to attempt another monotherapy prior to augmenting for ADHD
• Possibly combination with stimulants with caution (not licensed for combination therapy)
• Combinations for ADHD should be for the expert, while monitoring the patient closely, and when other treatment options have failed

Tests
• Baseline evaluation to identify increased risk of somnolence and sedation, hypotension and bradycardia, QT-prolongation arrhythmia and weight increase

- Blood pressure, heart rate, and BMI should be reviewed every 3 months during the first year of treatment, as guanfacine can cause hypotension and bradycardia
- Monitor for signs of adverse effects on a weekly basis whilst titrating up the dose, and then every 3 months for the first year, and every 6 months after that

SIDE EFFECTS

How Drug Causes Side Effects
- Excessive actions on alpha 2A receptors, non-selective actions on alpha 2B and alpha 2C receptors

Notable Side Effects
- Sedation, dizziness
- Dry mouth, constipation, abdominal pain
- Fatigue, weakness
- Hypotension

Common or very common
- CNS/PNS: altered mood, anxiety, depression, dizziness, drowsiness, headache, sleep disorders
- CVS: arrhythmias, hypotension
- GIT: constipation, decreased appetite, diarrhoea, dry mouth, gastrointestinal discomfort, nausea, vomiting, weight increased
- Other: asthenia, skin reactions, urinary disorders

Uncommon
- CNS: hallucination, loss of consciousness, seizure
- CVS: atrioventricular block, chest pain, syncope
- Other: asthma, pallor

Rare or very rare
- Feeling of malaise, high BP (including hypertensive encephalopathy)

Frequency not known
- Impotence

 Life-Threatening or Dangerous Side Effects
- Sinus bradycardia, hypotension (dose-related)

Weight Gain

- Reported but not expected

Sedation

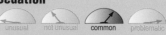
- Many experience and/or can be significant in amount
- Some patients may not tolerate it
- Can abate with time

What to Do About Side Effects
- Wait
- Adjust dose
- Adjust time of day dosing for once-daily dosing (e.g. where sedation is a persistent problem)
- If side effects persist, discontinue use

Best Augmenting Agents for Side Effects
- Dose reduction or switching to another agent may be more effective since most side effects cannot be improved with an augmenting agent

DOSING AND USE

Usual Dosage Range
- Modified-release: 1–7 mg/day

Dosage Forms
- Modified-release: 1 mg, 2 mg, 3 mg, 4 mg

How to Dose
- Modified-release: initial dose 1 mg/day; can increase by 1 mg/week; maintenance 0.05–0.12 mg/kg once daily. Dosed once daily, either in the morning or in the evening
- Child 6–12 years (body weight 25 kg and above) max dose 4 mg/day
- Child 13–17 years (body weight 34 kg to 41.4 kg) max dose 4 mg/day
- Child 13–17 years (body weight 41.5 kg to 49.4 kg) max dose 5 mg/day
- Child 13–17 years (body weight 49.5 kg to 58.4 kg) max dose 6 mg/day
- Child 13–17 years (body weight 58.5 kg and above) max dose 7 mg/day

 Dosing Tips
- Adverse effects are dose-related and usually transient
- Doses greater than 2 mg/day are associated with increased side effects

- If guanfacine is terminated abruptly, rebound hypertension may occur within 2–4 days
- Do not administer modified-release formulations with high-fat meals because this increases exposure
- Modified-release tablets should not be crushed, chewed, or broken
- Consider dosing on a mg/kg basis (0.05 mg/kg to 0.12 mg/kg)

Overdose
- Drowsiness, lethargy, bradycardia, hypotension, respiratory depression

Long-Term Use
- Studies of up to 2 years in children with ADHD show it is safe

Habit Forming
- No

How to Stop
- Taper to avoid rebound effects (nervousness, increased blood pressure)

Pharmacokinetics
- Elimination half-life of guanfacine is about 18 hours
- Metabolised by CYP450 3A4

 Drug Interactions
- CYP450 3A4 inhibitors such as fluoxetine, fluvoxamine, and ketoconazole may decrease clearance of guanfacine and raise guanfacine levels significantly, so a decrease in the guanfacine dose is recommended
- CYP450 3A4 inducers may increase clearance of guanfacine and lower guanfacine levels significantly
- Do not administer modified-release preparation with high-fat meals, because this increases exposure
- Combined use with valproate may increase plasma concentrations of valproate
- Increased depressive effects when taken with other CNS depressants
- Phenobarbital and phenytoin may reduce plasma concentrations of guanfacine
- Caution should be used administering with antihypertensives, as there is an increased risk of additive adverse effects including hypotension and syncope

 Other Warnings/Precautions
- Excessive heat (e.g. saunas) may exacerbate some of the side effects, such as dizziness and drowsiness
- Use with caution in patients with severe coronary insufficiency, recent myocardial infarction, cerebrovascular disease, or chronic renal or hepatic failure
- Risk of torsade de pointes in patients with bradycardia, heart block, hypokalaemia
- Use with caution in patients with history of QT-interval prolongation

Do Not Use
- If there is a proven allergy to guanfacine

SPECIAL POPULATIONS
Renal Impairment
- Patients with severe or end-stage renal disease should receive lower doses

Hepatic Impairment
- Use with caution
- 50% of clearance is hepatic so dose reduction should be considered

Cardiac Impairment
- Use with caution in patients with recent myocardial infarction, severe coronary insufficiency, cerebrovascular disease
- Use with caution in patients with bradycardia (risk of torsade de pointes), heart block (risk of torsade de pointes), history of QT-interval prolongation, hypokalaemia (risk of torsade de pointes)
- Use with caution in patients at risk for hypotension or syncope

Elderly
- Elimination half-life may be longer in elderly patients
- Elderly patients may be more sensitive to sedative effects
- Safety and efficacy not established in adults over 65

 Children and Adolescents
- Licensed for use for the treatment of ADHD for children aged 6–17

- Safety and efficacy not established in children under age 6

Before you prescribe:

- Diagnosis of ADHD should only be made by an appropriately qualified healthcare professional, e.g. specialist psychiatrist, paediatrician, and after full clinical and psychosocial assessment in different domains, full developmental and psychiatric history, observer reports across different settings and opportunity to speak to the child and carer on their own
- Children and adolescents with untreated anxiety, PTSD and mood disorders, or those who do not have a psychiatric diagnosis but social or environmental stressors, may present with anger, irritability, motor agitation, and concentration problems
- Consider undiagnosed learning disability or specific learning difficulties and sensory impairments that may potentially cause or contribute to inattention and restlessness, especially in school
- ADHD-specific advice on symptom management and environmental adaptations should be offered to all families and teachers, including reducing distractions, seating, shorter periods of focus, movement breaks and teaching assistants
- For children older than 5 years of age and young people with moderate ADHD pharmacological treatment should be considered if they continue to show significant impairment in at least one setting after symptom management and environmental adaptations have been implemented
- For severe ADHD, behavioural symptom management may not be effective until pharmacological treatment has been established

Practical notes:

ADHD

- Guanfacine may be offered where parents or the young person do not want stimulant medication. Depending on the child's profile, it may be a second- or third-line treatment in children, where other treatments have not been effective, or where stimulants not tolerated, or where there is co-morbid severely impairing tic disorder, or where stimulant medication has led to sustained and impairing exacerbation of tics

- Consider a course of cognitive behavioural therapy (CBT) for young people with ADHD who have benefited from medication but whose symptoms are still causing a significant impairment in at least one domain, addressing the following areas: social skills with peers, problem-solving, self-control, active listening skills, dealing with and expressing feelings
- Medication for ADHD for a child under 5 years should only be considered on specialist advice from an ADHD service with expertise in managing ADHD in young children (ideally a tertiary service). Use of medicines for treating ADHD is off-label in children aged less than 5 years of age
- Offer the same medication choices to people with ADHD and anxiety disorder, tic disorder or autism spectrum disorder as other people with ADHD
- Monitor behavioural response. If no change or behaviour worsens, adjust medication and/or review diagnosis, formulation and care-plan implementation

Tic disorders

- Transient tics occur in up to 20% of children. Tourette syndrome occurs in 1% of children
- Tics wax and wane over time and may be exacerbated by factors such as fatigue, inactivity, stress
- Tics are a lifelong disorder, but often get better over time. As many as 65% of young people with Tourette syndrome have only mild tics in adult life
- Co-morbid OCD, ADHD, depression, anxiety and behavioural problems should be treated first
- Most people don't require pharmacological intervention
- Psychoeducation and comprehensive behavioural interventions are recommended as first-line treatments
- It can be used as monotherapy or as adjunct

General

- Monitor patients face-to-face regularly, particularly during the first several weeks of treatment
- Children are more sensitive to side effects. Therefore: start slow and go slow with titration
- Children may be more sensitive to hypertensive effects of withdrawing treatment. Frequency and severity of

withdrawal symptoms may be less than with clonidine

*Because children commonly have gastrointestinal illnesses that lead to vomiting, they may be more likely to abruptly discontinue guanfacine and therefore be more susceptible to hypertensive episodes resulting from abrupt inability to take medication
* Children may be more likely to experience CNS depression with overdose and may even exhibit signs of toxicity with guanfacine
* Re-evaluate the need for continued treatment regularly
* Some reports of mania and aggressive behaviour in ADHD patients taking guanfacine

Pregnancy

* Controlled studies have not been conducted in pregnant women
* Very limited data on use during pregnancy
* Animal studies do not show adverse effects
* Use in women of childbearing potential requires weighing potential benefits to the mother against potential risks to the foetus

Breastfeeding

* Unknown if guanfacine is secreted in human breast milk, but all psychotropics assumed to be secreted in breast milk
* Recommended either to discontinue drug or bottle feed
* Infants of women who choose to breastfeed while on guanfacine should be monitored for possible adverse effects
* If irritability, sleep disturbance, or poor weight gain develop in nursing infant, may need to discontinue drug or bottle feed

THE ART OF PSYCHOPHARMACOLOGY

Potential Advantages

* No known abuse potential; not a controlled substance
* Not a stimulant
* For oppositional behaviour associated with ADHD
* Less sedation than clonidine
* Not been linked to any liver injury

Potential Disadvantages

* Not well studied in adults with ADHD

Primary Target Symptoms

* Concentration
* Motor hyperactivity
* Oppositional and impulsive behaviour
* High blood pressure

Pearls

* Guanfacine has been shown to be effective in both children and adults, and guanfacine modified-release is approved for ADHD in children aged 6–17 years
* Guanfacine can also be used to treat tic disorders, including Tourette syndrome, though there is less evidence than for clonidine
* Although both guanfacine and clonidine are alpha 2 adrenergic agonists, guanfacine is relatively selective for alpha 2A receptors, whereas clonidine binds not only alpha 2A, 2B, and 2C receptors but also imidazoline receptors, causing more sedation, hypotension, and side effects than guanfacine
* May be used as monotherapy or in combination with stimulants for the treatment of oppositional behaviour in children with or without ADHD

Guanfacine (Continued)

 Suggested Reading

Arnsten AF, Scahill L, Findling RL. Alpha2-adrenergic receptor agonists for the treatment of attention-deficit/hyperactivity disorder: emerging concepts from new data. J Child Adolesc Psychopharmacol 2007;17(4):393–406.

Biederman J, Melmed RD, Patel A, et al. Long-term, open-label extension study of guanfacine extended-release in children and adolescents with ADHD. CNS Spectr 2008;13(12):1047–55.

Cutler AJ, Mattingly GW, Jain R, et al. Current and future nonstimulants in the treatment of pediatric ADHD: monoamine reuptake inhibitors, receptor modulators, and multimodal agents. CNS Spectr 2022;27(2):199–207.

Mechler K, Banaschewski T, Hohmann S, et al. Evidence-based pharmacological treatment options for ADHD in children and adolescents. Pharmacol Ther 2022;230:107940.

Posey DJ, McDougal CJ. Guanfacine and guanfacine extended-release: treatment for ADHD and related disorders. CNS Drug Rev 2007;13(4):465–74.

Sallee FR, Lyne A, Wigal T, et al. Long-term safety and efficacy of guanfacine extended-release in children and adolescents with attention-deficit/hyperactivity disorder. J Child Adolesc Psychopharmacol 2009;19(3):215–26.

Sallee FR, McGough J, Wigal T, et al. Guanfacine extended-release in children and adolescents with attention-deficit/hyperactivity disorder: a placebo-controlled trial. J Am Acad Child Adolesc Psychiatry 2009;48(2):155–65.

Spencer TJ, Greenbaum M, Ginsberg LD, et al. Safety and effectiveness of coadministration of guanfacine extended-release and psychostimulants in children and adolescents with attention-deficit/hyperactivity disorder. J Child Adolesc Psychopharmacol 2009;19(5):501–10.

Haloperidol

Brands
- Haldol
- Halkid
- Haldol decanoate

Generic?
Yes

Class
- Neuroscience-based nomenclature: pharmacology domain – dopamine; mode of action – antagonist
- Conventional antipsychotic (neuroleptic, butyrophenone, dopamine 2 antagonist)

Commonly Prescribed for
(bold for BNF indication)
- **Schizophrenia and schizoaffective disorder [oral]**
- **Maintenance in schizophrenia and schizoaffective disorder (in patients currently stabilised on oral haloperidol) [long-acting IM injection]**
- **Acute delirium (where non-pharmacological treatments are ineffective) [oral, immediate-action IM injection]**
- **Moderate-to-severe manic episodes associated with bipolar I disorder [oral]**
- **Acute psychomotor agitation associated with psychotic disorder or manic episodes of bipolar I disorder [oral]**
- **Rapid control of severe acute psychomotor agitation associated with psychotic disorder or manic episodes of bipolar I disorder (when oral therapy is not appropriate) [immediate-action IM injection]**
- **Persistent aggression and psychotic symptoms in moderate to severe Alzheimer's dementia and vascular dementia (when non-pharmacological treatments are ineffective and there is risk of harm to self or others) [oral]**
- **Severe tic disorders, including Tourette syndrome (when educational, psychological, and other pharmacological treatments are ineffective) [oral]**
- **Mild-to-moderate chorea in Huntington's disease (when alternatives ineffective or not tolerated) [oral, immediate-action IM injection]**
- **Prophylaxis of postoperative nausea and vomiting (in patients at moderate to high risk and when alternatives ineffective or not tolerated)**
- **Combination treatment of postoperative nausea and vomiting (when alternatives ineffective or not tolerated)**
- Nausea and vomiting in palliative care (unlicensed)
- Restlessness and confusion in palliative care (unlicensed)

In children (under expert supervision):
- **Schizophrenia, 13–17 years old (when alternatives ineffective or not tolerated) [oral]**
- **Persistent, severe aggression in autism or pervasive developmental disorder, 6–17 years old (when other treatments ineffective or not tolerated)**
- **Severe tic disorders, including Tourette syndrome, 10–17 years old (when educational, psychological and other pharmacological treatments are ineffective)**
- Nausea and vomiting in palliative care (unlicensed)
- Restlessness and confusion in palliative care (unlicensed)

 ## How the Drug Works
- Blocks dopamine 2 receptors, reducing positive symptoms of psychosis and possibly combative, explosive, and hyperactive behaviours
- Blocks dopamine 2 receptors in the nigrostriatal pathway, improving tics and other symptoms in Tourette syndrome

How Long Until It Works
- Psychotic symptoms can improve within 1 week, but it may take several weeks for full effect on behaviour

If It Works
- Most often reduces positive symptoms in schizophrenia but does not eliminate them
- Most patients with schizophrenia do not have a total remission of symptoms but rather a reduction of symptoms by about a third
- Continue treatment in schizophrenia until reaching a plateau of improvement

Haloperidol (Continued)

- After reaching a satisfactory plateau, continue treatment for at least a year after first episode of psychosis in schizophrenia
- For second and subsequent episodes of psychosis in schizophrenia, treatment may need to be indefinite
- Reduces symptoms of acute psychotic mania but not proven as a mood stabiliser or as an effective maintenance treatment in bipolar disorder
- After reducing acute psychotic symptoms in mania, switch to a mood stabiliser and/or an atypical antipsychotic for mood stabilisation and maintenance

If It Doesn't Work

- Consider trying one of the first-line atypical antipsychotics (risperidone, olanzapine, quetiapine, aripiprazole, amisulpride)
- Consider trying another conventional antipsychotic
- If 2 or more antipsychotic monotherapies do not work, consider clozapine

Best Augmenting Combos for Partial Response or Treatment Resistance

- Augmentation of conventional antipsychotics has not been systematically studied
- Addition of a mood-stabilising anticonvulsant such as valproate, carbamazepine, or lamotrigine may be helpful in both schizophrenia and bipolar mania
- Augmentation with lithium in bipolar mania may be helpful
- Addition of a benzodiazepine, especially short-term for agitation

Tests

Baseline

*Measure weight, BMI, and waist circumference
- Get baseline personal and family history of diabetes, obesity, dyslipidaemia, hypertension, and cardiovascular disease
- Check for personal history of drug-induced leucopenia/neutropenia
*Check pulse and blood pressure, fasting plasma glucose or glycosylated haemoglobin (HbA1c), fasting lipid profile, and prolactin levels
- Full blood count (FBC)

- Assessment of nutritional status, diet, and level of physical activity
- Determine if the patient:
  - is overweight (BMI 25.0–29.9)
  - is obese (BMI ≥30)
  - has pre-diabetes – fasting plasma glucose: 5.5 mmol/L to 6.9 mmol/L or HbA1c: 42 to 47 mmol/mol (6.0 to 6.4%)
  - has diabetes – fasting plasma glucose: >7.0 mmol/L or HbA1c: ≥48 mmol/L (≥6.5%)
  - has hypertension (BP >140/90 mm Hg)
  - has dyslipidaemia (increased total cholesterol, LDL cholesterol, and triglycerides; decreased HDL cholesterol)
- Treat or refer such patients for treatment, including nutrition and weight management, physical activity counselling, smoking cessation, and medical management
- Baseline ECG for: inpatients; those with a personal history or risk factor for cardiac disease

Children and adolescents:
- As for adults
- Also check history of congenital heart problems, history of dizziness when stressed or on exertion, history of long-QT syndrome, family history of long-QT syndrome, bradycardia, myocarditis, family history of cardiac myopathies, low K+/low Mg++/low Ca++
- Measure weight, BMI, and waist circumference plotted on a growth chart
- Pulse, BP plotted on a percentile chart
- ECG: note for QTc interval – machine-generated may be incorrect in children as different formula needed if HR <60 or >100
- Baseline prolactin levels

Monitoring

- Monitor weight and BMI during treatment
- Consider monitoring fasting triglycerides monthly for several months in patients at high risk for metabolic complications and when initiating or switching antipsychotics
- While giving a drug to a patient who has gained >5% of initial weight, consider evaluating for the presence of pre-diabetes, diabetes, or dyslipidaemia, or consider switching to a different antipsychotic
- Patients with low white blood cell count (WBC) or history of drug-induced leucopenia/neutropenia should have full blood count (FBC) monitored frequently during the first few months and haloperidol should be discontinued at the first sign

of decline of WBC in the absence of other causative factors
* Monitor prolactin levels and for signs and symptoms of hyperprolactinaemia

Children and adolescents:
* As for adults
* Weight/BMI/waist circumference, weekly for the first 6 weeks, then at 12 weeks, then every 6 months, plotted on a growth/percentile chart
* Height every 6 months, plotted on a growth chart
* Pulse and blood pressure at 12 weeks, then every 6 months plotted on a percentile chart
* ECG prior to starting and after 2 weeks after dose increase for monitoring of QTc interval. Machine-generated may be incorrect in children as different formula needed if HR <60 or >100
* Prolactin levels: prior to starting and after 12 weeks, 24 weeks, and 6-monthly thereafter. Consider additional monitoring in young adults (under 25) who have not yet reached peak bone mass. In comparison quetiapine is only associated with marginal increase of prolactin
* In prepubertal children monitor sexual maturation
* In post-pubertal children and young person monitor sexual side effects (both sexes: loss of libido, sexual dysfunction, galactorrhoea, infertility; male: diminished ejaculate, gynaecomastia; female: oligorrhoea/amenorrhoea, reduced vaginal lubrication, dyspareunia, acne, hirsutism)

SIDE EFFECTS
How Drug Causes Side Effects
* By blocking dopamine 2 receptors in the striatum, it can cause motor side effects
* By blocking dopamine 2 receptors in the pituitary, it can cause elevations in prolactin
* By blocking dopamine 2 receptors excessively in the mesocortical and mesolimbic dopamine pathways, especially at high doses, it can cause worsening of negative and cognitive symptoms (neuroleptic-induced deficit syndrome)
* By blocking alpha 1 adrenergic receptors, it can cause dizziness, sedation, and hypotension

* Mechanism of weight gain and any possible increased incidence of diabetes or dyslipidaemia with conventional antipsychotics is unknown

Notable Side Effects
* Neuroleptic-induced deficit syndrome
* Akathisia
* Extrapyramidal symptoms, parkinsonism, tardive dyskinesia, tardive dystonia, hypersalivation
* Galactorrhoea, amenorrhoea
* Dizziness, sedation
* Dry mouth, constipation, urinary retention, blurred vision
* Decreased sweating
* Hypotension, tachycardia, hypertension
* Weight gain or decrease

Common or very common
* CNS/PNS: depression, eye and vision disorders, headache, neuromuscular dysfunction, psychosis
* GIT: increased salivation, nausea, weight loss

Uncommon
* CNS/PNS: abnormal gait, confusion, muscular rigidity, restlessness
* Other: breast abnormalities, dyspnoea, excessive sweating, hepatic disorders, menstrual cycle abnormalities, oedema, photosensitivity, sexual dysfunction, skin reactions, temperature dysregulation

Rare or very rare
* Hypoglycaemia, respiratory disorders, SIADH, trismus

Frequency not known
* Hypersensitivity vasculitis, pancytopenia, rhabdomyolysis, thrombocytopenia
* With oral use: angioedema
* With parenteral use: hypertension, severe cutaneous adverse reactions (SCARs)

 Life-Threatening or Dangerous Side Effects
* Rare neuroleptic malignant syndrome
* Rare seizures
* Rare jaundice, agranulocytosis, leucopenia, pancytopenia, thrombocytopenia
* Increased risk of death and cerebrovascular events in elderly patients with dementia-related psychosis
* Hypersensitivity vasculitis

Haloperidol (Continued)

Weight Gain

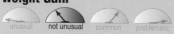

- Occurs in significant minority

Sedation

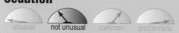

- Sedation is usually transient

What to Do About Side Effects

- Wait
- Wait
- Wait
- Reduce the dose
- Low-dose benzodiazepine or beta blocker may reduce akathisia
- Take more of the dose at bedtime to help reduce daytime sedation
- Weight loss, exercise programmes, and medical management for high BMIs, diabetes, and dyslipidaemia
- Switch to another antipsychotic (atypical) – quetiapine or clozapine are best in cases of tardive dyskinesia

Best Augmenting Agents for Side Effects

- Dystonia: antimuscarinic drugs (e.g. procyclidine) as oral or IM depending on the severity; botulinum toxin if antimuscarinics not effective
- Parkinsonism: antimuscarinic drugs (e.g. procyclidine)
- Akathisia: beta blocker propranolol (30–80 mg/day) or low-dose benzodiazepine (e.g. 0.5–3.0 mg/day of clonazepam) may help; other agents that may be tried include the 5HT2 antagonists such as cyproheptadine (16 mg/day) or mirtazapine (15 mg at night – caution in bipolar disorder); clonidine (0.2–0.8 mg/day) may be tried if the above ineffective
- Tardive dyskinesia: stop any antimuscarinic, consider tetrabenazine

DOSING AND USE

Usual Dosage Range

- Schizophrenia and schizoaffective disorder: orally 1–20 mg/day
- Acute delirium: orally 1–10 mg/day in 1–3 divided doses; by IM injection 1–10 mg/day at 2–4 hourly intervals

- Moderate to severe manic episodes associated with bipolar I disorder: orally 2–15 mg/day in divided doses
- Acute psychomotor agitation associated with psychotic disorder or manic episodes of bipolar I disorder: 5–10 mg orally prn (max 20 mg in 24 hours). Severe cases: 5 mg by IM injection prn (max 20 mg in 24 hours)
- Persistent aggression and psychotic symptoms in moderate to severe Alzheimer's dementia and vascular dementia: orally 0.5–5 mg/day in 1–2 divided doses (dose adjusted according to response)
- Severe tic disorders, including Tourette syndrome: orally 0.5–5 mg/day in 1–2 divided doses, dose adjusted according to response
- Mild to moderate chorea in Huntington's disease: orally 2–10 mg/day in 1–2 divided doses, dose adjusted according to response. When oral tablets not appropriate: by IM injection 2–5 mg prn (max 10 mg in 24 hours)
- Decanoate injection 25–300 mg every 4 weeks (see Haloperidol Decanoate section after Pearls for dosing and use)

Dosage Forms

- Tablet 0.5 mg, 1.5 mg, 5 mg, 10 mg
- Solution 200 mcg/mL, 1 mg/mL, 5 mg/5 mL, 2 mg/mL, 10 mg/5 mL
- Injection 5 mg/mL (immediate-release)
- Decanoate injection 50 mg/mL, 100 mg/mL

How to Dose

*Schizophrenia and schizoaffective disorder:
- Orally 2–10 mg/day in 1–2 divided doses
- Usual dose 2–4 mg/day in first-episode schizophrenia
- Up to 10 mg/day, in subsequent episodes
- Dose adjusted to response at intervals of 1–7 days
- Balance benefits versus risks for doses above 10 mg/day; max 20 mg per day
*Acute delirium:
- Orally 1–10 mg/day in 1–3 divided doses, start at lowest possible dose and adjust by increments every 2–4 hours as required; max 10 mg in 24 hours
- By IM injection 1–10 mg, start at lowest possible dose and adjust by increments at every 2–4 hours as required; max 10 mg in 24 hours
*Moderate to severe manic episodes associated with bipolar I disorder:
- Orally 2–10 mg/day in 1–2 divided doses, dose adjusted according to response at

intervals of 1–3 days. Balance benefit versus risk for doses above 10 mg/day; max 15 mg/day

＊Acute psychomotor agitation associated with psychotic disorder or manic episodes of bipolar I disorder:
- Orally 5–10 mg, may be repeated after 12 hours as needed; max 20 mg/day
- Severe cases: by IM injection 5 mg, dose may be repeated every hour – usually up to 15 mg/day; max 20 mg/day

＊Persistent aggression and psychotic symptoms in moderate to severe Alzheimer's dementia and vascular dementia:
- Orally 0.5–5 mg/day in 1–2 divided doses, adjusted according to response at intervals of 1–3 days. Reassess at 6 weeks

＊Severe tic disorders, including Tourette syndrome:
- Orally 0.5–5 mg/day in 1–2 divided doses, dose adjusted according to response at intervals of 1–7 days. Reassess every 6–12 months

＊Mild to moderate chorea in Huntington's disease:
- Orally 2–10 mg/day in 1–2 divided doses, dose adjusted according to response at intervals of 1–3 days. When IM injection required 2–5 mg, dose may be repeated every hour; max 10 mg/day

Dosing Tips

- Haloperidol is frequently dosed too high
- Some studies suggest that patients who respond well to low doses of haloperidol (e.g. about 2 mg/day) may have efficacy similar to atypical antipsychotics for both positive and negative symptoms of schizophrenia
- Higher doses may actually induce or worsen negative symptoms of schizophrenia
- Low doses, however, may not have beneficial actions for treatment-resistant cases or violence
- One of the few antipsychotics with a depot formulation lasting for up to a month
- Treatment should be suspended if absolute neutrophil count falls below 1.5×10^9/L

Overdose

- Fatalities have been reported; extrapyramidal symptoms, hypotension, sedation, respiratory depression, shock-like state, sinus tachycardia, arrhythmia, hypothermia

Long-Term Use

- Often used for long-term maintenance
- Some side effects may be irreversible (e.g. tardive dyskinesia)

Habit Forming

- No

How to Stop

- Slow down-titration of oral formulation (over 6–8 weeks), especially when simultaneously beginning a new antipsychotic while switching (i.e. cross-titration)
- Rapid oral discontinuation may lead to rebound psychosis and worsening of symptoms
- If anti-Parkinson agents are being used, they should be continued for a few weeks after haloperidol is discontinued

Pharmacokinetics

- Decanoate half-life is about 3 weeks
- Oral half-life about 12–38 hours (average 24 hours). Peak plasma level reached in 2–6 hours. Steady state reached within 1 week of initiation

Drug Interactions

- May decrease the effects of levodopa, dopamine agonists
- May increase the effects of antihypertensive drugs except for guanethidine, whose antihypertensive actions haloperidol may antagonise
- Additive effects may occur if used with CNS depressants; dose of other agent should be reduced
- Some pressor agents (e.g. adrenaline) may interact with haloperidol to lower blood pressure
- Haloperidol and anticholinergic agents together may increase intraocular pressure
- Reduces effects of anticoagulants
- Plasma levels of haloperidol may be lowered by rifampicin
- Some patients taking haloperidol and lithium have developed an encephalopathic syndrome similar to neuroleptic malignant syndrome
- May enhance effects of antihypertensive drugs

Other Warnings/Precautions

- All antipsychotics should be used with caution in patients with angle-closure glaucoma, blood disorders, cardiovascular disease, depression, diabetes, epilepsy and susceptibility to seizures, history of jaundice, myasthenia gravis, Parkinson's disease, photosensitivity, prostatic hypertrophy, severe respiratory disorders
- If signs of neuroleptic malignant syndrome develop, treatment should be immediately discontinued
- Use with caution in patients with respiratory disorders
- Avoid extreme heat exposure
- If haloperidol is used to treat mania, patients may experience a rapid switch to depression
- Patients with thyrotoxicosis may experience neurotoxicity
- Higher doses and parenteral administration may be associated with increased risk of QT prolongation and torsades de pointes
- Use with caution in patients with underlying cardiac abnormalities, bradycardia, electrolyte disturbances (correct before treatment initiation), personal or family history of QTc-interval prolongation including familial long-QT syndrome, hypotension (including orthostatic hypotension), hypothyroidism, risk factors for stroke
- Use with caution in patients taking a drug known to prolong QT interval
- Use with caution in patients with a history of heavy alcohol use
- Use with caution in patients with prolactin-dependent tumours or hyperprolactinaemia

Do Not Use

- If patient is in comatose state or has CNS depression
- If patient has Lewy body disease or progressive supranuclear palsy
- If there is congenital long-QT syndrome, history of torsade de pointes, history of ventricular arrhythmia, QTc-interval prolongation, recent acute myocardial infarction, decompensated heart failure, uncorrected hypokalaemia
- If there is a proven allergy to haloperidol

SPECIAL POPULATIONS

Renal Impairment

- Use with caution: consider lower dose and adjust with smaller increments at longer intervals

Hepatic Impairment

- Use with caution: halve initial dose and adjust with smaller increments at longer intervals

Cardiac Impairment

- Use with caution because of risk of orthostatic hypertension
- Possible increased risk of QT prolongation or torsades de pointes at higher doses or with IV administration

Elderly

- Lower doses should be used and patient should be monitored closely
- Elderly patients may be more susceptible to respiratory side effects and hypotension
- Elderly patients with dementia-related psychosis treated with antipsychotics are at an increased risk of death compared to placebo, and also have an increased risk of cerebrovascular events
- Schizophrenia and schizoaffective disorder: initially, use half the lowest adult dose and adjust gradually according to response to max 5 mg/day. Increases beyond 5 mg/day after full individual risk-benefit analysis if tolerated higher doses
- Acute delirium: orally – initially, use half the lowest adult dose, then adjust gradually according to response up to max 5 mg/day, doses above 5 mg/day should only be considered in patients who have tolerated higher doses and after reassessment of the individual benefit-risk. By IM injection – initially 500 mcg, dose adjusted gradually according to response up to max 5 mg/day, doses above 5 mg/day should only be considered in patients who have tolerated higher doses and after reassessment of the individual benefit-risk
- Moderate to severe manic episodes associated with bipolar I disorder: orally initially, use half the lowest adult dose, then adjust gradually according to response up to max 5 mg/day, doses above 5 mg/day should only be considered in patients who have tolerated higher doses and after reassessment of the individual benefit-risk;

continued use should be evaluated early in treatment
- Acute psychomotor agitation associated with psychotic disorder or manic episodes of bipolar I disorder: orally initial dose 2.5 mg, may be repeated after 12 hours if required up to max 5 mg/day, doses above 5 mg/day should only be considered in patients who have tolerated higher doses and after reassessment of the individual benefit-risk; continued use should be evaluated early in treatment. Severe cases: by IM injection 2.5 mg, dose may be repeated after an hour if required up to max 5 mg/day, doses above 5 mg/day should only be considered in patients who have tolerated higher doses and after reassessment of the individual benefit-risk; continued use should be evaluated early in treatment
- Persistent aggression and psychotic symptoms in moderate to severe Alzheimer's dementia and vascular dementia: orally 500 mcg/day, reassess treatment after no more than 6 weeks
- Severe tic disorders, including Tourette syndrome: orally initially, use half the lowest adult dose, then adjust gradually according to response up to max 5 mg/day. Reassess treatment every 6–12 months
- Mild to moderate chorea in Huntington's disease: orally initially, use half the lowest adult dose, then adjust gradually according to response up to max 5 mg/day, doses above 5 mg/day should only be considered in patients who have tolerated higher doses and after reassessment of the individual benefit-risk. When oral therapy inappropriate: by IM injection initially 1 mg, dose may be repeated hourly if required up to max 5 mg/day, doses above 5 mg/day should only be considered in patients who have tolerated higher doses and after reassessment of the individual benefit-risk

Children and Adolescents

- Generally considered second-line or third-line after atypical antipsychotics
- Safety and efficacy have not been established; not intended for use under age 3
- Should only be prescribed under expert supervision
- Not licensed for use in palliative care

Before you prescribe:
- Do not offer antipsychotic medication when transient or attenuated psychotic symptoms or other mental state changes associated with distress, impairment, or help-seeking behaviour are not sufficient for a diagnosis of psychosis or schizophrenia. Consider individual CBT with or without family therapy and other treatments recommended for anxiety, depression, substance use, or emerging personality disorder
- For first-episode psychosis (FEP) antipsychotic medication should only be started by a specialist following a comprehensive multidisciplinary assessment and in conjunction with recommended psychological interventions (CBT, family therapy)
- As first-line treatment: allow patient to choose from aripiprazole, olanzapine, or risperidone. As second-line treatment switch to alternative from list. Consider quetiapine depending on desired profile. Haloperidol only to be considered if other antipsychotic treatments ineffective or not tolerated
- Choice of antipsychotic medication should be an informed choice depending on individual factors and side-effect profile (metabolic, cardiovascular, extrapyramidal, hormonal, other)
- All children and young people with FEP/bipolar should be supported with sleep management, anxiety management, exercise and activation schedules, and healthy diet
- Where a child or young person presents with self-harm and suicidal thoughts the immediate risk management may take first priority
- Persistent severe aggression in children with autism or pervasive developmental disorders, when other treatments are ineffective or not tolerated. There are many reasons for challenging behaviours in autism spectrum disorder (ASD) and consideration should be given to possible physical, psychosocial, environmental or ASD-specific causes (e.g. sensory processing difficulties, communication). These should be addressed first. Consider behavioural interventions and family support. Pharmacological treatment can be offered alongside the above. It may be prudent to periodically discontinue prescriptions if symptoms are well controlled, and as irritability may

Haloperidol (Continued)

lessen as the patient is going through neurodevelopmental changes

- Severe tic disorder including Tourette syndrome under expert supervision, when educational, psychological and other pharmacological treatments are ineffective or not tolerated: transient tics occur in up to 20% of children. Tourette syndrome occurs in 1% of children. Tics wax and wane over time and are variably exacerbated by external factors such as stress, inactivity, fatigue. Tics are a lifelong disorder, but often get better over time. As many as 65% of young people with Tourette syndrome have only mild tics in adult life. Psychoeducation and evidence-based psychological interventions such as habit reversal therapy (HRT) or exposure and response prevention (ERP) should be offered first. Pharmacological treatment may be considered in conjunction with psychological interventions where tics result in significant impairment or psychosocial consequences, and/or where psychological interventions have been ineffective. If co-morbid with ADHD other choices (clonidine/guanfacine) may be better options to avoid polypharmacy
- A risk management plan is important prior to start of medication because of the possible increase in suicidal ideation and behaviours in adolescents and young adults

Practical notes:
- Carefully weigh the risks and benefits of pharmacological treatment against the risks and benefits of non-treatment and make sure to document this in the patient's chart
- Monitor weight, weekly for the first 6 weeks, then at 12 weeks, and then every 6 months (plotted on a growth chart)
- Monitor height every 6 months (plotted on a growth chart)
- Monitor waist circumference every 6 months (plotted on a percentile chart)
- Monitor pulse and blood pressure (plotted on a percentile chart) at 12 weeks and then every 6 months
- Monitor fasting blood glucose, HbA1c, blood lipid and prolactin levels at 12 weeks and then every 6 months
- Monitor for activation of suicidal ideation at the beginning of treatment. Inform parents or guardians of this risk so they can help observe child or adolescent patients

If it does not work:

- Review child's/young person's profile, consider new/changing contributing individual or systemic factors such as peer or family conflict. Consider drug/substance misuse. Consider dose adjustment before switching or augmentation. Be vigilant of polypharmacy especially in complex and highly vulnerable children/adolescents
- Consider non-concordance by parent or child, consider non-concordance in adolescents, address underlying reasons for non-concordance
- Children are more sensitive to most side effects
  - There is an inverse relationship between age and incidence of EPS
  - Exposure to antipsychotics during childhood and young age is associated with a three-fold increase of diabetes mellitus
  - Treatment with all second-generation antipsychotics has been associated with changes in most lipid parameters
  - Weight gain correlates with time on treatment. Any childhood obesity is associated with obesity in adults
- Dose adjustments may be necessary in the presence of interacting drugs
- Schizophrenia (child 13–17 years): oral 0.5–3.0 mg/day in 2–3 divided doses; increased up to 5 mg/day
- Persistent, severe aggression in autism or pervasive developmental disorders (child 6–11 years): oral 0.5–3.0 mg/day in 2–3 divided doses, the need for continued treatment must be reassessed after maximum of 6 weeks and regularly thereafter
- Persistent, severe aggression in autism or pervasive developmental disorder (child 12–17 years): oral 0.5–5.0 mg/day in 2–3 divided doses, the need for continued treatment must be reassessed after maximum of 6 weeks and regularly thereafter
- Severe tic disorders, including Tourette syndrome (child 1–17 years): oral 0.5–3.0 mg/day in 2–3 divided doses, the need for continued treatment must be reassessed every 6–12 months
- Re-evaluate the need for continued treatment regularly
- Monitoring of endocrine function (weight, height, sexual maturation and menses) is required when a child is taking an antipsychotic drug that is known to cause hyperprolactinaemia

Pregnancy

- Very limited safety data for the use of haloperidol in pregnancy
- There is a risk of abnormal muscle movements and withdrawal symptoms in newborns whose mothers took an antipsychotic during the third trimester; symptoms may include agitation, abnormally increased or decreased muscle tone, tremor, sleepiness, severe difficulty breathing, and difficulty feeding
- Reports of extrapyramidal symptoms, jaundice, hyperreflexia, hyporeflexia in infants whose mothers took a conventional antipsychotic during pregnancy
- Psychotic symptoms may worsen during pregnancy and some form of treatment may be necessary
- Switching antipsychotics may increase the risk of relapse
- Haloperidol may be preferable to anticonvulsant mood stabilisers if treatment or prophylaxis are required during pregnancy
- Effects of hyperprolactinaemia on the foetus are unknown
- Depot antipsychotics should only be used when there is a good response to the depot and a history of non-concordance with oral medication

Breastfeeding

- Small amounts expected in mother's breast milk
- Risk of accumulation in infant due to long half-life
- Haloperidol is considered to be the preferred first-generation antipsychotic, and quetiapine the preferred second-generation antipsychotic
- Infants of women who choose to breastfeed should be monitored for possible adverse effects

THE ART OF PSYCHOPHARMACOLOGY
Potential Advantages

- Intramuscular formulation for emergency use
- 4-week depot formulation for better adherence
- Low-dose responders may have comparable positive and negative symptom efficacy to atypical antipsychotics
- Low-cost, effective treatment
- Less sedating

Potential Disadvantages

- Patients with tardive dyskinesia or who wish to avoid tardive dyskinesia and extrapyramidal symptoms
- Vulnerable populations such as children or elderly
- Patients with notable cognitive or mood symptoms

Primary Target Symptoms

- Positive symptoms of psychosis
- Violent or aggressive behaviour

Pearls

- Prior to the introduction of atypical antipsychotics, haloperidol was one of the most preferred antipsychotics
- Haloperidol may still be a useful antipsychotic, especially at low doses for those patients who require management with a conventional antipsychotic
- Low doses may not induce negative symptoms, but high doses may
- Not clearly effective for improving cognitive or affective symptoms of schizophrenia
- May be effective for bipolar maintenance, but there may be more tardive dyskinesia when affective disorders are treated with a conventional antipsychotic long-term
- Less sedating than many other conventional antipsychotics, especially "low potency" phenothiazines
- Haloperidol may be used to treat delirium in combination with lorazepam
- Haloperidol's long-acting intramuscular formulation lasts up to 4 weeks, whereas some other long-acting intramuscular antipsychotics may last only up to 2 weeks
- Decanoate administration is intended for patients with chronic schizophrenia who have been stabilised on oral antipsychotic medication
- Patients have very similar antipsychotic responses to any conventional antipsychotic, which is different from atypical antipsychotics where antipsychotic responses of individual patients can occasionally vary greatly from one atypical antipsychotic to another
- Patients receiving atypical antipsychotics may occasionally require a "top up" of a conventional antipsychotic such as

haloperidol to control aggression or violent behaviour
- Patients with inadequate responses to atypical antipsychotics may benefit from a trial of augmentation with a conventional antipsychotic such as haloperidol or from switching to a conventional antipsychotic such as haloperidol
- However, long-term polypharmacy with a combination of a conventional antipsychotic such as haloperidol with an atypical antipsychotic may combine their side effects without clearly augmenting the efficacy of either
- For treatment-resistant patients, especially those with impulsivity, aggression, violence, and self-harm, long-term polypharmacy with 2 atypical antipsychotics or with 1 atypical antipsychotic and 1 conventional antipsychotic may be useful or even necessary while closely monitoring
- In such cases, it may be beneficial to combine 1 depot antipsychotic with 1 oral antipsychotic
- Subcutaneous haloperidol can be used for managing restlessness and confusion in palliative care

HALOPERIDOL DECANOATE

Haloperidol Decanoate Properties

Vehicle	Sesame oil/benzyl alcohol
Duration of action	6 weeks
Tmax	3–9 days (average 7 days)
T1/2 with single dosing	18–21 days
T1/2 with multiple dosing	18–21 days
Time to reach steady state	10–14 weeks
Dosing schedule (maintenance)	4 weeks
Injection site	Intramuscular (gluteal)
Needle gauge	21
Dosage forms	50 mg, 100 mg
Injection volume	50 mg/mL or 100 mg/mL; not to exceed 3 mL

Usual Dosage Range

- Maintenance in schizophrenia and paranoid psychoses
- Adult: 10–15 times the previous oral dose, typically 50–200 mg every 4 weeks. Max per dose 300 mg every 4 weeks

- Elderly: a quarter to half usual starting dose to be used (typically 12.5–75 mg every 4 weeks)
- Test doses: 50 mg (adult), 12.5–25 mg (elderly)

How to Dose

Adult:
- Transition from oral haloperidol: a haloperidol decanoate dose of 10 to 15 times the previous daily dose of oral haloperidol is recommended; thus the haloperidol decanoate dose will be 25 to 150 mg for most patients
- Continuation of treatment: recommended to adjust the haloperidol decanoate dose by up to 50 mg every 4 weeks (based on individual patient response) until an optimal therapeutic effect is obtained; the most effective dose is expected to range between 50 and 200 mg; assess the individual benefit-risk when considering doses above 200 mg every 4 weeks; max dose of 300 mg every 4 weeks must not be exceeded as safety concerns outweigh any clinical benefits of treatment
- Dosing interval: usually 4 weeks between injections; adjustment of the dosing interval may be required (based on individual patient response)
- Supplementation with non-decanoate haloperidol: supplementation with non-decanoate haloperidol may be considered during transition to Haldol decanoate, dose adjustment or episodes of exacerbation of psychotic symptoms (based on individual patient response); the combined total dose of haloperidol from both formulations must not exceed the corresponding max oral haloperidol dose of 20 mg/day

Elderly:
- Transition from oral haloperidol: a low haloperidol decanoate dose of 12.5 to 25 mg is recommended
- Continuation of treatment: recommended only to adjust the haloperidol decanoate dose if required (based on individual patient response) until an optimal therapeutic effect is obtained; the most effective dose is expected to range between 25 and 75 mg; doses above 75 mg every 4 weeks should only be considered in patients who have tolerated higher doses and after reassessment of the patient's individual benefit-risk profile

- Dosing interval: usually 4 weeks between injections; adjustment of the dosing interval may be required (based on individual patient response)
- Supplementation with non-decanoate haloperidol: supplementation with non-decanoate haloperidol may be considered during transition to Haldol decanoate, dose adjustment or episodes of exacerbation of psychotic symptoms (based on individual patient response); the combined total dose of haloperidol from both formulations must not exceed the corresponding max oral haloperidol dose of 5 mg/day or the previously administered oral haloperidol dose in patients who have received long-term treatment with oral haloperidol

Dosing Tips

- With depot injections, the absorption rate constant is slower than the elimination rate constant, thus resulting in "flip-flop" kinetics – i.e. time to steady state is a function of absorption rate, while concentration at steady state is a function of elimination rate
- The rate-limiting step for plasma drug levels for depot injections is not drug metabolism, but rather slow absorption from the injection site
- In general, 5 half-lives of any medication are needed to achieve 97% of steady-state levels
- The long half life of depot antipsychotics means that one must either adequately load the dose (if possible) or provide oral supplementation
- The failure to adequately load the dose leads either to prolonged cross-titration from oral antipsychotic or to sub-therapeutic antipsychotic plasma levels for weeks or months in patients who are not receiving (or adhering to) oral supplementation
- Because plasma antipsychotic levels increase gradually over time, dose requirements may ultimately decrease from initial; if possible obtaining periodic

plasma levels can be beneficial to prevent unnecessary plasma level creep
- The time to get a blood level for patients receiving depot is the morning of the day they will receive their next injection
- Therapeutic plasma concentrations range between 1–10 ng/mL; plasma levels greater than 20 ng/mL are generally not well tolerated
- Single injection volumes greater than 300 mg (3 mL) are not well tolerated, so patients who require higher doses typically receive the monthly dose as split injections every 2 weeks
- A loading strategy advocated by some is to give 300 mg depot every 1–2 weeks for 2 doses and then measure plasma drug concentrations just prior to a third loading dose to see if a third dose is necessary

THE ART OF SWITCHING

Switching from Oral Antipsychotics to Haloperidol Decanoate

- Discontinuation of oral antipsychotic can begin immediately if adequate loading is pursued; however, oral coverage may still be necessary for the first week
- How to discontinue oral formulations:
  - Down-titration is not required for: amisulpride, aripiprazole, cariprazine, paliperidone
  - 1-week down-titration is required for: lurasidone, risperidone
  - 3–4-week down-titration is required for: asenapine, olanzapine, quetiapine
  - 4+-week down-titration is required for: clozapine
  - For patients taking benzodiazepine or anticholinergic medication, this can be continued during cross-titration to help alleviate side effects such as insomnia, agitation, and/or psychosis. Once the patient is stable on the depot, these can be tapered one at a time as appropriate

Suggested Reading

Cipriani A, Rendell JM, Geddes JR. Haloperidol alone or in combination for acute mania. Cochrane Database Syst Rev 2006;19(3):CD004362.

Huf G, Alexander J, Allen MH, et al. Haloperidol plus promethazine for psychosis-induced aggression. Cochrane Database Syst Rev 2009;8(3):CD005146.

Huhn M, Nikolakopoulou A, Schneider-Thoma J, et al. Comparative efficacy and tolerability of 32 oral antipsychotics for the acute treatment of adults with multi-episode schizophrenia: a systematic review and network meta-analysis. Lancet 2019;394(10202):939–51.

Joy CB, Adams CE, Lawrie SM. Haloperidol versus placebo for schizophrenia. Cochrane Database Syst Rev 2006;18(4):CD003082.

Leucht C, Kitzmantel M, Chua L, et al. Haloperidol versus chlorpromazine for schizophrenia. Cochrane Database Syst Rev 2008;23(1):CD004278.

Meyer JM. Converting oral to long-acting injectable antipsychotics: a guide for the perplexed. CNS Spectr 2017;22(S1):14–28.

Patel MX, Sethi FN, Barnes TR, et al. Joint BAP NAPICU evidence-based consensus guidelines for the clinical management of acute disturbance: De-escalation and rapid tranquillisation. J Psychopharmacol 2018;32(6):601–40.

Pillinger T, McCutcheon RA, Vano L, et al. Comparative effects of 18 antipsychotics on metabolic function in patients with schizophrenia, predictors of metabolic dysregulation, and association with psychopathology: a systematic review and network meta-analysis. Lancet Psychiatry 2020;7(1):64–77.

Hydroxyzine hydrochloride

Brands
- Non-proprietary

Generic?
Yes

Class
- Neuroscience-based nomenclature: pharmacology domain – histamine; mode of action – antagonist
- Antihistamine (anxiolytic, hypnotic, antiemetic)

Commonly Prescribed for
(bold for BNF indication)
- **Pruritus**
- Anxiety and tension associated with psychoneurosis
- Adjunct in organic disease states in which anxiety is manifested
- Premedication sedation
- Sedation following general anaesthesia
- Acute disturbance/hysteria
- Anxiety withdrawal symptoms in alcoholics or patients with delirium tremens
- Adjunct in pre/post-operative and pre/post-partum patients to allay anxiety, control emesis, and reduce narcotic dose
- Nausea and vomiting
- Insomnia

 How the Drug Works
- Blocks histamine 1 receptors

How Long Until It Works
- 15–20 minutes
- Some immediate relief with first dosing is common; can take several weeks with daily dosing for maximal therapeutic benefit in chronic conditions

If It Works
- For short-term symptoms of anxiety: after a few weeks, discontinue use or use on an "as needed" basis
- For chronic anxiety disorders, the goal of treatment is complete remission of symptoms as well as prevention of future relapses
- For chronic anxiety disorders, treatment most often reduces or even eliminates symptoms, but is not a cure since symptoms can recur after medicine stopped

- For long-term symptoms of anxiety, consider switching to an SSRI or SNRI for long-term maintenance
- If long-term maintenance is necessary, continue treatment for 6 months after symptoms resolve, and then taper dose slowly
- If symptoms re-emerge, consider treatment with an SSRI or SNRI, or consider restarting hydroxyzine

If It Doesn't Work
- Consider switching to another agent, or adding an appropriate augmenting agent

 Best Augmenting Combos for Partial Response or Treatment Resistance
- Hydroxyzine can be used as an adjunct to SSRIs or SNRIs in treating anxiety disorders

Tests
- None for healthy individuals
- Hydroxyzine may cause falsely elevated urinary concentrations of 17-hydroxycorticosteroids in certain lab tests (e.g. Porter-Silber reaction, Glenn-Nelson method)
- May interfere with methacholine test – manufacturer advises to stop treatment 96 hours prior to test
- May interfere with skin testing for allergy – stop treatment 1 week prior to test

How Drug Causes Side Effects
- Blocking histamine 1 receptors can cause sedation
- Anticholinergic activity may lead to cognitive-related adverse effects particularly in the elderly

Notable Side Effects
- Anticholinergic effects: dry mouth, blurred vision, urinary retention, constipation
- Sedation
- Tremor
- Fatigue
- Headache

Rare or very rare
- Severe cutaneous adverse reactions (SCARs), skin reactions

Hydroxyzine hydrochloride (Continued)

Frequency not known
- Blood disorders: agranulocytosis, haemolytic anaemia, leucopenia, thrombocytopenia
- CNS/PNS: anxiety, coma, confusion, depression, dizziness, drowsiness, dyskinesia (on discontinuation), hallucination, headache, impaired concentration, irritability, labyrinthitis, movement disorders, paraesthesia, seizure (with high doses), sleep disorders, slurred speech, tinnitus, tremor (with high doses), vertigo, vision disorders
- CVS: arrhythmias, hypotension, palpitations, QT interval prolongation
- GIT: abnormal hepatic function, bitter taste, constipation, decreased appetite, diarrhoea, dry mouth, epigastric pain, gastrointestinal disorders, nausea, vomiting
- Resp: increased bronchial viscosity, chest tightness, dry throat, nasal congestion, respiratory disorders, respiratory tract dryness
- Other: alopecia, anticholinergic syndrome, asthenia, chills, fever, flushing, hyperhidrosis, malaise, menstruation irregular, myalgia, sexual dysfunction, urinary disorders

 ### Life-Threatening or Dangerous Side Effects
- Rare convulsions (generally at high doses)
- Torsades de pointes, cardiac arrest and death
- Bronchospasm
- Respiratory depression
- Paradoxical stimulation at high doses in the elderly

Weight Gain

- Reported but not expected

Sedation

- Many experience and/or can be significant in amount
- Sedation is usually transient

What To Do About Side Effects
- Wait
- Switch to another agent

Best Augmenting Agents for Side Effects
- Many side effects cannot be improved with an augmenting agent

DOSING AND USE
Usual Dosage Range
- Pruritus: 25 mg 3–4 times per day (adult)
- Anxiety: 50–100 mg/day in divided doses

Dosage Forms
- Tablet 10 mg, 25 mg
- Oral solution 10 mg/5 mL

How to Dose
*Pruritus:
- Initial dose 25 mg at night; increase as needed to 25 mg 3–4 times per day
*Anxiety:
- 50 mg/day in 3 separate administrations; in severe cases doses up to 100 mg/day may be used
See also The Art of Switching, after Pearls

 ### Dosing Tips
- Tolerance usually develops to sedation, allowing higher dosing over time
- Hydroxyzine should be administered cautiously in patients with increased potential for convulsions
- Dosing adjustments may be required if hydroxyzine is used simultaneously with other CNS-depressant drugs or with drugs having anticholinergic properties

Overdose
- Sedation, hypotension, possible QT prolongation, nausea, vomiting

Long-Term Use
- Evidence of efficacy for up to 16 weeks

Habit Forming
- No

How to Stop
- Taper generally not necessary

Pharmacokinetics

- Rapidly absorbed from gastrointestinal tract
- Mean elimination half-life about 20 hours

Drug Interactions

- Increased risk of antimuscarinic side effects when antihistamines given with antimuscarinics
- Increased sedative effect when alcohol given with antihistamines
- Potentially serious increase in sedative effects when opioid analgesics given with sedating antihistamines – avoid concomitant administration, or undertake with caution and monitoring
- Increased sedative effect when anxiolytics and hypnotics given with antihistamines
- Increased antimuscarinic and sedative effects when tricyclics given with antihistamines
- Increased antimuscarinic and sedative effects when MAOIs given with antihistamines – avoidance of MAOIs advised by manufacturer of hydroxyzine
- Plasma concentration of hydroxyzine increased by cimetidine

Other Warnings/Precautions

- Hydroxyzine may impair the ability to react and concentrate; patients should be warned of this possibility and cautioned against driving a car or operating machinery
- Use with caution in patients with bladder outflow obstruction, decreased gastrointestinal mobility, dementia, prostatic hypertrophy, pyloroduodenal obstruction, stenosing peptic ulcer, susceptibility to angle-closure glaucoma, urinary retention
- Use with caution in patients with breathing problems, cardiovascular disease, epilepsy, hypertension, hyperthyroidism, myasthenia gravis

Do Not Use

- In patients with acquired or congenital QT interval prolongation, or predisposition to QT interval prolongation
- In acute porphyrias
- In patients with previous hypersensitivity to cetirizine or other piperazine derivatives, and aminophylline

Renal Impairment

- Reduce the daily dose by 50% in moderate-severe renal impairment

Hepatic Impairment

- Reduce daily dose by one-third
- Avoid in severe liver disease – increased risk of coma

Cardiac Impairment

- Hydroxyzine is associated with a small risk of QT interval prolongation and torsade de pointes
- These events are most likely to occur in patients who have risk factors for QT prolongation (e.g. concomitant use of drugs that prolong the QT interval, cardiovascular disease, family history of sudden cardiac death, significant electrolyte imbalance, or significant bradycardia)

Elderly

- Elderly patients may be more sensitive to sedative and anticholinergic effects; avoid use in the elderly, or use a lower dose
- Max daily dose in the elderly is 50 mg (if use of hydroxyzine cannot be avoided)

Children and Adolescents

- Dosing in child 6 months–5 years: 5–15 mg/day in divided doses, dose adjusted according to weight; max 2 mg/kg
- Dosing in child 6–17 years (body weight up to 40 kg): Initial dose 15–25 mg/day in divided doses, dose increased as required; max 2 mg/kg
- Dosing in child 6–17 years (body weight 40 kg and above): initial dose 5–25 mg/day in divided doses, increased as required to 50–100 mg/day in divided doses, dose adjusted according to weight
- Children have an increased susceptibility to side effects, particularly CNS effects
- Ucerax preparations not licensed for use in children less than 1 year of age

Pregnancy

- Hydroxyzine is contraindicated in pregnancy
- In animal studies, hydroxyzine at high doses was teratogenic in mice, rats and rabbits

- Withdrawal effects in the infant have been reported including hypotonia, movement disorders, clonic movements, tachypnoea, irritability, and poor feeding

Breastfeeding

- Unknown if hydroxyzine is secreted in human breast milk, but all psychotropics assumed to be secreted in breast milk
- *Recommended either to discontinue drug or bottle feed

THE ART OF PSYCHOPHARMACOLOGY

Potential Advantages

- No abuse liability, dependence, or withdrawal

Potential Disadvantages

- Patients with severe anxiety disorders
- Elderly patients
- Dementia patients

Primary Target Symptoms

- Anxiety
- Skeletal muscle tension
- Itching
- Nausea, vomiting

Pearls

- Promethazine has replaced hydroxyzine for treatment of short-term periods of agitation or anxiety
- A preferable anxiolytic for patients with dermatitis or skin symptoms such as pruritis
- Anxiolytic actions may be proportional to sedating actions
- Hydroxyzine tablets are made with 1,1,1-trichloroethane, which destroys the ozone
- Hydroxyzine may not be as effective as benzodiazepines or newer agents in the management of anxiety

THE ART OF SWITCHING

Switching

- When switching consider the fact that hydroxyzine has a half-life of 20 hours in adults, 29 hours in the elderly and 37 hours in patients with hepatic dysfunction

Suggested Reading

Diehn F, Tefferi A. Pruritus in polycythaemia vera: prevalence, laboratory correlates and management. Br J Haematol 2001;115(3):619–21.

Ferreri M, Hantouche EG. Recent clinical trials of hydroxyzine in generalized anxiety disorder. Acta Psychiatr Scand Suppl 1998;393:102–8.

Guaiana G, Barbui C, Cipriani A. Hydroxyzine for generalised anxiety disorder. Cochrane Database Syst Rev 2010;(12):CD006815.

Paton DM, Webster DR. Clinical pharmacokinetics of H1-receptor antagonists (the antihistamines). Clin Pharmacokinet 1985;10(6):477–97.

Hyoscine hydrobromide

Brands
- Kwells
- Travel Calm
- Joy-Rides
- Kwells Kids

Generic?
Yes

Class
- Neuroscience-based nomenclature: antimuscarinic; anticholinergic

Commonly Prescribed for
(bold for BNF indication)
- **Motion sickness**
- **Hypersalivation associated with clozapine therapy (unlicensed use)**
- **Palliative care (excessive respiratory secretion; bowel colic; bowel colic pain)**
- **Premedication before induction of anaesthesia**
- Major depressive disorder (experimental)
- Bipolar disorder (experimental)

How the Drug Works
- Hyoscine hydrobromide is a centrally and peripherally acting antimuscarinic antagonist, with high potency for all five subtypes (M1–5)
- Small doses effectively inhibit salivary and bronchial secretions and sweating, provide a degree of amnesia, and prevent motion sickness
- Intravenous hyoscine may have rapid antidepressant effects, consistent with the hypothesis that hypersensitivity of the cholinergic system may play a role in pathophysiology of mood disorders
- Immediate antidepressant effects are likely due to muscarinic antagonism
- Abnormal glutamate transmission has been implicated in the pathophysiology of depression, so longer-lasting antidepressant effects may be due to reduced NMDA receptor expression; induction of the mTOR pathway may also be present

How Long Until It Works
- For oral, intramuscular, or subcutaneous administration, effects occur within 15–30 minutes
- Antidepressant effects occur within 3 days, possibly within 24 hours

If It Works
- For depression, can rapidly alleviate depressed mood and may last several weeks beyond the final administration
- Unclear whether persistence of the antidepressant response depends on repeated administration, although it is suggested to provide additional benefit
- Hyoscine may be used to provide immediate antidepressant relief in the weeks before conventional therapies reach their maximal therapeutic benefit
- For other indications, can continue to use as long as it is beneficial

If It Doesn't Work
- Try an antihistamine with or without sedative effects for motion sickness
- Ketamine and esketamine have also been reported to have immediate antidepressant effects
- Try a traditional antidepressant or electro-convulsive therapy (ECT) for treatment-resistant depression
- Commonly used alternatives to hyoscine for hypersalivation associated with clozapine therapy include trihexyphenidyl, pirenzepine or amisulpride; increasing interest and anecdotal evidence found for botulinum toxin

Best Augmenting Combos for Partial Response or Treatment Resistance
- Best to switch to an alternative than augment in motion sickness or for the treatment of hypersalivation associated with clozapine therapy
- Hyoscine has been tried as an adjunct to SSRI therapy for treatment of patients with depression

Tests
- None for healthy individuals

SIDE EFFECTS

How Drug Causes Side Effects

- Many side effects can be attributed to the anticholinergic properties of hyoscine
- Direct effect on both central and peripheral muscarinic receptors (M1–5)
- Penetrates the blood–brain barrier easily

Notable Side Effects

- Blurred vision
- Constipation
- Dry mouth
- Urinary retention

Common or very common

- CNS/PNS: dizziness, drowsiness, headache, vision disorders
- CVS: palpitations, tachycardia
- GIT: constipation, dry mouth, dyspepsia, nausea, vomiting
- Other: flushing, skin reactions, urinary disorders
- With transdermal use: eye disorders, eyelid irritation

Rare or very rare

- Angioedema, confusion (more common in elderly)
- With transdermal use: glaucoma, hallucinations, impaired concentration, memory loss, restlessness

Frequency not known

With oral use:
- CNS/PNS: CNS stimulation, hallucination, mydriasis, restlessness, seizure
- CVS: cardiovascular disorders
- GIT: gastrointestinal disorders
- Resp: asthma, respiratory tract reaction
- Other: hypersensitivity, hyperthermia, hypohidrosis, oedema

With parenteral use:
- CNS: agitation, delirium, exacerbation of epilepsy, hallucination, loss of consciousness, mydriasis, psychosis
- CVS: arrhythmias
- GIT: dysphagia, thirst
- Resp: dyspnoea
- Other: angle-closure glaucoma, hypersensitivity, idiosyncratic drug reaction, neuroleptic malignant syndrome

With transdermal use:
- Impaired balance

 ### Life-Threatening or Dangerous Side Effects

- Angle-closure glaucoma
- Increased seizure frequency in epileptic patients
- Use in patients with ulcerative colitis may lead to ileus or megacolon
- Pyrexia at high ambient temperatures due to decreased sweating

Weight Gain

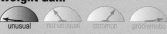

- Not reported

Sedation

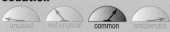

- Many experience and/or can be significant in amount
- Sedative effects may be enhanced with alcohol or CNS depressants

What To Do About Side Effects

- If patients experience drowsiness, they should not drive or operate machinery
- Avoid alcohol
- Side effects are generally transient and well tolerated
- For glaucoma, pilocarpine can be given locally

Best Augmenting Agents for Side Effects

- Many side effects cannot be improved with an augmenting agent

DOSING AND USE

Usual Dosage Range

- Motion sickness (child 4–9 years): oral 75–450 mcg/day in divided doses; 1 patch
- Motion sickness (adult and child 10–17 years): oral 150–900 mcg/day in divided doses; 1 patch
- Hypersalivation associated with clozapine therapy: oral 300–900 mcg/day in divided doses or patch 1.5 mg/72 hours
- Excessive respiratory secretion in palliative care: subcutaneous injection 400–2400 mcg/day in divided doses; subcutaneous infusion 1.2–2 mg/24 hours

- Bowel colic in palliative care: subcutaneous injection 400–2400 mcg/day in divided doses; subcutaneous infusion 1.2–2 mg/24 hours
- Bowel colic pain in palliative care: sublingual 300–900 mcg/day in divided doses
- Premedication: subcutaneous or IM injection 200–600 mcg
- Depression: IV infusion 4.0 mcg/kg/15 minutes; administer 3 times, with each infusion separated by 3–5 days (specialist clinics only)

Dosage Forms

- Tablet 150 mcg, 300 mcg
- Chewable tablet 150 mcg
- Transdermal patch 1.5 mg (1 mg absorbed per 72 hours)
- Injection 400 mcg/mL, 600 mcg/mL (specialist clinics only)

How to Dose

*Motion sickness:
- Child 4–9 years: oral 75–150 mcg 30 minutes before journey, then every 6 hours if needed; max 450 mcg/day
- Adult or child 10–17 years: oral 150–300 mcg 30 minutes before journey, then every 6 hours as required; max 900 mcg/day; transdermal patch apply 1 patch behind ear 5–6 hours before journey, then apply second patch behind other ear 72 hours later if needed (remove old patch)

*Hypersalivation associated with clozapine therapy:
- Oral 300 mcg up to 3 times per day; max 900 mcg/day

*Excessive respiratory secretion in palliative care:
- Subcutaneous injection: 400 mcg every 4 hours as required; hourly use may be necessary
- Subcutaneous infusion: 1.2–2 mg/24 hours

*Bowel colic in palliative care:
- Subcutaneous injection: 400 mcg every 4 hours as required; hourly use may be necessary
- Subcutaneous infusion: 1.2–2 mg/24 hours

*Bowel colic pain in palliative care:
- Oral (sublingual as Kwells) 300 mcg 3 times per day

*Premedication:
- Subcutaneous or IM injection: 200–600 mcg 30–60 minutes before induction of anaesthesia

*Depression:
- IV infusion: 4.0 mcg/kg over 15 minutes; administer 3 times, with each infusion separated by 3–5 days (specialist clinics only)

 Dosing Tips

- Long-term use may facilitate tolerance, requiring an increase in dosage
- The antidepressant and anti-anxiety effect is greater in women than men
- Transdermal and oral hyoscine may improve depressive symptoms for some patients

Overdose

- Dry mouth, drowsiness, delirium, restlessness, hallucination, nausea, vomiting, constipation, urinary retention, blurred vision, mydriasis, tachycardia, arrhythmia, hyperpyrexia
- Severe overdose: paranoia and psychosis, seizures, coma, circulatory/respiratory failure and death

Management:
- Physostigmine 1–4 mg by slow IV injection to reverse anticholinergic effects (hazardous so generally not recommended)
- Catheterisation for urinary retention
- Consider gastric lavage or induced emesis in cases of oral ingestion; charcoal may be used to prevent further absorption
- Diazepam may be used to control excitement
- Cardiovascular and respiratory complications should be treated according to usual therapeutic principles
- Otherwise, treatment should be symptomatic and supportive

Long-Term Use

- Safe
- Long-term use may facilitate tolerance, requiring an increase in dosage

Habit Forming

- No

How to Stop

- Taper not necessary
- Withdrawal-type symptoms such as dizziness, nausea, headache and vertigo have been reported following removal of patches, after several days of use

Hyoscine hydrobromide (Continued)

Pharmacokinetics
- Rapidly absorbed from the gastro-intestinal tract and following IV or IM injection
- Circulates bound to plasma proteins
- Almost completely metabolised by the liver and excreted in the urine (only a small proportion unchanged)
- Half-life 8 hours

 Drug Interactions
- Concurrent use alongside other anticholinergic/antimuscarinic drugs increases the risk of these side effects
- May be an increased risk of side effects when given with MAOIs due to inhibition of drug-metabolising enzymes
- May increase absorption of levodopa
- May reduce effect of sublingual nitrates (failure to dissolve under the tongue due to dry mouth)
- May enhance tachycardic effects of beta-adrenergic agents
- Effects may be potentiated by phenothiazines, tricyclic antidepressants or alcohol; hyoscine may potentiate effects of tricyclic antidepressants
- Use of hyoscine alongside dopamine antagonists may reduce effects of both drugs on the gastrointestinal tract
- Reduction in gastric motility may affect absorption of other drugs
- Increased sedative effect when taken with alcohol or CNS depressants

 Other Warnings/Precautions
- Use with caution in patients with acute myocardial infarction, arrhythmias, cardiac insufficiency, undergoing cardiac surgery, conditions associated with tachycardia, congestive heart failure, coronary artery disease or hypertension
- Use with caution in patients with diarrhoea, gastro-oesophageal reflux disease, hiatus hernia with reflux oesophagitis or ulcerative colitis (may lead to ileus or megacolon)
- Use with caution in patients with hyperthyroidism (due to associated tachycardia)
- Use with caution in patients susceptible to acute angle-closure glaucoma

- Use with caution in patients with prostatic hyperplasia
- Patients should avoid alcohol due to enhanced sedative effects, and should not drive or operate machinery
- May increase frequency of seizures in epileptic patients
- Use with caution in patients with Down's syndrome or in the elderly
- Use with caution in patients with pyrexia as hyoscine can decrease sweating
- Avoid giving IM to patients being treated with anticoagulant drugs since intramuscular haematoma may occur

Do Not Use
- If patient has acute-angle glaucoma
- If patient has gastrointestinal obstruction, intestinal atony, paralytic ileus, pyloric stenosis, severe ulcerative colitis or toxic megacolon
- If patient has myasthenia gravis
- If patient has significant bladder outflow obstruction or urinary retention
- If there is a proven allergy to hyoscine

Renal Impairment
- Use with caution

Hepatic Impairment
- Use with caution

Cardiac Impairment
- Use with caution in patients with acute myocardial infarction, arrhythmias, cardiac insufficiency, undergoing cardiac surgery, conditions associated with tachycardia, congestive heart failure, coronary artery disease or hypertension

Elderly
- Potentially inappropriate due to increased risk of adverse side effects, particularly cognitive impairment, delirium and constipation
- Research into efficacy in treating depression has not included elderly populations

 Children and Adolescents
- Indicated for use in motion sickness
- Indicated for use as premedication

- Indicated for use in palliative care (excessive respiratory secretion; bowel colic)
- Unlicensed use for excessive respiratory secretion and clozapine-induced hypersalivation
- Use with caution as children may be at increased risk of adverse side effects
- Injection solution may be given orally

Pregnancy

- Controlled studies have not been conducted in pregnant women
- Use of centrally acting drugs throughout pregnancy or around time of delivery is associated with an increased risk of poor neonatal adaptation syndrome
- Maternal exposure prior to delivery may cause anticholinergic side effects in the newborn

Breastfeeding

- Small amounts expected to be secreted in human breast milk
- *Recommended either to discontinue drug or bottle feed unless the potential benefit to the mother justifies the potential risk to the child
- Infants of women who choose to breastfeed while on hyoscine should be monitored for possible adverse effects

THE ART OF PSYCHOPHARMACOLOGY
Potential Advantages

- Very effective treatment for motion sickness
- Commonly used practice for reducing hyersalivation associated with clozapine therapy
- Promising immediate treatment for resistant depression, with lasting effects (still experimental)

Potential Disadvantages

- Potentially serious adverse effects
- Repeated intravenous administration may be required for continuous antidepressant effects

Primary Target Symptoms

- Motion sickness
- Hypersalivation due to clozapine
- Depression

Pearls

- Hyoscine is also known as scopolamine
- Hyoscine is a commonly prescribed medication in UK to counter the hypersalivation encountered with clozapine therapy; it is an unlicensed indication
- For hypersalivation patients need to be advised to either chew or suck on the tablet rather than swallow
- Some patients may prefer, tolerate better or respond better to the patch formulation instead
- A slightly lowered and clinically effective dose of clozapine may also help
- Alternative unlicensed treatments may be tried if hyoscine fails in reducing hypersalivation; these commonly include trihexyphenidyl, pirenzepine or amisulpride
- The use of hyoscine as an antidepressant or as an augmenting agent in depression is not licensed in UK and should only be used for this purpose in specialist services, e.g. resistant depression clinics
- Use in older people is limited due to increased risk of confusion and hallucinations

Suggested Reading

Drevets WC, Bhattacharya A, Furey ML.The antidepressant efficacy of the muscarinic antagonist scopolamine: past findings and future directions. Adv Pharmacol 2020;89:357–86.

Drevets WC, Zarate Jr CA, Furey ML. Antidepressant effects of the muscarinic cholinergic receptor antagonist scopolamine: a review. Biol Psychiatry 2013;73(12):1156–63.

Furey ML, Zarate Jr CA. Pulsed intravenous administration of scopolamine produces rapid antidepressant effects and modest side effects. J Clin Psychiatry 2013;74(8):850–1.

Jaffe RJ, Novakovic V, Peselow ED. Scopolamine as an antidepressant: a systematic review. Clin Neuropharmacol 2013;36(1):24–6.

Imipramine hydrochloride

Brands
• Non-proprietary

Generic?
Yes

Class
• Neuroscience-based nomenclature: pharmacology domain – serotonin, norepinephrine; mode of action – reuptake inhibitor
• Tricyclic antidepressant (TCA)
• Serotonin and noradrenaline reuptake inhibitor

Commonly Prescribed for
(bold for BNF indication)
• **Depressive illness (especially for inpatients)**
• **Nocturnal enuresis**
• **Attention deficit hyperactivity disorder (unlicensed use in children under expert supervision)**
• Anxiety
• Insomnia
• Neuropathic pain/chronic pain
• Treatment-resistant depression
• Cataplexy syndrome
• Panic disorder
• Post-traumatic stress disorder (PTSD)

 ## How the Drug Works
• Boosts neurotransmitters serotonin and noradrenaline
• Blocks serotonin reuptake pump (serotonin transporter), presumably increasing serotonergic neurotransmission
• Blocks noradrenaline reuptake pump (noradrenaline transporter), presumably increasing noradrenergic neurotransmission
• Presumably desensitises both serotonin 1A receptors and beta-adrenergic receptors
• Since dopamine is inactivated by noradrenaline reuptake in frontal cortex, which largely lacks dopamine transporters, imipramine can increase dopamine neurotransmission in this part of the brain
• May be effective in treating enuresis because of its anticholinergic properties

How Long Until It Works
• May have immediate effects in treating insomnia or anxiety
• Onset of therapeutic actions with some antidepressants can be seen within 1–2 weeks, but often delayed 2–4 weeks
• If it is not working within 3–4 weeks for depression, it may require a dosage increase or it may not work at all
• By contrast, for generalised anxiety, onset of response and increases in remission rates may still occur after 8 weeks, and for up to 6 months after initiating dosing
• May continue to work for many years to prevent relapse of symptoms

If It Works
• The goal of treatment is complete remission of current symptoms as well as prevention of future relapses
• Treatment most often reduces or even eliminates symptoms, but is not a cure since symptoms can recur after medicine is stopped
• Continue treatment until all symptoms are gone (remission), especially in depression and whenever possible in anxiety disorders
• Once symptoms are gone, continue treating for at least 6–9 months for the first episode of depression or >12 months if relapse indicators present
• If >5 episodes and/or 2 episodes in the last few years then need to continue for at least 2 years or indefinitely
• The goal of treatment of chronic neuropathic pain is to reduce symptoms as much as possible, especially in combination with other treatments
• Treatment of chronic neuropathic pain may reduce symptoms, but rarely eliminates them completely, and is not a cure since symptoms can recur after medicine has been stopped
• Use in anxiety disorders and chronic pain may also need to be indefinite, but long-term treatment is not well studied in these conditions

If It Doesn't Work
• Important to recognise non-response to treatment early on (3–4 weeks)
• Many patients have only a partial response where some symptoms are improved but others persist (especially insomnia, fatigue, and problems concentrating)

Imipramine hydrochloride (Continued)

- Other patients may be non-responders, sometimes called treatment-resistant or treatment-refractory
- Some patients who have an initial response may relapse even though they continue treatment
- Consider increasing dose, switching to another agent, or adding an appropriate augmenting agent
- Lithium may be added for suicidal patients or those at high risk of relapse
- Consider psychotherapy
- Consider ECT
- Consider evaluation for another diagnosis or for a co-morbid condition (e.g. medical illness, substance abuse, etc.)
- Some patients may experience a switch into mania and so would require antidepressant discontinuation and initiation of a mood stabiliser
- For children and adolescents, irrespective of indication for prescribing (enuresis or ADHD) re-consider diagnosis. Consider evaluation for another diagnosis or for a co-morbid condition (e.g. bipolar disorder, substance abuse, medical illness, etc.). In children consider other important factors, such as ongoing conflicts, family psychopathology, adverse environment, maltreatment, for which alternate interventions might be more appropriate (e.g. social care referral, trauma-informed care)

⚖️ Best Augmenting Combos for Partial Response or Treatment Resistance

- Mood stabilisers or atypical antipsychotics for bipolar depression
- Atypical antipsychotics for psychotic depression
- Atypical antipsychotics as first-line augmenting agents (quetiapine MR 300 mg/day or aripiprazole at 2.5–10 mg/day) for treatment-resistant depression
- Atypical antipsychotics as second-line augmenting agents (risperidone 0.5–2 mg/day or olanzapine 2.5–10 mg/day) for treatment-resistant depression
- Mirtazapine at 30–45 mg/day as another second-line augmenting agent (a dual serotonin and noradrenaline combination, but observe for switch into mania, increase in suicidal ideation or serotonin syndrome)

- Although T3 (20–50 mcg/day) is another second-line augmenting agent the evidence suggests that it works best with tricyclic antidepressants
- Other augmenting agents but with less evidence include bupropion (up to 400 mg/day), buspirone (up to 60 mg/day) and lamotrigine (up to 400 mg/day)
- Benzodiazepines if agitation present
- Hypnotics or trazodone for insomnia (but beware of serotonin syndrome with trazodone)
- Augmenting agents reserved for specialist use include: modafinil for sleepiness, fatigue and lack of concentration; stimulants, oestrogens, testosterone
- Lithium is particularly useful for suicidal patients and those at high risk of relapse including with factors such as severe depression, psychomotor retardation, repeated episodes (>3), significant weight loss, or a family history of major depression (aim for lithium plasma levels 0.6–1.0 mmol/L)
- For elderly patients lithium is a very effective augmenting agent
- For severely ill patients other combinations may be tried especially in specialist centres
- Augmenting agents that may be tried include omega-3, SAM-e, L-methylfolate
- Additional non-pharmacological treatments such as exercise, mindfulness, CBT, and IPT can also be helpful
- If present after treatment response (4–8 weeks) or remission (6–12 weeks), the most common residual symptoms of depression include cognitive impairments, reduced energy and problems with sleep
- Gabapentin, tiagabine, other anticonvulsants, even opiates if done by experts while monitoring carefully in difficult cases (for chronic pain)

Tests

- Baseline ECG is useful for patients over age 50
- ECGs may be useful for selected patients (e.g. those with personal or family history of QTc prolongation; cardiac arrhythmia; recent myocardial infarction; decompensated heart failure; or taking agents that prolong QTc interval such as pimozide, thioridazine, selected antiarrhythmics, moxifloxacin etc.)

*Since tricyclic and tetracyclic antidepressants are frequently associated with weight gain, before starting treatment, weigh all patients and determine if the patient is already overweight (BMI 25.0–29.9) or obese (BMI ≥30)
• Before giving a drug that can cause weight gain to an overweight or obese patient, consider determining whether the patient already has:
  • Pre-diabetes – fasting plasma glucose: 5.5 mmol/L to 6.9 mmol/L or HbA1c: 42 to 47 mmol/mol (6.0 to 6.4%)
  • Diabetes – fasting plasma glucose: >7.0 mmol/L or HbA1c: ≥48 mmol/L (≥6.5%)
  • Hypertension (BP >140/90 mm Hg)
  • Dyslipidaemia (increased total cholesterol, LDL cholesterol, and triglycerides; decreased HDL cholesterol)
• Treat or refer such patients for treatment, including nutrition and weight management, physical activity counselling, smoking cessation, and medical management
*Monitor weight and BMI during treatment
*While giving a drug to a patient who has gained >5% of initial weight, consider evaluating for the presence of pre-diabetes, diabetes, dyslipidaemia, or consider switching to a different antidepressant
• Patients at risk for electrolyte disturbances (e.g. patients aged >60, patients on diuretic therapy) should have baseline and periodic serum potassium and magnesium measurements

SIDE EFFECTS

How Drug Causes Side Effects
• Anticholinergic activity may explain sedative effects, dry mouth, constipation, and blurred vision
• Sedative effects and weight gain may be due to antihistamine properties
• Blockade of alpha adrenergic 1 receptors may explain dizziness, sedation, and hypotension
• Cardiac arrhythmias and seizures, especially in overdose, may be caused by blockade of ion channels

Notable Side Effects
• Blurred vision, constipation, urinary retention, increased appetite, dry mouth, nausea, diarrhoea, heartburn, unusual taste in mouth, weight gain

• Fatigue, weakness, dizziness, sedation, headache, anxiety, nervousness, restlessness
• Sexual dysfunction, sweating

Common or very common
• CNS/PNS: altered mood, anxiety, confusion, delirium, depression, dizziness, drowsiness, epilepsy, hallucinations, headache, paraesthesia, sleep disorders, tremor
• CVS: arrhythmias, cardiac conduction disorders, hypotension, palpitations
• GIT: decreased appetite, hepatic disorders, nausea, vomiting, weight changes
• Other: asthenia, sexual dysfunction, skin reactions

Uncommon
• Psychosis

Rare or very rare
• Blood disorders: agranulocytosis, eosinophilia, leucopenia, thrombocytopenia, bone marrow depression
• CNS: aggression, movement disorders, mydriasis, speech disorder
• Endocrine: enlarged mammary gland, galactorrhoea,
• GIT: oral and gastrointestinal disorders
• Other: alopecia, glaucoma, fever, heart failure, oedema, peripheral vasospasm, photosensitivity, respiratory disorders, SIADH

Frequency not known
• CNS: exacerbation of paranoid delusions, neurological effects, psychiatric disorders, suicidal behaviours, tinnitus
• Other: anticholinergic syndrome, cardiovascular effects, drug fever, hyponatraemia; increased risk of fracture, urinary disorder, withdrawal syndrome

 Life-Threatening or Dangerous Side Effects
• Paralytic ileus, hyperthermia (TCAs + anticholinergic agents)
• Lowered seizure threshold and rare seizures
• Orthostatic hypotension, sudden death, arrhythmias, tachycardia
• QTc prolongation
• Hepatic failure, extrapyramidal symptoms
• Increased intraocular pressure, increased psychotic symptoms
• Rare induction of mania

Imipramine hydrochloride (Continued)

- Rare increase in suicidal ideation and behaviours in adolescents and young adults (up to age 25), hence patients should be warned of this potential adverse event

Weight Gain

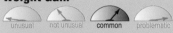

- Many experience and/or can be significant in amount
- Can increase appetite and carbohydrate craving

Sedation

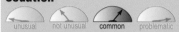

- Many experience and/or can be significant in amount
- Tolerance to sedative effects may develop with long-term use

What to Do About Side Effects

- Wait
- Wait
- Wait
- The risk of side effects is reduced by titrating slowly to the minimum effective dose (every 2–3 days)
- Consider using a lower starting dose in elderly patients
- Manage side effects that are likely to be transient (e.g. drowsiness) by explanation, reassurance and, if necessary, dose reduction and re-titration
- Giving patients simple strategies for managing mild side effects (e.g. dry mouth) may be useful

For persistent, severe or distressing side effects the options are:

- Dose reduction and re-titration if possible
- Switching to an antidepressant with a lower propensity to cause that side effect
- Non-drug management of the side effect (e.g. diet and exercise for weight gain)

Best Augmenting Agents for Side Effects

- Many side effects cannot be improved with an augmenting agent

DOSING AND USE

Usual Dosage Range

- Depression: 75–200 mg/day in divided doses (elderly 10–50 mg/day in divided doses); inpatients 75–300 mg/day in divided doses
- Enuresis: 25–75 mg at bedtime depending on the age of the child

Dosage Forms

- Tablet 10 mg, 25 mg
- Oral solution 25 mg/5 mL (150 mL bottle)

How to Dose

∗Depression:
- Adults – initial dose 75 mg/day in divided doses, then increased to 150–200 mg/day. Up to 150 mg may be given as a single dose at night
- Elderly – initial dose 10 mg/day, increased gradually to 30–50 mg/day
- Inpatient adults – initial dose 75 mg/day in divided doses, can be increased up to 300 mg/day in divided doses
∗Nocturnal enuresis:
- Initial period of treatment (including gradual withdrawal) is 3 months – full physical examination needed before further course
- For child 6–7 years: 25 mg at bedtime
- For child 8–10 years: 25–50 mg at bedtime
- For child 11–17 years: 50–75 mg at bedtime

 Dosing Tips

- Dose at bedtime for insomnia
- If given in a single dose, should generally be administered at bedtime because of its sedative properties
- If given in split doses, largest dose should generally be given at bedtime because of its sedative properties
- If patients experience nightmares, split dose and do not give large dose at bedtime
- Patients treated for chronic pain may only require lower doses
- If intolerable anxiety, insomnia, agitation, akathisia, or activation occur either upon dosing initiation or discontinuation, consider the possibility of activated bipolar disorder, and switch to a mood stabiliser or an atypical antipsychotic

Overdose

- Can be fatal
- Dry mouth, convulsions, CNS depression, extensor plantar response, respiratory failure, coma of varying degree, cardiac dysrhythmias, severe hypotension, hypothermia, conduction abnormalities, ECG changes. Dilated pupils and urinary retention may also occur

Long-Term Use

- Safe

Habit Forming

- No

How to Stop

- Taper gradually to avoid withdrawal effects
- Even with gradual dose reduction some withdrawal symptoms may appear within the first 2 weeks
- It is best to reduce the dose gradually over 4 weeks or longer if withdrawal symptoms emerge
- If severe withdrawal symptoms emerge during discontinuation, raise dose to stop symptoms and then restart withdrawal much more slowly (over at least 6 months in patients on long-term maintenance treatment)

Pharmacokinetics

- Mean elimination half-life about 19 hours
- Substrate for CYP450 2D6 and 1A2
- Metabolised to an active metabolite, desipramine, a predominantly noradrenaline reuptake inhibitor, by demethylation via CYP450 1A2
- Food does not affect absorption

 Drug Interactions

- Tramadol increases the risk of seizures and serotonin syndrome in patients taking TCAs
- Use of TCAs with anticholinergic drugs may result in paralytic ileus or hyperthermia
- Fluoxetine, paroxetine, bupropion, duloxetine, and other CYP450 2D6 inhibitors may increase TCA concentrations and increase the risk of serotonin syndrome. Monitor for toxicity and adjust dose
- Studies suggest cinacalcet and terbinafine might increase exposure to imipramine.

Dronedarone is theoretically predicted to increase exposure to imipramine
- Fluvoxamine, a CYP450 1A2 inhibitor, can decrease the conversion of imipramine to desmethylimipramine (desipramine) and increase imipramine plasma concentrations and the risk of serotonin syndrome
- Cimetidine may increase plasma concentrations of TCAs and cause anticholinergic symptoms
- Phenothiazines or haloperidol may raise TCA blood concentrations
- May alter effects of antihypertensive drugs; may inhibit hypotensive effects of clonidine and increase the risk of hypotension when used in combination with other antihypertensives
- Use with sympathomimetic agents may increase sympathetic activity
- Methylphenidate may inhibit metabolism of TCAs
- Activation and agitation, especially following switching or adding antidepressants, may represent the induction of a bipolar state, especially a mixed dysphoric bipolar condition sometimes associated with suicidal ideation, and require the addition of lithium, a mood stabiliser or an atypical antipsychotic, and/or discontinuation of imipramine
- There is anecdotal evidence to suggest combined use of imipramine and lithium increases risk of neurotoxicity

 Other Warnings/Precautions

- Add or initiate other antidepressants with caution for up to 2 weeks after discontinuing imipramine
- Generally, do not use with MAO inhibitors, including 14 days after MAOIs are stopped; do not start an MAOI for at least 5 half-lives (5 to 7 days for most drugs) after discontinuing imipramine, but see Pearls
- Use with caution in patients with history of seizures, psychosis or bipolar disorder, or presenting with a significant risk of suicide
- Warn patients and their caregivers about the possibility of activating side effects and advise them to report such symptoms immediately

Imipramine hydrochloride (Continued)

- Treatment should be stopped if the patient enters a manic phase
- Monitor patients for activation of suicidal ideation
- Use with caution in patients with diabetes
- Use with caution in patients with chronic constipation, urinary retention, prostatic hypertrophy, susceptibility to angle-closure glaucoma, raised intraocular pressure
- Use with caution in patients with cardiovascular disease, hyperthyroidism and phaeochromocytoma due to increased risk of arrhythmias
- TCAs can increase QTc interval, especially at toxic doses, which can be attained not only by overdose but also by combining with drugs that inhibit its metabolism via CYP450 2D6, potentially causing torsade de pointes-type arrhythmia or sudden death
- Because TCAs can prolong QTc interval, use with caution in patients who have bradycardia or who are taking drugs that can induce bradycardia (e.g. beta blockers, calcium channel blockers, clonidine, digitalis)
- Because TCAs can prolong QTc interval, use with caution in patients who have hypokalaemia and/or hypomagnesaemia or who are taking drugs that can induce hypokalaemia and/or hypomagnesaemia (e.g. diuretics, stimulant laxatives, intravenous amphotericin B, glucocorticoids, tetracosactide)

Do Not Use

- If patient enters a manic phase
- If there is a history of cardiac arrhythmia, recent acute myocardial infarction, heart block
- If patient is taking agents capable of significantly prolonging QTc interval (e.g. pimozide, selected antiarrhythmics, moxifloxacin)
- If there is a history of QTc prolongation or cardiac arrhythmia, recent acute myocardial infarction, decompensated heart failure
- In acute porphyrias
- If patient is taking drugs that inhibit TCA metabolism, including CYP450 2D6 inhibitors, except by an expert
- If there is reduced CYP450 2D6 function, such as patients who are poor 2D6

metabolisers, except by an expert and at low doses
- If there is a proven allergy to imipramine, desipramine, or lofepramine

Renal Impairment

- Caution especially in severe impairment

Hepatic Impairment

- Cautious use; may need lower dose, avoid in severe impairment

Cardiac Impairment

- Baseline ECG is recommended
- TCAs have been reported to cause arrhythmias, prolongation of conduction time, orthostatic hypotension, sinus tachycardia, and heart failure, especially in the diseased heart
- Myocardial infarction and stroke have been reported with TCAs
- TCAs produce QTc prolongation, which may be enhanced by the existence of bradycardia, hypokalaemia, congenital or acquired long QTc interval, which should be evaluated prior to administering imipramine
- Use with caution if treating concomitantly with a medication likely to produce prolonged bradycardia, hypokalaemia, slowing of intracardiac conduction, or prolongation of the QTc interval
- Avoid TCAs in patients with a known history of QTc prolongation, recent acute myocardial infarction, and decompensated heart failure
- TCAs may cause a sustained increase in heart rate in patients with ischaemic heart disease and may worsen (decrease) heart rate variability, an independent risk of mortality in cardiac populations
- Since SSRIs may improve (increase) heart rate variability in patients following a myocardial infarct and may improve survival as well as mood in patients with acute angina or following a myocardial infarction, these are more appropriate agents for cardiac population than tricyclic/tetracyclic antidepressants
- *Risk/benefit ratio may not justify use of TCAs in cardiac impairment

Elderly

- Baseline ECG required
- May be sensitive to anticholinergic, cardiovascular, hypotensive, and sedative effects
- Low initial doses should be used, with close monitoring, particularly for psychiatric and cardiac side effects
- Reduction in the risk of suicidality with antidepressants compared to placebo in adults age 65 and older

Children and Adolescents

Before you prescribe:
- Third-line treatment for treatment-refractory ADHD should be reserved for the expert
- Nocturnal enuresis if organic causes excluded and other behavioural interventions unsuccessful
- Second-line pharmacological treatment for enuresis

For enuresis:
- Irrespective of the child's age consider underlying organic causes (including urinary tract infection, constipation, diabetes type 1 and 2, diabetes insipidus) and emotional or behavioural problems (including anxiety, PTSD, sleep disorders). Consider child maltreatment
- Address underlying causes
- Children are expected to be dry at night by about 5 years. Interventions in practice often not commenced till 7 years
- For children of all ages try behavioural interventions first (e.g. diary, toileting before bed, fluid restriction before bed); consider bed alarm if other interventions fail

For ADHD:
- Diagnosis of ADHD should only be made by an appropriately qualified healthcare professional, e.g. specialist psychiatrist, paediatrician, and after full clinical and psychosocial assessment in different domains, full developmental and psychiatric history, observer reports across different settings and opportunity to speak to the child and carer on their own
- Children and adolescents with untreated anxiety, PTSD and mood disorders, or those who do not have a psychiatric diagnosis but social or environmental stressors, may present with anger, irritability, motor agitation, and concentration problems
- Consider undiagnosed learning disability or specific learning difficulties, and sensory impairments that may potentially cause or contribute to inattention and restlessness, especially in school
- ADHD-specific advice on symptom management and environmental adaptations should be offered to all families and teachers, including reducing distractions, seating, shorter periods of focus, movement breaks and teaching assistants
- For children above 5 years of age and young people with ADHD pharmacological treatment should be considered if they continue to show significant impairment in at least one setting after symptom management and environmental adaptations have been implemented
- For severe ADHD, behavioural symptom management may not be effective until pharmacological treatment has been established

Practical notes:
- Only consider after first- and second-line options have been tried; initiation and monitoring by expert only
- Monitor patients face-to-face regularly, particularly during the first several weeks of treatment
- Monitor for activation of suicidal ideation at the beginning of treatment
- Consider a course of cognitive behavioural therapy (CBT) for young people with ADHD who have benefited from medication, but whose symptoms are still causing a significant impairment in at least one domain, addressing the following areas: social skills with peers, problem-solving, self-control, active listening skills, dealing with and expressing feelings
- Medication for ADHD for a child under 5 years should only be considered on specialist advice from an ADHD service with expertise in managing ADHD in young children (ideally a tertiary service). Use of all medicines for treating ADHD is off-label in children aged under 5
- Offer the same medication choices to people with ADHD and anxiety disorder, tic disorder or autism spectrum disorder as other people with ADHD

Imipramine hydrochloride (Continued)

- Limited quantities should be prescribed at any time because of their potentially lethal cardiovascular and epileptogenic effects in overdose
- Parents and children need to be advised that drowsiness may affect performance in skilled tasks (e.g. sport, driving, operating machinery)
- Blurred vision might affect school performance
- Imipramine is associated with weight gain. Weight and height should be monitored using a growth chart
- Do not use in children with structural cardiac abnormalities or other serious cardiac problems
- Sudden death in children and adolescents with serious heart problems has been reported
- American Heart Association recommends ECG prior to initiating stimulant treatment in children, although not all experts agree, and it is not usual practice in UK
- Dosing for nocturnal enuresis once daily at bedtime, for ADHD 10–30 mg twice daily
- Re-evaluate the need for continued treatment regularly
- Provide the Medicines for Children leaflet: Imipramine-various-conditions (https:www.medicinesforchildren.org.uk/imipramine-various-conditions)

Pregnancy

- No strong evidence of TCA maternal use during pregnancy being associated with an increased risk of congenital malformations
- Risk of malformations cannot be ruled out due to limited information on specific TCAs
- Poor neonatal adaptation syndrome and/or withdrawal has been reported in infants whose mothers took a TCA during pregnancy or near delivery
- Maternal use of more than one CNS-acting medication is likely to lead to more severe symptoms in the neonate
- Must weigh the risk of treatment (first trimester foetal development, third trimester newborn delivery) to the child against the risk of no treatment (recurrence of depression, maternal health, infant bonding) to the mother and child
- For many patients this may mean continuing treatment during pregnancy

Breastfeeding

- Small amounts found in mother's breast milk
- Infant should be monitored for sedation and poor feeding
- Immediate postpartum period is a high-risk time for depression, especially in women who have had prior depressive episodes; antidepressants may need to be reinstituted late in the third trimester or shortly after childbirth to prevent a recurrence during the postpartum period
- Must weigh benefits of breastfeeding with risks and benefits of antidepressant treatment versus nontreatment to both the infant and the mother
- For many patients this may mean continuing treatment during breastfeeding
- Imipramine and nortriptyline are preferred TCAs for depression in breastfeeding mothers

THE ART OF PSYCHOPHARMACOLOGY

Potential Advantages
- Patients with insomnia
- Severe or treatment-resistant depression
- Patients with enuresis

Potential Disadvantages
- Elderly patients more prone to side effects
- Patients concerned with weight gain
- Cardiac patients

Primary Target Symptoms
- Depressed mood
- Chronic pain

Pearls
- Was once one of the most widely prescribed agents for depression
- Evaluate risks and benefits carefully before prescribing to a patient with suicidal ideation as it can be potentially lethal in overdose
- *Probably the most preferred TCA for treating enuresis in children
- *Preference of some prescribers for imipramine over other TCAs for the treatment of enuresis is based more upon art and anecdote and empiric clinical experience than comparative clinical trials with other TCAs

- TCAs are no longer generally considered a first-line treatment option for depression because of their side-effect profile
- TCAs may aggravate psychotic symptoms
- Alcohol should be avoided because of additive CNS effects
- Underweight patients may be more susceptible to adverse cardiovascular effects
- Children, patients with inadequate hydration, and patients with cardiac disease may be more susceptible to TCA-induced cardiotoxicity than healthy adults
- For the expert only: although generally prohibited, a heroic but potentially dangerous treatment for severely treatment-resistant patients is to give a tricyclic/tetracyclic antidepressant other than clomipramine simultaneously with an MAOI for patients who fail to respond to numerous other antidepressants
- If this option is elected, start the MAOI with the tricyclic/tetracyclic antidepressant simultaneously at low doses after appropriate drug washout, then alternately increase doses of these agents every few days to a week as tolerated
- Although very strict dietary and concomitant drug restrictions must be observed to prevent hypertensive crises and serotonin syndrome, the most common side effects of MAOI/tricyclic or tetracyclic combinations may be weight gain and orthostatic hypotension
- Patients on TCAs should be aware that they may experience symptoms such as photosensitivity or blue-green urine
- SSRIs may be more effective than TCAs in women, and TCAs may be more effective than SSRIs in men
- Since tricyclic/tetracyclic antidepressants are substrates for CYP450 2D6, and 7% of the population (especially Whites) may have a genetic variant leading to reduced activity of 2D6, such patients may not safely tolerate normal doses of tricyclic/tetracyclic antidepressants and may require dose reduction
- Phenotypic testing may be necessary to detect this genetic variant prior to dosing with a tricyclic/tetracyclic antidepressant, especially in vulnerable populations such as children, elderly, cardiac populations, and those on concomitant medications
- Patients who seem to have extraordinarily severe side effects at normal or low doses may have this phenotypic CYP450 2D6 variant and require low doses or switching to another antidepressant not metabolised by 2D6

 Suggested Reading

Anderson IM. Selective serotonin reuptake inhibitors versus tricyclic antidepressants: a meta-analysis of efficacy and tolerability. J Affect Disord 2000;58(1):19–36.

Anderson IM. Meta-analytical studies on new antidepressants. Br Med Bull 2001;57:161–78.

Preskorn SH. Comparison of the tolerability of bupropion, fluoxetine, imipramine, nefazodone, paroxetine, sertraline, and venlafaxine. J Clin Psychiatry 1995;56(Suppl 6):12–21.

Workman EA, Short DD. Atypical antidepressants versus imipramine in the treatment of major depression: a meta-analysis. J Clin Psychiatry 1993;54(1):5–12.

Isocarboxazid

Brands
• Non-proprietary

Generic?
Yes

 Class

• Neuroscience-based nomenclature: pharmacology domain – serotonin, norepinephrine, dopamine; mode of action – enzyme inhibitor
• Monoamine oxidase inhibitor (MAOI)

Commonly Prescribed for
(bold for BNF indication)
• **Depressive illness (in adults)**
• Treatment-resistant depression
• Treatment-resistant panic disorder
• Treatment-resistant social anxiety disorder

 How the Drug Works

• Irreversibly blocks monoamine oxidase (MAO) from breaking down noradrenaline, serotonin, and dopamine
• This presumably boosts noradrenergic, serotonergic, and dopaminergic neurotransmission

How Long Until It Works
• Onset of therapeutic actions with some antidepressants can be seen within 1–2 weeks, but often delayed 2–4 weeks
• If it is not working within 3–4 weeks for depression, it may require a dosage increase or it may not work at all
• May continue to work for many years to prevent relapse of symptoms

If It Works
• The goal of treatment is complete remission of current symptoms as well as prevention of future relapses
• Treatment most often reduces or even eliminates symptoms, but is not a cure since symptoms can recur after medicine is stopped
• Continue treatment until all symptoms are gone (remission), especially in depression and whenever possible in anxiety disorders
• Once symptoms are gone, continue treating for at least 6–9 months for the first episode

of depression or >12 months if relapse indicators present
• If >5 episodes and/or 2 episodes in the last few years then need to continue for at least 2 years or indefinitely
• Use in anxiety disorders may also need to be indefinite

If It Doesn't Work
• Important to recognise non-response to treatment early on (3–4 weeks)
• Many patients have only a partial response where some symptoms are improved but others persist (especially insomnia, fatigue, and problems concentrating)
• Other patients may be non-responders, sometimes called treatment-resistant or treatment-refractory
• Some patients who have an initial response may relapse even though they continue treatment
• Consider increasing dose, switching to another agent, or adding an appropriate augmenting agent
• Lithium may be added for suicidal patients or those at high risk of relapse
• Consider psychotherapy
• Consider ECT
• Consider evaluation for another diagnosis or for a co-morbid condition (e.g. medical illness, substance abuse, etc.)
• Some patients may experience a switch into mania and so would require antidepressant discontinuation and initiation of a mood stabiliser

Best Augmenting Combos for Partial Response or Treatment Resistance
∗Augmentation of MAOIs has not been systematically studied, and this is something for the expert, to be done with caution and with careful monitoring
• Lithium is particularly useful for suicidal patients and those at high risk of relapse including with factors such as severe depression, psychomotor retardation, repeated episodes (>3), significant weight loss, or a family history of major depression (aim for lithium plasma levels 0.6–1.0 mmol/L)
• Atypical antipsychotics (with special caution for those agents with monoamine reuptake blocking properties)

- Mood-stabilising anticonvulsants
* A stimulant such as dexamfetamine or methylphenidate (with caution; may activate bipolar disorder and suicidal ideation; may elevate blood pressure)

Tests

- Patients should be monitored for changes in blood pressure
- Patients receiving high doses or long-term treatment should have hepatic function evaluated periodically
* Since MAOIs are frequently associated with weight gain, before starting treatment, weigh all patients and determine if the patient is already overweight (BMI 25.0–29.9) or obese (BMI ≥30)
- Before giving a drug that can cause weight gain to an overweight or obese patient, consider determining whether the patient already has pre-diabetes (fasting plasma glucose 5.5–6.9 mmol/L), diabetes (fasting plasma glucose >7 mmol/L), or dyslipidaemia (increased total cholesterol, LDL cholesterol, and triglycerides; decreased HDL cholesterol), and treat or refer such patients for treatment, including nutrition and weight management, physical activity counselling, smoking cessation, and medical management
* Monitor weight and BMI during treatment
* While giving a drug to a patient who has gained >5% of initial weight, consider evaluating for the presence of pre-diabetes, diabetes, or dyslipidaemia, or consider switching to a different antidepressant

SIDE EFFECTS

How Drug Causes Side Effects

- Theoretically due to increases in monoamines in parts of the brain and body and at receptors other than those that cause therapeutic actions (e.g. unwanted actions of serotonin in sleep centres causing insomnia, unwanted actions of norepinephrine on vascular smooth muscle causing hypertension, etc.)
- Side effects are generally immediate, but immediate side effects often disappear in time

Notable Side Effects

- Dizziness, sedation, headaches, sleep disturbances, fatigue, weakness, tremor, movement problems, blurred vision, increased sweating
- Constipation, dry mouth, nausea, change in appetite, weight gain
- Sexual dysfunction
- Orthostatic hypotension (dose-related); syncope may develop at high doses

Frequency not known

- Granulocytopenia, peripheral oedema, sexual dysfunction

Life-Threatening or Dangerous Side Effects

- Hypertensive crisis (especially when MAOIs are used with certain tyramine-containing foods or prohibited drugs)
- Granulocytopenia
- Induction of mania
- Rare increase in suicidal ideation and behaviours in adolescents and young adults (up to age 25), hence patients should be warned of this potential adverse event
- Seizures
- Hepatotoxicity

Weight Gain

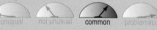

- Many experience and/or can be significant in amount

Sedation

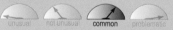

- Many experience and/or can be significant in amount
- Can also cause activation

What to Do About Side Effects

- Wait
- Wait
- Wait
- Lower the dose
- Take at night if daytime sedation
- Switch after appropriate washout to an SSRI or newer antidepressant

Best Augmenting Agents for Side Effects

- Trazodone (with caution) for insomnia
- Benzodiazepines for insomnia
- Many side effects cannot be improved with an augmenting agent

DOSING AND USE

Usual Dosage Range
- Depressive illness: 30–60 mg/day (elderly 5–10 mg/day)

Dosage Forms
- Tablet 10 mg

How to Dose
- Initial dose 10 mg twice per day, then 30 mg/day in single or divided doses (it may be increased after 4 weeks as required to max 60 mg/day for 4–6 weeks), then reduce to usual maintenance dose 10–20 mg/day (but up to 40 mg/day may be required)

Dosing Tips
- Orthostatic hypotension, especially at high doses, may require splitting into 3 or 4 daily doses
- Patients receiving high doses may need to be evaluated periodically for effects on the liver

Overdose
- Dizziness, sedation, ataxia, headache, insomnia, restlessness, anxiety, irritability; cardiovascular effects, confusion, respiratory depression, or coma may also occur

Long-Term Use
- May require periodic evaluation of hepatic function
- MAOIs may lose some efficacy long-term

Habit Forming
- Some patients have developed dependence to MAOIs

How to Stop
- Generally no need to taper as drug wears off slowly over 2–3 weeks

Pharmacokinetics
- Clinical duration of action may be up to 14 days due to irreversible enzyme inhibition

Drug Interactions
- Tramadol may increase the risk of seizures in patients taking an MAOI

- Can cause a fatal "serotonin syndrome" when combined with drugs that block serotonin reuptake, so do not use with a serotonin reuptake inhibitor or for 5 half-lives of the SSRI after stopping the serotonin reuptake inhibitor (see Table 1 after Pearls)
- Hypertensive crisis with headache, intracranial bleeding, and death may result from combining MAOIs with sympathomimetic drugs (e.g. amfetamines, methylphenidate, cocaine, dopamine, adrenaline and related compounds, methyldopa, L-dopa, L-tryptophan, L-tyrosine, and phenylalanine)
- Do not combine with another MAOI, alcohol, or guanethidine
- Adverse drug reactions can result from combining MAOIs with tricyclic/tetracyclic antidepressants and related compounds, including carbamazepine and mirtazapine, and should be avoided except by experts to treat difficult cases (see Pearls)
- MAOIs in combination with spinal anaesthesia may cause combined hypotensive effects
- Combination of MAOIs and CNS depressants may enhance sedation and hypotension

Other Warnings/Precautions
- Use requires low-tyramine diet (see Table 2 after Pearls)
- Patient and prescriber must be vigilant to potential interactions with any drug, including antihypertensives and over-the-counter cough/cold preparations
- Over-the-counter medications to avoid include cough and cold preparations, including those containing dextromethorphan, nasal decongestants (tablets, drops, or spray), hay-fever medications, sinus medications, asthma inhalant medications, anti-appetite medications, weight-reducing preparations, "pep" pills (see Table 3 after Pearls)
- Use cautiously in patients receiving reserpine, anaesthetics, disulfiram, anticholinergic agents
- Isocarboxazid is not recommended for use in patients who cannot be monitored closely
- Use with caution in acute porphyrias, blood disorders, cardiovascular disease, diabetes, epilepsy

- Use with caution in patients undergoing ECT
- Use with great caution in the elderly
- Use with caution in patients undergoing surgery
- When treating children, carefully weigh the risks and benefits of pharmacological treatment against the risks and benefits of nontreatment with antidepressants and make sure to document this in the patient's record
- Warn patients and their caregivers about the possibility of activating side effects and advise them to report such symptoms immediately
- Monitor patients for activation of suicidal ideation, especially those up to the age of 25

Do Not Use

- In agitated patients or in the manic phase
- If patient is taking pethidine
- If patient is taking a sympathomimetic agent or taking guanethidine
- If patient is taking another MAOI
- If patient is taking any agent that can inhibit serotonin reuptake (e.g. SSRIs, sibutramine, tramadol, duloxetine, venlafaxine, clomipramine, etc.)
- If patient is taking diuretics
- If patient is taking medications containing morphinan compounds
- If patient has phaeochromocytoma
- If patient has severe cardiovascular disease or cerebrovascular disease
- If patient has frequent or severe headaches
- If patient needs surgery with general anaesthesia
- If patient has a history of liver disease or abnormal liver function tests
- If patient is taking a prohibited drug
- If patient cannot adhere to a low-tyramine diet
- If there is a proven allergy to isocarboxazid

Renal Impairment

- Use with caution – drug may accumulate in plasma
- May require lower than usual adult dose

Hepatic Impairment

- Not for use in hepatic impairment

Cardiac Impairment

- Contraindicated in patients with congestive heart failure or hypertension
- Any other cardiac impairment may require lower than usual adult dose
- Patients with angina pectoris or coronary artery disease should limit their exertion

Elderly

- Take great caution in elderly (increased risk of postural hypotension)
- Initial dose lower than usual adult dose
- Elderly patients may have greater sensitivity to adverse effects
- Reduction in the risk of suicidality with antidepressants compared to placebo in adults age 65 and older

Children and Adolescents

- Not recommended for use in children and adolescents

Pregnancy

- Controlled studies have not been conducted in pregnant women
- Not generally recommended for use during pregnancy, especially during first and third trimesters
- Should evaluate patient for treatment with an antidepressant with a better risk/benefit ratio

Breastfeeding

- Some drug is found in mother's breast milk
- Effects on infant unknown
- Immediate postpartum period is a high-risk time for depression, especially in women who have had prior depressive episodes, so drug may need to be reinstituted shortly after childbirth to prevent a recurrence during the postpartum period
- Should evaluate patient for treatment with an antidepressant with a better risk/benefit ratio

THE ART OF PSYCHOPHARMACOLOGY

Potential Advantages

- Atypical depression
- Severe depression
- Treatment-resistant depression or anxiety disorders

Potential Disadvantages

- Requires adherence to dietary restrictions and concomitant drug restrictions
- Patients with cardiac problems or hypertension
- Multiple daily doses

Primary Target Symptoms

- Depressed mood
- Somatic symptoms
- Sleep and eating disturbances
- Psychomotor retardation
- Morbid preoccupation

 Pearls

- MAOIs are generally reserved for use after SSRIs, SNRIs, TCAs or combinations of newer antidepressants have failed
- Despite little utilisation, some patients respond to isocarboxazid who do not respond to other antidepressants including other MAOIs
- Patient should be advised not to take any prescription or over-the-counter drugs without consulting their doctor because of possible drug interactions with the MAOI
- Headache is often the first symptom of hypertensive crisis
- The rigid dietary restrictions may reduce concordance (see Table 2 after Pearls)
- Mood disorders can be associated with eating disorders (especially in adolescent females), and isocarboxazid can be used to treat both depression and bulimia

- MAOIs are viable treatment options in depression when other classes of antidepressants have not worked, but they are not frequently used
- *Myths about the danger of dietary tyramine can be exaggerated, but prohibitions against concomitant drugs often not followed closely enough
- *Postural hypotension can be a good marker for adequate MAO blockade
- Orthostatic hypotension, insomnia, and sexual dysfunction are often the most troublesome common side effects
- *MAOIs should be for the expert, especially if combining with agents of potential risk (e.g. stimulants, trazodone, TCAs)
- *MAOIs should not be neglected as therapeutic agents for the treatment-resistant
- Although generally prohibited, a heroic but potentially dangerous treatment for severely treatment-resistant patients is for an expert to give a tricyclic/tetracyclic antidepressant other than clomipramine simultaneously with an MAOI for patients who fail to respond to numerous other antidepressants
- Use of MAOIs with clomipramine is always prohibited because of the risk of serotonin syndrome and death
- Start the MAOI with the tricyclic/tetracyclic antidepressant simultaneously at low doses after appropriate drug washout, then alternately increase doses of these agents every few days to a week as tolerated
- Although very strict dietary and concomitant drug restrictions must be observed to prevent hypertensive crises and serotonin syndrome, the most common side effects of MAOI and tricyclic/tetracyclic combinations may be weight gain and orthostatic hypotension

Isocarboxazid (Continued)

Table 1. Drugs contraindicated due to risk of serotonin syndrome/toxicity

Do Not Use:			
Antidepressants	**Drugs of Abuse**	**Opioids**	**Other**
SSRIs	MDMA (ecstasy)	Pethidine	Non-subcutaneous sumatriptan
SNRIs	Cocaine	Tramadol	Chlorphenamine
Clomipramine	Metamfetamine	Methadone	Procarbazine?
St. John's wort	High-dose or injected amfetamine	Fentanyl	Morphinan-containing compounds

Table 2. Dietary guidelines for patients taking MAOIs

Foods to avoid*	Foods allowed
Dried, aged, smoked, fermented, spoiled, or improperly stored meat, poultry, and fish including game	Fresh or processed meat, poultry, and fish; properly stored pickled or smoked fish
Broad bean pods	All other vegetables
Aged cheeses	Processed cheese slices, cottage cheese, ricotta cheese, yoghurt, cream cheese
Tap and unpasteurised beer	Canned or bottled beer and alcohol
Marmite	Brewer's and baker's yeast
Sauerkraut, kimchi	
Soy products/tofu	Peanuts
Banana peel	Bananas, avocados, raspberries
Tyramine-containing nutritional supplement	

*Not necessary for 6-mg transdermal or low-dose oral selegiline

Table 3. Drugs that boost norepinephrine: should only be used with caution with MAOIs

Use With Caution:			
Decongestants	**Stimulants**	**Antidepressants with norepinephrine reuptake inhibition**	**Other**
Phenylephrine	Amfetamines	Most tricyclics	Local anaesthetics containing vasoconstrictors
Pseudoephedrine	Methylphenidate	NRIs	Tapentadol
	Cocaine	NDRIs	
	Metamfetamine		
	Modafinil		

 Suggested Reading

Amsterdam JD, Kim TT. Relative effectiveness of monoamine oxidase inhibitor and tricyclic antidepressant combination therapy for treatment-resistant depression. J Clin Psychopharmacol 2019;39(6):649–52.

Gillman PK. A reassessment of the safety profile of monoamine oxidase inhibitors: elucidating tired old tyramine myths. J Neural Transm (Vienna) 2018;125(11):1707–17.

Kennedy SH. Continuation and maintenance treatments in major depression: the neglected role of monoamine oxidase inhibitors. J Psychiatry Neurosci 1997;22(2):127–31.

Kim T, Xu C, Amsterdam JD. Relative effectiveness of tricyclic antidepressant versus monoamine oxidase inhibitor monotherapy for treatment-resistant depression. J Affect Disord 2019;250:199–203.

Larsen JK, Rafaelsen OJ. Long-term treatment of depression with isocarboxazide. Acta Psychiatr Scand 1980;62(5):456–63.

Lippman SB, Nash K. Monoamine oxidase inhibitor update. Potential adverse food and drug interactions. Drug Saf 1990;5(3):195–204.

Lamotrigine

Brands
- Lamictal

Generic?
Yes

Class
- Neuroscience-based nomenclature: pharmacology domain – glutamate; mode of action – channel blocker
- Anticonvulsant, mood stabiliser, voltage-sensitive sodium channel antagonist

Commonly Prescribed for
(bold for BNF indication)
- **Monotherapy (or adjunctive therapy) of bipolar disorder**
- **Seizures (monotherapy in children over 12 years and adults or adjunctive therapy in children aged 2 years and above and adults): for focal seizures; for primary and secondary generalised tonic-clonic seizures; for seizures associated with Lennox-Gastaut syndrome**
- Bipolar depression
- Bipolar mania (adjunctive and second-line)
- Psychosis, schizophrenia (adjunctive)
- Neuropathic pain/chronic pain
- Major depressive disorder (adjunctive)
- Other seizure types and as initial monotherapy for epilepsy

How the Drug Works
* Acts as a use-dependent blocker of voltage-sensitive sodium channels
* Interacts with the open channel conformation of voltage-sensitive sodium channels
* Interacts at a specific site of the alpha pore-forming subunit of voltage-sensitive sodium channels
- Inhibits release of glutamate and aspartate

How Long Until It Works
- May take several weeks to improve bipolar depression
- May take several weeks to months to optimise an effect on mood stabilisation
- Can reduce seizures by 2 weeks, but may take several weeks to months to reduce seizures

If It Works
- The goal of treatment is complete remission of symptoms (e.g. seizures, depression, pain)
- Continue treatment until all symptoms are gone or until improvement is stable and then continue treating indefinitely as long as improvement persists
- Continue treatment indefinitely to avoid recurrence of depression, mania, and/or seizures
- Treatment of chronic neuropathic pain may reduce but does not eliminate pain symptoms and is not a cure since pain usually recurs after medicine stopped

If It Doesn't Work (for bipolar disorder)
* Many patients have only a partial response where some symptoms are improved but others persist or continue to wax and wane without stabilisation of mood
- Other patients may be non-responders, sometimes called treatment-resistant or treatment-refractory
- Consider increasing dose, switching to another agent, or adding an appropriate augmenting agent
- Consider adding psychotherapy
- Consider biofeedback or hypnosis for pain
- Consider the presence of non-concordance and counsel patient
- Switch to another mood stabiliser (in particular consider lithium)
- Consider evaluation for another diagnosis or for a co-morbid condition (e.g. medical illness, substance abuse, etc.)

Best Augmenting Combos for Partial Response or Treatment Resistance (for bipolar disorder)
- Lithium
- Atypical antipsychotics (especially quetiapine, risperidone, olanzapine or aripiprazole)
* Valproate (with caution and at half dose of lamotrigine in the presence of valproate, because valproate can double lamotrigine levels)
* Antidepressants (with caution because antidepressants can destabilise mood in some patients, including induction of rapid

cycling or suicidal ideation; in particular consider bupropion; also SSRIs, SNRIs, others; generally avoid TCAs, MAOIs)

Tests
- None required
- The value of monitoring plasma concentrations of lamotrigine has not been established
- Because lamotrigine binds to melanin-containing tissues, ophthalmological checks may be considered

SIDE EFFECTS

How Drug Causes Side Effects
- CNS side effects theoretically due to excessive actions at voltage-sensitive sodium channels
- Rash hypothetically an allergic reaction

Notable Side Effects
* Benign rash (about 10%)
- Dose-dependent: blurred or double vision, dizziness, ataxia
- Sedation, headache, tremor, insomnia, poor coordination, fatigue
- Nausea (dose-dependent), vomiting, dyspepsia, rhinitis
- Additional effects in paediatric patients with epilepsy: infection, pharyngitis, asthenia

Common or very common
- CNS: aggression, agitation, dizziness, drowsiness, headache, irritability, sleep disorders, tremor
- GIT: diarrhoea, dry mouth, nausea, vomiting
- Other: arthralgia, fatigue, pain

Uncommon
- Alopecia, movement abnormalities, visual problems

Rare or very rare
- CNS/PNS: aseptic meningitis, confusion, hallucination, nystagmus, seizure, tic
- Other: conjunctivitis, disseminated intravascular coagulation, facial oedema, fever, hepatic disorders, lupus-like syndrome, lymphadenopathy, multi-organ failure, severe cutaneous adverse reactions (SCARs)

Frequency not known
- Suicidal behaviours

 Life-Threatening or Dangerous Side Effects
* Rare serious rash (risk may be greater in paediatric patients but still rare)
- Rare multi-organ failure associated with Stevens-Johnson syndrome, toxic epidermal necrolysis, or drug hypersensitivity syndrome
- Rare blood dyscrasias
- Rare aseptic meningitis
- Rare sudden unexplained deaths have occurred in epilepsy (unknown if related to lamotrigine use)
- Withdrawal seizures upon abrupt withdrawal
- Rare activation of suicidal ideation and behaviour (suicidality)

Weight Gain

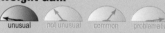

- Reported but not expected

Sedation

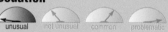

- Reported but not expected
- Dose-related
- Can wear off with time

What to Do About Side Effects
- Warn patients and carers to see their doctor immediately if rash or signs or symptoms of hypersensitivity syndrome develop
- Wait
- Take at night to reduce daytime sedation
- Divide dosing to twice daily
* If patient develops signs of a rash with benign characteristics (i.e. a rash that peaks within days, settles in 10–14 days, is spotty, nonconfluent, nontender, has no systemic features, and laboratory tests are normal):
  - Reduce lamotrigine dose or stop dosage increase
  - Warn patient to stop drug and contact physician if rash worsens or new symptoms emerge
  - Prescribe antihistamine and/or topical corticosteroid for pruritis
  - Monitor patient closely

*If patient develops signs of a rash with serious characteristics (i.e. a rash that is confluent and widespread, or purpuric or tender; with any prominent involvement of neck or upper trunk; any involvement of eyes, lips, mouth, etc.; any associated fever, malaise, pharyngitis, anorexia, or lymphadenopathy; abnormal blood tests for FBC, liver function, urea, creatinine):
• Stop lamotrigine (and valproate if administered)
• Monitor and investigate organ involvement (hepatic, renal, haematologic)
• Patient may require admission
• Monitor patient very closely

Best Augmenting Agents for Side Effects
• Antihistamines and/or topical corticosteroid for rash, pruritis
• Many side effects cannot be improved with an augmenting agent

DOSING AND USE

Usual Dosage Range
• Monotherapy or adjunctive therapy of bipolar disorder (without enzyme-inducing drugs, e.g. carbamazepine, phenobarbital, phenytoin, and primidone) and without valproate: 200–400 mg/day in 1–2 divided doses
• Adjunctive therapy of bipolar disorder with valproate: 100–200 mg/day in 1–2 divided doses
• Monotherapy for seizures in patients over age 12: 100–500 mg/day in 1–2 divided doses
• Adjunctive treatment for seizures in patients over age 12: for regimens containing valproate (100–200 mg/day in 1–2 divided doses); in regimens with enzyme-inducing drugs without valproate (200–700 mg/day in 1–2 divided doses); regimens without enzyme-inducing drugs and without valproate (100–200 mg/day in 1–2 divided doses)
• Patients aged 2–12 with epilepsy are dosed based on body weight and concomitant medications

Dosage Forms
• Tablet 25 mg, 50 mg, 100 mg, 200 mg
• Dispersible tablet 2 mg, 5 mg, 25 mg, 100 mg
• Can get oral suspension and oral solution from special order manufacturers

How to Dose
*Bipolar disorder (monotherapy):
• 25 mg/day; at week 3 increase to 50 mg/day; from week 5 onwards, you can increase by increments of up to 100 mg every 7–14 days. Maintenance dose is 100–200 mg/day in 1–2 divided doses; max 500 mg/day. Repeat dose titration if restarting after an interval of more than 5 days
*Bipolar disorder (adjunct to valproate):
• For adults: for the first 2 weeks administer 25 mg/day on alternate days for 2 weeks; at week 3 increase to 25 mg/day for next 2 weeks in 1–2 divided doses, then at week 5, administer 50 mg/day in 1–2 divided doses. Maintenance: 100 mg/day in 1–2 divided doses; max 200 mg/day. Repeat dose titration if restarting after an interval of more than 5 days
*When used as an adjunct with enzyme-inducing drugs and without valproate for bipolar disorder:
• For adults: for the first 2 weeks administer 50 mg/day for 2 weeks; at week 3 increase to 50 mg twice per day for next 2 weeks, then at week 5, administer 100 mg twice per day, then at week 6, increase to 150 mg twice per day for 7 days. Maintenance: 200 mg twice per day. Repeat dose titration if restarting after an interval of more than 5 days
*When used in monotherapy or an adjunct without valproate or any enzyme-inducing drug for bipolar disorder:
• For adults: for the first 2 weeks administer 25 mg/day for 2 weeks; at week 3 increase to 50 mg/day for next 2 weeks in 1–2 divided doses, then at week 5, administer 100 mg/day in 1–2 divided doses. Maintenance: 200 mg/day in 1–2 divided doses. Max 400 mg/day. Repeat dose titration if restarting after an interval of more than 5 days

Lamotrigine (Continued)

＊When used as an adjunct with valproate for focal seizures, or primary and secondary generalised tonic-clonic seizures or for Lennox-Gastaut syndrome (children 2–17 years and adults):
- For children 2–11 years (body weight up to 13 kg): for the first 2 weeks, administer 2 mg/day on alternate days, then at week 3, give 300 mcg/kg once daily, from week 5, you can increase by increments of up to 300 mcg/kg every 7–14 days. Maintenance dose: 1–5 mg/kg in 1–2 divided doses. Repeat dose titration if restarting after an interval of more than 5 days. Max 200 mg/day
- For children 2–11 years (body weight 13 kg and above): for the first 2 weeks, administer 150 mcg/kg once daily for 2 weeks, then at week 3, give 300 mcg/kg once daily, from week 5, you can increase by increments of up to 300 mcg/kg every 7–14 days. Maintenance dose: 1–5 mg/kg in 1–2 divided doses. Repeat dose titration if restarting after an interval of more than 5 days. Max 200 mg/day
- For children 12–17 and adults: for the first 2 weeks administer 25 mg every other day; at week 3 increase to 25 mg/day; every 1–2 weeks can increase by increments of up to 50 mg/day. Maintenance dose 100–200 mg/day in 1–2 divided doses. Repeat dose titration if restarting after an interval of more than 5 days

＊When used as an adjunct with enzyme-inducing drugs (without valproate) for focal seizures, or primary and secondary generalised tonic-clonic seizures or for Lennox-Gastaut syndrome (children 2–17 years and adults):
- For children 2–11 years: for the first 2 weeks, administer 300 mcg/kg twice daily for 2 weeks, then at week 3, give 600 mcg/kg twice daily, from week 5, you can increase by increments of up to 1.2 mg/kg every 7–14 days. Maintenance dose: 5–15 mg/kg in 1–2 divided doses. Repeat dose titration if restarting after an interval of more than 5 days. Max 400 mg/day
- For children 12–17 and adults: for the first 2 weeks administer 50 mg every other day; at week 3 increase to 50 mg twice per day; from week 5, you can increase by increments of up to 100 mg/day every 7–14 days. Maintenance dose 200–400 mg/day in 2 divided doses. Max 700 mg/day.

Repeat dose titration if restarting after an interval of more than 5 days
＊When used as an adjunct without enzyme-inducing drugs (without valproate) for focal seizures, or primary and secondary generalised tonic-clonic seizures or for Lennox-Gastaut syndrome (children 2–17 years and adults):
- For children 2–11 years: for the first 2 weeks, administer 300 mcg/kg/day in 1–2 divided doses for 2 weeks, then at week 3, give 600 mcg/kg daily in 1–2 divided doses for further 2 weeks, from week 5, you can increase by increments of up to 600 mcg/kg every 7–14 days. Maintenance dose: 1–10 mg/kg in 1–2 divided doses. Repeat dose titration if restarting after an interval of more than 5 days. Max 200 mg/day
- For children 12–17 and adults: for the first 2 weeks administer 25 mg once daily for 2 weeks; at week 3 increase to 50 mg once daily; from week 5, you can increase by increments of up to 100 mg/day every 7–14 days. Maintenance dose 100–200 mg/day in 1–2 divided doses. Repeat dose titration if restarting after an interval of more than 5 days

 Dosing Tips

＊Very slow dose titration may reduce the incidence of skin rash
- Therefore, dose should not be titrated faster than recommended because of possible risk of increased side effects, including rash
- If patient stops taking lamotrigine for 5 days or more it is necessary to restart the drug with the initial dose titration, as rashes have been reported on re-exposure
- Advise patient to avoid new medications, foods, or products during the first 3 months of lamotrigine treatment in order to decrease the risk of unrelated rash; patient should also not start lamotrigine within 2 weeks of a viral infection, rash, or vaccination
＊If lamotrigine is added to patients taking valproate, remember that valproate inhibits lamotrigine metabolism and therefore titration rate and ultimate dose of lamotrigine should be reduced by 50% to reduce the risk of rash
＊Thus, if concomitant valproate is discontinued after lamotrigine dose is stabilised, then the lamotrigine dose should

be cautiously doubled over at least 2 weeks in equal increments each week following discontinuation of valproate
- Also, if concomitant enzyme-inducing antiepileptic drugs such as carbamazepine, phenobarbital, phenytoin, and primidone are discontinued after lamotrigine dose is stabilised, then the lamotrigine dose should be maintained for 1 week following discontinuation of the other drug and then reduced by half over 2 weeks in equal decrements each week
- Since oral contraceptives and pregnancy can decrease lamotrigine levels, adjustments to the maintenance dose of lamotrigine are recommended in women taking, starting, or stopping oral contraceptives, becoming pregnant, or after delivery
- Orally disintegrating tablet should be placed onto the tongue and moved around in the mouth; the tablet will disintegrate rapidly and can be swallowed with or without food or water

Overdose
- Lamotrigine has low toxicity in overdose. Smallest dose likely to cause death is at least 4 g
- Signs and symptoms of overdose are drowsiness, vomiting, ataxia, seizures, tachycardia, dyskinesia and QT prolongation. Some fatalities have occurred

Long-Term Use
- Safe

Habit Forming
- No

How to Stop
- Taper over at least 2 weeks
*Rapid discontinuation can increase the risk of relapse in bipolar disorder
- Patients with epilepsy may seize upon withdrawal, especially if withdrawal is abrupt
- Discontinuation symptoms uncommon

Pharmacokinetics
- Elimination half-life in healthy volunteers about 33 hours (range 14–103 hours) after a single dose of lamotrigine
- Elimination half-life in patients receiving concomitant valproate treatment about 70 hours after a single dose of lamotrigine

- Elimination half-life in patients receiving concomitant enzyme-inducing antiepileptic drugs (such as carbamazepine, phenobarbital, phenytoin, and primidone) about 14 hours after a single dose of lamotrigine
- Metabolised in the liver through glucuronidation not through the CYP450 enzyme system
- Inactive metabolite
- Renally excreted
- Lamotrigine inhibits dihydrofolate reductase and may therefore reduce folate concentrations
- Rapidly and completely absorbed; bioavailability not affected by food

 ## Drug Interactions
*Valproate increases plasma concentrations and half-life of lamotrigine, requiring lower doses of lamotrigine (half or less)
*Use of lamotrigine with valproate may be associated with an increased incidence of rash
- Enzyme-inducing antiepileptic drugs (e.g. carbamazepine, phenobarbital, phenytoin, primidone) may increase the clearance of lamotrigine and lower its plasma levels
- Oral contraceptives may decrease plasma levels of lamotrigine
- No likely pharmacokinetic interactions of lamotrigine with lithium. May increase levels of atypical antipsychotics or oxcarbazepine
- False-positive urine immunoassay screening tests for phencyclidine (PCP) have been reported in patients taking lamotrigine due to a lack of specificity of the screening tests

 ## Other Warnings/Precautions
*Life-threatening rashes have developed in association with lamotrigine use; lamotrigine should generally be discontinued at the first sign of serious rash
*Risk of rash may be increased with higher doses, faster dose escalation, concomitant use of valproate, or in children under age 12
- Patient should be instructed to report any symptoms of hypersensitivity immediately (fever; flu-like symptoms; rash; blisters on skin or in eyes, mouth, ears, nose,

Lamotrigine (Continued)

or genital areas; swelling of eyelids, conjunctivitis, lymphadenopathy)
- Aseptic meningitis has been reported rarely in association with lamotrigine use
- Patients should be advised to report any symptoms of aseptic meningitis immediately; these include headache, chills, fever, vomiting and nausea, a stiff neck, and sensitivity to light
- Depressive effects may be increased by other CNS depressants (alcohol, MAOIs, other anticonvulsants, etc.)
- Some people may experience a worsening of myoclonic seizures
- Use with caution in Brugada syndrome
- Parkinson's disease in adults may be exacerbated by lamotrigine
- May cause photosensitivity
- Lamotrigine binds to tissue that contains melanin, so for long-term treatment ophthalmological checks may be considered
- Warn patients and their caregivers about the possibility of activation of suicidal ideation and advise them to report such side effects immediately

Do Not Use
- If there is a proven allergy to lamotrigine

Renal Impairment
- Lamotrigine is renally excreted, so the maintenance dose may need to be lowered
- Can be removed by haemodialysis; patients receiving haemodialysis may require supplemental doses of lamotrigine

Hepatic Impairment
- Dose adjustment not necessary in mild impairment
- Initial, escalation, and maintenance doses should be reduced by 50% in patients with moderate and severe liver impairment without ascites and 75% in patients with severe liver impairment with ascites

Cardiac Impairment
- Clinical experience is limited
- Drug should be used with caution

Elderly
- Some patients may tolerate lower doses better
- Elderly patients may be more susceptible to adverse effects

 Children and Adolescents
- Monotherapy of focal seizures (child 12–17 years)
- Monotherapy of primary and secondary generalised tonic-clonic seizures (child 12–17 years)
- Monotherapy of seizures associated with Lennox-Gastaut syndrome (child 12–17 years)
- Monotherapy of typical absence seizures (child 2–11 years)
- Adjunctive therapy of focal seizures (child 2–17 years)
- Adjunctive therapy of primary and secondary generalised tonic-clonic seizures (child 2–17 years)
- Adjunctive therapy of seizures associated with Lennox-Gastaut syndrome (child 2–17 years)
- Dose adjustment necessary dependent on the presence or absence of valproate or enzyme-inducing drugs
- Clearance of lamotrigine may be influenced by weight
- *Risk of rash is increased in paediatric patients, especially in children under 12 and in children taking valproate

Pregnancy
- Majority of data does not show increased risk of overall malformation or specific malformations
- Not associated with increased rates of perinatal death, low weight for gestational age or preterm delivery
- Evidence does not suggest increased rates of neurodevelopmental delay, but data too limited to exclude risk completely
- Use in women of childbearing potential requires weighing potential benefits to the mother against the risks to the foetus
- *If treatment with lamotrigine is continued, plasma concentrations may be reduced during pregnancy. Plasma levels should be monitored before, during and after pregnancy. The dose should be adjusted as necessary to maintain plasma levels and clinical response
- Taper drug if discontinuing
- Seizures, even mild seizures, may cause harm to the embryo/foetus

- Recurrent bipolar illness during pregnancy can be quite disruptive
* If drug is continued, start on folate 5 mg/ day early in pregnancy to reduce risk of neural tube defects
* For bipolar patients in whom treatment is discontinued, given the risk of relapse in the postpartum period, lamotrigine should generally be restarted immediately after delivery
* Antipsychotics may be preferable to lamotrigine if treatment of bipolar disorder is required during pregnancy, but lamotrigine is preferable to other anticonvulsants such as valproate if anticonvulsant treatment is required during pregnancy
- Bipolar symptoms may recur or worsen during pregnancy and some form of treatment may be necessary

Breastfeeding

- Significant amount found in mother's breast milk
- If drug is continued while breastfeeding, infant should be monitored for possible adverse effects, including haematological effects and rash
- If infant shows signs of irritability, sedation, or rash, drug may need to be discontinued
- Withdrawal effects may occur in the infant if the mother suddenly stops breastfeeding
* Bipolar disorder may recur during the postpartum period, particularly if there is a history of prior postpartum episodes of either depression or psychosis
* Relapse rates may be lower in women who receive prophylactic treatment for postpartum episodes of bipolar disorder
- Antipsychotics and carbamazepine may be safer than lamotrigine during the postpartum period when breastfeeding

THE ART OF PSYCHOPHARMACOLOGY
Potential Advantages

- Depressive stages of bipolar disorder (bipolar depression)
- To prevent recurrences of both depression and possibly mania in bipolar disorder

Potential Disadvantages

- Not as effective in the manic stage of bipolar disorder

Primary Target Symptoms

- Incidence of seizures
- Unstable mood, especially depression, in bipolar disorder
- Pain

Pearls

* Lamotrigine is a first-line treatment option that may be best for patients with bipolar depression as part of bipolar condition. These patients have usually had experience of ineffective antidepressant medication
* Seems to be more effective in treating depressive episodes than manic episodes in bipolar disorder (treats from below better than it treats from above)
* It is better for preventing depressive relapses than for preventing manic relapses
- For maintenance in bipolar I disorder lamotrigine should be combined with a long-term antimanic agent
* Despite evidence of efficacy in bipolar disorder, lamotrigine is not used commonly outside specialist centres
* Low levels of use may be based upon exaggerated fears of skin rashes or lack of knowledge about how to manage skin rashes if they occur
* May actually be one of the best-tolerated mood stabilisers with little weight gain or sedation
- Actual risk of serious skin rash may be comparable to agents erroneously considered "safer" including carbamazepine, phenytoin, phenobarbital, and zonisamide
- Rashes are common even in placebo-treated patients in clinical trials of bipolar patients (5–10%) due to non-drug-related causes including eczema, irritant and allergic contact dermatitis, such as poison ivy and insect bite reactions
* To manage rashes in bipolar patients receiving lamotrigine, realise that rashes that occur within the first 5 days or after 8–12 weeks of treatment are rarely drug-related, and learn the clinical distinctions between a benign rash and a serious rash (see What to Do About Side Effects section)
- Rash, including serious rash, appears riskiest in younger children, in those who are receiving concomitant valproate, and/or in those receiving rapid lamotrigine titration and/or high dosing

Lamotrigine (Continued)

- Risk of serious rash is less than 1% and has been declining since slower titration, lower dosing, adjustments to use of concomitant valproate administration, and limitations on use in children under 12 have been implemented
- Incidence of serious rash is very low (approaching zero) in recent studies of bipolar patients
- Benign rashes related to lamotrigine may affect up to 10% of patients and resolve rapidly with drug discontinuation
- *Given the limited treatment options for bipolar depression, patients with benign rashes can even be re-challenged with lamotrigine 5–12 mg/day with very slow titration after risk/benefit analysis if they are informed, reliable, closely monitored, and warned to stop lamotrigine and contact their physician if signs of hypersensitivity occur

- Only a third of bipolar patients experience adequate relief with a monotherapy, so most patients need multiple medications for best control
- Lamotrigine is useful in combination with atypical antipsychotics and/or lithium for acute mania
- Usefulness for bipolar disorder in combination with anticonvulsants other than valproate is not well demonstrated; such combinations can be expensive and are possibly ineffective or even irrational
- May be useful as an adjunct to atypical antipsychotics for rapid onset of action in schizophrenia
- May be useful as an adjunct to antidepressants in unipolar depression
- Early studies suggest possible utility for patients with neuropathic pain such as diabetic peripheral neuropathy, HIV-associated neuropathy, and other pain conditions including migraine

 ## Suggested Reading

Calabrese JR, Bowden CL, Sachs GS, et al. A double-blind placebo-controlled study of lamotrigine monotherapy in outpatients with bipolar I depression. Lamictal 602 Study Group. J Clin Psychiatry 1999;60(2):79–88.

Calabrese JR, Sullivan JR, Bowden CL, et al. Rash in multicenter trials of lamotrigine in mood disorders: clinical relevance and management. J Clin Psychiatry 2002;63(11):1012–19.

Culy CR, Goa KL. Lamotrigine. A review of its use in childhood epilepsy. Paediatr Drugs 2000;2(4):299–330.

Cunnington M, Tennis P, International Lamotrigine Pregnancy Registry Scientific Advisory Committee. Lamotrigine and the risk of malformations in pregnancy. Neurology 2005;64(6):955–60.

Geddes JR, Gardiner A, Rendell J, et al. Comparative evaluation of quetiapine plus lamotrigine combination versus quetiapine monotherapy (and folic acid versus placebo) in bipolar depression (CEQUEL): a 2 × 2 factorial randomised trial. Lancet Psychiatry 2016;3(1):31–9.

Goodwin GM, Bowden CL, Calabrese JR, et al. A pooled analysis of 2 placebo-controlled 18-month trials of lamotrigine and lithium maintenance treatment in bipolar I disorder. J Clin Psychiatry 2004;65(3):432–41.

Green B. Lamotrigine in mood disorders. Curr Med Res Opin 2003;19(4):272–7.

Levomepromazine

Brands
• Nozinan

Generic?
Yes

Class
• Neuroscience-based nomenclature:
pharmacology domain – dopamine,
serotonin; mode of action – antagonist
• Conventional antipsychotic (neuroleptic,
phenothiazine, dopamine 2 antagonist,
antiemetic)

Commonly Prescribed for
(bold for BNF indication)
• **Schizophrenia**
• **Palliative care (for pain; for restlessness
and confusion; for nausea and vomiting)**
• Acute behavioural disturbance

 ## How the Drug Works
• Blocks dopamine 2 receptors, reducing
positive symptoms of psychosis
• Antagonistic effects at adrenergic,
dopamine, histamine, muscarinic, and
serotonin receptors exerting antiemetic,
analgesic and sedative effects

How Long Until It Works
• Further research is required to guide the
length of an adequate trial of treatment
• Psychotic symptoms can improve within 1
week, but it may take several weeks for full
effect on behaviour

If It Works
For schizophrenia:
• Most often reduces positive symptoms in
schizophrenia but does not eliminate them
• Most patients with schizophrenia do not
have a total remission of symptoms but
rather a reduction of symptoms by about
a third
• Continue treatment in schizophrenia until
reaching a plateau of improvement
• After reaching a satisfactory plateau,
continue treatment for at least a year after
first episode of psychosis in schizophrenia
• For second and subsequent episodes of
psychosis in schizophrenia, treatment may
need to be indefinite

If It Doesn't Work
• Consider trying one of the first-line atypical
antipsychotics (risperidone, olanzapine,
quetiapine, aripiprazole, paliperidone,
amisulpride)
• Consider trying another conventional
antipsychotic
• If two or more antipsychotic monotherapies
do not work, consider clozapine

 ## Best Augmenting Combos
for Partial Response or Treatment
Resistance
• Augmentation of conventional
antipsychotics has not been systematically
studied
• Addition of a mood-stabilising
anticonvulsant such as valproate,
carbamezapine, or lamotrigine may be
helpful in schizophrenia
• Addition of a benzodiazepine, especially
short-term for agitation

Tests
Baseline
＊Measure weight, BMI, and waist
circumference
• Get baseline personal and family history
of diabetes, obesity, dyslipidaemia,
hypertension, and cardiovascular disease
• Check for personal history of drug-induced
leucopenia/neutropenia
＊Check pulse and blood pressure,
fasting plasma glucose or glycosylated
haemoglobin (HbΛ1c), fasting lipid profile,
and prolactin levels
• Full blood count (FBC)
• Assessment of nutritional status, diet, and
level of physical activity
• Determine if the patient:
  • is overweight (BMI 25.0–29.9)
  • is obese (BMI ≥30)
  • has pre-diabetes – fasting plasma
  glucose: 5.5 mmol/L to 6.9 mmol/L or
  HbA1c: 42 to 47 mmol/mol (6.0 to 6.4%)
  • has diabetes – fasting plasma glucose: >7.0
  mmol/L or HbA1c: ≥48 mmol/L (≥6.5%)
  • has hypertension (BP >140/90 mm Hg)
  • has dyslipidaemia (increased total
  cholesterol, LDL cholesterol, and
  triglycerides; decreased HDL cholesterol)
• Treat or refer such patients for
treatment, including nutrition and weight

management, physical activity counselling, smoking cessation, and medical management
- Baseline ECG for: inpatients; those with a personal history or risk factor for cardiac disease

Monitoring
- Monitor weight and BMI during treatment
- Consider monitoring fasting triglycerides monthly for several months in patients at high risk for metabolic complications and when initiating or switching antipsychotics
- While giving a drug to a patient who has gained >5% of initial weight, consider evaluating for the presence of pre-diabetes, diabetes, or dyslipidaemia, or consider switching to a different antipsychotic
- Patients with low white blood cell count (WBC) or history of drug-induced leucopenia/neutropenia should have full blood count (FBC) monitored frequently during the first few months and levomepromazine should be discontinued at the first sign of decline of WBC in the absence of other causative factors
- Monitor prolactin levels and for signs and symptoms of hyperprolactinaemia

SIDE EFFECTS

How Drug Causes Side Effects
- Exerts antagonistic effects at adrenergic, dopamine, histamine, muscarinic, and serotonin receptors
- By blocking dopamine 2 receptors in the striatum, it can cause motor side effects
- By blocking dopamine 2 receptors in the pituitary, it can cause elevations in prolactin
- By blocking dopamine 2 receptors excessively in the mesocortical and mesolimbic dopamine pathways, especially at high doses, it can cause worsening of negative and cognitive symptoms (neuroleptic-induced deficit syndrome)
- By blocking dopamine 2 receptors in the chemoreceptor trigger zone it can have an antiemetic effect
- By blocking muscarinic receptors it is thought this helps to maintain the dopamine/acetylcholine balance reducing extrapyramidal side effects
- By blocking alpha 1 adrenergic receptors, it can cause dizziness, sedation, and hypotension

- By blocking histamine 1 receptors levomepromazine exerts its sedative effect and contributes to its antiemetic effect
- Mechanism of weight gain and any possible increased incidence of diabetes or dyslipidaemia with conventional antipsychotics is unknown

Notable Side Effects
- Dry mouth
- Somnolence
- QT prolongation
- Asthenia
- Heat stroke
- Hypotension – particularly in the elderly

Common or very common
- Asthenia, heat stroke

Rare or very rare
- Cardiac arrest, hepatic disorders

Frequency not known
- Allergic dermatitis, confusion, delirium, gastrointestinal disorders, hyperglycaemia, hyponatraemia, impaired glucose tolerance, photosensitivity, priapism, SIADH

 Life-Threatening or Dangerous Side Effects
- Hypotension in the elderly, debilitated, or those with cardiac disease
- Rare agranulocytosis
- Rare neuroleptic malignant syndrome
- Rare seizures
- Rare jaundice
- Increased risk of death and cerebrovascular events in elderly patients with dementia-related psychosis
- Sudden cardiac death
- Necrotising enterocolitis

Weight Gain
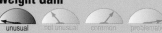
- Reported but not expected
- Weight gain including hyperglycaemia may be seen

Sedation
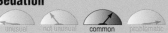
- Frequent and can be significant in amount
- Strong sedative effect

What To Do About Side Effects

- Wait
- Wait
- Wait
- Reduce the dose
- Low-dose benzodiazepine or beta blocker may reduce akathisia
- Take more of the dose at bedtime to help reduce daytime sedation
- Weight loss, exercise programmes, and medical management for high BMIs, diabetes, and dyslipidaemia
- Switch to another antipsychotic (atypical) – quetiapine or clozapine are best in cases of tardive dyskinesia

Best Augmenting Agents for Side Effects

- Dystonia: antimuscarinic drugs (e.g. procyclidine) as oral or IM depending on the severity; botulinum toxin if antimuscarinics not effective
- Parkinsonism: antimuscarinic drugs (e.g. procyclidine)
- Akathisia: beta blocker propranolol (30–80 mg/day) or low-dose benzodiazepine (e.g. 0.5–3.0 mg/day of clonazepam) may help; other agents that may be tried include the 5HT2 antagonists such as cyproheptadine (16 mg/day) or mirtazapine (15 mg at night – caution in bipolar disorder); clonidine (0.2–0.8 mg/day) may be tried if the above ineffective
- Tardive dyskinesia: stop any antimuscarinic, consider tetrabenazine

DOSING AND USE

Usual Dosage Range

- 25–1000 mg/day

Dosage Forms

- Tablet 6 mg, 25 mg, 100 mg
- Solution for injection 25 mg/mL solution (can be given IV or IM)
- Oral solution and oral suspension available by special order from manufacturers
- Only oral levomepromazine is licensed for the treatment of schizophrenia

How to Dose

- For ambulant adults – initial dosing should be 25–50 mg/day in divided doses. Titrate to response and side effects
- For non-ambulant adults – initial dosing may be 100–200 mg/day in three divided doses increased up to 1000 mg/day as required

 ### Dosing Tips

- Low doses for nausea/vomiting and higher doses for delirium/agitation
- Patients receiving large initial doses should remain supine

Overdose

- Drowsiness, loss of consciousness, hypotension, tachycardia, ECG changes, ventricular arrhythmias, hypothermia, seizures, and extrapyramidal dyskinesias may occur in levomepromazine overdose
- Treatment is supportive but if seen within 6 hours of overdose gastric lavage may be attempted and activated charcoal should be given. Arrhythmia usually responds to restoration of circulatory or metabolic disturbance and normothermia. Severe dystonia responds to procyclidine. Circulatory collapse may require intravenous fluids or inotropic agents (adrenaline should be avoided in neuroleptic overdose)

Long-Term Use

- There is high risk of relapse if levomepromazine is stopped after 1–2 years
- Some side effects may be irreversible (e.g. tardive dyskinesia)

Habit Forming

- No

How to Stop

- High risk of relapse if stopped after 1–2 years thus there should be slow down-titration of medication with clinical monitoring for 2 years after cessation
- Rapid oral discontinuation may lead to rebound psychosis and worsening of symptoms

Pharmacokinetics

- Maximum serum concentrations achieved in 2–3 hours depending on the route of administration
- Half-life about 15–30 hours
- Maximum concentration reached in 30–90 minutes via intramuscular route

Levomepromazine (Continued)

Drug Interactions

- Levomepromazine may antagonise the effects of levodopa and dopamine agonists
- Levomepromazine is a potent inhibitor of cytochrome P450 2D6 causing increased serum levels of drugs metabolised by the CYP450 2D6 system
- Increased risk of arrhythmias when used with medications which also prolong the QT interval
- Anticholinergic effect is enhanced by other anticholinergic drugs
- Avoid other neuroleptics and drugs causing electrolyte imbalance
- Avoid diuretics; if necessary there is a preference for potassium-sparing agents
- Theoretical serious interaction with desferrioxamine causing transient metabolic encephalopathy and loss of consciousness for 48 to 72 hours

Other Warnings/Precautions

- All antipsychotics should be used with caution in patients with angle-closure glaucoma, blood disorders, cardiovascular disease, depression, diabetes, epilepsy and susceptibility to seizures, history of jaundice, myasthenia gravis, Parkinson's disease, photosensitivity, prostatic hypertrophy, severe respiratory disorders
- If signs of neuroleptic malignant syndrome develop, treatment should be immediately discontinued
- Ensure appropriate glycaemic monitoring in those with or at risk of diabetes mellitus
- Risk of postural hypotension especially in children and those over 50 years of age
- Caution in liver disease

Do Not Use

- If there is CNS depression
- If the patient is in a comatose state
- If the patient has phaeochromocytoma
- If there is a proven allergy to levomepromazine
- If there is a known sensitivity to any phenothiazine

Renal Impairment

- Start with small doses in severe renal impairment because of increased cerebral sensitivity

Hepatic Impairment

- Avoid in liver dysfunction, or use with caution

Cardiac Impairment

- Avoid in cardiac disease, or use with caution

Elderly

- Not advised in ambulant patients over the age of 50 unless the risk of hypotensive reaction has been assessed
- Relatively high degree of antimuscarinic action with implications in the elderly

Children and Adolescents

- Parenteral levomepromazine is used in children to treat restlessness and confusion in palliative care, and to treat nausea and vomiting in palliative care
- Levomepromazine is not licensed for the treatment of schizophrenia in children and adolescents
- Children are very sensitive to the hypotensive and soporific effects of levomepromazine

Pregnancy

- Controlled studies have not been conducted in pregnant women
- There is a risk of abnormal muscle movements and withdrawal symptoms in newborns whose mothers took an antipsychotic during the third trimester; symptoms may include agitation, abnormally increased or decreased muscle tone, tremor, sleepiness, severe difficulty breathing, and difficulty feeding
- Reports of extrapyramidal symptoms, jaundice, hyperreflexia, hyporeflexia in infants whose mothers took a phenothiazine during pregnancy

- Psychotic symptoms may worsen during pregnancy and some form of treatment may be necessary
- Switching antipsychotics may increase the risk of relapse
- Effects of hyperprolactinaemia on the foetus are unknown

Breastfeeding

- Small amounts expected in mother's breast milk
- Risk of accumulation in infant due to long half-life
- Haloperidol is considered to be the preferred first-generation antipsychotic, and quetiapine the preferred second-generation antipsychotic
- Infants of women who choose to breastfeed should be monitored for possible adverse effects

THE ART OF PSYCHOPHARMACOLOGY

Potential Advantages

- Less extrapyramidal side effects compared to haloperidol and chlorpromazine
- In the context of rapid tranquillisation, levomepromazine is more sedative than haloperidol but IM olanzapine is safer and better at improving symptoms

Potential Disadvantages

- Highly sedating
- Risk of hypotensive reaction, particularly concerning in the ambulant elderly patient
- No depot formulation available
- Higher doses required for antipsychotic effect are more likely than lower doses to cause significant sedation or postural hypotension
- Relatively high degree of antimuscarinic action with implications in the elderly

Primary Target Symptoms

- Positive symptoms of schizophrenia

Pearls

- Levomepromazine can be used as an alternative to chlorpromazine in schizophrenia especially when it is desirable to reduce psychomotor activity
- Levomepromazine is a low-potency phenothiazine
- Sedative actions of low-potency phenothiazines are an important aspect of their therapeutic actions in some patients and side-effect profile in others
- Low-potency phenothiazines like levomepromazine have a greater risk of cardiovascular side effects
- Patients have very similar antipsychotic responses when treated with any of the conventional antipsychotics, which is different from atypical antipsychotics where antipsychotic responses of individual patients can occasionally vary greatly from one atypical to another
- Patients with inadequate responses to atypical antipsychotics may benefit from a trial of augmentation with a conventional antipsychotic such as levomepromazine or from switching to a conventional antipsychotic such as levomepromazine
- However, long-term polypharmacy with a combination of a conventional antipsychotic such as levomepromazine with an atypical antipsychotic may combine their side effects without clearly augmenting the efficacy of either
- For treatment-resistant patients, especially those with impulsivity, aggression, violence, and self-harm, long-term polypharmacy with 2 atypical antipsychotics and 1 conventional antipsychotic may be useful or even necessary while closely monitoring
- In such cases, it may be beneficial to combine 1 depot antipsychotic with 1 oral antipsychotic

Levomepromazine (Continued)

 Suggested Reading

Green B, Pettit T, Faith L, et al. Focus on levomepromazine. Curr Med Res Opin 2004;20(12):1877–81.

Higashima M, Takeda T, Nagasawa T, et al. Combined therapy with low-potency neuroleptic levomepromazine as an adjunct to haloperidol for agitated patients with acute exacerbation of schizophrenia. Eur Psychiatry 2004 Sep;19(6):380–1.

Huhn M, Nikolakopoulou A, Schneider-Thoma J, et al. Comparative efficacy and tolerability of 32 oral antipsychotics for the acute treatment of adults with multi-episode schizophrenia: a systematic review and network meta-analysis. Lancet 2019;394(10202):939–51.

Sivaraman P, Rattehalli RD, Jayaram M. Levomepromazine for schizophrenia. Schizophr Bull 2012;38(2):219–20.

Lisdexamfetamine mesilate

Brands
• Elvanse

Generic?
No, not in UK

Class
• Neuroscience-based nomenclature: pharmacology domain – dopamine, norepinephrine; mode of action domain – multimodal
• Stimulant; dopamine and noradrenaline reuptake inhibitor and releaser (DN-RIRe)

Commonly Prescribed for
(bold for BNF indication)
• **Attention deficit hyperactivity disorder (ADHD) (age 6 years and older)**
• Narcolepsy

 How the Drug Works

∗Lisdexamfetamine is a prodrug of dexamfetamine and is thus not active until after it has been absorbed by the intestinal tract and converted to dexamfetamine (active component) and L-lysine
∗Once converted to dexamfetamine, it increases noradrenaline and especially dopamine actions by blocking their reuptake and facilitating their release
• Enhancement of dopamine and noradrenaline signalling in certain brain regions (e.g. dorsolateral prefrontal cortex) may improve attention, concentration, executive dysfunction, and wakefulness
• Enhancement of dopamine-mediated signalling in other brain regions (e.g. basal ganglia) may improve hyperactivity
• Enhancement of dopamine and noradrenaline signalling in yet other brain regions (e.g. medial prefrontal cortex, hypothalamus) may improve depression, fatigue, and sleepiness

How Long Until It Works
• Some immediate effects can be seen with first dosing
• Can take several weeks to attain maximum therapeutic benefit

If It Works (for ADHD)
• The goal of treatment of ADHD is reduction of symptoms of inattentiveness, motor hyperactivity, and/or impulsiveness that disrupt social, school, and/or occupational functioning
• Continue treatment until all symptoms are under control or improvement is stable and then continue treatment indefinitely as long as improvement persists
• Re-evaluate the need for treatment periodically
• Treatment for ADHD begun in childhood may need to be continued into adolescence and adulthood if continued benefit is documented

If It Doesn't Work (for ADHD)
• Inform patient it may take several weeks for full effects to be seen
• Consider adjusting dose or switching to another formulation or another agent. It is important to consider if maximal dose has been achieved before deciding there has not been an effect and switching
• Consider behavioural therapy or cognitive behavioural therapy if appropriate – to address issues such as social skills with peers, problem-solving, self-control, active listening and dealing with and expressing emotions
• Consider the possibility of non-concordance and counsel patients and parents
• Consider evaluation for another diagnosis or for a co-morbid condition (e.g. bipolar disorder, substance abuse, medical illness, etc.)
• In children consider other important factors, such as ongoing conflicts, family psychopathology, adverse environment, for which alternate interventions might be more appropriate (e.g. social care referral, trauma-informed care)
∗Some ADHD patients and some depressed patients may experience lack of consistent efficacy due to activation of latent or underlying bipolar disorder, and require either augmenting with a mood stabiliser or switching to a mood stabiliser

Best Augmenting Combos for Partial Response or Treatment Resistance

* Best to attempt other monotherapies prior to augmenting
* For the expert, can combine with modafinil or atomoxetine for ADHD, though there is little evidence about the efficacy or safety of this combination
* For the expert, can occasionally combine with atypical antipsychotics in highly treatment-resistant cases of ADHD

Tests

* Before treatment, assess for presence of cardiac disease (history, family history, physical exam)
* Pulse, BP, appetite, weight, height, psychiatric symptoms should be recorded at initiation of therapy, following every dose change and every 6 months after that
* In children, pulse, BP, height and weight should be recorded on percentile charts; observe growth trajectory by plotting a graph
* Monitor for aggressive behaviour or hostility during initial treatment

SIDE EFFECTS

How Drug Causes Side Effects

* Increases in noradrenaline especially peripherally can cause autonomic sympathetic side effects, including tremor, tachycardia, hypertension, and cardiac arrhythmias
* Increases in noradrenaline and dopamine centrally can cause CNS side effects such as insomnia, agitation, psychosis, and substance abuse

Notable Side Effects

* Insomnia, headache, exacerbation of tics, nervousness, irritability, overstimulation, tremor, dizziness
* Anorexia, nausea, dry mouth, constipation, diarrhoea, weight loss
* Can temporarily slow normal growth in children (controversial)

* Sexual dysfunction long-term (impotence, libido changes), but can also improve sexual dysfunction short-term

Common or very common

* CNS/PNS: abnormal behaviour, altered mood, anxiety, dizziness, headache, insomnia, jitteriness, movement disorders (uncommon in children), tremor
* GIT: constipation, decreased appetite, decreased weight, diarrhoea, dry mouth, nausea, upper abdominal pain
* Other: dyspnoea, fatigue, hyperhidrosis (uncommon in children), palpitations, sexual dysfunction (uncommon in children), tachycardia

Uncommon

* CNS/PNS: altered taste, blurred vision, depression (very common in children), drowsiness (very common in children), logorrhoea, psychiatric disorders (very common in children)
* Other: fever (very common in children), skin reactions (very common in children), vomiting (very common in children)

Frequency not known

* CNS/PNS: drug dependence; hallucination (uncommon in children), mydriasis (uncommon in children), psychotic disorder, seizure
* Other: allergic hepatitis, angioedema, cardiomyopathy (uncommon in children), Raynaud's phenomenon (uncommon in children), Stevens-Johnson syndrome

 Life-Threatening or Dangerous Side Effects

* Psychotic episodes
* Seizures
* Palpitations, tachycardia, hypertension
* Rare activation of hypomania, mania, or suicidal ideation (controversial)
* Cardiovascular adverse effects, sudden death in patients with pre-existing cardiac abnormalities or long-QT syndrome

Weight Gain

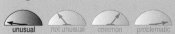

* Reported but not expected
* Some patients may experience weight loss

Sedation

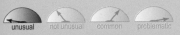

unusual not unusual common problematic

- Reported but not expected
- Activation much more common than sedation

What to Do About Side Effects

- Wait
- Can usually be managed by symptomatic management and/or dose reduction
- If lack of appetite and weight is a clinical concern suggest taking medication with or after food and offer high calorie food or snacks early morning or late evening when stimulant effects have worn off
- If child or young person on ADHD medication shows persistent resting heart rate >120 bpm, arrhythmia, or systolic BP (measured on 2 occasions) with clinically significant increase or >95th percentile, then reduce medication dose and refer to specialist physician
- If a person taking stimulants develops tics, consider: are the tics related to the stimulant (tics naturally wax and wane)? Observe tic evolution over 3 months. Consider if the impairment associated with the tics outweighs the benefits of ADHD treatment
- If tics are stimulant related, reduce the stimulant dose, or consider changing to guanfacine (in children aged 5 years and over and young people only), atomoxetine, clonidine or stopping medication
- If a person with ADHD presents with seizures (new or worsening), review and stop any ADHD medication that could reduce the seizure threshold. Cautiously reintroduce the ADHD medication after completing necessary tests and confirming it as non-contributory towards the cause of the seizures
- If sleep becomes a problem: assess sleep at baseline. Monitor changes in sleep pattern (for example, with a sleep diary). Adjust medication accordingly. Advise on sleep hygiene as appropriate. Prescription of melatonin may be helpful to promote sleep onset where behavioural and environmental adjustments have not been effective
- Consider drug holidays to prevent growth retardation in children
- Switch to another agent, e.g. atomoxetine or guanfacine

Best Augmenting Agents for Side Effects

- Beta blockers for peripheral autonomic side effects
- Beta blockers or pregabalin for anxiety; do not prescribe benzodiazepines
- SSRIs or SNRIs for depression
- If psychosis develops, stop lisdexamfetamine and add antipsychotics such as olanzapine or quetiapine, consider a switch to atomoxetine
- Consider melatonin for insomnia in children
- Dose reduction or switching to another agent may be more effective

DOSING AND USE

Usual Dosage Range
- ADHD: 30–70 mg/day

Dosage Forms
- Capsule 20 mg, 30 mg, 40 mg, 50 mg, 60 mg, 70 mg

How to Dose
- Child 6–17 years: initial dose either 30 mg/day or 20 mg/day in the morning; increase by increments of 10–20 mg each week as needed; max dose generally 70 mg/day. Discontinue after 1 month if response insufficient
- Adult: initial dose 30 mg/day in the morning; increase by 20 mg each week as needed; max dose generally 70 mg/day. Discontinue after 1 month if response insufficient

Dosing Tips
- 10–12 hour duration of clinical action
- Capsules can either be taken whole or they can be opened and the contents mixed with soft food such as yoghurt or dissolved in water or orange juice; contents should be dispersed completely and consumed immediately
- Dose of a single capsule should not be divided
- Once-daily dosing can be an important practical element in stimulant use, eliminating the hassle and pragmatic difficulties of lunchtime dosing at school, including storage problems, potential diversion, and the need for a medical professional to supervise dosing away from home

Lisdexamfetamine mesilate (Continued)

- Avoid dosing after the morning because of the risk of insomnia
- *May be possible to dose only during the school week for some ADHD patients
- *May be able to give drug holidays for patients with ADHD over the summer in order to reassess therapeutic utility and effects on growth suppression as well as to assess any other side effects and the need to reinstitute stimulant treatment for the next school term

Overdose

- Rarely fatal; panic, hyperreflexia, rhabdomyolysis, rapid respiration, confusion, coma, hallucination, convulsion, arrhythmia, change in blood pressure, circulatory collapse

Long-Term Use

- Can be used long-term for ADHD when ongoing monitoring documents continued efficacy
- Dependence and/or abuse may develop
- Tolerance to therapeutic effects may develop in some patients
- Long-term stimulant use may be associated with growth suppression in children (controversial)
- Important to periodically monitor weight, blood pressure and psychiatric symptoms
- Cardiomyopathy has been reported with chronic amfetamine use

Habit Forming

- Lisdexamfetamine is a Class B/Schedule 2 drug
- Patients may develop tolerance and psychological dependence
- Theoretically less abuse potential than other stimulants when taken as directed because it is inactive until it reaches the gut and thus has delayed time to onset as well as long duration of action

How to Stop

- Taper to avoid withdrawal effects
- Withdrawal following chronic therapeutic use may unmask symptoms of the underlying disorder and may require follow-up and reinstitution of treatment
- Careful supervision is required during withdrawal from abuse use since severe depression may occur

Pharmacokinetics

- Lisdexamfetamine dimesylate is converted to dexamfetamine and L-lysine by metabolism in red blood cells
- Lisdexamfetamine is not metabolised by cytochrome P450 enzymes
- 1 hour to maximum concentration of lisdexamfetamine, 3.5 hours to maximum concentration of dexamfetamine
- Onset of action <2 hours
- Duration of clinical action 10–12 hours
- The plasma elimination half-life of lisdexamfetamine typically is less than 1 hour. The half-life of dexamfetamine is about 11 hours

 Drug Interactions

- May affect blood pressure and should be used cautiously with agents used to control blood pressure
- Gastrointestinal acidifying agents (guanethidine, reserpine, glutamic acid, ascorbic acid, fruit juices, etc.) and urinary acidifying agents (ammonium chloride, sodium phosphate, etc.) lower amfetamine plasma levels, so such agents can be useful to administer after an overdose but may also lower therapeutic efficacy of amfetamines
- Gastrointestinal alkalinising agents (sodium bicarbonate, etc.) and urinary alkalinising agents (acetazolamide, some thiazides) increase amfetamine plasma levels and potentiate amfetamine's actions
- Theoretically, agents with noradrenaline reuptake blocking properties, such as venlafaxine, duloxetine, atomoxetine, and reboxetine, could add to amfetamine's CNS and cardiovascular effects
- Amfetamines may counteract the sedative effects of antihistamines
- Haloperidol, chlorpromazine, and lithium may inhibit stimulatory effects of amfetamine
- Theoretically, atypical antipsychotics should also inhibit stimulatory effects of amfetamines
- Theoretically, amfetamines could inhibit the antipsychotic actions of antipsychotics
- Theoretically, amfetamines could inhibit the mood-stabilising actions of atypical antipsychotics in some patients

- Combinations of amfetamines with mood stabilisers (lithium, anticonvulsants, atypical antipsychotics) is generally something for experts only, when monitoring patients closely and when other options fail
- Absorption of phenobarbital, phenytoin, and ethosuximide is delayed by amfetamines
- Amfetamines inhibit adrenergic blockers and enhance adrenergic effects of noradrenaline
- Amfetamines may antagonise hypotensive effects of Veratrum alkaloids and other antihypertensives
- Amfetamines can raise plasma corticosteroid levels
- MAOIs slow absorption of amfetamines and thus potentiate their actions, which can cause headache, hypertension, and rarely hypertensive crisis and malignant hyperthermia, sometimes with fatal results
- Use with MAOIs, including within 14 days of MAOI use, is not advised
- There is a risk of serotonin syndrome if lisdexamfetamine combined with serotonergic drugs, or other agents that increase the risk of serotonin syndrome (St John's wort, bupropion, linezolid, granisetron, ondansetron, opiates, SSRIs, SNRIs, TCAs, MAOIs, lithium, or triptans)

 Other Warnings/Precautions

- Use with caution in patients with a history of cardiovascular disease
- Caution if patient has or is susceptible to angle-closure glaucoma
- Children who are not growing or not gaining weight should stop treatment, at least temporarily
- May worsen motor and phonic tics
- Caution if patient has motor tics or Tourette syndrome or if there is a family history of Tourette syndrome
- May worsen symptoms of thought disorder and behaviour disturbance in psychotic patients, special caution advised with bipolar disorder
- Stimulants have a high potential for abuse and must be used with caution in anyone with a current or past history of substance abuse or alcoholism or in emotionally unstable patients
- Administration of stimulants for prolonged periods of time should be avoided

whenever possible or done only with close monitoring, as it may lead to marked tolerance and drug dependence, including psychological dependence with varying degrees of abnormal behaviour
- Particular attention should be paid to the possibility of subjects obtaining stimulants for non-therapeutic use or distribution to others and the drugs should in general be prescribed sparingly with documentation of appropriate use
- Usual dosing with amfetamine has been associated with sudden death in children with cardiac rhythm abnormalities, e.g. long QT
- Not a recommended treatment for depression or for normal fatigue
- May lower the seizure threshold (discontinue if seizures occur)
- Emergence or worsening of activation and agitation may represent the induction of a bipolar state, especially a mixed dysphoric bipolar condition sometimes associated with suicidal ideation, and requires the addition of a mood stabiliser and/or discontinuation of lisdexamfetamine

Do Not Use

- If patient is in an agitated state
- Should generally not be administered with an MAOI, including within 14 days of MAOI use
- If patient has advanced arteriosclerosis, symptomatic cardiovascular disease, or moderate/severe hypertension
- If patient has hyperthyroidism
- If there is a proven allergy to any sympathomimetic agent

SPECIAL POPULATIONS

Renal Impairment

- Severe impairment: max dose 50 mg/ day
- End-stage renal disease: max dose 30 mg/ day

Hepatic Impairment

- Use with caution

Cardiac Impairment

- Use with caution, particularly in patients with recent myocardial infarction or other conditions that could be negatively affected by increased blood pressure

- Do not use in patients with cardiac rhythm abnormalities, cardiac myopathy, serious heart arrhythmia, or coronary artery disease

Elderly

- Some patients may tolerate lower doses better

Children and Adolescents

Before you prescribe:

- Safety and efficacy not established in children under age 6
- Use in young children should be reserved for the expert
- Diagnosis of ADHD should only be made by an appropriately qualified healthcare professional, e.g. specialist psychiatrist, paediatrician, and after full clinical and psychosocial assessment in different domains, full developmental and psychiatric history, observer reports across different settings and opportunity to speak to the child and carer on their own
- Children and adolescents with untreated anxiety, PTSD and mood disorders, or those who do not have a psychiatric diagnosis but social or environmental stressors, may present with anger, irritability, motor agitation, and concentration problems
- Consider undiagnosed learning disability or specific learning difficulties, and sensory impairments that may potentially cause or contribute to inattention and restlessness, especially in school
- ADHD-specific advice on symptom management and environmental adaptations should be offered to all families and teachers, including reducing distractions, seating, shorter periods of focus, movement breaks and teaching assistants
- For children >5 years and young people with moderate ADHD pharmacological treatment should be considered if they continue to show significant impairment in at least one setting after symptom management and environmental adaptations have been implemented
- For severe ADHD, behavioural symptom management may not be effective until pharmacological treatment has been established

Practical notes:

- Consider when single-day dosage and longer cover is needed; may improve adherence, reduce stigma, acceptability to schools
- Monitor patients face-to-face regularly, particularly during the first several weeks of treatment
- Monitor for activation of suicidal ideation at the beginning of treatment
- Consider cognitive behavioural therapy (CBT) for those whose ADHD symptoms are still causing significant difficulties in one or more domains, addressing emotion regulation, problem-solving, self-control, and social skills (including active listening skills and interactions with peers)
- Medication for ADHD for a child under 5 years should only be considered on specialist advice from an ADHD service with expertise in managing ADHD in young children (ideally a tertiary service). Use of medicines for treating ADHD is off-label in children aged <5 years
- Same medication choices should be offered to patients with co-morbidities (e.g. anxiety, tic disorders, or autism spectrum disorders) as to patients with ADHD alone
- Insomnia is common
- Dexamfetamine may worsen symptoms of behavioural disturbance and thought disorder in psychotic children
- Dexamfetamine has acute effects on growth hormone; long-term effects are unknown but weight and height should be monitored 6-monthly using a growth chart
- Do not use in children with structural cardiac abnormalities or other serious cardiac problems
- Sudden death in children and adolescents with serious heart problems has been reported
- American Heart Association recommends ECG prior to initiating stimulant treatment in children, although not all experts agree, and it is not usual practice in UK
- Re-evaluate the need for continued treatment regularly

Pregnancy

- Possible increased risk of premature birth, low birth weight and neurodevelopmental

delay in infants whose mothers take lisdexamfetamine during pregnancy
- Infants whose mothers take lisdexamfetamine during pregnancy may experience withdrawal symptoms
- In animal studies, dexamfetamine caused delayed skeletal ossification and decreased postweaning weight gain in rats; no major malformations occurred in rat or rabbit studies
- Use in women of childbearing potential requires weighing potential benefits to the mother against potential risks to the foetus
＊For ADHD patients, lisdexamfetamine should generally be discontinued before anticipated pregnancies

Breastfeeding

- Small amounts found in mother's breast milk
- Infants of women who choose to breastfeed while on lisdexamfetamine should be monitored for possible adverse effects
- If irritability, sleep disturbance, or poor weight gain develop in nursing infant, may need to discontinue drug or bottle feed

THE ART OF PSYCHOPHARMACOLOGY

Potential Advantages

- Although restricted as a Schedule 2 controlled substance like other major stimulants, as a prodrug lisdexamfetamine may have less propensity for abuse, intoxication, or dependence than other stimulants
- May be particularly useful in adult patients without prior diagnosis and treatment of ADHD as a child to prevent abuse and diversion since lisdexamfetamine may be less abusable than other stimulants

Potential Disadvantages

- Patients with current or past substance abuse
- Patients with current or past bipolar disorder or psychosis

Primary Target Symptoms

- Concentration, attention span
- Motor hyperactivity
- Impulsivity
- Physical and mental fatigue
- Daytime sleepiness
- Depression

 Pearls

- Approved for the treatment of binge eating disorder in USA, but not UK
- Can be used to potentiate opioid analgesia and reduce sedation, particularly in end-of-life management
- Some patients respond to or tolerate lisdexamfetamine better than methylphenidate or amfetamine and vice versa
＊Can reverse sexual dysfunction caused by psychiatric illness and by some drugs such as SSRIs, including decreased libido, erectile dysfunction, delayed ejaculation, and anorgasmia
- Atypical antipsychotics may be useful in treating stimulant or psychotic consequences of overdose
- Half-life and duration of clinical action tend to be shorter in younger children
- Drug abuse may actually be lower in ADHD adolescents treated with stimulants than in ADHD adolescents who are not treated

Suggested Reading

Biederman J, Boellner SW, Childress A, et al. Lisdexamfetamine dimesylate and mixed amphetamine salts extended-release in children with ADHD: a double-blind, placebo-controlled, crossover analog classroom study. Biol Psychiatry 2007;62(9):970–6.

Biederman J, Krishnan S, Zhang Y, et al. Efficacy and tolerability of lisdexamfetamine dimesylate (NRP-104) in children with attention-deficit/hyperactivity disorder: a phase III, multicenter, randomized, double-blind, forced dose, parallel-group study. Clin Ther 2007;29(3):450–63.

Castells X, Blanco-Silvente L, Cunhill R. Amphetamines for attention deficit hyperactivity disorder (ADHD) in adults. Cochrane Database Syst Rev 2018;8(8):CD007813.

Lithium

Brands
- Priadel
- Camcolit
- Liskonum
- Li-Liquid

Generic?
Yes

Class
- Neuroscience-based nomenclature: pharmacology domain – lithium; mode of action – enzyme modulator
- Mood stabiliser

Commonly Prescribed for
(bold for BNF indication)
- **Treatment and prophylaxis of mania (adults; children > 12 years)**
- **Treatment and prophylaxis of bipolar disorder (adults; children > 12 years)**
- **Treatment and prophylaxis of recurrent depression (adults; children > 12 years)**
- **Treatment and prophylaxis of aggressive or self-harming behaviour (adults; children > 12 years)**
- Neutropenia (to raise white blood cell count in patients receiving clozapine)

 How the Drug Works
- Unknown and complex
- Alters sodium transport across cell membranes in nerve and muscle cells
- Alters metabolism of neurotransmitters including catecholamines and serotonin
- *May alter intracellular signalling through actions on second messenger systems
- Specifically, inhibits inositol monophosphatase, possibly affecting neurotransmission via phosphatidyl inositol second messenger system
- Also reduces protein kinase C activity, possibly affecting genomic expression associated with neurotransmission
- Increases cytoprotective proteins, activates signalling cascade utilised by endogenous growth factors, and increases grey matter content, possibly by activating neurogenesis and enhancing trophic actions that maintain synapses

How Long Until It Works
- 1–3 weeks for mania
- Judge over at least 3 months for maintenance

If It Works
- The goal of treatment is complete remission of symptoms (i.e. mania and/or depression) and prevention of recurrence
- Continue treatment until all symptoms are gone or until improvement is stable and then continue treating indefinitely as long as improvement persists
- Continue treatment indefinitely to avoid recurrence of mania or depression

If It Doesn't Work
- *Many patients have only a partial response where some symptoms are improved, but others persist or continue to wax and wane without stabilisation of mood
- Other patients may be non-responders, sometimes called treatment-resistant or treatment-refractory
- Consider checking serum lithium concentrations, increasing dose, switching to another mood stabiliser, or adding an appropriate augmenting agent
- Consider additional psychoeducation or psychotherapy
- Consider the presence of non-concordance and discuss with patient
- Consider evaluation for another diagnosis or for a co-morbid condition (e.g. medical illness, substance abuse, anxiety disorder etc.)

 Best Augmenting Combos for Partial Response or Treatment Resistance
- Atypical antipsychotics (especially quetiapine, olanzapine, aripiprazole, risperidone)
- Lamotrigine
- Valproate
- *Antidepressants (with caution because antidepressants can destabilise mood in some patients, including induction of rapid cycling or suicidal ideation; in particular SSRIs, SNRIs; generally avoid TCAs, MAOIs)

Lithium

Tests

- Lithium salts have a narrow therapeutic/toxic ratio and should be prescribed only when facilities for monitoring serum Li concentrations are available
- *Before initiating treatment, kidney function tests with estimated glomerular filtration rate (eGFR), calcium and thyroid function tests; electrocardiogram for patients over 50 and for those with cardiac disease or risk factors for it; urea and electrolytes and full blood count should also be checked
- *Since lithium is associated with weight gain, before starting treatment, weigh all patients and determine if the patient is already overweight (BMI 25.0–29.9) or obese (BMI ≥30)
- Before giving a drug that can cause weight gain to an overweight or obese patient, consider determining whether the patient already has pre-diabetes – fasting plasma glucose: 5.5 mmol/L to 6.9 mmol/L or HbA1c: 42 to 47 mmol/mol (6.0 to 6.4%), diabetes – fasting plasma glucose: >7.0 mmol/L or HbA1c: ≥48 mmol/L (≥6.5%), or dyslipidaemia (increased total cholesterol, LDL cholesterol, and triglycerides; decreased HDL cholesterol), and treat or refer such patients for treatment, including nutrition and weight management, physical activity counselling, smoking cessation, and medical management
- Samples to monitor lithium level should be taken 12 hours after the last dose to achieve a serum Li concentration of 0.6–1.0 mmol/L (a lower range from 0.4 for elderly patients)
- A target serum Li concentration of 0.8–1.2 mmol/L is recommended for acute episodes of mania, and for patients who have previously relapsed
- Routine serum Li monitoring should be performed weekly after initiation and after each dose change until concentrations are stable, then every 3 months for the first year, and then every 6 months thereafter
- Additional serum Li measurements should be made after dose change, if a patient develops significant intercurrent disease or if there is a significant change in a patient's sodium or fluid intake
- Monitor body weight or BMI, serum electrolytes, eGFR, and thyroid function every 6 months during treatment, and more often if there is evidence of impaired renal or thyroid function, or raised calcium levels
- *While giving a drug to a patient who has gained >5% of initial weight, consider evaluating for the presence of pre-diabetes, diabetes, or dyslipidaemia, or consider switching to a different agent

SIDE EFFECTS

How Drug Causes Side Effects

- Unknown and complex
- CNS side effects theoretically due to excessive actions at the same or similar sites that mediate its therapeutic actions
- Some renal side effects theoretically due to lithium's actions on ion transport

Notable Side Effects

- *Essential tremor (usually mild)
- *Thirst, polyuria, polydipsia (nephrogenic diabetes insipidus)
- *Diarrhoea, nausea
- *Weight gain
- Euthyroid goitre or hypothyroid goitre, possibly with increased TSH and reduced thyroxine levels
- Acne, rash, alopecia, worsening of psoriasis
- Leucocytosis
- Side effects are typically dose-related

Rare or very rare

- Nephropathy

Frequency not known

- CNS/PNS: abnormal reflexes, cerebellar syndrome, coma, delirium, dizziness, encephalopathy, idiopathic intracranial hypertension, memory loss, movement disorders, muscle weakness, myasthenia gravis, nystagmus, peripheral neuropathy, seizure, speech impairment, tremor, vertigo, vision disorders
- CVS: arrhythmias, atrioventricular block, cardiomyopathy, circulatory collapse, hypotension, QT interval prolongation
- Endocrine: goitre, hyperglycaemia, hyperparathyroidism, hypothyroidism, nausea, thyrotoxicosis
- GIT: abdominal discomfort, altered taste, decreased appetite, diarrhoea, dry mouth, gastritis, hypersalivation, increased weight, vomiting
- Renal: polyuria, renal disorders, renal impairment

- Other: alopecia, angioedema, electrolyte imbalance, folliculitis, leucocytosis, neoplasms, peripheral oedema, rhabdomyolysis, sexual dysfunction, skin reactions, skin ulcer

Life-Threatening or Dangerous Side Effects

- Lithium toxicity with vomiting, diarrhoea, ataxia and confusion
- Renal impairment (interstitial nephritis)
- Nephrogenic diabetes insipidus
- Arrhythmia, cardiovascular changes, sick sinus syndrome, bradycardia, hypotension
- T-wave flattening and inversion
- Rare pseudotumour cerebri
- Seizures

Weight Gain

- Many experience and/or can be significant in amount
- Can become a health problem in some
- May be associated with increased appetite or thirst

Sedation

- Some experience and/or can be significant in amount
- May wear off with time

What to Do About Side Effects

- Wait
- Check lithium level is accurate (ensure 12 hours post dose)
- Wait
- Lower the dose
- Usually the entire dose is taken at night with a modified-release preparation
- *Split doses may reduce side effects such as diuresis at night
- *Change to a different lithium preparation (but ensure bioequivalence)
- If signs of lithium toxicity occur, discontinue immediately and check lithium level
- For stomach upset, take with food
- For tremor, avoid caffeine
- Switch to another agent

Best Augmenting Agents for Side Effects

- *Propranolol 20–30 mg 2–3 timer per day may reduce tremor
- Many side effects cannot be improved with an augmenting agent

DOSING AND USE

Usual Dosage Range

- Doses adjusted according to serum lithium concentration; doses are initially divided throughout the day, but once-daily administration is preferred when serum lithium concentration stabilised
- Maintenance in bipolar: recommended 0.6–1.0 mmol/L (lower end of the range safer, but higher end of the range more effective)
- Acute mania: recommended 0.8–1.2 mmol/L (in some cases may need levels as high as 1.5 mmol/L)
- Depression: recommended 0.6–1.0 mmol/L

Dosage Forms

- Tablet (lithium carbonate) 250 mg
- Tablet modified-release (lithium carbonate) 200 mg, 400 mg, 450 mg
- Oral solution (lithium citrate) 509 mg/5 mL, 520 mg/5 mL, 1.018 g/5 mL
- For Li-Liquid: lithium citrate tetrahydrate 509 mg is equivalent to lithium carbonate 200 mg
- For Priadel liquid: lithium citrate tetrahydrate 520 mg is equivalent to lithium carbonate 204 mg

How to Dose

- Start at 400 mg at night (200 mg in the elderly)
- Monitor plasma levels after 7 days, then 7 days after every dose change until the desired level is reached
- Take care when prescribing liquid preparations to clearly specify the strength required
- For Li-Liquid: initial dose 509 mg/day in 2 divided doses (adults < 50 kg) or 1.018–3.054 g/day in 2 divided doses (adults > 50 kg), then adjust dose according to serum levels

Lithium (Continued)

- For Priadel liquid: initial dose 520 mg twice per day (adults < 50 kg) or 1.04–3.12 g/day in 2 divided doses (adults > 50 kg), then adjust dose according to serum levels. Once-daily administration is preferred when serum levels stabilised

Dosing Tips

* Modified-release formulations are standard and may reduce gastric irritation, lower peak lithium plasma levels, and diminish peak dose side effects (i.e. side effects occurring 1–2 hours after each dose of standard lithium carbonate may be improved by modified-release formulation)
- Therapeutic blood levels are standardised to be taken about 12 (10–14) hours after the last dose
- After stabilisation, most patients do best with a once-daily dose at night
- Responses in acute mania may take 7–14 days even with adequate plasma lithium levels
* Some patients apparently respond to plasma lithium levels below 0.5 mmol/L
- Use the lowest dose of lithium associated with adequate therapeutic response
- Lower doses and lower plasma lithium levels (<0.6 mmol/L) are often adequate and advisable in the elderly
* Rapid discontinuation increases the risk of relapse and possibly suicide; this is a rebound effect, so lithium needs to be tapered over at least 4 weeks and preferably slowly over 2–3 months if possible
- Note that changing the preparation requires the same precautions as at the initiation of treatment

Overdose

- Symptoms and signs of intoxication include increasing gastrointestinal disturbances, visual disturbances, polyuria, muscle weakness, tremors, CNS disturbances, abnormal reflexes, myoclonus, incontinence and hypernatraemia
- With severe overdosage seizures, cardiac arrhythmias, autonomic instability, renal failure, coma and sudden death could occur

Long-Term Use

- The most effective medication for prevention of relapse in bipolar disorder and should be considered for all patients with this diagnosis

- May cause reduced kidney function
- Requires regular therapeutic monitoring of lithium levels (3–6-monthly) as well as of kidney function and thyroid function (annually)
- Calcium levels should also be checked before and annually

Habit Forming

- No

How to Stop

- Intermittent treatment with lithium may worsen the natural course of bipolar illness
- Taper gradually over at least 4 weeks (preferably over 3 months) to avoid relapse, but warn patients of potential for relapse
- Rapid discontinuation increases the risk of relapse and possibly suicide
- If lithium is to be discontinued abruptly, consider changing therapy to an atypical antipsychotic or valproate
- Discontinuation symptoms uncommon

Pharmacokinetics

- Lithium is primarily excreted by the kidneys (>95% of the dose)
- Half-life varies with the formulation, but ranges from 12–24 hours following a single dose
- Can be eliminated by haemodialysis
- Lower absorption on empty stomach

Drug Interactions

- Most clinically significant interactions are with drugs that alter renal sodium handling
* Non-steroidal anti-inflammatory agents, including ibuprofen and selective COX-2 inhibitors (cyclooxygenase 2), can <u>increase</u> plasma lithium concentrations; add with caution to patients stabilised on lithium
* Diuretics, especially thiazides, can <u>increase</u> plasma lithium concentrations; add with caution to patients stabilised on lithium
- Angiotensin-converting enzyme inhibitors can <u>increase</u> plasma lithium concentrations; add with caution to patients stabilised on lithium
- Metronidazole can lead to lithium toxicity through decreased renal clearance
- Acetazolamide, alkalising agents, xanthine preparations, and urea may <u>lower</u> lithium plasma concentrations

- Methyldopa, carbamazepine, and phenytoin may interact with lithium to increase its toxicity
- Use lithium cautiously with calcium channel blockers, which may also increase lithium toxicity
- Use of lithium with an SSRI may raise risk of dizziness, confusion, diarrhoea, agitation, tremor
- Some patients taking haloperidol and lithium have developed an encephalopathic syndrome similar to neuroleptic malignant syndrome
- Lithium may prolong effects of neuromuscular blocking agents
- No likely pharmacokinetic interactions of lithium with mood-stabilising anticonvulsants or atypical antipsychotics

 Other Warnings/Precautions

*Toxic levels are near therapeutic levels; signs of toxicity include tremor, ataxia, diarrhoea, vomiting, sedation
- Monitor for dehydration; lower dose if patient exhibits signs of infection, excessive sweating, diarrhoea
- Closely monitor patients with thyroid disorders
- Lithium may cause unmasking of Brugada syndrome; consultation with a cardiologist is recommended if patients develop unexplained syncope or palpitations after starting lithium

Do Not Use

- If patient has Addison's disease
- If patient has severe kidney disease
- If patient has severe cardiovascular disease especially with a rhythm disorder or cardiac insufficiency
- If patient has personal or family history of Brugada syndrome
- If patient has severe dehydration
- If patient has sodium depletion
- If the patient has untreated hypothyroidism
- If there is a proven allergy to lithium

Renal Impairment

- Not recommended for use in patients with severe impairment
- Caution in mild to moderate impairment – monitor serum-lithium concentration closely and adjust dose accordingly

Hepatic Impairment

- No special indications

Cardiac Impairment

- Not recommended for use in patients with severe impairment
- Lithium can cause reversible T-wave changes, sinus bradycardia, sick sinus syndrome, or heart block

Elderly

- Likely that elderly patients will require lower doses to achieve therapeutic serum levels
- Elderly patients may be more sensitive to adverse effects
*Neurotoxicity, including delirium and other mental status changes, may occur even at therapeutic doses in elderly and organically compromised patients
- Lower doses and lower plasma lithium levels (0.4 to 0.6 mmol/L) are often adequate and advisable in the elderly

 Children and Adolescents

- Lithium citrate is not licensed for use in children
- Lithium carbonate: Camcolit brand immediate and modified-release tablet is not licensed for use in children
- Lithium carbonate is not licensed for the prophylaxis of aggressive or self-harming behaviour in children
- Safety and efficacy not established in children under age 12
- Use only with caution
- Prescribing only by expert
Before you prescribe:
- For bipolar disorder: if bipolar disorder is suspected in primary care in children or adolescents refer them to a specialist service with expertise in the assessment and management of bipolar disorder. Management of bipolar disorder should include assertive outreach approaches, family involvement, access to structured psychological interventions and psychologically informed care, vocational and educational interventions
- As first-line treatment for acute mania: consider decision-making capacity and involve parents in decision about medication. Allow to choose from aripiprazole, olanzapine or risperidone.

Lithium (Continued)

Lithium is not recommended as first-line option for management of acute manic episodes in children and adolescents
- Lithium may be considered for longer-term prophylaxis of bipolar disorder or prophylaxis of recurrent depression in children or adolescents with bipolar disorder. Choice should be given between continued antipsychotic medication and lithium. The decision should involve parents or carers. Lithium should not be prescribed unless facilities for monitoring are available
- For bipolar depression offer structured psychological intervention first. This should be of at least 3 months. If ineffective, consider alternative individual or family interventions. If the bipolar depression is moderate to severe, consider a pharmacological intervention in addition to psychological interventions
- Where a child or young person presents with self-harm and suicidal thoughts the immediate risk management may take first priority
- All children and young people with FEP/bipolar should be supported with sleep management, anxiety management, exercise and activation schedules, and healthy diet
- A risk management plan is important prior to start of medication because of the possible risks in overdose

Practical notes:
- Carefully weigh the risks and benefits of pharmacological treatment against the risks and benefits of non-treatment and make sure to document this in the patient's chart
- Monitoring of plasma levels similar to that for adults: weekly until lithium plasma levels stable then every 2–3 months for the first 6 months, then every 6 months. However, consider growth might affect dosing needs
- Monitoring as with adults. Monitor weight (plotted on a growth chart)
- Younger children tend to have more frequent and severe side effects
- The child, adolescent and parent should be advised to report signs and symptoms of lithium toxicity (including diarrhoea, tremor, ataxia, vomiting, sedation), hypothyroidism, renal dysfunction and benign intracranial hypertension (persistent headache and visual disturbance)
- Advise parent and child on the importance of adequate fluid intake by the child

- Dose adjustments may be necessary in the presence of interacting drugs
- Children are more sensitive to most side effects
  - Lithium is associated with weight gain
  - Weight gain correlates with time on treatment. Any childhood obesity is associated with obesity in adults

If it does not work:
- Review child's/young person's profile, consider new/changing contributing individual or systemic factors such as peer or family conflict. Consider drug/substance misuse. Consider dose adjustment before switching or augmentation. Be vigilant of polypharmacy especially in complex and highly vulnerable children/adolescents
- Consider non-concordance by parent or child, consider non-concordance in adolescents, address underlying reasons for non-concordance
- Re-evaluate the need for continued treatment regularly
- A lithium treatment pack should be given to patient and parents on initiation of treatment with lithium. The pack consists of information booklet, lithium alert card, and a record book for tracking serum-lithium concentration. These can be purchased from nhsforms@mmm.uk.com

Pregnancy
- Data suggests no increased risk of major congenital malformations
- Early study suggested increased risk in cardiac anomalies (especially Ebstein's anomaly) in infants whose mothers took lithium during pregnancy; not replicated by further studies
- Not associated with increased rates of perinatal death, low weight for gestational age or preterm delivery, but evidence too limited to completely exclude risk
- Very limited evidence suggests lack of association between lithium use during pregnancy and adverse neurodevelopmental effects in the neonate
- If lithium is continued, monitor serum lithium levels every 4 weeks, then every week beginning at 36 weeks
- Dehydration due to morning sickness may cause rapid increases in lithium levels

- If lithium is continued during pregnancy hospital birth is advised
- Monitoring during delivery should include fluid balance
- Lithium should be stopped during labour and levels should be checked
- Infants exposed to lithium during pregnancy should have serum lithium levels measured shortly after birth
- Should not be offered to women planning a pregnancy or pregnant unless antipsychotics have been shown to be ineffective
- Use in pregnancy may be justified if the benefit of continued treatment exceeds any associated risk
- Recurrent bipolar illness during pregnancy can be quite disruptive
- Taper drug if discontinuing
- Given the risk of bipolar relapse in the postpartum period, lithium should generally be restarted immediately after delivery
- This may mean no breastfeeding, since lithium can be found in breast milk, possibly at full therapeutic levels
- Pre-pregnancy lithium dose may be sufficient, higher doses used during pregnancy risk toxicity
- *Atypical antipsychotics may be preferable to lithium or anticonvulsants if treatment of bipolar disorder is required during pregnancy
- Bipolar symptoms may recur or worsen during pregnancy and some form of treatment may be necessary

Breastfeeding

- Significant amounts found in mother's breast milk, possibly at full therapeutic levels since lithium is soluble in breast milk
- Case reports of lithium toxicity in breastfed infants
- *Recommended either to discontinue drug or bottle feed
- *Bipolar disorder may recur during the postpartum period, particularly if there is a history of prior postpartum episodes of either depression or psychosis
- *Relapse rates may be lower in women who receive prophylactic treatment for postpartum episodes of bipolar disorder
- Antipsychotics and carbamazepine may be safer than lithium during the postpartum period when breastfeeding

THE ART OF PSYCHOPHARMACOLOGY
Potential Advantages
- Euphoric mania and episodic pattern with good inter-episode function
- Treatment-resistant depression
- Reduces suicide risk
- Works well in combination with atypical antipsychotics and/or mood-stabilising anticonvulsants such as valproate

Potential Disadvantages
- Dysphoric mania
- Mixed mania, rapid-cycling mania
- Those with poor concordance (may worsen illness course)
- Depressed phase of bipolar disorder
- Patients unable to tolerate tremor, gastrointestinal effects, renal effects, weight gain and other side effects
- Requires blood monitoring

Primary Target Symptoms
- Relapsing bipolar episodes
- Mania

 Pearls

*Lithium was the original mood stabiliser and is a first-line treatment option for prevention of recurrence in bipolar disorder. It is underutilised since it is an older agent and is less promoted for use in bipolar disorder than newer agents. Some doctors are concerned about the complications of monitoring and it does require an experienced and confident psychiatrist to initiate lithium
*Seems to be more effective in treating manic episodes than depressive episodes in bipolar disorder (treats from above better than it treats from below)
*Prevents both manic and depressive episodes, but may be more effective in preventing manic relapses (stabilises from above better than it stabilises from below)
*Good evidence of reduced suicide and suicide attempts in both bipolar disorder and unipolar depression
- Poor concordance can radically reduce the potential effectiveness
*Due to its narrow therapeutic index, lithium's toxic side effects occur at doses close to its therapeutic effects

Lithium (Continued)

* May be best for euphoric mania and an episodic pattern; patients with rapid-cycling and mixed-state types of bipolar disorder generally do less well on lithium
* Close therapeutic monitoring of plasma drug levels is required during lithium treatment; lithium is the first psychiatric drug that required blood level monitoring
* Probably less effective than antipsychotics for severe, excited, disturbed, hyperactive, or psychotic patients with mania
* Due to delayed onset of action, lithium monotherapy may not be the first choice in acute mania, but rather may be used as an adjunct to atypical antipsychotics, benzodiazepines, and/or valproate loading
* After acute symptoms of mania are controlled, some patients can be maintained on lithium monotherapy
* One in three bipolar patients experience a major benefit from lithium treatment; one in three experiences little change; many patients need multiple medications for best control
* Lithium is not a convincing augmentation agent to atypical antipsychotics for the treatment of schizophrenia

* Lithium is one of the most useful adjunctive agents to augment antidepressants for treatment-resistant unipolar depression
* Lithium may be useful for a number of patients with episodic, recurrent symptoms with or without affective illness, including episodic rage, anger or violence, and self-destructive behaviour; such symptoms may be associated with psychotic or non-psychotic illnesses, personality disorders, organic disorders, or mental retardation
* Lithium is better tolerated during acute manic phases than when manic symptoms have abated
* Adverse effects generally increase in incidence and severity as lithium serum levels increase
* Although not recommended for use in patients with severe renal or cardiovascular disease, dehydration, or sodium depletion, lithium can be administered cautiously in a hospital setting to such patients, with lithium serum levels determined daily
* Lithium-induced weight gain may be more common in women than in men

 ## Suggested Reading

Baldessarini RJ, Tondo L, Davis P, et al. Decreased risk of suicides and attempts during long-term lithium treatment: a meta-analytic review. Bipolar Disord 2006;8(5 Pt 2):625–39.

Findling RL, Robb A, McNamara NK, et al. Lithium in the acute treatment of bipolar I disorder: a double-blind, placebo-controlled study. Pediatrics 2015;136(5):885–94.

Goodwin FK. Rationale for using lithium in combination with other mood stabilizers in the management of bipolar disorder. J Clin Psychiatry 2003;64(Suppl 5):18–24.

Goodwin GM. Recurrence of mania after lithium withdrawal. Br J Psychiatry 1994;164(2):149–52.

Goodwin GM, Bowden CL, Calabrese JR, et al. A pooled analysis of 2 placebo-controlled 18-month trials of lamotrigine and lithium maintenance treatment in bipolar I disorder. J Clin Psychiatry 2004;65(3):432–41.

Malhi GS, Tanious M. Optimal frequency of lithium administration in the treatment of bipolar disorder: clinical and dosing considerations. CNS Drugs 2011;25(4):289–98.

Severus WE, Kleindienst N, Seemueller F, et al. What is the optimal serum lithium level in the long-term treatment of bipolar disorder–a review? Bipolar Disord 2008;10(2):231–7.

Tueth MJ, Murphy TK, Evans DL. Special considerations: use of lithium in children, adolescents, and elderly populations. J Clin Psychiatry 1998;59(Suppl 6):66–73.

Lofepramine

THERAPEUTICS

Brands
• Non-proprietary

Generic?
Yes

Class
• Neuroscience-based nomenclature: pharmacology domain – norepinephrine, serotonin; mode of action – reuptake inhibitor
• Tricyclic antidepressant (TCA)
• Predominantly a noradenraline reuptake inhibitor

Commonly Prescribed for
(bold for BNF indication)
• **Depressive illness**
• Anxiety
• Insomnia
• Neuropathic pain/chronic pain

 ### How the Drug Works
• Boosts neurotransmitter noradrenaline
• Blocks noradrenaline reuptake pump (noradrenaline transporter), presumably increasing noradrenergic neurotransmission
• Since dopamine is inactivated by noradrenaline reuptake in frontal cortex, which largely lacks dopamine transporters, lofepramine can increase dopamine neurotransmission in this part of the brain
• A more potent inhibitor of noradrenaline reuptake pump than serotonin reuptake pump (scrotonin transporter)
• At high doses may also boost neurotransmitter serotonin and presumably increase serotonergic neurotransmission

How Long Until It Works
• May have immediate effects in treating insomnia or anxiety
• Onset of therapeutic actions with some antidepressants can be seen within 1–2 weeks, but often delayed up to 2–4 weeks
• If it is not working within 3–4 weeks for depression, it may require a dosage increase or it may not work at all
• By contrast, for generalised anxiety, onset of response and increases in remission rates may still occur after 8 weeks, and for up to 6 months after initiating dosing

If It Works
• The goal of treatment is complete remission of current symptoms as well as prevention of future relapses
• Treatment often reduces or even eliminates symptoms, but it is not a cure since symptoms can recur after medicine stopped
• Continue treatment until all symptoms are gone (remission), especially in depression and whenever possible in anxiety disorders
• Once symptoms are gone, continue treating for at least 6–9 months for the first episode of depression or >12 months if relapse indicators present
• If >5 episodes and/or 2 episodes in the last few years then need to continue for at least 2 years or indefinitely
• The goal of treatment of chronic pain conditions such as neuropathic pain, fibromyalgia, headaches, low back pain, and neck pain is to reduce symptoms as much as possible, especially in combination with other treatments
• Treatment of chronic pain conditions such as neuropathic pain, fibromyalgia, headache, low back pain, and neck pain may reduce symptoms, but rarely eliminates them completely, and is not a cure since symptoms can recur after medicine is stopped
• Use in anxiety disorders and chronic pain conditions such as neuropathic pain, fibromyalgia, headache, low back pain, and neck pain may also need to be indefinite, but long-term treatment is not well studied in these conditions

If It Doesn't Work
• Depressed patients may have only a partial response where some symptoms are improved but others persist
• Other depressed patients may be non-responsive
• It is important to recognise non-response to treatment early on (3–4 weeks)
• Some patients who have an initial response may relapse even though they continue treatment
• Consider increasing dose, switching to another agent, or adding an appropriate augmenting agent
• Lithium may be added for suicidal patients or those at high risk of relapse
• Consider psychotherapy
• Consider ECT

- Consider evaluation for another diagnosis or for a co-morbid condition (e.g. medical illness, substance abuse, etc.)
- Some patients may experience a switch into mania and so would require antidepressant discontinuation and initiation of a mood stabiliser

Best Augmenting Combos for Partial Response or Treatment Resistance

- Mood stabilisers or atypical antipsychotics for bipolar depression
- Atypical antipsychotics for psychotic depression
- Atypical antipsychotics as first-line augmenting agents (quetiapine MR 300 mg/day or aripiprazole at 2.5–10 mg/day) for treatment-resistant depression
- Atypical antipsychotics as second-line augmenting agents (risperidone 0.5–2 mg/day or olanzapine 2.5–10 mg/day) for treatment-resistant depression
- Mirtazapine at 30–45 mg/day as another second-line augmenting agent (a dual serotonin and noradrenaline combination, but observe for switch into mania, increase in suicidal ideation or serotonin syndrome)
- T3 (20–50 mcg/day) is another second-line augmenting agent that works best with tricyclic antidepressants
- Other augmenting agents but with less evidence include bupropion (up to 400 mg/day), buspirone (up to 60 mg/day) and lamotrigine (up to 400 mg/day)
- Benzodiazepines if agitation present
- Hypnotics or trazodone for insomnia (but beware of serotonin syndrome with trazodone)
- Augmenting agents reserved for specialist use include: modafinil for sleepiness, fatigue and lack of concentration; stimulants, oestrogens, testosterone
- Lithium is particularly useful for suicidal patients and those at high risk of relapse including with factors such as severe depression, psychomotor retardation, repeated episodes (>3), significant weight loss, or a family history of major depression (aim for lithium plasma levels 0.6–1.0 mmol/L)
- For elderly patients lithium is a very effective augmenting agent

- For severely ill patients other combinations may be tried especially in specialist centres
- Augmenting agents that may be tried include omega-3, SAM-e, L-methylfolate
- Additional non-pharmacological treatments such as exercise, mindfulness, CBT, and IPT can also be helpful
- If present after treatment response (4–8 weeks) or remission (6–12 weeks), the most common residual symptoms of depression include cognitive impairments, reduced energy and problems with sleep
- For chronic pain: gabapentin, other anticonvulsants, or opiates if done by experts while monitoring carefully in difficult cases

Tests

- Baseline ECG is useful for patients over age 50
- ECGs may be useful for selected patients (e.g. those with personal or family history of QTc prolongation; cardiac arrhythmia; recent myocardial infarction; decompensated heart failure; or taking agents that prolong QTc interval such as pimozide, thioridazine, selected antiarrhythmics, moxifloxacin etc.)
- *Since tricyclic and tetracyclic antidepressants are frequently associated with weight gain, before starting treatment, weigh all patients and determine if the patient is already overweight (BMI 25.0–29.9) or obese (BMI ≥30)
- Before giving a drug that can cause weight gain to an overweight or obese patient, consider determining whether the patient already has:
  - Pre-diabetes – fasting plasma glucose: 5.5 mmol/L to 6.9 mmol/L or HbA1c: 42 to 47 mmol/mol (6.0 to 6.4%)
  - Diabetes – fasting plasma glucose: >7.0 mmol/L or HbA1c: ≥48 mmol/L (≥6.5%)
  - Hypertension (BP >140/90 mm Hg)
  - Dyslipidaemia (increased total cholesterol, LDL cholesterol, and triglycerides; decreased HDL cholesterol)
- Treat or refer such patients for treatment, including nutrition and weight management, physical activity counselling, smoking cessation, and medical management
- *Monitor weight and BMI during treatment
- *While giving a drug to a patient who has gained >5% of initial weight, consider evaluating for the presence of pre-diabetes,

diabetes, dyslipidaemia, or consider switching to a different antidepressant
- Patients at risk for electrolyte disturbances (e.g. patients aged >60, patients on diuretic therapy) should have baseline and periodic serum potassium and magnesium measurements

SIDE EFFECTS

How Drug Causes Side Effects
- Anticholinergic activity may explain sedative effects, dry mouth, constipation, and blurred vision
- Sedative effects and weight gain may be due to antihistamine properties
- Blockade of alpha adrenergic 1 receptors may explain dizziness, sedation, and hypotension
- Cardiac arrhythmias and seizures, especially in overdose, may be caused by blockade of ion channels

Notable Side Effects
- Blurred vision, constipation, urinary retention, increased appetite, dry mouth, nausea, diarrhoea, heartburn, unusual taste in mouth, weight gain
- Fatigue, weakness, dizziness, sedation, headache, anxiety, nervousness, restlessness
- Sexual dysfunction, sweating

Frequency not known
- Blood disorders: agranulocytosis, eosinophilia, granulocytopenia, leucopenia, thrombocytopenia
- CNS/PNS: abnormal coordination, agitation, altered mood, confusion, dizziness, drowsiness, hallucination, headache, paraesthesia, paranoid delusions, psychosis, seizure, sleep disorder, suicidal tendencies, tinnitus, tremor
- CVS: arrhythmias, cardiac conduction disorder, heart failure aggravated, hypotension
- Endocrine: galactorrhoea, gynaecomastia
- GIT: altered taste, constipation, dry mouth, hepatic disorders, mucositis, nausea, vomiting
- Other: accommodation disorder, bone marrow disorders, facial oedema, glaucoma, hyperhidrosis (on discontinuation), hyponatraemia; increased risk of fracture, malaise, photosensitivity, respiratory depression, sexual dysfunction, SIADH, skin haemorrhage, skin reactions, testicular disorders, urinary disorders, withdrawal syndrome

 Life-Threatening or Dangerous Side Effects
- Paralytic ileus, hyperthermia (TCAs + anticholinergic agents)
- Lowered seizure threshold and rare seizures
- Orthostatic hypotension, sudden death, arrhythmias, tachycardia
- QTc prolongation
- Hepatic failure, extrapyramidal symptoms
- Increased intraocular pressure
- Rare induction of mania and paranoid delusions
- Rare increase in suicidal ideation and behaviours in adolescents and young adults (up to age 25), hence patients should be warned of this potential adverse event

Weight Gain

- Many experience and/or can be significant in amount
- Can increase appetite and carbohydrate craving

Sedation
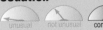
- Many experience and/or can be significant in amount
- Tolerance to sedative effect may develop with long-term use
- Sedative effects increased in hepatic impairment

What To Do About Side Effects
- Wait
- Wait
- Wait
- The risk of side effects is reduced by titrating slowly to the minimum effective dose (every 2–3 days)
- Consider using a lower starting dose in elderly patients
- Manage side effects that are likely to be transient (e.g. drowsiness) by explanation, reassurance and, if necessary, dose reduction and re-titration

Lofepramine (Continued)

- Giving patients simple strategies for managing mild side effects (e.g. dry mouth) may be useful
- For persistent, severe or distressing side effects the options are:
  - Dose reduction and re-titration if possible
  - Switching to an antidepressant with a lower propensity to cause that side effect
  - Non-drug management of the side effect (e.g. diet and exercise for weight gain)

Best Augmenting Agents for Side Effects

- Many side effects cannot be improved with an augmenting agent

DOSING AND USE

Usual Dose Range

- Adult: 140–210 mg/day in divided doses
- Elderly may respond to lower doses (70–140 mg/day at night or in divided doses)

Dosage Forms

- Tablet 70 mg
- Oral suspension 70 mg/5 mL

How to Dose

- Initial dose either 70 mg/day once daily or in divided doses; gradually increase daily dose to achieve desired therapeutic effects with a dose of up to 210 mg/day in divided doses

 Dosing Tips

- The risk of side effects is reduced by titrating slowly to the minimum effective dose (every 2–3 days)
- Consider using a lower starting dose in elderly patients; recommended starting dose 35 mg nocte, usual maintenance dose 70 mg nocte, max recommended dose in elderly 140 mg nocte or in divided doses
- For panic disorder, can dose at 70–140 mg/day in divided doses
- Usually safe to restart lofepramine at the previous dose after a period of non-concordance

Overdose

- Tricyclic and related antidepressants can cause arrhythmias, cardiac conduction

defects, coma, dilated pupils, dry mouth, extensor plantar responses, hyperreflexia, hypotension, hypothermia, respiratory failure, seizures, tachycardia and urinary retention
- Lofepramine is associated with the lowest risk of death in overdose when compared to other TCA drugs
- Lofepramine lacks the overdose arrhythmogenicity of other TCAs, despite its major metabolite, desipramine, being a potent potassium channel blocker
- Lofepramine is less cardiotoxic than other TCAs for unclear reasons

Long-Term Use

- Safe

Habit Forming

- No

How to Stop

- Taper gradually to avoid withdrawal effects
- Even with gradual dose reduction some withdrawal symptoms may appear within the first 2 weeks
- It is best to reduce the dose gradually over 4 weeks or longer if withdrawal symptoms emerge
- If severe withdrawal symptoms emerge during discontinuation, raise dose to stop symptoms and then restart withdrawal much more slowly (over at least 6 months in patients on long-term maintenance treatment)

Pharmacokinetics

- Substrate for CYP450 2D6
- Half-life of parent compound about 1.5–6 hours
- Major metabolite is the antidepressant desipramine, with a half-life of about 12–24 hours

 Drug Interactions

- Tramadol increases the risk of seizure in patients taking TCAs
- Use of TCAs with anticholinergic drugs may result in paralytic ileus or hyperthermia
- Fluoxetine, paroxetine, bupropion, duloxetine, terbinafine and other CYP450 2D6 inhibitors may increase TCA concentrations

- Cimetidine may increase plasma concentrations of TCAs and cause anticholinergic symptoms
- Phenothiazines or haloperidol may raise TCA blood concentrations
- May alter effects of antihypertensive drugs; may inhibit hypotensive effects of clonidine
- Use with sympathomimetic agents may increase sympathetic activity
- Methylphenidate may inhibit metabolism of TCAs
- Lofepramine can increase the effects of adrenaline/epinephrine
- Carbamazepine decreases the exposure to lofepramine
- Lofepramine is predicted to increase the risk of severe toxic reaction when given with MAOIs; avoid and for 14 days after stopping the MAOI
- Both lofepramine and MAOIs can increase the risk of hypotension
- Do not start an MAOI for at least 5 half-lives (5 to 7 days for most drugs) after discontinuing lofepramine
- Activation and agitation, especially following switching or adding antidepressants, may represent the induction of a bipolar state, especially a mixed dysphoric bipolar condition sometimes associated with suicidal ideation, and require the addition of lithium, a mood stabiliser or an atypical antipsychotic, and/or discontinuation of lofepramine

 Other Warnings/Precautions

- Can possibly increase QTc interval at higher doses
- Arrhythmias may occur at higher doses, but are rare
- Increased risk of arrhythmias in patients with hyperthyroidism or phaeochromocytoma
- In one study, clinical use of lofepramine was associated with an increased risk of myocardial infarction whereas other antidepressants were not
- Caution if patient is taking agents capable of significantly prolonging QTc interval or if there is a history of QTc prolongation
- Caution if the patient is taking drugs that inhibit TCA metabolism, including CYP450 2D6 inhibitors
- Because TCAs can prolong QTc interval, use with caution in patients who have bradycardia or who are taking drugs that can induce bradycardia (e.g. beta blockers, calcium channel blockers, clonidine, digitalis)
- Because TCAs can prolong QTc interval, use with caution in patients who have hypokalaemia and/or hypomagnesaemia or who are taking drugs that can induce hypokalaemia and/or hypomagnesaemia (e.g. diuretics, stimulant laxatives, intravenous amphotericin B, glucocorticoids, tetracosactide)
- Caution if there is reduced CYP450 2D6 function, such as patients who are poor 2D6 metabolisers
- Can exacerbate chronic constipation
- Use caution when treating patients with epilepsy
- Use caution in patients with diabetes
- Use with caution in patients with a history of bipolar disorder, psychosis or significant risk of suicide
- Use with caution in patients with increased intra-ocular pressure or susceptibility to angle-closure glaucoma
- Use with caution in patients with prostatic hypertrophy or urinary retention

Do Not Use

- In patients during a manic phase
- If there is a history of cardiac arrhythmia, recent acute myocardial infarction, heart block
- In patients with acute porphyrias
- If there is a proven allergy to lofepramine, desipramine, imipramine

Renal Impairment

- Use with caution; avoid in severe renal impairment
- Little information is available about lofepramine use in renal impairment; less than 5% is excreted unchanged in urine

Hepatic Impairment

- Use with caution
- Sedative effects are increased in hepatic impairment
- Avoid in severe liver disease

Cardiac Impairment

- Baseline ECG is recommended
- TCAs have been reported to cause arrhythmias, prolongation of conduction

Lofepramine (Continued)

time, orthostatic hypotension, sinus tachycardia, and heart failure, especially in the diseased heart
- Myocardial infarction and stroke have been reported with TCAs
- TCAs produce QTc prolongation, which may be enhanced by the existence of bradycardia, hypokalaemia, congenital or acquired long QTc interval, which should be evaluated prior to administering lofepramine
- Use with caution if treating concomitantly with a medication likely to produce prolonged bradycardia, hypokalaemia, slowing of intracardiac conduction, or prolongation of the QTc interval
- Avoid TCAs in patients with a known history of QTc prolongation, recent acute myocardial infarction, and decompensated heart failure
- TCAs may cause a sustained increase in heart rate in patients with ischaemic heart disease and may worsen (decrease) heart rate variability, an independent risk of mortality in cardiac populations
- Since SSRIs may improve (increase) heart rate variability in patients following a myocardial infarct and may improve survival as well as mood in patients with acute angina or following a myocardial infarction, these are more appropriate agents for cardiac population than tricyclic/tetracyclic antidepressants
- *Risk/benefit ratio may not justify use of TCAs in cardiac impairment

Elderly
- Baseline ECG is useful for patients over the age of 50
- May be more sensitive to anticholinergic, cardiovascular, hypotensive, and sedative effects
- Constipation/sweating side effects may be severe
- Reduction in the risk of suicidality with antidepressants compared to placebo in adults age 65 and older
- Postural hypertension can be a problem, but generally better tolerated than other tricyclics
- Minimal side effects of sedation
- Relatively safe in overdose
- May cause raised LFTs in elderly

Children and Adolescents
- Not licensed for use in children and adolescents

Pregnancy
- No strong evidence of TCA maternal use during pregnancy being associated with an increased risk of congenital malformations
- Risk of malformations cannot be ruled out due to limited information on specific TCAs
- Poor neonatal adaptation syndrome and/or withdrawal has been reported in infants whose mothers took a TCA during pregnancy or near delivery
- Maternal use of more than one CNS-acting medication is likely to lead to more severe symptoms in the neonate
- Must weigh the risk of treatment (first trimester foetal development, third trimester newborn delivery) to the child against the risk of no treatment (recurrence of depression, maternal health, infant bonding) to the mother and child
- For many patients this may mean continuing treatment during pregnancy

Breastfeeding
- Some drug is found in mother's breast milk
- Infant should be monitored for sedation and poor feeding
- Immediate postpartum period is a high-risk time for depression, especially in women who have had prior depressive episodes; antidepressants may need to be reinstituted late in the third trimester or shortly after childbirth to prevent a recurrence during the postpartum period
- Must weigh benefits of breastfeeding with risks and benefits of antidepressant treatment versus nontreatment to both the infant and the mother
- For many patients this may mean continuing treatment during breastfeeding
- Other antidepressants may be preferable, e.g. imipramine or nortriptyline

THE ART OF PSYCHOPHARMACOLOGY

Potential Advantages
- Patients with insomnia
- Severe or treatment-resistant depression
- Anxious depression

Potential Disadvantages
- Elderly patients
- Patients concerned with weight gain
- Cardiac patients

Primary Target Symptoms
- Depressed mood

Pearls
- TCAs are often a first-line treatment option for chronic pain
- TCAs are no longer generally considered a first-line option for depression, because of their side-effect profile
- TCAs continue to be useful for severe or treatment-resistant depression
- Noradrenergic reuptake inhibitors such as lofepramine may be used as a second-line treatment for smoking cessation, cocaine dependence, and attention deficit disorder
- *Lofepramine is a short-acting prodrug of the TCA desipramine
- *Fewer anticholinergic side effects, particularly sedation, than some other tricyclics
- Once a popular TCA in UK, but not widely marketed throughout the world
- TCAs may aggravate psychotic symptoms
- Use with alcohol can cause additive CNS-depressant effects
- Underweight patients may be more susceptible to adverse cardiovascular effects

- Patients with inadequate hydration and patients with cardiac disease may be more susceptible to TCA-induced cardiotoxicity than healthy adults
- Patients on TCAs should be aware that they may experience symptoms such as photosensitivity or blue-green urine
- SSRIs may be more effective than TCAs in women, and TCAs may be more effective than SSRIs in men
- Since tricyclic/tetracyclic antidepressants are substrates for CYP450 2D6, and 7% of the population (especially Whites) may have a genetic variant leading to reduced activity of 2D6; such patients may not safely tolerate normal doses of tricyclic/tetracyclic antidepressants and may require dose reduction
- Patients who seem to have extraordinarily severe side effects at normal or low doses may have this phenotypic CYP450 2D6 variant and require low doses or switching to another antidepressant not metabolised by 2D6

THE ART OF SWITCHING

 ### Switching
- Consider switching to another agent or adding an appropriate augmenting agent if it doesn't work
- Consider switching to a different antidepressant if the patient has gained >5% of initial weight
- With patients with significant side effects at normal or low doses, they may have the phenotypic CYP450 2D6 variant; consider low doses or switching to another antidepressant not metabolised by 2D6

Suggested Reading

Coupland C, Hill T, Morriss R, et al. Antidepressant use and risk of cardiovascular outcomes in people aged 20–64: cohort study using primary care database. BMJ 2016;352:i1350.

Fahy TJ, O'Rourke D, Brophy J, et al. The Galway Study of Panic Disorder. I: clomipramine and lofepramine in DSM III-R panic disorder: a placebo controlled trial. J Affect Disord 1992;25(1):63–75.

Lofepramine (Continued)

Lancaster SG, Gonzalez JP. Lofepramine. A review of its pharmacodynamic and pharmacokinetic properties, and therapeutic efficacy in depressive illness. Drugs 1989;37(2):123–40.

Stern H, Konetschny J, Herrmann L, et al. Cardiovascular effects of single doses of the antidepressants amitriptyline and lofepramine in healthy subjects. Pharmacopsychiatry 1985;18(4):272–7.

Warrington SJ, Padgham C, Lader M. The cardiovascular effects of antidepressants. Psychol Med Monogr Suppl 1989;16:i-iii,1–40.

Loprazolam

THERAPEUTICS

Brands
- Non-proprietary

Generic?
Yes

Class
- Positive modulator of GABA-A receptor complex
- Benzodiazepine

Commonly Prescribed for
(bold for BNF indication)
- **Insomnia (short-term use)**

How the Drug Works
- Benzodiazepines have a widespread action as a result of their enhancing the release of gamma-aminobutyric acid (GABA)
- They are effective as anticonvulsants, muscle relaxants, anti-anxiety agents, pre-medications and sedative hypnotics
- Binds to benzodiazepine receptors at the GABA-A ligand-gated chloride channel complex
- Enhances the inhibitory effects of GABA
- Boosts chloride conductance through GABA-regulated channels
- Inhibits neuronal activity presumably in amygdala-centred fear circuits to provide therapeutic benefits in anxiety disorders
- Inhibitory actions in cerebral cortex may provide therapeutic benefits in seizure disorders

How Long Until It Works
- Loprazolam is slowly and variably absorbed following oral ingestion, peak plasma concentrations usually being reached at 2 to 5 hours in non-fasting subjects

If It Works
- Faster sleep onset
- Improves quality of sleep
- Reduced nocturnal awakenings

If It Doesn't Work
- Increase the dose
- Improve sleep hygiene
- Switch to another agent

Best Augmenting Combos for Partial Response or Treatment Resistance
- Generally best to switch to another agent
- RCTs support the effectiveness of Z-hypnotics
- Trazodone
- Agents with antihistamine actions (e.g. promethazine, TCAs)
- Use melatonin and melatonin-related drugs (adults over age 55)

SIDE EFFECTS

How Drug Causes Side Effects
- Inhibitory actions in sleep centres may provide sedative hypnotic effects
- Same mechanism for side effects as for therapeutic effects – namely due to excessive actions at benzodiazepine receptors
- Actions at benzodiazepine receptors that carry over to the next day can cause daytime sedation, amnesia, and ataxia
- Long-term adaptations in benzodiazepine receptors may explain the development of dependence, tolerance, and withdrawal

Notable Side Effects
- Sedation, fatigue, depression
- Vertigo, ataxia, slurred speech
- Forgetfulness, confusion
- Agitation or aggression
- Hypotension
- Uncommon hallucinations

Frequency not known
- Adjustment disorder, cognitive disorder, decreased muscle tone, speech disorder

Life-Threatening or Dangerous Side Effects
- Respiratory depression

Weight Gain

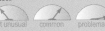

unusual   not unusual   common   problematic

- Reported but not expected

Loprazolam (Continued)

Sedation

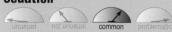

- Many experience and/or can be significant in amount
- Attention should be drawn to the risk of drowsiness, sedation, amnesia, impaired concentration and muscular weakness, especially in drivers of vehicles and operators of machinery

What To Do About Side Effects

- Lower the dose
- Switch to a shorter-acting sedative hypnotic
- Switch to a non-benzodiazepine hypnotic
- Administer flumazenil if side effects are severe or life-threatening

Best Augmenting Agents for Side Effects

- Many side effects cannot be improved with an augmenting agent

DOSING AND USE

Usual Dosage Range

- Insomnia: 1–2 mg at bedtime

Dosage Forms

- Tablet 1 mg

How to Dose

*Insomnia (short-term use):
- Adult: 1 mg at bedtime, increased to 1.5–2 mg at bedtime as required
- Debilitated patients and elderly: 0.5–1 mg at bedtime

 Dosing Tips

- Dosage should not exceed 2 mg/day
- Treatment should if possible be intermittent
- The lowest dose to control symptoms should be used
- Treatment should not normally be continued beyond 4 weeks
- Long-term chronic use is not recommended
- Treatment should always be tapered off gradually
- Patients who have taken benzodiazepines for a long time may require a longer period during which doses are reduced

Overdose

- Overdose not usually fatal
- Treatment is symptomatic and gastric lavage helpful
- Use of a specific antidote such as flumazenil in association with symptomatic treatment in hospital should be considered

Long-Term Use

- Long-term chronic use is not recommended

Habit Forming

- Yes
- Loprazolam is a Class C/Schedule 4 drug

How to Stop

- Systematic reduction over 1–2 weeks

Pharmacokinetics

- Half-life about 8 hours (6–12 hours)
- Liver metabolism
- Excretion via kidneys
- Delay in action: 2 hours for it to reach a peak in serum concentrations

 **Drug Interactions**

- Increased depressive effects when taken with other CNS depressants

 Other Warnings/Precautions

- Warning regarding the increased risk of CNS-depressant effects (especially alcohol) when benzodiazepines and opioid medications are used together, including specifically the risk of slowed or difficulty breathing and death
- If alternatives to the combined use of benzodiazepines and opioids are not available, clinicians should limit the dosage and duration of each drug to the minimum possible while still achieving therapeutic efficacy
- Patients and their caregivers should be warned to seek medical attention if unusual dizziness, light-headedness, sedation, slowed or difficulty breathing, or unresponsiveness occur
- Dosage changes should be made in collaboration with prescriber
- History of drug or alcohol abuse often creates greater risk for dependency

- Some depressed patients may experience a worsening of suicidal ideation
- Some patients may exhibit abnormal thinking or behavioural changes similar to those caused by other CNS depressants (i.e. either depressant actions or disinhibiting actions)
- Avoid prolonged use and abrupt cessation
- Use lower doses in debilitated patients and the elderly
- Use with caution in patients with myasthenia gravis; respiratory disease
- Use with caution in patients with acute porphyrias; hypoalbuminaemia
- Use with caution in patients with personality disorder (dependent/avoidant or anankastic types) as may increase risk of dependence
- Use with caution in patients with a history of alcohol or drug dependence/abuse
- Benzodiazepines may cause a range of paradoxical effects including aggression, antisocial behaviours, anxiety, overexcitement, perceptual abnormalities and talkativeness. Adjustment of dose may reduce impulses
- Use with caution as loprazolam can cause muscle weakness
- Insomnia may be a symptom of a primary disorder, rather than a primary disorder itself
- Loprazolam should be administered only at bedtime

Do Not Use

- In patients with acute pulmonary insufficiency, respiratory depression, significant neuromuscular respiratory weakness, sleep apnoea syndrome or unstable myasthenia gravis
- Alone in chronic psychosis in adults
- On its own to try to treat depression, anxiety associated with depression, obsessional states or phobic states
- If patient has angle-closure glaucoma
- If there is a proven allergy to loprazolam or any benzodiazepine

Renal Impairment

- Increased cerebral sensitivity to benzodiazepines
- Start with small doses in severe impairment

Hepatic Impairment

- Use with caution in mild to moderate impairment; avoid in severe impairment

- Benzodiazepines with a shorter half-life are considered safer in hepatic impairment

Cardiac Impairment

- Benzodiazepines have been used to treat insomnia associated with acute myocardial infarction

Elderly

- Due to its pharmacological properties, loprazolam can cause drowsiness and a decreased level of consciousness, which may lead to falls and consequently to severe injuries, especially in elderly

Children and Adolescents

- There is insufficient evidence to recommend the use of loprazolam in children

Pregnancy

- Possible increased risk of birth defects when benzodiazepines taken during pregnancy
- Because of the potential risks, loprazolam is not generally recommended as treatment for insomnia during pregnancy, especially during the first trimester
- Drug should be tapered if discontinued
- Infants whose mothers received a benzodiazepine late in pregnancy may experience withdrawal effects
- Neonatal flaccidity has been reported in infants whose mothers took a benzodiazepine during pregnancy
- Seizures, even mild seizures, may cause harm to the embryo/foetus

Breastfeeding

- Unknown if loprazolam is secreted in human breast milk, but all psychotropics assumed to be secreted in breast milk
- Effects on infant have been observed and include feeding difficulties, sedation, and weight loss
- Caution should be taken with the use of benzodiazepines in breastfeeding mothers; seek to use low doses for short periods to reduce infant exposure
- Use of shorter-acting 'Z' drugs zopiclone or zolpidem preferred
- Mothers taking hypnotics should be warned about the risks of co-sleeping

Loprazolam (Continued)

Potential Advantages

- Patients with insomnia

Potential Disadvantages

- Rebound insomnia
- Residual drowsiness
- Changes in mood, anxiety and restlessness

Primary Target Symptoms

- Quicker sleep onset
- Reducing nocturnal awakenings
- Increasing total sleep duration and quality

 Pearls

- NICE Guidelines recommend medication for insomnia only as a second-line treatment after non-pharmacological treatment options have been tried (e.g. cognitive behavioural therapy for insomnia)

- Loprazolam is a short-acting hypnotic
- It causes little or no hangover effects
- Paradoxical effects such as hostility and aggression may be seen in some patients
- In hepatic impairment start with a lower dose or reduce dose
- Loprazolam in comparison with other benzodiazepines has a delay in its action: 2 hours for it to reach a peak in serum concentrations

 **Switching**

- Substitute with equivalent dose of diazepam which has a longer half-life and thus less severe withdrawal
- Precautions apply in patients with hepatic dysfunction as diazepam can accumulate to toxic levels

Suggested Reading

Clark BG, Jue SG, Dawson GW et al. Loprazolam. A preliminary review of its pharmacodynamic and pharmacokinetic properties and therapeutic efficacy in insomnia. Drugs 1986;31(6):500–16.

Markota M, Rummans TA, Bostwick JM, et al. Benzodiazepine use in older adults: dangers, management, and alternative therapies. Mayo Clin Proc 2016;91(11):1632–9.

Matheson E, Hainer BL. Insomnia: pharmacologic therapy. Am Fam Physician 2017;96(1):29–35.

Lorazepam

Brands
• Ativan

Generic?
Yes

Class
• Neuroscience-based nomenclature: pharmacology domain – GABA; mode of action – positive allosteric modulator (PAM)
• Benzodiazepine (anxiolytic, anticonvulsant)

Commonly Prescribed for
(bold for BNF indication)
• **Anxiety (short-term use, oral)**
• **Insomnia associated with anxiety (short-term, oral)**
• **Acute panic attacks**
• **Convulsions (status epilepticus; febrile convulsions; convulsions caused by poisoning)**
• **Conscious sedation for procedures**
• **Premedication (unlicensed for IV use in children less than 12 years of age; unlicensed for oral use in children less than 5 years of age)**
• **In children: status epilepticus**
• **In children: unlicensed use in febrile convulsions and in convulsions caused by poisoning**
• Anxiety associated with depressive symptoms (oral)
• Muscle spasm
• Alcohol withdrawal psychosis
• Headache
• Panic disorder
• Acute mania (adjunctive)
• Acute psychosis (adjunctive)
• Delirium (with haloperidol)
• Catatonia

How the Drug Works
• Binds to benzodiazepine receptors at the GABA-A ligand-gated chloride channel complex
• Enhances the inhibitory effects of GABA
• Boosts chloride conductance through GABA-regulated channels
• Inhibits neuronal activity presumably in amygdala-centred fear circuits to provide therapeutic benefits in anxiety disorders
• Inhibitory actions in cerebral cortex may provide therapeutic benefits in seizure disorders

How Long Until It Works
• Some immediate relief with first dosing is common; can take several weeks for maximal therapeutic benefit with daily dosing

If It Works
• For short-term symptoms of anxiety – after a few weeks, discontinue use or use on an "as-needed" basis
• For chronic anxiety disorders, the goal of treatment is complete remission of symptoms as well as prevention of future relapses
• For chronic anxiety disorders, treatment most often reduces or even eliminates symptoms, but is not a cure since symptoms can recur after medicine stopped
• For long-term symptoms of anxiety, consider switching to an SSRI or SNRI for long-term maintenance
• Avoid long-term maintenance with a benzodiazepine
• If symptoms re-emerge after stopping a benzodiazepine, consider treatment with an SSRI or SNRI, or consider restarting the benzodiazepine; sometimes benzodiazepines have to be used in combination with SSRIs or SNRIs at the start of treatment for best results

If It Doesn't Work
• Consider switching to another agent or adding an appropriate augmenting agent
• Consider psychotherapy, especially cognitive behavioural psychotherapy
• Consider presence of concomitant substance abuse
• Consider presence of lorazepam abuse
• Consider another diagnosis such as a co-morbid medical condition

Best Augmenting Combos for Partial Response or Treatment Resistance
• Benzodiazepines are frequently used as augmenting agents for antipsychotics and mood stabilisers in the treatment of psychotic and bipolar disorders

- Benzodiazepines are frequently used as augmenting agents for SSRIs and SNRIs in the treatment of anxiety disorders
- Not generally rational to combine with other benzodiazepines
- Caution if using as an anxiolytic concomitantly with other sedative hypnotics for sleep

Tests

- In patients with seizure disorders, concomitant medical illness, and/or those with multiple concomitant long-term medications, periodic liver tests and blood counts may be prudent

---

SIDE EFFECTS

How Drug Causes Side Effects

- Same mechanism for side effects as for therapeutic effects – namely due to excessive actions at benzodiazepine receptors
- Long-term adaptations in benzodiazepine receptors may explain the development of dependence, tolerance, and withdrawal
- Side effects are generally immediate, but immediate side effects often disappear in time

Notable Side Effects

*Sedation, fatigue, depression
*Dizziness, ataxia, slurred speech, weakness
*Forgetfulness, confusion
*Hyperexcitability, nervousness
*Pain at injection site
- Rare hallucination, mania
- Rare hypotension
- Hypersalivation, dry mouth

Common or very common
- CNS/PNS: coma, disinhibition, extrapyramidal symptoms, memory loss, slurred speech, suicide attempt
- Other: apnoea, asthenia, hypothermia

Uncommon
- Allergic dermatitis, constipation, sexual dysfunction

Rare or very rare
- Blood disorders: agranulocytosis, pancytopenia, thrombocytopenia
- Other: altered saliva, hyponatraemia, SIADH

Frequency not known
- Drug dependence, leucopenia (with parenteral use)

- Paradoxical effects: increased hostility, aggression and psychomotor agitation. These effects are seen more commonly with lorazepam than with other benzodiazepines

 ### Life-Threatening or Dangerous Side Effects

- Respiratory depression, especially when taken with CNS depressants in overdose
- Rare hepatic dysfunction, renal dysfunction, blood dyscrasias

Weight Gain

- Reported but not expected

Sedation

  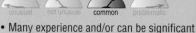

- Many experience and/or can be significant in amount
- Especially at initiation of treatment or when dose increases
- Tolerance often develops over time

What to Do About Side Effects

- Wait
- Wait
- Wait
- Lower the dose
- Take largest dose at bedtime to avoid sedative effects during the day
- Switch to another agent
- Administer flumazenil if side effects are severe or life-threatening

Best Augmenting Agents for Side Effects

- Many side effects cannot be improved with an augmenting agent

---

DOSING AND USE

Usual Dosage Range

- Short-term use in anxiety (adults): 1–4 mg in divided doses (oral)
- Short-term use in anxiety (elderly/debilitated): 0.5–2 mg in divided doses (oral)
- Short-term use in insomnia with anxiety: 1–2 mg at bedtime (oral)
- Acute panic attacks: 25–30 mcg/kg every 6 hours as needed, usual dose 1.5–2.5 mg

per 6 hours (by intravenous injection into large vein, only use IM route when oral and intravenous not available)
- Conscious sedation for procedures: 2–3 mg the night before operation (oral); 2–4 mg about 1–2 hours before operation (oral); 50 mcg/kg to be administered 30–45 minutes before operation (slow intravenous injection); 50 mcg/kg, to be administered 60–90 minutes before operation (IM injection)
- Premedication: 2–3 mg the night before operation; 2–4 mg about 1–2 hours before operation (oral); 50 mcg/kg, to be administered 30–45 minutes before operation (slow intravenous injection); 50 mcg/kg, to be administered 60–90 minutes before operation (IM injection)
- Status epilepticus, febrile convulsions, convulsions caused by poisoning: for adults, 4 mg for 1 dose, then 4 mg after 10 minutes if required for 1 dose, to be administered into a large vein

Dosage Forms
- Tablet 0.5 mg, 1 mg, 2.5 mg
- Oral solution 1 mg/1 mL
- Solution for injection 2 mg/mL, 4 mg/mL

How to Dose
- Oral: initial dose 1–4 mg/day in 2–3 doses; increase as needed, starting with evening dose; max generally 10 mg/day
- Injection: initial dose 1–2.5 mg administered slowly; after 10–15 minutes may administer again
- Take liquid formulation with water, juice, or pudding
- Catatonia: initial dose 1–2 mg; can repeat in 3 hours and then again in another 3 hours if necessary

 Dosing Tips

∗One of the few benzodiazepines available in an oral liquid formulation
∗One of the few benzodiazepines available in an injectable formulation
- Lorazepam injection is intended for acute use; patients who require longer treatment should be switched to the oral formulation
- Use lowest possible effective dose for the shortest possible period of time (a benzodiazepine-sparing strategy)
- Assess need for continued treatment regularly

- Risk of dependence may increase with dose and duration of treatment
- For inter-dose symptoms of anxiety, can either increase dose or maintain same total daily dose but divide into more frequent doses
- Can also use an as-needed occasional "top up" dose for inter-dose anxiety
- Because panic disorder may require higher doses, the risk of dependence may be greater in these patients
- Frequency of dosing in practice is often greater than predicted from half-life, as duration of biological activity is often shorter than pharmacokinetic terminal half-life

Overdose
- Fatalities can occur; signs of overdose may include mental confusion, dysarthria, paradoxical reactions, drowsiness, hypotonia, ataxia, hypotension, hypnotic state, coma, cardiovascular depression, respiratory depression, and death
- In cases of a suspected overdose, it is important to establish whether the person is a regular user of lorazepam or other benzodiazepines since regular use causes tolerance to develop

Long-Term Use
- Some evidence of efficacy up to 16 weeks, but long-term use should be avoided
- Risk of dependence, particularly for treatment periods longer than 12 weeks and especially in patients with past or current polysubstance abuse

Habit Forming
- Lorazepam is a Class C/Schedule 4 drug
- Patients may develop dependence and/or tolerance with long-term use

How to Stop
- Patients with history of seizure may seize upon withdrawal, especially if withdrawal is abrupt
- Taper by 0.5 mg every 3 days to reduce chances of withdrawal effects
- For difficult-to-taper cases, consider reducing dose much more slowly once reaching 3 mg/day, perhaps by as little as 0.25 mg per week or less
- For other patients with severe problems discontinuing a benzodiazepine, dosing may need to be tapered over many months

Lorazepam (Continued)

(i.e. reduce dose by 1% every 3 days by crushing tablet and suspending or dissolving in 100 mL of fruit juice and then disposing of 1 mL while drinking the rest; 3–7 days later, dispose of 2 mL, and so on). This is both a form of very slow biological tapering and a form of behavioural desensitisation

- Be sure to differentiate re-emergence of symptoms requiring reinstitution of treatment from withdrawal symptoms
- Benzodiazepine-dependent anxiety patients and insulin-dependent diabetics are not addicted to their medications. When benzodiazepine-dependent patients stop their medication, disease symptoms can re-emerge, disease symptoms can worsen (rebound), and/or withdrawal symptoms can emerge

Pharmacokinetics

- Food does not affect absorption
- Onset of action 1–5 min (IV), 15–30 min (IM)
- Elimination half-life is about 12 hours (10–20 hours)
- No active metabolites
- Duration of action 12–24 hours (IV, IM)
- Excretion via kidneys

 Drug Interactions

- Increased depressive effects when taken with other CNS depressants (see Warnings below)
- Valproate and probenecid may reduce clearance and raise plasma concentrations of lorazepam
- Oral contraceptives may increase clearance and lower plasma concentrations of lorazepam
- Flumazenil (used to reverse the effects of benzodiazepines) may precipitate seizures and should not be used in patients treated for seizure disorders with lorazepam

 Other Warnings/Precautions

- Warning regarding the increased risk of CNS-depressant effects (especially alcohol) when benzodiazepines and opioid medications are used together, including specifically the risk of slowed or difficulty breathing and death
- If alternatives to the combined use of benzodiazepines and opioids are not available, clinicians should limit the dosage and duration of each drug to the minimum possible while still achieving therapeutic efficacy
- Patients and their caregivers should be warned to seek medical attention if unusual dizziness, light-headedness, sedation, slowed or difficulty breathing, or unresponsiveness occur
- Dosage changes should be made in collaboration with prescriber
- History of drug or alcohol abuse often creates greater risk for dependency
- Some depressed patients may experience a worsening of suicidal ideation
- Some patients may exhibit abnormal thinking or behavioural changes similar to those caused by other CNS depressants (i.e. either depressant actions or disinhibiting actions)
- Avoid prolonged use and abrupt cessation
- Use lower doses in debilitated patients and the elderly
- Use with caution in patients with myasthenia gravis; respiratory disease
- Use with caution in patients with personality disorder (dependent/avoidant or anankastic types) as may increase risk of dependence
- Use with caution in patients with a history of alcohol or drug dependence/abuse
- Benzodiazepines may cause a range of paradoxical effects including aggression, antisocial behaviours, anxiety, overexcitement, perceptual abnormalities and talkativeness. Adjustment of dose may reduce impulses
- Use with caution in patients with muscle weakness or organic brain changes
- With parenteral administration close observation is required until full recovery achieved from sedation
- When given intravenously, facilities for reversing respiratory depression with mechanical ventilation must be immediately available

Do Not Use

- If patient has acute pulmonary insufficiency, respiratory depression, significant

neuromuscular respiratory weakness, sleep apnoea syndrome or unstable myasthenia gravis
- In patients with CNS depression, compromised airway
- Alone in chronic psychosis in adults
- On its own to treat depression, anxiety associated with depression, obsessional states or phobic states
- If patient has angle-closure glaucoma
- Injections containing benzyl alcohol in neonates
- Intra-arterially as may cause arteriospasm and result in gangrene
- If there is a proven allergy to lorazepam or any benzodiazepine

SPECIAL POPULATIONS

Renal Impairment
- Increased cerebral sensitivity to benzodiazepines
- Start with small doses in severe impairment
- 1–2 mg/day in 2–3 doses

Hepatic Impairment
- Because of its short half-life and inactive metabolites, lorazepam may be a preferred benzodiazepine in some patients with liver disease
- Caution in mild to moderate impairment; avoid in severe impairment
- 1–2 mg/day in 2–3 doses

Cardiac Impairment
- Benzodiazepines have been used to treat anxiety associated with acute myocardial infarction
- Rare reports of QTc prolongation in patients with underlying arrhythmia
- Lorazepam may be used as an adjunct to control drug-induced cardiovascular emergencies

Elderly
- 1–2 mg/day in 2–3 doses
- May be more sensitive to sedative or respiratory effects

Children and Adolescents
- May be used for premedication for children 1 month–17 years
- May be used by slow intravenous injection in status epilepticus, febrile convulsions, and convulsions caused by poisoning in neonates and children up to the age of 17
- Long-term effects of lorazepam in children/adolescents are unknown
- Should generally receive lower doses and be more closely monitored

Pregnancy
- Possible increased risk of birth defects when benzodiazepines taken during pregnancy
- Because of the potential risks, lorazepam is not generally recommended as treatment for anxiety during pregnancy, especially during the first trimester
- Drug should be tapered if discontinued
- Infants whose mothers received a benzodiazepine late in pregnancy may experience withdrawal effects
- Neonatal flaccidity has been reported in infants whose mothers took a benzodiazepine during pregnancy
- Seizures, even mild seizures, may cause harm to the embryo/foetus

Breastfeeding
- Small amounts found in mother's breast milk
- Effects of benzodiazepines on infant have been observed and include feeding difficulties, sedation, and weight loss
- Caution should be taken with the use of benzodiazepines in breastfeeding mothers; seek to use low doses for short periods to reduce infant exposure
- Use of short-acting agents, e.g. oxazepam or lorazepam, preferred
- Considered not to pose a risk to the infant when given as a single dose (e.g. for premedication)

THE ART OF PSYCHOPHARMACOLOGY
Potential Advantages
- Rapid onset of action
- Availability of oral liquid as well as injectable dosage formulations

Potential Disadvantages
- Euphoria may lead to abuse
- Abuse especially risky in past or present substance abusers
- Possibly more sedation than some other benzodiazepines commonly used to treat anxiety

Lorazepam (Continued)

Primary Target Symptoms
- Panic attacks
- Anxiety
- Muscle spasms
- Incidence of seizures (adjunct)

Pearls
- NICE Guidelines recommend medication for insomnia only as a second-line treatment after non-pharmacological treatment options have been tried (e.g. cognitive behavioural therapy for insomnia)
- *One of the most popular and useful benzodiazepines for treatment of agitation associated with psychosis, bipolar disorder, and other disorders, especially in the inpatient setting; this is due in part to useful sedative properties and flexibility of administration with oral tablets, oral liquid, or injectable formulations, which can be used for rapid tranquillisation
- Is a very useful adjunct to SSRIs and SNRIs in the treatment of numerous anxiety disorders
- Though not systematically studied, benzodiazepines, and lorazepam in particular, have been used effectively to treat catatonia and are the initial recommended treatment
- Not effective for treating psychosis as a monotherapy, but can be used as an adjunct to antipsychotics
- Not effective for treating bipolar disorder as a monotherapy, but can be used as an adjunct to mood stabilisers and antipsychotics
- Because of its short half-life and inactive metabolites, lorazepam may be preferred over some benzodiazepines for patients with liver disease
- *Lorazepam may be preferred over other benzodiazepines for the treatment of delirium
- When treating delirium, lorazepam is often combined with haloperidol, with the haloperidol dose 2.5 times the lorazepam dose
- *Lorazepam is often used to induce pre-operative anterograde amnesia to assist in anaesthesia
- May both cause depression and treat depression in different patients
- Clinical duration of action may be shorter than plasma half-life, leading to dosing more frequently than 2–3 times daily in some patients
- When using to treat insomnia, remember that insomnia may be a symptom of some other primary disorder itself, and thus warrants assessment for co-morbid psychiatric and/or medical conditions

 Suggested Reading

Bonnet MH, Arand DL. The use of lorazepam TID for chronic insomnia. Int Clin Psychopharmacol 1999;14(2):81–9.

Edinoff AN, Kaufman SE, Hollier JW, et al. Catatonia: clinical overview of the diagnosis, treatment, and clinical challenges. Neurol Int 2021;13(4):570–86.

Greenblatt DJ. Clinical pharmacokinetics of oxazepam and lorazepam. Clin Pharmacokinet 1981;6(2):89–105.

Mancuso CE, Tanzi MG, Gabay M. Paradoxical reactions to benzodiazepines: literature review and treatment options. Pharmacotherapy 2004;24(9):1177–85.

Patel MX, Sethi FN, Barnes TR, et al. Joint BAP NAPICU evidence-based consensus guidelines for the clinical management of acute disturbance: de-escalation and rapid tranquillisation. J Psychopharmacol 2018;32(6):601–40.

Pietras CJ, Lieving LM, Cherek DR, et al. Acute effects of lorazepam on laboratory measures of aggressive and escape responses of adult male parolees. Behav Pharmacol 2005;16(4):243–51.

Starreveld E, Starreveld AA. Status epilepticus. Current concepts and management. Can Fam Physician 2000;46:1817–23.

Wagner BK, O'Hara DA, Hammond JS. Drugs for amnesia in the ICU. Am J Crit Care 1997;6(3):192–201; quiz 202–3.

Loxapine

Brands
• Adasuve (inhaled loxapine)

Generic?
No, not in UK

Class
• Neuroscience-based nomenclature: pharmacology domain – dopamine, serotonin; mode of action – antagonist
• Conventional antipsychotic (neuroleptic, dopamine 2 antagonist, serotonin dopamine antagonist)

Commonly Prescribed for
(bold for BNF indication)
• **Rapid control of mild-moderate agitation in patients with schizophrenia or bipolar disorder (specialist supervision in hospital)**

 ## How the Drug Works
• Blocks dopamine 2 receptors, reducing positive symptoms of psychosis
∗Although classified as a conventional antipsychotic, loxapine is a potent serotonin 2A antagonist with its receptor spectrum close to an atypical profile (D2/5HT2A ratio 1.14). These properties might be relevant at low doses, but generally are overwhelmed by high dosing
• Also binds with noradrenergic, histaminergic, and cholinergic receptors
• Changes in the level of excitability of subcortical inhibitory areas have been observed in several animal species, associated with calming effects and suppression of aggressive behaviour

How Long Until It Works
• Rapid onset of action due to inhalational form, with Tmax of 2 minutes and reduction in agitation by 10 minutes
• Works faster than IM aripiprazole

If It Works
• Once the period of agitation has settled, then patients with schizophrenia or bipolar disorder still need oral treatment with an atypical antipsychotic or mood stabiliser for maintenance treatment

If It Doesn't Work
• Can give another dose after 2 hours
• Consider standard choices of lorazepam, haloperidol and promethazine or buccal midazolam, as well as a number of oral antipsychotics in addition to parenteral options of IM aripiprazole or IM olanzapine

 ## Best Augmenting Combos for Partial Response or Treatment Resistance
• Risk of CNS-depressant effects when combined with a benzodiazepine
• Risk of anti-muscarinic effects when combined with an antihistamine

Tests
Baseline
∗Measure weight, BMI, and waist circumference
• Get baseline personal and family history of diabetes, obesity, dyslipidaemia, hypertension, and cardiovascular disease
• Check for personal history of drug-induced leucopenia/neutropenia
∗Check pulse and blood pressure, fasting plasma glucose or glycosylated haemoglobin (HbA1c), fasting lipid profile, and prolactin levels
• Full blood count (FBC)
• Assessment of nutritional status, diet, and level of physical activity
• Determine if the patient:
  • is overweight (BMI 25.0–29.9)
  • is obese (BMI ≥30)
  • has pre-diabetes – fasting plasma glucose: 5.5 mmol/L to 6.9 mmol/L or HbA1c: 42 to 47 mmol/mol (6.0 to 6.4%)
  • has diabetes – fasting plasma glucose: >7.0 mmol/L or HbA1c: ≥48 mmol/L (≥6.5%)
  • has hypertension (BP >140/90 mm Hg)
  • has dyslipidaemia (increased total cholesterol, LDL cholesterol, and triglycerides; decreased HDL cholesterol)
• Treat or refer such patients for treatment, including nutrition and weight management, physical activity counselling, smoking cessation, and medical management
• Baseline ECG for: inpatients; those with a personal history or risk factor for cardiac disease

Specifically for inhalational loxapine
- ECG and check for history of cardiovascular disease
- Check for history of asthma, COPD, other lung disease associated with bronchospasm, acute respiratory signs/symptoms, current use of medications to treat airways, history of bronchospasm following treatment with loxapine inhalation powder
- Blood pressure
- Hydration status
- After administering inhalation powder, monitor patients for signs and symptoms of bronchospasm at least every 15 minutes for at least an hour

---

SIDE EFFECTS

How Drug Causes Side Effects
- By blocking dopamine 2 receptors in the striatum, it can cause motor side effects
- By blocking dopamine 2 receptors in the pituitary, it can cause elevations in prolactin
- By blocking dopamine 2 receptors excessively in the mesocortical and mesolimbic dopamine pathways, especially at high doses, it can cause worsening of negative and cognitive symptoms (neuroleptic-induced deficit syndrome)
- Anticholinergic actions may cause sedation, blurred vision, constipation, dry mouth
- Antihistaminergic actions may cause sedation, weight gain
- By blocking alpha 1 adrenergic receptors, it can cause dizziness, sedation, and hypotension
- Mechanism of weight gain and any possible increased incidence of diabetes or dyslipidaemia with conventional antipsychotics is unknown

Notable Side Effects
*Neuroleptic-induced deficit syndrome
*Galactorrhoea, amenorrhoea, erectile dysfunction, gynaecomastia, hyperprolactinaemia
- Constipation, vision disturbance, urinary retention, tachycardia
- Rash, vomiting, hyperglycaemia

Common or very common
- CNS: dizziness, sedation
- GIT: altered taste, dry mouth

- Resp: irritation of throat
- Other: fatigue

Uncommon
- CNS: akathisia, dystonia, dyskinesis, oculogyric crisis, restlessness, tremor
- Other: bronchospasm, hypotension

Frequency not known
- Blurred vision, dry eye, hypertension, syncope

Life-Threatening or Dangerous Side Effects
- Bronchospasm, with the potential to lead to respiratory distress and respiratory arrest
- Rare neuroleptic malignant syndrome
- Rare agranulocytosis
- Rare hepatocellular injury
- Rare seizures
- Increased risk of death and cerebrovascular events in elderly patients with dementia-related psychosis

Weight Gain

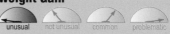
unusual   not unusual   common   problematic

- Reported but not expected

Sedation

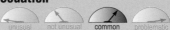
unusual   not unusual   common   problematic

- Many experience and/or can be significant in amount
- Sedation is usually transient

What to Do About Side Effects
- Bronchospasm after administration should be treated with a short-acting bronchodilator, although staff trained in airway management should be available
- Wait
- Wait
- Wait
- Reduce the dose
- Low-dose benzodiazepine or beta blocker may reduce akathisia
- Take more of the dose at bedtime to help reduce daytime sedation
- Weight loss, exercise programmes, and medical management for high BMIs, diabetes, and dyslipidaemia
- Switch to another antipsychotic (atypical) – quetiapine or clozapine are best in cases of tardive dyskinesia

Best Augmenting Agents for Side Effects

- Dystonia: antimuscarinic drugs (e.g. procyclidine) as oral or IM depending on the severity; botulinum toxin if antimuscarinics not effective
- Parkinsonism: antimuscarinic drugs (e.g. procyclidine)
- Akathisia: beta blocker propranolol (30–80 mg/day) or low-dose benzodiazepine (e.g. 0.5–3.0 mg/day of clonazepam) may help; other agents that may be tried include the 5HT2 antagonists such as cyproheptadine (16 mg/day) or mirtazapine (15 mg at night – caution in bipolar disorder); clonidine (0.2–0.8 mg/day) may be tried if the above ineffective
- Tardive dyskinesia: stop any antimuscarinic, consider tetrabenazine

DOSING AND USE

Usual Dosage Range
- 4.5–18.2 mg/day in divided doses

Dosage Forms
- Inhalant 10 mg unit (supplies 9.1 mg) in a single-use inhaler
- Should be stored in original pouch to protect from light and moisture. Does not require any special temperature storage conditions

How to Dose
- By inhalation: either 9.1 mg as a single dose, followed by 9.1 mg after 2 hours if required, or 4.5 mg as a single dose, followed by 4.5 mg after 2 hours if required – lower dose may be given if appropriate or if higher dose not previously tolerated
- Inhalation powder: 10 mg by oral inhalation using an inhaler
- Remove pull-tab and wait for green light to turn on (product must be used within 15 minutes of pulling tab); instruct patient to inhale through mouthpiece and then hold breath briefly. When green light turns off, the dose has been delivered
- Must be administered by a healthcare professional in a setting with immediate onsite access to equipment and personnel trained to manage acute bronchospasm, including advanced airway management. After administering inhalation powder, monitor patients for signs and symptoms

of bronchospasm at least every 15 minutes for at least an hour. Can be treated with a short-acting beta-agonist bronchodilator

 Dosing Tips

- Prior to administering inhalation powder, screen all patients for a history of pulmonary disease, and examine patients (including chest auscultation) for respiratory abnormalities (e.g. wheezing)
- Correct use of inhaler is important for administration of the full dose. Patient acceptance is thus necessary. Ultimately patient preference needs to be considered in order to establish good therapeutic relationships, but it has been shown that patients prefer the inhalation route versus drugs via the IM route
- Patients receiving atypical antipsychotics may occasionally require a "top up" of a conventional antipsychotic to control aggression or violent behaviour

Overdose
- Signs and symptoms will depend on the number of units taken and individual patient tolerance
- Deaths have occurred
- Extrapyramidal symptoms, CNS depression, cardiovascular effects (including sinus tachycardia and arrhythmia), hypotension, hypothermia, seizures, respiratory depression, renal failure, coma
- Treatment is essentially symptomatic and supportive. Severe hypotension might respond to noradrenaline or phenylephrine (not adrenaline). Severe extrapyramidal reactions should be treated with anticholinergic anti-Parkinson medicinal products or diphenhydramine hydrochloride, and anticonvulsant therapy should be initiated as indicated. Additional measures include oxygen and intravenous fluids

Long-Term Use
- Some side effects may be irreversible (e.g. tardive dyskinesia)

Habit Forming
- No

How to Stop
- Not a problem to stop as used in the short term

Pharmacokinetics

- Rapid absorption with median time of maximum plasma concentration by 2 minutes
- Rapidly distributed in tissues; 96.6% bound to human plasma proteins
- Metabolised extensively in the liver, with multiple metabolites formed with longer half-lives than the parent drug
- * *N*-desmethyl loxapine is amoxapine, an antidepressant
- 8-hydroxyloxapine and 7-hydroxyloxapine are also serotonin-dopamine antagonists
- 8-hydroxyamoxapine and 7-hydroxyamoxapine are also serotonin-dopamine antagonists
- Terminal elimination half-life of 6–8 hours
- Excretion mostly occurs in the first 24 hours

Drug Interactions

- Loxapine may antagonise the effects of levodopa and dopamine agonists
- Respiratory depression may occur when loxapine is combined with lorazepam
- Additive effects may occur if used with CNS depressants
- Some patients taking a neuroleptic and lithium have developed an encephalopathic syndrome similar to neuroleptic malignant syndrome
- Combined use with adrenaline may lower blood pressure since beta-adrenoceptor stimulation may worsen hypotension in the setting of loxapine-induced partial alpha-adrenoceptor blockade
- May increase the effects of antihypertensive drugs causing hypotension (except for guanethidine, whose antihypertensive actions loxapine may antagonise)
- May increase antimuscarinic side effects of other drugs
- Effects of alcohol are enhanced
- Predicted to decrease effects of amantadine, apomorphine, bromocriptine, cabergoline, rotigotine, ropinirole, quinagolide, pramipexole, pergolide. Manufacturer makes no recommendations
- Ciprofloxacin, combined hormonal contraceptives and fluvoxamine are predicted to increase the exposure to loxapine and the manufacturer advises to avoid

 Other Warnings/Precautions

- All antipsychotics should be used with caution in patients with angle-closure glaucoma, blood disorders, cardiovascular disease, depression, diabetes, epilepsy and susceptibility to seizures, history of jaundice, myasthenia gravis, Parkinson's disease, photosensitivity, prostatic hypertrophy, severe respiratory disorders
- If signs of neuroleptic malignant syndrome develop, treatment should be immediately discontinued
- Use cautiously in patients with alcohol withdrawal or convulsive disorders because of possible lowering of seizure threshold
- Antiemetic effect can mask signs of other disorders or overdose
- Do not use adrenaline in event of overdose
- Observe for signs of ocular toxicity (pigmentary retinopathy, lenticular pigmentation)
- Avoid extreme heat exposure
- Use only with caution if at all in Lewy body disease

Do Not Use

- If patient is in a comatose state or has CNS depression
- If patient has asthma or history of asthma, COPD, other lung disease associated with bronchospasm, acute respiratory signs/symptoms, current use of medications to treat airways, history of bronchospasm following treatment with loxapine inhalation powder (inhalant only)
- If patient has cardiovascular or cerebrovascular disease
- In elderly patients (especially those with dementia-related psychosis)
- If patient is hypovolaemic (risk of hypotension)
- If patient is dehydrated (risk of hypotension)
- If there is a proven allergy to loxapine or to amoxapine
- If there is a known sensitivity to any dibenzoxazepine

SPECIAL POPULATIONS

Renal Impairment
- Use with caution
- Not been studied; no data available

Hepatic Impairment
- Use with caution
- Not been studied; no data available

Cardiac Impairment
- No data are available, but is contraindicated in those with known cardiovascular disease. Clinically relevant QT prolongation does not appear to be associated with single and repeat doses, but the potential risk of QTc prolongation due to interaction with medicinal products known to prolong QTc interval is unknown

Elderly
- Contraindicated in the elderly, especially those with dementia-related psychosis
- Safety and efficacy have not been established; no data available

 ### Children and Adolescents
- Not for use in children and adolescents
- Safety and efficacy not established

 ### Pregnancy
- Controlled studies have not been conducted in pregnant women
- There is a risk of abnormal muscle movements and withdrawal symptoms in newborns whose mothers took an antipsychotic during the third trimester; symptoms may include agitation, abnormally increased or decreased muscle tone, tremor, sleepiness, severe difficulty breathing, and difficulty feeding
- Renal papillary abnormalities have been seen in rats during pregnancy
- Psychotic symptoms may worsen during pregnancy and some form of treatment may be necessary
- Use in pregnancy may be justified if the benefit of continued treatment exceeds any associated risk
- Switching antipsychotics may increase the risk of relapse

- Antipsychotics may be preferable to anticonvulsant mood stabilisers if treatment is required for mania during pregnancy
- Olanzapine and clozapine have been associated with maternal hyperglycaemia which may lead to developmental toxicity, risk may also apply for other atypical antipsychotics

Breastfeeding
- Unknown if loxapine is secreted in human breast milk, but all psychotropics assumed to be secreted in breast milk
- Haloperidol is considered to be the preferred first-generation antipsychotic, and quetiapine the preferred second-generation antipsychotic
- Infants of women who choose to breastfeed should be monitored for possible adverse effects

THE ART OF PSYCHOPHARMACOLOGY

Potential Advantages
- Inhalational formulation for rapid use

Potential Disadvantages
- Patients with tardive dyskinesia

Primary Target Symptoms
- Positive symptoms of psychosis
- Motor and autonomic hyperactivity
- Violent or aggressive behaviour

 ### Pearls
- *Recently discovered to be a serotonin dopamine antagonist (binding studies and PET scans)
- Developed as a conventional antipsychotic; i.e. reduces positive symptoms, but causes extrapyramidal symptoms and prolactin elevations
- Lower extrapyramidal symptoms than haloperidol in some studies, but no fixed-dose studies and no low-dose studies
- For previously stabilised patients with "breakthrough" agitation or incipient decompensation, "top-up" the atypical antipsychotic with as-needed inhalational loxapine

Loxapine (Continued)

- Several studies have corroborated the benefits of inhaled loxapine. PANSS-EC score which measures behaviour such as excitement, tension, hostility and uncooperativeness was reported to decrease compared to placebo. Behavioural activity rating (BAR) scores were also shown to decrease following treatment compared to placebo. Moreover, Clinical Global Impression (CGI) scores improved and there was less need for rescue medication after treatment compared to placebo

- Inhaled loxapine may provide a good alternative to treat mild-moderate agitation in a clinical setting due to its rapid effects and non-invasive method over the traditional IM injections
- Due to the risk of bronchospasm, loxapine inhalation powder should be administered only in an enrolled healthcare facility that has immediate onsite access to equipment and personnel trained to manage acute bronchospasm, including advanced airway management (intubation and mechanical ventilation)

 ## Suggested Reading

Allen MH, Feifel D, Lesem MD, et al. Efficacy and safety of loxapine for inhalation in the treatment of agitation in patients with schizophrenia: a randomized, double-blind, placebo-controlled trial. J Clin Psychiatry 2011;72(10):1313–21.

de Beradis D, Fornaro M, Orsolini L, et al. The role of inhaled loxapine in the treatment of acute agitation in patients with psychiatric disorders: a clinical review. Int J Mol Sci 2017;18(2):349.

Ferreri F, Drapier D, Baloche E, et al. The in vitro actions of loxapine on dopaminergic and serotonergic receptors. Time to consider atypical classification of this antipsychotic drug? Int J Neuropsychopharmacol 2018;21(4):355–60.

Gil E, Garcia-Alonso F, Boldeanu A, et al. Loxapine Inhaled Home Use study investigator's team. Safety and efficacy of self-administered inhaled loxapine (ADASUVE) in agitated patients outside the hospital setting: protocol for a phase IV, single-arm, open-label trial. BMJ Open 2018;8(10):e020242.

Huhn M, Nikolakopoulou A, Schneider-Thoma J, et al. Comparative efficacy and tolerability of 32 oral antipsychotics for the acute treatment of adults with multi-episode schizophrenia: a systematic review and network meta-analysis. Lancet 2019;394(10202):939–51.

Jorgensen TR, Emborg C, Dahlen K, et al. Patient preferences for medicine administration for acute agitation: results from an internet-based survey of patients diagnosed with bipolar disorder or schizophrenia in two Nordic countries. Psychol Health Med 2018;23(1):30–8.

Lesem M, Tran-Johnson T, Riesenberg R, et al. Rapid acute treatment of agitation in individuals with schizophrenia: multicentre, randomised, placebo-controlled study of inhaled loxapine. Br J Psychiatry 2011;198(1):51–8.

McDowell M, Nitti K, Kulstad E, et al. Clinical outcomes in patients taking inhaled loxapine, haloperidol, or ziprasidone in the emergency department. Clin Neuropharmacol 2019;42(2):23–6.

Patel M, Sethi F, Barnes TR, et al. Joint BAP NAPICU evidence-based consensus guidelines for the clinical management of acute disturbance: de-escalation and rapid tranquillisation. J Psychopharmacol 2018;32(6):601–40.

Patrizi B, Navarro-Haro MV, Gasol M. Inhaled loxapine for agitation in patients with personality disorder: an initial approach. Eur Neuropsychopharmacol 2019;29(1):122–6.

San L, Estrada G, Oudovenko N, et al. PLACID study: a randomized trial comparing the efficacy and safety of inhaled loxapine versus intramuscular aripiprazole in acutely agitated patients with schizophrenia or bipolar disorder. Eur Neuropsychopharmacol 2018;28(6):710–18.

Lurasidone hydrochloride

Brands
• Latuda

Generic?
No, not in UK

Class
• Neuroscience-based nomenclature: pharmacology domain – dopamine, serotonin; mode of action – antagonist
• Atypical antipsychotic (serotonin-dopamine antagonist; second-generation antipsychotic; also a potential mood stabiliser)

Commonly Prescribed for
(bold for BNF indication)
• **Schizophrenia**
• **Schizophrenia when given with moderate CYP3A4 inhibitors (e.g. diltiazem, erythromycin, fluconazole, verapamil)**
• Bipolar depression
• Acute mania/mixed mania
• Other psychotic disorders
• Bipolar maintenance
• Treatment-resistant depression
• Behavioural disturbances in dementia
• Behavioural disturbances in children and adolescents
• Disorders associated with problems with impulse control

How the Drug Works
• Blocks dopamine 2 receptors, reducing positive symptoms of psychosis and stabilising affective symptoms
• Blocks serotonin 2A receptors, causing enhancement of dopamine release in certain brain regions and thus reducing motor side effects and possibly improving cognition and affective symptoms
• Potently blocks serotonin 7 receptors, which may be beneficial for mood, sleep, cognitive impairment, and negative symptoms in schizophrenia, and also in bipolar disorder and major depressive disorder
• Partial agonist at 5HT1A receptors, and antagonist actions at serotonin 7 and alpha 2A and alpha 2 C receptors, which may be beneficial for mood, anxiety and cognition in a number of disorders
• Lacks potent actions at dopamine D1, muscarinic M1, and histamine H1 receptors, theoretically suggesting less propensity for inducing cognitive impairment, weight gain, or sedation compared to other agents with these properties

How Long Until It Works
• Psychotic symptoms can improve within 1 week, but it may take several weeks for full effect on behaviour as well as on cognition
• Classically recommended to wait at least 4–6 weeks to determine efficacy of drug, but in practice some patients may require up to 16–20 weeks to show a good response, especially on cognitive impairment and functional outcome
• Patients should be closely monitored during this period, particularly if high-risk for suicide

If It Works
• Most often reduces positive symptoms but does not eliminate them
• Can improve negative symptoms, as well as aggressive, cognitive, and affective symptoms in schizophrenia
• Most patients with schizophrenia do not have a total remission of symptoms but rather a reduction of symptoms by about a third
• Perhaps 5–15% patients with schizophrenia can experience an overall improvement of >50–60%, especially when receiving stable treatment for >1 year
• Such patients are considered super-responders or "awakeners" since they may be well enough to be employed, live independently, and sustain long-term relationships
• Continue treatment until reaching a plateau of improvement
• After reaching a satisfactory plateau, continue treatment for at least 1 year after first episode of psychosis, but it may be preferable to continue treatment indefinitely to avoid subsequent episodes
• After any subsequent episodes of psychosis, treatment may need to be indefinite

If It Doesn't Work
• Try one of the other atypical antipsychotics (risperidone or olanzapine should be considered first before considering other agents such as quetiapine, amisulpride, or aripiprazole)

Lurasidone hydrochloride (Continued)

- If 2 or more antipsychotic monotherapies do not work, consider clozapine
- Some patients may require treatment with a conventional antipsychotic
- If no first-line atypical antipsychotic is effective, consider higher doses or augmentation with valproate or lamotrigine
- Consider non-concordance and switch to another antipsychotic with fewer side effects or to an antipsychotic that can be given by depot injection
- Consider initiating rehabilitation and psychotherapy
- Consider presence of concomitant drug abuse

⚖ Best Augmenting Combos for Partial Response or Treatment Resistance

- Valproic acid (Depakote or Epilim)
- Mood-stabilising anticonvulsants (see Drug interactions)
- Lithium
- Benzodiazepines

Tests

Before starting an atypical antipsychotic

* Measure weight, BMI, and waist circumference (lurasidone is not clearly associated with weight gain, but monitoring recommended nonetheless as obesity prevalence is high in this patient group)
- Get baseline personal and family history of diabetes, obesity, dyslipidaemia, hypertension, and cardiovascular disease
* Check pulse and blood pressure, fasting plasma glucose or glycosylated haemoglobin (HbA1c), fasting lipid profile, and prolactin levels
- Full blood count (FBC), urea and electrolytes (including creatinine and eGFR), liver function tests (LFTs)
- Assessment of nutritional status, diet, and level of physical activity
- Determine if the patient:
  - is overweight (BMI 25.0–29.9)
  - is obese (BMI ≥30)
  - has pre-diabetes – fasting plasma glucose: 5.5 mmol/L to 6.9 mmol/L or HbA1c: 42 to 47 mmol/mol (6.0 to 6.4%)
  - has diabetes – fasting plasma glucose: >7.0 mmol/L or HbA1c: ≥48 mmol/L (≥6.5%)
  - has hypertension (BP >140/90 mm Hg)

- has dyslipidaemia (increased total cholesterol, LDL cholesterol, and triglycerides; decreased HDL cholesterol)
- Treat or refer such patients for treatment, including nutrition and weight management, physical activity counselling, smoking cessation, and medical management
- Baseline ECG for: inpatients; those with a personal history or risk factor for cardiac disease

Monitoring after starting an atypical antipsychotic

- FBC annually to detect chronic bone marrow suppression, stop treatment if neutrophils fall below 1.5x10⁹/L and refer to specialist care if neutrophils fall below 0.5x10⁹/L
- Urea and electrolytes (including creatinine and eGFR) annually
- LFTs annually
- Prolactin levels at 6 months and then annually (prolactin elevations low and generally transient with lurasidone)
* Weight/BMI/waist circumference, weekly for the first 6 weeks, then at 12 weeks, at 1 year, and then annually
* Pulse and blood pressure at 12 weeks, 1 year, and then annually
* Fasting blood glucose, HbA1c, and blood lipids at 12 weeks, at 1 year, and then annually
* For patients with type 2 diabetes, measure HbA1c at 3–6 month intervals until stable, then every 6 months
* Even in patients without known diabetes, be vigilant for the rare but life-threatening onset of diabetic ketoacidosis, which always requires immediate treatment, by monitoring for the rapid onset of polyuria, polydipsia, weight loss, nausea, vomiting, dehydration, rapid respiration, weakness and clouding of sensorium, even coma
- If HbA1c remains ≥48 mmol/mol (6.5%) then drug therapy should be offered, e.g. metformin
- Treat or refer for treatment or consider switching to another atypical antipsychotic for patients who become overweight, obese, pre-diabetic, diabetic, hypertensive, or dyslipidaemic while receiving an atypical antipsychotic (these problems are relatively less likely with lurasidone)

SIDE EFFECTS

How Drug Causes Side Effects

- By blocking dopamine 2 receptors in the striatum, it can cause motor side effects
- By blocking dopamine 2 receptors in the pituitary, it can cause elevations in prolactin
- Mechanism of weight gain and increased incidence of diabetes and dyslipidaemia with atypical antipsychotics is unknown

Notable Side Effects

- Dose-dependent sedation
- Akathisia
- Nausea
- Dose-dependent hyperprolactinaemia
- Rare tardive dyskinesia (much reduced risk compared to conventional antipsychotics)

Common or very common

- CNS/PNS: akathisia, anxiety, musculoskeletal stiffness, oculogyric crisis, psychiatric disorders, sleep disorders
- GIT: drooling, gastrointestinal discomfort, nausea, oral disorders
- Other: fatigue, pain

Uncommon

- Abnormal gait, blurred vision, decreased appetite, dysarthria, dysuria, hot flush, hyperhidrosis, hypertension, nasopharyngitis

Rare or very rare

- Eosinophilia, tardive dyskinesia

Frequency not known

- CNS: suicidal behaviour, vertigo
- Endocrine: dose-dependent hyperprolactinaemia (breast abnormalities, dysmenorrhea), diabetes and dyslipidaemia (however relatively better metabolic profile compared to others)
- Other: anaemia, angina pectoris, angioedema, dysphagia, pruritus, renal failure, Stevens-Johnson syndrome

 Life-Threatening or Dangerous Side Effects

- Tachycardia, first-degree AV block
- Hyperglycaemia, in some cases extreme and associated with ketoacidosis or hyperosmolar coma or death, has been reported in patients taking atypical antipsychotics
- Increased risk of death and cerebrovascular events in elderly patients with dementia-related psychosis

- Rare neuroleptic malignant syndrome (much reduced risk compared to conventional antipsychotics)
- Rare seizures

Weight Gain

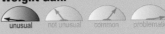

unusual   not unusual   common   problematic

Short Term
- Many experience about 0.5–1.0 kg weight gain greater than placebo in short-term 6-week trials

Long Term
- Patients in long-term 52-week trials actually lost about 0.5 kg on average
- However, clinical experience in UK is still limited
- Appears to be less weight gain than observed with some antipsychotics
- Many patients lost weight in long-term trials when switching from olanzapine to lurasidone

Sedation

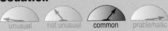

unusual   not unusual   common   problematic

- May be higher in short-term trials than in long-term use
- Dose dependent

What to Do About Side Effects

- Wait
- Wait
- Wait
- Reduce the dose
- Low-dose benzodiazepine or beta blocker may reduce akathisia
- Take more of the dose at night time (with evening meal) to help reduce daytime sedation
- Weight loss, exercise programmes, and medical management for high BMIs, diabetes, and dyslipidaemia
- Switch to another antipsychotic (atypical) – quetiapine or clozapine are best in cases of tardive dyskinesia

Best Augmenting Agents for Side Effects

- Dystonia: antimuscarinic drugs (e.g. procyclidine) as oral or IM depending on the severity; botulinum toxin if antimuscarinics not effective
- Parkinsonism: antimuscarinic drugs (e.g. procyclidine)

Lurasidone hydrochloride (Continued)

- Akathisia: beta blocker propranolol (30–80 mg/day) or low-dose benzodiazepine (e.g. 0.5–3.0 mg/day of clonazepam) may help; other agents that may be tried include the 5HT2 antagonists such as cyproheptadine (16 mg/day) or mirtazapine (15 mg at night – caution in bipolar disorder); clonidine (0.2–0.8 mg/day) may be tried if the above ineffective
- Tardive dyskinesia: stop any antimuscarinic, consider tetrabenazine

DOSING AND USE

Usual Dosage Range
- Schizophrenia: 37–148 mg/day
- Schizophrenia when given with moderate CYP450 3A4 inhibitors: 18.5–74 mg/day
- Bipolar depression (off-label use): 18.5–111 mg/day

Dosage Forms
- Tablet 18.5 mg, 37 mg, 74 mg

How to Dose
* Schizophrenia:
- Initial dose 37 mg/day with food
- Dose titration to initial dose is not required
- Consider dose increases up to 148 mg/day as necessary and as tolerated
- Where treatment has been interrupted for more than 3 days: for patients on doses less than 111 mg/day can restart on usual dose; for patients on doses higher than 111 mg/day should restart on 111 mg/day and then titrate up to usual dose
* Schizophrenia when given with moderate CYP450 3A4 inhibitors:
- Initial dose 18.5 mg/day (max per dose 74 mg/day)
* Bipolar depression (off-label use):
- Initial dose 18.5 mg/day with food
- Consider dose increases up to 111 mg/day as necessary and as tolerated

 Dosing Tips
- Lurasidone should be taken with food (at least a small meal of >350 calories). Absorption can be decreased by up to 50% on an empty stomach and more consistent efficacy will be seen if dosing is done regularly with food

- Should be swallowed whole without chewing or crushing
- Once-daily dosing
- Should be taken at the same time every day to aid concordance
- Giving lurasidone at bedtime can greatly reduce daytime sedation, akathisia, and EPS
- The starting dose may be an adequate dose for some patients with schizophrenia, especially first-episode and early-onset psychosis cases
- 37–74 mg/day was suggested by controlled clinical trials as adequate for many patients with schizophrenia
- Some patients benefit from higher dosing, with controlled clinical trials up to 148 mg/day
- Higher doses than 148 mg/day may benefit more difficult patients with treatment non-responsiveness to other agents
- Higher dosing, however, may cause more side effects
- Found to have higher rate of discontinuation than risperidone (64% compared to 52%) due to perceived ineffectiveness or adverse effects
- 18.5–55.5 mg/day may be adequate for many patients with bipolar depression

Overdose
- Limited data
- No specific antidote available, therefore, supportive measures including cardiovascular monitoring and support required
- Gastric lavage, administration of activated charcoal and a laxative may be required
- If antiarrhythmic administered, there is a risk of QT-prolongation
- Do not use adrenaline or dopamine
- Anticholinergics useful against severe extrapyramidal symptoms
- Seizures or dystonias may lead to aspiration

Long-Term Use
- Not extensively studied past 52 weeks, but long-term maintenance treatment is often necessary for schizophrenia
- Should periodically re-evaluate long-term usefulness in individual patients, but treatment may need to continue for many years in patients with schizophrenia

Habit Forming
- No

How to Stop

- Down-titration, especially when simultaneously beginning a new antipsychotic while switching (i.e. cross-titration)
- Rapid discontinuation could theoretically lead to rebound psychosis and worsening of symptoms. Withdrawal should always be gradual and closely monitored
- There is a high risk of relapse if medication is stopped after 1–2 years. After withdrawal of an antipsychotic, patients should be monitored for signs and symptoms of relapse for 2 years

Pharmacokinetics

- Reaches peak serum concentration in 1–3 hours
- Half-life 20–40 hours (shorter half-life better documented at the 40 mg dose)
- Metabolised by CYP450 3A4
- Lurasidone and its active metabolite ID-14283 both contribute to the pharmacodynamic effect at the dopaminergic and serotonergic receptors
- Cmax and bioavailability are reduced if taken without food

 Drug Interactions

- Inhibitors of CYP450 3A4 may increase plasma levels of lurasidone
- Co-administration with a strong CYP450 3A4 inhibitor (atazanavir, clarithromycin, cobicistat, darunavir, fosamprenavir, idelalisib, itraconazole, ketoconazole, lopinavir, ritonavir, saquinavir, tipranavir, voriconazole) including grapefruit juice is contraindicated
- Co-administration with moderate CYP450 3A4 inhibitors (fluvoxamine, fluoxetine, ketoconazole, aprepitant, crizotinib, diltiazem, dronedarone, erythromycin, fluconazole, imatinib, isavuconazole, netupitant, nilotinib, posaconazole, St John's wort, verapamil) can be considered; recommended starting dose is 18.5 mg/day; recommended maximum dose is 74 mg/day
- Inducers of CYP450 3A4 may decrease plasma levels of lurasidone
- Co-administration with a strong CYP450 3A4 inducer (e.g. fosphenytoin, mitotane, phenobarbital, phenytoin, primidone, rifampicin) is contraindicated
- Co-administration with moderate inducers of CYP450 3A4 (bosentan, carbamazepine, efavirenz, enzalutamide, nevirapine) may decrease plasma levels of lurasidone. Monitor and adjust dose
- May antagonise levodopa, dopamine agonists
- May increase effects of antihypertensive agents
- May have additive effect with CNS depressants
- Caution advised when prescribing with medicinal products known to prolong the QT interval – class IA and III antiarrhythmics, some antihistamines, some other antipsychotics and some antimalarials

 Other Warnings/Precautions

- All antipsychotics should be used with caution in patients with angle-closure glaucoma, blood disorders, cardiovascular disease, depression, diabetes, epilepsy and susceptibility to seizures, history of jaundice, myasthenia gravis, Parkinson's disease, photosensitivity, prostatic hypertrophy, severe respiratory disorders
- Use with caution in patients with conditions that predispose to hypotension (dehydration, overheating)
- Dysphagia has been associated with antipsychotic use, and lurasidone should be used cautiously in patients at risk for aspiration pneumonia
- Caution in elderly patients with dementia who have risk factors for stroke
- Caution in patients with Parkinson's disease – the benefits should outweigh the risks
- Caution in patients with a history of seizures or other conditions that potentially lower the seizure threshold
- Caution in those with a high risk of suicide
- Caution in patients with known cardiovascular disease or family history of QT prolongation, hypokalaemia, and in concomitant use with other medicinal products thought to prolong the QT interval
- Performance of skilled tasks (e.g. driving/operating machinery) may be affected by drowsiness especially at start of treatment; an enhancement of the effects of alcohol can occur

Lurasidone hydrochloride (Continued)

Do Not Use
- If patient is taking a strong CYP450 3A4 inhibitor or inducer
- If there is a proven allergy to lurasidone

Renal Impairment
- Use only if potential benefit outweighs risk if eGFR less than 15 mL/minute/1.73 m^2
- Initial dose 18.5 mg/day, up to max 74 mg/day if eGFR less than 50 mL/minute/1.73 m^2

Hepatic Impairment
- Moderate impairment (Child-Pugh Class B): initial dose 18.5 mg/day, up to max 74 mg/day
- Severe impairment (Child-Pugh Class C): use with caution – initial dose 18.5 mg/day, up to max 37 mg/day

Cardiac Impairment
- Should be used with caution because of theoretical risk of orthostatic hypotension, although low potency at alpha 1 receptors suggests this risk may be less than for some other antipsychotics
- Caution if susceptibility to QT interval prolongation

Elderly
- In general, no dose adjustment is necessary for elderly patients
- However, some elderly patients may tolerate lower doses better and may have diminished renal function requiring lower doses
- Also, there should be caution with higher doses as there is limited data available
- Although atypical antipsychotics are commonly used for behavioural disturbances in dementia, no agent has been approved for treatment of elderly patients with dementia-related psychosis
- Elderly patients with dementia-related psychosis treated with atypical antipsychotics are at an increased risk of death compared to placebo, and also have an increased risk of cerebrovascular events

Children and Adolescents
- Schizophrenia (child 13–17 years): initial dose 37 mg/day, increased as needed up to 74 mg/day – should be prescribed by a specialist
- Schizophrenia [when given with moderate CYP450 3A4 inhibitors such as diltiazem, erythromycin, fluconazole, verapamil] (child 13–17 years): initial dose 18.5 mg/day (max per dose 74 mg once daily), treatment should be prescribed by a specialist
- Lurasidone is also approved in several other countries for use in schizophrenia and has some of the best long-term (up to 2 years) data in children and adolescents for any atypical antipsychotic

Pregnancy
- Controlled studies have not been conducted in pregnant women
- Animal studies do not show adverse effects but data is limited
- There is a risk of abnormal muscle movements and withdrawal symptoms in newborns whose mothers took an antipsychotic during the third trimester; symptoms may include agitation, abnormally increased or decreased muscle tone, tremor, sleepiness, severe difficulty breathing, and difficulty feeding
- Psychotic symptoms may worsen during pregnancy and some form of treatment may be necessary
- Use in pregnancy may be justified if the benefit of continued treatment exceeds any associated risk
- Switching antipsychotics may increase the risk of relapse
- Antipsychotics may be preferable to anticonvulsant mood stabilisers if treatment is required for mania during pregnancy
- Olanzapine and clozapine have been associated with maternal hyperglycaemia which may lead to developmental toxicity; risk may also apply for other atypical antipsychotics

Breastfeeding
- Unknown if lurasidone is secreted in human breast milk, but all psychotropics assumed to be secreted in breast milk

- Risk of accumulation in infant due to long half-life
- Haloperidol is considered to be the preferred first-generation antipsychotic, and quetiapine the preferred second-generation antipsychotic
- Infants of women who choose to breastfeed should be monitored for possible adverse effects

THE ART OF PSYCHOPHARMACOLOGY

Potential Advantages

- Patients requiring rapid onset of antipsychotic action without dosage titration
- Patients who wish to take an antipsychotic once a day
- Patients experiencing weight gain from other antipsychotics or who wish to avoid weight gain

Potential Disadvantages

- Patients who cannot take a medication consistently with food

Primary Target Symptoms

- Positive symptoms of psychosis
- Negative symptoms of psychosis
- Cognitive symptoms
- Unstable mood (both depression and mania)
- Aggressive symptoms

Pearls

- Clinical trials suggest that lurasidone is well tolerated with a favourable balance of efficacy and safety
- One of the few "metabolically friendly" antipsychotics
- Neutral for weight gain (1–2 pounds weight gain in short-term studies, with 1–2 pounds weight loss in long-term studies)
- Neutral for lipids (triglycerides and cholesterol)
- Neutral for glucose
- Only atypical antipsychotic documented not to cause QTc prolongation, and one of the few atypical antipsychotics without a QTc warning
- Seems to have low-level EPS, especially when dosed at bedtime

- Somnolence and akathisia are the most common side effects in short-term clinical trials of schizophrenia that dosed lurasidone in the daytime, but these adverse effects were reduced in a controlled study of lurasidone administered at night with food
- Nausea and occasional vomiting occurred in bipolar depression studies especially at higher doses
- Nausea and vomiting generally rapidly abates within a few days or can be avoided by slow dose titration and giving lower doses
- Prolactin elevations low and generally transient
- Agitation experienced by some patients
- Receptor binding profile suggests favourable potential as an antidepressant
- 5HT7 antagonism is antidepressant in animal models and has pro-cognitive actions in animal models
- 5HT7 antagonism and 5HT1A partial agonism enhance serotonin levels in animals treated with SSRIs/SNRIs, suggesting use for lurasidone as an augmenting agent to SSRIs/SNRIs in depression
- 5HT7 antagonism plus the absence of D1, H1, and M1 antagonism suggest potential for cognitive improvement
- Lack of D1 antagonist, anticholinergic, and antihistamine properties may explain relative lack of cognitive side effects in most patients
- One of the best-studied agents for depression with mixed features, showing efficacy in a large randomised controlled trial
- Not approved for mania, but almost all atypical antipsychotics approved for acute treatment of schizophrenia have proven effective in the acute treatment of mania as well
- Patients with inadequate responses to atypical antipsychotics may benefit from determination of plasma drug levels and, if low, a dosage increase even beyond the usual prescribing limits
- Patients with inadequate responses to atypical antipsychotics may also benefit from a trial of augmentation with a conventional antipsychotic or switching to a conventional antipsychotic
- However, long-term polypharmacy with a combination of a conventional antipsychotic with an atypical antipsychotic may combine

Lurasidone hydrochloride (Continued)

their side effects without clearly augmenting the efficacy of either
- For treatment-resistant patients, especially those with impulsivity, aggression, violence, and self-harm, long-term polypharmacy with 2 atypical antipsychotics or with 1 atypical antipsychotic and 1 conventional antipsychotic may be useful or even necessary while closely monitoring

- In such cases, it may be beneficial to combine 1 depot antipsychotic with 1 oral antipsychotic
- Lurasidone is approved in several countries for use in schizophrenia and has some of the best long-term (up to 2 years) data in children and adolescents for any atypical antipsychotic

THE ART OF SWITCHING

 Switching from Oral Antipsychotics to Lurasidone
- With aripiprazole, amisulpride, and paliperidone, immediate stop is possible; begin lurasidone at an intermediate dose
- Clinical experience has shown that quetiapine, olanzapine, and asenapine should be tapered off slowly over a period of 3–4 weeks, to allow patients to readapt to the withdrawal of blocking cholinergic, histaminergic, and alpha 1 receptors
- Clozapine should always be tapered off slowly, over a period of 4 weeks or more
∗Benzodiazepine or anticholinergic medication can be administered during cross-titration to help alleviate side effects such as insomnia, agitation, and/or psychosis

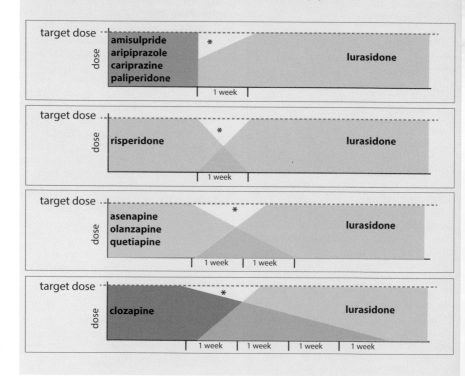

Suggested Reading

Arango C, Ng-Mak D, Finn E, et al. Lurasidone compared to other atypical antipsychotic monotherapies for adolescent schizophrenia: a systematic literature review and network meta-analysis. Eur Child Adolesc Psychiatry 2020;29(9):1195–205.

Citrome L, Cucchiaro J, Kaushnik S, et al. Long-term safety and tolerability of lurasidone in schizophrenia; a 12-month, double-blind, active-controlled study. Int Clin Psychopharmacol 2012;27(3):165–76.

Huhn M, Nikolakopoulou A, Schneider-Thoma J, et al. Comparative efficacy and tolerability of 32 oral antipsychotics for the acute treatment of adults with multi-episode schizophrenia: a systematic review and network meta-analysis. Lancet 2019;394(10202):939–51.

Leucht S, Cipriani A, Spineli L, et al. Comparative efficacy and tolerability of 15 antipsychotic drugs in schizophrenia: a multiple-treatments meta-analysis. Lancet 2013;382(9896):951–62.

Loebel A, Cucchiaro J, Xu J, et al. Effectiveness of lurasidone vs. quetiapine XR for relapse prevention in schizophrenia: a 12-month, double-blind, noninferiority study. Schizophr Res 2013;147(1):95–102.

McEvoy JP, Citrome L, Hernandez D, et al. Effectiveness of lurasidone in patients with schizophrenia or schizoaffective disorder switched from other antipsychotics: a randomized, six week, open-label study. J Clin Psychiatry 2013;74(2):170–9.

Nasrallah HA, Cucchiaro JB, Mao Y, et al. Lurasidone for the treatment of depressive symptoms in schizophrenia: analysis of four pooled, six week, placebo-controlled studies. CNS Spectr 2015;20(2):140–7.

Osborne IJ, Mace S, Taylor D. A prospective year-long follow-up of lurasidone use in clinical practice: factors predicting treatment persistence. Ther Adv Psychopharmacol 2018;8(4):117–25.

Ostacher M, Ng-Mak D, Patel P, et al. Lurasidone compared to other atypical antipsychotic monotherapies for bipolar depression: a systematic review and network meta-analysis. World J Biol Psychiatry 2018;19(8):586–601.

Pillinger T, McCutcheon RA, Vano L, et al. Comparative effects of 18 antipsychotics on metabolic function in patients with schizophrenia, predictors of metabolic dysregulation, and association with psychopathology: a systematic review and network meta-analysis. Lancet Psychiatry 2020;7(1):64–77.

Suppes T, Silva R, Cucchiaro J, et al. Lurasidone for the treatment of major depressive disorder with mixed features: a randomized, double-blind, placebo-controlled study. Am J Psychiatry 2016;173(4):400–7.

Wang H, Xiao L, Wang H-L, et al. Efficacy and safety of lurasidone versus placebo as adjunctive to mood stabilizers in bipolar I depression: a meta-analysis. J Affect Disord 2020;264:227–33.

Melatonin

Brands
- Vespro Melatonin
- Ceyesto
- Syncordin
- Slenyto
- Circadin

Generic?
Yes

Class
- Neuroscience-based nomenclature: pharmacology domain – melatonin; mode of action – agonist
- Hormone; hypnotic; melatonin receptor agonist

Commonly Prescribed for
(bold for BNF indication)
- **Insomnia in adults >55 years (short-term use)**
- **Jet lag (short-term use)**
- **Sleep onset insomnia in children (unlicensed use initiated under specialist supervision)**
- **Delayed sleep phase syndrome in children (unlicensed use initiated under specialist supervision)**
- **Insomnia in patients with learning disabilities – where sleep hygiene measures have been insufficient (unlicensed use initiated under specialist supervision)**
- **Insomnia in adolescents and children with autism and ADHD (where sleep hygiene measures have been insufficient)**
- Parasomnias
- Tardive dyskinesia
- Antipsychotic-induced weight gain

How the Drug Works
- Melatonin is a natural hormone which is produced by the pineal gland in the brain
- The secretion of melatonin is under control of the suprachiasmatic nucleus (SCN) in the hypothalamus in a negative feedback manner. The SCN is the circadian pacemaker
- Physiologically the SCN triggers the pineal gland to synthesise and secrete melatonin soon after darkness
- Melatonin levels peak at 2–4 am and then decline throughout the rest of the night

- Melatonin has direct sleep-facilitating and phase-shifting effects (shifts biological clock) within the brain
- Exogenous melatonin promotes sleep onset. It does this by acting at MT1 and MT2 receptors which are involved in the regulation of circadian rhythms and sleep regulation
- Overall, when administered, it works to decrease sleep latency in individuals with a primary sleep disorder

How Long Until It Works
- Licensed for up to 13 weeks use in adults > 55 years for the treatment of insomnia, however it should only be used in the short term
- Positive effects should be seen by at least 3 weeks in adults with insomnia

If It Works
- Continue at minimal effective dose for a maximum of 13 weeks

If It Doesn't Work
- If not working increase the dose up to a max of 12 mg
- If still not working discontinue melatonin
- Consider other factors that may interfere with sleep such as other prescribed medications, drug and alcohol use, physical causes such as pain, restless leg syndrome, sleep apnoea
- Give sleep hygiene advice and offer behavioural interventions
- Consider short course of benzodiazepines if not tried already

Best Augmenting Combos for Partial Response or Treatment Resistance
- Melatonin is used as an adjunct therapy when discontinuing benzodiazepines in adults
- If the patient does not respond to melatonin it should be discontinued
- Refer to specialist services and offer CBT and sleep hygiene advice such as:
  - The environment should be conducive to sleep; sleep in cool, dark and comfortable environment
  - Establish bedtime routine; relax before bedtime and sleep and wake at the same time each day
  - Regular exercise (not before bedtime), exposure to sunlight

- Only stay in bed when sleeping
- Avoid caffeine late in the day
- Reduce screen-time in evening or switch on night-mode
- Avoid smoking and excessive alcohol
- Avoid napping during the day

Tests

- Review efficacy of melatonin after 3 weeks of therapy
- Although unlikely, monitor patient for significant adverse drug reactions throughout therapy
- After a maximum of 13 weeks discontinue and trial sleep without melatonin

SIDE EFFECTS

How Drug Causes Side Effects

- MT1 receptors are expressed in the SCN, hippocampus, substantia nigra, cerebellum, central dopaminergic pathways, ventral tegmental area and nucleus accumbens
- MT1 is also expressed in the retina, ovary, testis, mammary gland, coronary circulation and aorta, gallbladder, liver, kidney, skin and the immune system
- MT2 receptors are expressed mainly in the CNS, also in the lung, cardiac, coronary and aortic tissue, myometrium and granulosa cells, immune cells, duodenum and adipocytes
- Activity in sites other than the pineal gland may lead to the manifestation of CNS, abdominal, cardiac and immune-related side effects

Notable Side Effects

- Headache
- Drowsiness
- Loss of concentration

Common or very common

- Arthralgia, headaches, increased risk of infection, pain

Uncommon

- CNS/PNS: altered mood, anxiety, dizziness, drowsiness, movement disorders, sleep disorders
- CVS: chest pain, hypertension
- GIT: dry mouth, gastrointestinal discomfort, hyperbilirubinaemia, nausea, oral disorders, weight increase
- Other: asthenia, menopausal symptoms, night sweats, skin reactions, urine abnormalities

Rare or very rare

- Blood disorders: leucopenia, thrombocytopenia
- CNS/PNS: aggression, crying, depression, disorientation, excessive tearing, impaired concentration, memory loss, paraesthesia, partial complex seizure, vertigo, vision disorders
- CVS: angina pectoris, palpitations, syncope
- GIT: gastrointestinal disorders, thirst, vomiting
- Other: arthritis, electrolyte imbalance, haematuria, hot flush, hypertriglyceridaemia, muscle complaints, nail disorder, prostatitis, sexual dysfunction, urinary disorders

 Life-Threatening or Dangerous Side Effects

- Drowsiness and loss of concentration: melatonin may make the patient sleepy, increase reaction times and reduce concentration
- These effects can be present in the first few days of treatment or all throughout the treatment
- The patient should not drive or use tools or machines to avoid injury to self and others until these side effects have worn off
- Patients should also avoid alcohol during treatment with melatonin as alcohol can enhance the drowsiness and loss of concentration experienced

Weight Gain

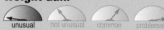
unusual | not unusual | common | problematic

- Reported but not expected

Sedation

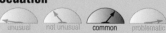
unusual | not unusual | common | problematic

- Many experience and/or can be significant in amount
- May experience sedation or sleepiness immediately after dosing, but not commonly after awakening from a night's sleep

What To Do About Side Effects

- Wait
- Lower the dose
- Switch to another hypnotic
- Refer to specialist service

Best Augmenting Agents for Side Effects

- Many side effects cannot be improved with an augmenting agent
- Encourage optimal sleep hygiene and CBT alongside melatonin treatment as this can lead to smaller doses being required

DOSING AND USE

Usual Dosage Range

- 2–12 mg/day

Dosage Forms

- Tablet 0.5 mg, 1 mg, 3 mg, 5 mg (import from USA)
- Tablet (modified-release) 1 mg, 2 mg, 3 mg, 5 mg
- Oral solution 1 mg/mL

How to Dose

Adults:

* For the treatment of insomnia in adults >55 yrs:
  - Modified-release tablet: 2 mg/day for up to 13 weeks, dose to be taken 1–2 hours before bedtime

* Jet lag (short-term use):
  - Immediate-release medicine: 3 mg/day, increased as required to 6 mg/day for up to 5 days, first dose should be taken at the habitual bedtime after arrival at destination. Doses should not be taken before 8 pm or after 4 am. Maximum of 16 treatment courses per year

* Insomnia in patients with learning disabilities – where sleep hygiene measures have been insufficient (unlicensed use initiated under specialist supervision):
  - Modified-release tablet: initial dose 2 mg/day, increased as required to 4–6 mg/day, dose to be taken 30–60 minutes before bedtime; max 10 mg/day

Children and adolescents:

* Insomnia:
  - 2 mg before bedtime for 1–2 weeks, increased as required to 4–6 mg/day; max 10 mg/day

Dosing Tips

- Dose can be increased steadily depending on response

- However additional benefit of doses above 6–9 mg uncertain
- If immediate-release form needed to reduce sleep latency, then licensed modified-release tablets can be opened and mixed with oral drink to be taken 1 hour before bedtime
- This is preferred to trying to obtain unlicensed oral solutions over the counter with unknown quantities of active ingredient
- Some patients may benefit from a mixture of both immediate-release and modified-release to help with reducing sleep latency and reducing night time waking respectively

Overdose

- Overdose uncommon and severe toxicity in overdose not yet reported
- Acute overdose may result in asthenia, confusion, dizziness, drowsiness, hallucinations, headache, lethargy, nightmares, slurred speech, tremors
- Plasma concentrations are not clinically useful in melatonin overdose
- Patient should be offered supportive treatment; vital signs and mental status should also be monitored
- Consider the possibility of multi-drug overdose

Long-Term Use

- Patients should be maintained on the lowest effective dose
- Can be used for a maximum of 13 weeks
- After 13 weeks patients should be trialled without melatonin
- For jet lag – maximum of 16 treatment courses per year

Habit Forming

- Unlike benzodiazepines, melatonin use carries a low risk of dependence, habituation and hangover effects

How to Stop

- Patients should taper off melatonin for 1–2 weeks depending on how high their maintenance dose is as a precaution
- Melatonin may very rarely cause short-term rebound insomnia
- A small percentage of patients may also experience withdrawal symptoms after high doses

Pharmacokinetics

Absorption:
- Oral melatonin is completely absorbed in adults, however decreased by as much as 50% in the elderly
- The kinetics of melatonin are linear over 2–8 mg
- Bioavailability is 15% as there is a significant first-pass effect (85%)
- The intake of food with immediate-release melatonin may increase the bioavailability of melatonin. In contrast, licensed immediate-release formulations should be taken on an empty stomach, 2 hours before or 2 hours after food – intake with carbohydrate-rich meals may impair blood glucose control

Distribution:
- Melatonin binds to albumin, alpha1-acid glycoprotein and high-density lipoprotein in the plasma

Biotransformation:
- CYP450 1A1, CYP450 1A2 and CYP450 2C19 systems are involved in metabolising melatonin in the liver
- The main metabolite of melatonin is the inactive 6-sulphatoxy-melatonin (6-S-MT)
- 6-S-MT is excreted completely within 12 hours of melatonin ingestion

Elimination:
- Plasma elimination half-life of immediate-release melatonin is about 45 minutes (range 30–60 minutes)
- Elimination of the inactive metabolite occurs via renal excretion
- About 1–2% is excreted as melatonin unchanged

 Drug Interactions

- Melatonin is mainly metabolised by the CYP450 1A family of enzymes. In addition to this it is also metabolised by CYP450 2C19. Drugs which affect the activity of these enzymes can therefore interfere with plasma levels of melatonin
- Anticoagulants and anti-platelet drugs: melatonin may slow blood clotting. Care should be taken when prescribing melatonin with medications that slow clotting as this may increase the risk of bruising and bleeding
- Anticonvulsants: melatonin may increase the frequency of seizures in some individuals, particularly children with a background of neuropsychiatric disorder
- Antidepressants: fluvoxamine increases melatonin levels by up to 17-fold by inhibiting CYP450 1A2 and CYP450 2C19 liver enzymes. This combination of medications should be avoided
- Antihypertensives: melatonin may make blood pressure worse in patients who are already taking antihypertensive medication, in particular nifedipine and other calcium channel blockers. Monitor blood pressure control when combining these drugs
- Oral contraceptive drugs: oral contraceptives are CYP450 1A2 enzyme inhibitors and may lead to increased plasma levels of melatonin. Be cautious when combining these drugs
- Diabetes medications: melatonin may directly affect blood sugar levels and impact the effectiveness of diabetes medications. Blood sugars should be monitored closely when combining melatonin with diabetes medications
- Immunosuppressants: melatonin may increase a patient's susceptibility to infection, care should be taken when prescribing melatonin to patients already on potentially immunosuppressive therapy
- Sedatives: melatonin may also enhance the sedative effects of benzodiazepines and other non-benzodiazepine hypnotics. They should not be concurrently prescribed
- Cigarette smoking may decrease melatonin levels due to induction of CYP450 1A2

 Other Warnings/Precautions

- Melatonin may cause drowsiness therefore care should be taken if driving or operating heavy machinery during the day
- Circadin contains lactose, patients with problems of galactose intolerance should not take this medicine
- When melatonin is prescribed a licensed preparation is preferred to an unlicensed preparation; the latter may be food supplements of uncertain quantity

Do Not Use
- In patients with autoimmune disorders
- If there is a proven allergy to melatonin

Renal Impairment
• Use with caution

Hepatic Impairment
• Avoid as clearance is reduced

Elderly
• Melatonin metabolism declines with age
• Elderly patients may benefit from smaller starting doses of melatonin
• When a hypnotic is indicated in patients over 55 years melatonin is a good option

Children and Adolescents

Before you prescribe:
• Sleep patterns change significantly during development. Careful assessment of history, expectations from child and parent, and exploration of possible causes are always required
• Sleep disturbance is often secondary to other issues such as psychiatric disorders, neurodevelopmental conditions (e.g. attention deficit hyperactivity disorder) or other psychiatric disorders (e.g. anxiety, depression), substance use physical disorders, or distress, lack of structure in family environment. Primary causes should be addressed first and concurrently
• Sleep hygiene and behavioural measures should be attempted first (see above) and continued when prescribing

Practical notes:
• Carefully weigh the risks and benefits of pharmacological treatment against the risks and benefits of non-treatment and make sure to document this in the patient's chart
• If it does not work: review child's/young person's profile, consider new/changing contributing individual or systemic factors such as peer or family conflict. Consider dose adjustment before switching or augmentation. Be vigilant of polypharmacy especially in complex and highly vulnerable children/adolescents
• Consider non-concordance by parent or child/adolescent, address underlying reasons for non-concordance
• Melatonin 2 mg should be prescribed. This is off-licence use

• If 2 mg is ineffective the dose can be sequentially increased. Continue medication at minimum effective dose
• Children and adolescents who cannot swallow tablets can be given crushed melatonin tablets mixed with water (becomes immediate-release). This is also off-licence
• 0.5 mg = physiological dose of melatonin in the blood for children and adolescents. Evidence suggests that a dose range of 1–10 mg is safe and effective
• Re-evaluate the need for continued treatment regularly
• If ineffective then discontinue melatonin
• Provide Medicines for Children leaflet: Melatonin for sleep disorders

Pregnancy
• Controlled studies have not been conducted in pregnant women
• Evidence from animal studies suggests possible foetal toxicity
• Not generally recommended in pregnancy
• If melatonin is used synthetic melatonin should be chosen as animal-derived products may pose infection risk

Breastfeeding
• Endogenous melatonin excreted in mother's breast milk therefore likely that exogenous melatonin also secreted
• Effects of increased levels due to exogenous melatonin unknown
• Not generally recommended for use in breastfeeding mothers
• Mothers taking hypnotics should be warned about the risks of co-sleeping

Potential Advantages
• Modified-release melatonin improves sleep onset latency and quality in patients over 55 years
• Melatonin reduces long sleep latency in children with sleep onset insomnia or delayed sleep phase syndrome, with autism or Smith-Magenis syndrome
• Melatonin has low risk of dependence, habituation and hangover effect, unlike benzodiazepines
• For circadian rhythm disturbances

Potential Disadvantages

- It is unknown whether improvement in insomnia lasts after treatment is stopped
- Currently the use of melatonin in children and adolescents is unlicensed
- The long-term effects of melatonin use in children are unknown

Primary Target Symptoms

- Sleep onset latency
- Sleep maintenance
- Early waking

Pearls

- NICE Guidelines recommend medication for insomnia only as a second-line treatment after non-pharmacological treatment options have been tried (e.g. cognitive behavioural therapy for insomnia)
- Improving sleep hygiene should be considered first before prescribing for insomnia
- Melatonin can act as an alternative hypnotic for adults with insomnia that are over the age of 55 years
- Melatonin is less likely to have hangover effects
- Can act by promoting the proper maintenance of circadian rhythms underlying a normal sleep-wake cycle
- Most adverse effects can likely be easily managed by dosing in accordance with natural circadian rhythms
- Melatonin does not cause dependency
- Lack of action on GABA systems may be related to lack of abuse potential
- Rebound insomnia not common
- Although use is off-label for children and adolescents, its short-term use under specialist supervision can be helpful in many cases

 Suggested Reading

Abad VC, Guilleminault C. Insomnia in elderly patients: recommendations for pharmacological management. Drugs Aging 2018;35(9):791–817.

Esposito S, Laino D, D'Alonzo R, et al. Pediatric sleep disturbances and treatment with melatonin. J Transl Med 2019;17(1):77.

Malow BA, Findling RL, Schroder CM, et al. Sleep, growth, and puberty after 2 years of prolonged-release melatonin in children with autism spectrum disorder. J Am Acad Child Adolesc Psychiatry 2021;60(2):252-61.e3.

Tordjman S, Chokron S, Delorme R, et al. Melatonin: pharmacology, functions and therapeutic benefits. Curr Neuropharmacol 2017;15(3):434–43.

Zisapel N. New perspectives on the role of melatonin in human sleep, circadian rhythms and their regulation. Br J Pharmacol 2018;175(16):3190–9.

Memantine hydrochloride

Brands
- Ebixa
- Marixino
- Valios

Generic?
Yes

Class
- Neuroscience-based nomenclature: pharmacology domain – glutamate; mode of action – antagonist (NMDA)
- NMDA receptor antagonist; N-methyl-d-aspartate (NMDA) subtype of glutamate receptor antagonist; cognitive enhancer

Commonly Prescribed for
(bold for BNF indication)
- **Moderate-severe Alzheimer's disease**
- **Oscillopsia in multiple sclerosis (unlicensed)**
- Parkinson's disease dementia and dementia with Lewy bodies (known together as Lewy body dementias)
- Mixed dementia

How the Drug Works
* Low to moderate affinity non-competitive antagonist at NMDA receptors; binds preferentially to the open NMDA receptor-operated cation channels
- NMDA receptors are thought to be persistently activated in Alzheimer's disease by the excessive release of glutamate, and memantine most likely works by interfering with this process

How Long Until It Works
- Memory improvement is not expected and it may take months before any stabilisation in degenerative course is evident

If It Works
- May slow progression of disease, but does not reverse the degenerative process

If It Doesn't Work
- Consider adjusting dose, switching to a cholinesterase inhibitor, or adding a cholinesterase inhibitor

- Reconsider diagnosis and rule out other conditions such as depression or a dementia other than Alzheimer's disease

Best Augmenting Combos for Partial Response or Treatment Resistance
* May be combined with cholinesterase inhibitors, and there is weak evidence to suggest that combination therapy is superior in moderate to severe Alzheimer's disease
* Atypical antipsychotics should only be used for severe aggression or psychosis when this is causing significant distress
- Careful consideration needs to be undertaken of co-morbid conditions and the benefits and risks of treatment in view of the increased risk of stroke and death with antipsychotic drugs in dementia
* Antidepressants if concomitant depression, apathy, or lack of interest, however efficacy may be limited

Tests
- No baseline or monitoring investigations required

How Drug Causes Side Effects
- Presumably due to excessive NMDA receptor antagonism

Notable Side Effects
- Dizziness, headache
- Constipation

Common or very common
- CNS: dizziness, drowsiness, headache, impaired balance
- Other: constipation, dyspnoea, hypersensitivity, hypertension

Uncommon
- CNS: confusion, hallucination
- CVS: embolism and thrombosis, heart failure
- GIT: vomiting
- Other: fatigue, fungal infection

Rare or very rare
- Seizures

Memantine hydrochloride (Continued)

Frequency not known
- Hepatitis, pancreatitis, psychosis

 Life-Threatening or Dangerous Side Effects
- Thromboembolism (uncommon)
- Heart failure (uncommon)
- Seizures (rare)

Weight gain

unusual / not unusual / common / problematic
- Reported but not expected

Sedation

unusual / not unusual / common / problematic
- Reported but not expected
- Fatigue may occur

What to Do About Side Effects
- Wait
- Wait
- Wait
- Consider lowering dose or switching to a different agent

Best Augmenting Agents for Side Effects
- Many side effects cannot be improved with an augmenting agent

DOSING AND USE

Usual Dosage Range
- Moderate-severe Alzheimer's disease: 10–20 mg/day

Dosage Forms
- Tablet 5 mg, 10 mg, 15 mg, 20 mg
- Orodispersible tablet 5 mg, 10 mg, 15 mg, 20 mg
- Oral solution 5 mg/0.5 mL, 10 mg/mL (50 ml, 100 mL bottle)

How to Dose
- Initial dose 5 mg/day; can increase by 5 mg each week; usual maintenance 20 mg/day; max 20 mg/day

 Dosing Tips
- Both patient and caregiver should be instructed on how to dose memantine since patients with moderate to severe dementia may require assistance
- *Memantine is unlikely to affect pharmacokinetics of acetylcholinesterase inhibitors
- Absorption not affected by food

Overdose
- No fatalities have been reported; restlessness, psychosis, visual hallucinations, sedation, stupor, loss of consciousness

Long-Term Use
- Drug may lose effectiveness in slowing degenerative course of Alzheimer's disease after 6 months

Habit Forming
- No

How to Stop
- No known withdrawal symptoms
- Theoretically, discontinuation could lead to notable deterioration in memory and behaviours which may not be restored when drug is restarted or a cholinesterase inhibitor is initiated

Pharmacokinetics
- Little metabolism; mostly excreted unchanged in the urine
- Terminal elimination half-life about 60–100 hours
- Minimal inhibition of CYP450 enzymes

 Drug Interactions
- No interactions with drugs metabolised by CYP450 enzymes
- Increased risk of CNS toxicity when memantine combined with amantadine; use with caution or avoid
- Memantine is predicted to increase the effects of dopamine receptor agonists (apomorphine, bromocriptine, cabergoline, pergolide, pramiprexole, quinaglide, ropinirole, rotigotine); use with caution
- Predicted to increase the effects of levodopa
- Avoid use with ketamine
- *No interactions with cholinesterase inhibitors

Other Warnings/Precautions

∗Increased risk of CNS toxicity if administered with other NMDA antagonists such as amantadine, ketamine, and dextromethorphan
• Use with caution in patients with epilepsy, history of convulsions, or with risk factors for epilepsy

Do Not Use

• If there is a proven allergy to memantine

SPECIAL POPULATIONS

Renal Impairment

• Avoid if eGFR less than 5 mL/minute/1.73 m^2
• Reduce dose to 10 mg/day if eGFR 5–49 mL/minute/1.73 m^2; if eGFR is 30–49 mL/minute/1.73 m^2 and the 10 mg dose is well tolerated after 7 days, then dosing may be incrementally increased back to 20 mg/day

Hepatic Impairment

• Avoid in severe impairment, otherwise not likely to require dosage adjustment in mild to moderate impairment

Cardiac Impairment

• Not likely to require dosage adjustment

Elderly

• Pharmacokinetics similar to younger adults

Children and Adolescents

• Memantine use has not been studied in children or adolescents

Pregnancy

• Controlled studies have not been conducted in pregnant women
• Animal studies do not show adverse effects
∗Not recommended for use in pregnant women or women of childbearing potential

Breastfeeding

• Unknown if memantine is secreted in human breast milk, but all psychotropics assumed to be secreted in breast milk

∗Recommended either to discontinue drug or bottle feed
• Memantine is not recommended for use in nursing women

THE ART OF PSYCHOPHARMACOLOGY

Potential Advantages

• In patients with more advanced Alzheimer's disease

Potential Disadvantages

• Unproven to be effective in mild Alzheimer's disease

Primary Target Symptoms

• Memory loss in Alzheimer's disease
• Behavioural symptoms in Alzheimer's disease
• Memory loss and behavioural symptoms in Lewy body dementias

Pearls

∗Memantine's actions are somewhat like the natural inhibition of NMDA receptors by magnesium, and thus memantine is a sort of "artificial magnesium"
• Theoretically, NMDA antagonism of memantine is strong enough to block chronic low-level overexcitation of glutamate receptors associated with Alzheimer's disease, but not strong enough to interfere with periodic high level utilisation of glutamate for plasticity, learning, and memory
• Structurally related to the antiparkinsonian and anti-influenza agent amantadine, which is also a weak NMDA antagonist
∗Memantine is well tolerated with a low incidence of adverse effects
• Antagonist actions at 5HT3 receptors have unknown clinical consequences but may contribute to low incidence of gastrointestinal side effects
• Treat the patient but ask the caregiver about efficacy
• Delay in progression of Alzheimer's disease is not evidence of disease-modifying actions of NMDA antagonism
• Not proven to be effective in vascular dementia

Memantine hydrochloride (Continued)

 Suggested Reading

Dudas R, Malouf R, McCleery J, et al. Antidepressants for treating depression in dementia. Cochrane Database Syst Rev 2018;8(8):CD003944.

Folch J, Busquets O, Ettcheto M, et al. Memantine for the treatment of dementia: a review on its current and future applications. J Alzheimers Dis 2018;62(3):1223–40.

McShane R, Westby MJ, Roberts E, et al. Memantine for dementia. Cochrane Database Syst Rev 2019;3(3):CD003154.

O'Brien JT, Holmes C, Jones M, et al. Clinical practice with anti-dementia drugs: a revised (third) consensus statement from the British Association for Psychopharmacology. J Psychopharmacol 2017;31(2):147–68.

Methadone hydrochloride

Brands

- Methadose
- Metharose
- Physeptone

Generic?

Yes

Class

- Neuroscience-based nomenclature: pharmacology domain – opioid; mode of action – agonist
- Opioid dependence adjunctive treatment; long-acting mu opioid receptor agonist; diphenylpropylamine derivative

Commonly Prescribed for

(bold for BNF indication)
- **Severe pain**
- **Adjunct in treatment of opioid dependence**
- **Cough in palliative care**
- **Neonatal opioid withdrawal**

 How the Drug Works

- Synthetic long-acting opioid analgesic that acts on the central nervous system and smooth muscles via the peripheral nervous system
- Primarily a mu-receptor agonist that may mimic endogenous opioids, thus providing analgesic properties
- It may also affect the release of other neurotransmitters, e.g. acetylcholine, noradrenaline and dopamine, which may account for its effects on respiratory rate, sedation, decrease in bowel motility and other autonomic effects

How Long Until It Works

- Analgesic effect occurs 10–20 minutes after intramuscular or subcutaneous injection, but there is a large amount of variation between individuals
- Effect can take 2–6 hours post oral dose (2–4 hours for first dose)
- It takes 4–5 days for methadone tissue and plasma levels to stabilise, but accumulation continues beyond this until a steady state is reached at 10 days
- Once a steady state is reached, variations in blood concentration levels are small

If It Works

- Treatment needs to be reviewed at every contact and re-examined formally every 3–4 months
- Any use of alcohol or drugs on top of methadone prescription needs to be monitored
- A drug screen needs to be taken frequently at the beginning of treatment and when the patient is stabilised, regularly (usually between 2–4 times a year) if continuing on to maintenance to confirm use of medication
- Positive screens for heroin and other drugs require a review of treatment and dose, but should not lead to cessation of treatment or dose reduction

If It Doesn't Work

- Increase maintenance dose up to 120 mg if tolerated
- If not tolerated, consider alternative methods of treatment:
  - Buprenorphine, a semi-synthetic opioid with mixed agonist-antagonist properties; its primary action is as a partial opiate agonist
  - There is a small evidence base for dihydrocodeine in opioid dependency and it was used in the recent past, however it is not currently licensed for this purpose
  - Morphine sulfate, not licensed for the treatment of drug dependency in UK and should only be used by specialists and in rare circumstances; it is used elsewhere in Europe in patients who fail to tolerate or stabilise on methadone
  - Diamorphine, a pharmaceutical form of heroin, can be used in patients where all other treatment has failed

 Best Augmenting Combos for Partial Response or Treatment Resistance

- Levomethadyl acetate hydrochloride (LAAM, a mu-opioid agonist) may be used instead of methadone if treatment-resistant
- LAAM may potentially be more effective than methadone at reducing heroin use

Tests

- Regular drug screen: urine and oral fluid swab
- Baseline ECG and electrolytes, and subsequent annual ECG monitoring for increased risk of QT interval prolongation, especially in individuals with risk factors, e.g. known heart disease and doses of methadone exceeding 100 mg

SIDE EFFECTS

How Drug Causes Side Effects

- Effects may be cumulative due to methadone being a long-acting opioid
- It may also have effects on the release of other neurotransmitters

Notable Side Effects

- Methadone is a long-acting opioid thus effects may be cumulative
- Arrhythmias, palpitations
- Confusion, dizziness, headache, vertigo, visual impairment
- Euphoric mood, hallucination
- Constipation, nausea, vomiting
- Drowsiness, dry mouth, flushing, hyperhidrosis, hypotension (with high doses), miosis, vertigo, urinary retention
- Skin reactions

Frequency not known

- Altered mood, dry eye, dysuria, exacerbation of asthma, hyperprolactinaemia, hypothermia, menstrual cycle irregularities, nasal dryness, QTc prolongation
- Specific to oral use: galactorrhoea, increased intracranial pressure
- Specific to parenteral use: biliary spasm, muscle rigidity, neonatal withdrawal syndrome, oedema, restlessness, sexual dysfunction, sleep disorder, ureteral spasm

 Life-Threatening or Dangerous Side Effects

- Respiratory depression (with high doses)
- QT interval prolongation
- Risk of increased use of cocaine needs to be carefully surveyed by clinicians

Weight Gain

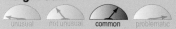

- Many experience and/or can be significant in amount

- More likely in women than men; may not be directly linked to methadone use but may represent disparity between levels of nutritional education

Sedation

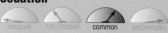

- Many experience and/or can be significant in amount
- Can be problematic if used concomitantly with other CNS depressants

What To Do About Side Effects

- Wait
- Adjust dose
- If side effects persist, consider reduction and switch to alternative treatment, e.g. buprenorphine

Best Augmenting Agents for Side Effects

- Dose reduction or switching to another agent may be more effective since most side effects cannot be improved with an augmenting agent

DOSING AND USE

Usual Dosage Range

- Adjunct in treatment of opioid dependence: 10–120 mg/day (oral solution)

Dosage Forms

- Solution for injection 10 mg/mL, 50 mg/mL
- Oral solution 1 mg/mL, 10 mg/mL, 20 mg/mL
- Tablet 5 mg (physeptone only, not licensed for the treatment of drug dependence)

How to Dose

See also The Art of Switching, after Pearls

- Starting dose should be low, usually in the form of an oral solution, at between 10–30 mg/day
- Dose depends on the amount of heroin, the length and method of use or other opioids being used due to the cumulative effect until steady state is reached
- The optimal daily dose is usually 60–120 mg, and the starting dose should be titrated slowly towards this
- Maximum increase of 5–10 mg/day, with a maximum of 30 mg increase each week for the first 2 weeks

- After the first 2 weeks, titration can be quicker
- Increases may be slower in those with a short history of dependence, young people, or unknown tolerance

 Dosing Tips

- Several missed doses may mean a loss of tolerance to opioids
- Three consecutive days missed should lead to a dose review and a possible reduction in dose
- Five consecutive days or more missed should lead to re-assessment and re-induction if there is likely to be a significant loss of tolerance
- Effective opioid maintenance doses provide important protection against overdose
- Doses between 60–120 mg may have effects for 24–36 hours, whereas low doses exert clinical effects for only a few hours
- Level of heroin use is not the only factor in determining the final dose of substitution that will be required due to differences in individual patients

Overdose

- Over 20% of all methadone deaths in treatment take place within 2 weeks of commencement of prescribing and most occur during sleep
- Risk of overdose is increased by low opioid tolerance, too high an initial dose, too rapid increases and concurrent use of other drugs, particularly alcohol, benzodiazepines and antidepressants
- Needs extensive monitoring after overdose due to long duration of action
- In the event of overdose, naloxone should be administered following BNF guidelines
- Naloxone is short-acting so its effect may reverse within 20 minutes to 1 hour, and so a patient can revert back into an overdose state

Long-Term Use

- Tolerance develops at a different speed in different individuals over time and develops differently for different effects
- With long-term use, neuro-adaptation occurs and involves changes in nerve and receptor function

Habit Forming

- Yes
- Methadone is a Class A/Schedule 2 drug

How to Stop

- Untreated methadone withdrawal typically reaches its peak between 4–6 days after last dose and symptoms do not substantially subside for 10–12 days
- The dose can be reduced at a rate to suit the patient
- Commonly, a reduction to zero takes 12 weeks and involves a reduction of 5 mg every 1–2 weeks
- It is important for patients to stay on their optimal dose until they have stopped using heroin completely and then reduce the dose at their own pace, which may take months or years
- There is little evidence to support slow detoxification regimes, but has been found effective in practice
- Careful monitoring of increased drug or alcohol use on top of medication is advisable during slower reductions
- Detoxification can improve a patient's confidence in their abilities to manage on lower opioid doses
- Lofexidine can be prescribed for the management of symptoms of opioid withdrawal
- Naltrexone is recommended as a treatment option in detoxified, formerly opioid-dependent people who want assistance to remain opioid-free, but it must be prescribed together with providing psychological support, including relapse prevention
- See Table 1 for drugs that may help to reduce symptoms observed in the end stages of detoxification

Pharmacokinetics

- The pharmacokinetic properties of methadone vary depending on the individual and their opioid-tolerance, as well as whether it is a single or maintenance dose
- The half-life of methadone in an opioid-tolerant patient is about 24 hours; the half-life in an opioid-naive patient is about 55 hours, which means there is a longer duration of effect in opioid-naive patients
- Methadone's long half-life means that its full analgesic effects may not be attained until after 3–5 days of use, and therefore

Table 1: Opioid withdrawal symptoms and their respective treatments

Symptom	Drug	Dose
Muscle cramps	Quinine sulfate	200–300 mg nocte
Gastrointestinal spasm/stomach cramps	Hyoscine butylbromide	10–20 mg QDS PRN
Diarrhoea	Loperamide hydrochloride	4 mg stat, then 2 mg after each loose stool
Nausea	Metoclopramide hydrochloride	10 mg TDS
Anxiety	Propranolol	10 mg PRN
Bone pain and headaches	Paracetamol	1 g QDS
	NSAIDs, e.g. ibuprofen	400 mg TDS after food
Sedation	Trazodone	100–150 mg nocte
	Diazepam	2–10 mg PRN day, 10 mg nocte for 3–5 days

the dose must be titrated more slowly than other opioids

- A single dose has a half-life of 12–18 hours, which stretches to 13–112 hours in the first few days
- Rapid onset of action
- Elimination half-life is normally 13–55 hours, but can range up to 91 hours for some individuals
- Optimal doses are usually between 24–36 hours
- Primarily metabolised by liver CYP450 3A4, 2B6 and 2D6
- Excretion: urine, faeces

 Drug Interactions

- CYP450 3A4 inhibitors, e.g. clarithromycin, idelalisib and anti-fungals (e.g. fluconazole) may increase methadone levels
- CYP450 3A4 inducers have been shown to decrease methadone levels, e.g. HIV medications (nevirapine, efavirenz), anti-epileptics (carbamazepine, phenytoin), St John's wort, bosentan, enzalutamide, mitotane, nalmefene, phenobarbital, primidone, rifampicin
- Drugs with a risk of QT interval prolongation may increase the same risk for methadone, e.g. SSRIs, tyrosine kinase inhibitors, anti-arrhythmics, beta blockers, D2 and 5-HT3 antagonists, antipsychotics (e.g. haloperidol, quetiapine)
- Drugs that may cause hypokalaemia could increase the risk of torsade de pointes if

given with methadone, e.g. steroids, loop and thiazide diuretics, beta blockers

- An increased risk of opiate withdrawal may be caused by buprenorphine and pentazocine
- Increased risk of CNS excitation or depression if given with isocarboxazid, phenelzine, tranylcypromine, benzodiazepines, alcohol
- Increased sedation and risk of overdose with antidepressants
- Cocaine is a common drug taken by polydrug users and increases the risk of cardiac rhythm abnormalities and overdose

 Other Warnings/Precautions

- Non-dependent adults are at risk of toxicity and dependent adults are at risk of tolerance if incorrectly assessed during induction
- Risk of fatal overdose is enhanced when methadone is taken concomitantly with alcohol and other respiratory depressant drugs
- Risk of QT prolongation in patients on doses above 100 mg/day as well as those with risk factors: history of cardiac conduction abnormalities, family history of sudden death, heart or liver disease, electrolyte abnormalities, concomitant medicines/drugs with increased risk of QT prolongation
- A reduced dose is recommended in adrenocortical insufficiency, elderly, debilitated patients, hypothyroidism

- Use with caution in patients with impaired respiratory function or central sleep apnoea
- Use with caution in patients with seizures
- Use with caution in patients with myasthenia gravis
- Use with caution in patients with current or a history of mental disorders or substance misuse
- Use with caution in patients with a disease of the biliary tracts, inflammatory or obstructive bowel disorders
- Take caution in patients with hypotension or shock
- Use with caution in patients with prostatic hypertrophy or urethral stenosis

Do Not Use
- In patients with acute respiratory depression
- In patients during an acute attack of asthma
- In patients with chronic obstructive pulmonary disease
- In patients with phaeochromocytoma
- In comatose patients
- In patients with head injury or raised intracranial pressure (due to interference with pupillary responses needed for assessment)
- In patients with risk of paralytic ileus
- If there is a proven allergy to methadone

Renal Impairment
- Avoid or reduce dose
- Effects are increased and prolonged in renal impairment, and increased cerebral sensitivity occurs
- Due to extended plasma half-life, the interval between assessments during initial dosing may need to be extended

Hepatic Impairment
- Avoid use or reduce dose
- May precipitate coma in patients with hepatic impairment
- Due to extended plasma half-life, the interval between assessments during initial dosing may need to be extended

Cardiac Impairment
- Caution and monitoring of ECG required due to increased risk of QT prolongation and precipitation of torsade de pointes, especially in patients with risk factors

Elderly
- Reduced dose recommended

 ## Children and Adolescents
- Not licensed for use in children, nevertheless indicated for use in neonatal opioid withdrawal
- Toxicity is a special hazard in children
- Methadone is not usually first-line treatment for heroin-using patients under the age of 18 as their drug use is often short-term and there tends to be less tolerance
- Detoxification, usually with buprenorphine, may be considered as first-line treatment and it is important that specialist young people services should be involved

 ## Pregnancy
- Pregnancy is not a contraindication under the UK MHRA licence
- Very limited data of methadone use in pregnancy
- Data confounded by possible underreporting of substance misuse
- Prolonged neonatal withdrawal has been reported following use of methadone during pregnancy
- Use of opioids during pregnancy, especially close to delivery, presents a risk of respiratory depression in the neonate
- Women dependent on opioids should be encouraged to use maintenance treatment
- Detoxification increases risk of relapse, but if requested is best managed in the second trimester (contraindicated during first trimester)
- Withdrawal during first trimester increases risk of spontaneous abortion
- Withdrawal during third trimester increases risk of foetal stress and stillbirth
- Metabolism may increase during the third trimester and require split dosing

Breastfeeding
- Small amounts found in mother's breast milk
- Infants of mothers taking methadone during pregnancy should breastfeed normally as methadone in the mother's milk may reduce risk of withdrawal symptoms

- Risk of withdrawal if the mother stops methadone suddenly or stops breastfeeding abruptly
- Infants of women who choose to breastfeed while on methadone should be monitored for possible adverse effects; the risk of adverse effects is higher in infants not exposed during pregnancy or when the mother is taking a high maintenance dose

THE ART OF PSYCHOPHARMACOLOGY

Potential Advantages

- Clinical effectiveness supported by extensive research
- Alleviates opioid withdrawal symptoms
- Oral use of methadone reduces risks associated with heroin injection
- Dosing can be carefully titrated to optimal level and blood levels kept stable, eliminating post-dose euphoria and pre-dose withdrawal
- High-dose methadone for those wishing to cease heroin use completely as blockade effects interfere with subjective effects of additional heroin use
- May be better than buprenorphine in treating those using high-dose heroin
- More suitable than buprenorphine for those with greater risk of diversion (previous history of diversion or treatment in prison)
- If relapse, lower mortality than buprenorphine

Potential Disadvantages

- Methadone can be abused
- Many patients report a "clouding" effect in the mind with methadone, compared to a "clear head" response with buprenorphine (whether this is an advantage or disadvantage depends on individual patients)
- The dry mouth caused by opiates can lead to poor oral health
- More interactions with enzyme inducers/inhibitors versus buprenorphine
- More sedating than buprenorphine

- Risks in overdose higher with methadone than buprenorphine

Primary Target Symptoms

- Targets opioid withdrawal symptoms
- Blocks effects of additional opioids
- Alleviates craving
- Can reduce the constant need to obtain illicit opioid drugs

Pearls

- Daily assessment by a pharmacist using supervised consumption is the best safeguard to prevent undetected over-sedation in a patient
- Methadone patients should be informed of the increasing effect of a dose as a steady state is achieved so that they do not excessively "top up" with street drugs
- During induction, psychological factors and psychiatric morbidity need to be taken into consideration on the premise that depression may contribute to suicidal ideation
- In patients with co-morbidity, good control of opioid dependence leads to stability and improvements in mental health
- For pain management in patients on methadone, non-opioid analgesics should be used in preference where appropriate
- If opioid analgesia is indicated due to the type and severity of pain, then this should be titrated accordingly for pain relief in line with usual analgesic protocols
- Titration of methadone dose to provide analgesia may be used in certain circumstances, but should only be carried out by experienced specialists

THE ART OF SWITCHING

 **Switching**

- Patients unable to reduce doses of methadone to <60 mg/day without becoming unstable cannot be easily transferred to buprenorphine without going into withdrawal

Suggested Reading

Anderson IB, Kearney TE. Use of methadone. West J Med 2000;172(1):43–6.

Brown R, Kraus C, Fleming M, et al. Methadone: applied pharmacology and use as adjunctive treatment in chronic pain. Postgrad Med J 2004;80(949):654–9.

Clark NC, Lintzeris N, Gijsbers A, et al. LAAM maintenance vs methadone maintenance for heroin dependence. Cochrane Database Syst Rev 2002;(2):CD002210.

Faggiano F, Vigna-Taglianti F, Versino E, et al. Methadone maintenance at different dosages for opioid dependence. Cochrane Database Syst Rev 2003;(3):CD002208.

Fenn JM, Laurent JS, Sigmon SC. Increases in body mass index following initiation of methadone treatment. J Subst Abuse Treat 2015;51:59–63.

Peles E, Schreiber S, Sason A, et al. Risk factors for weight gain during methadone maintenance treatment. Subst Abus 2016;37(4):613–18.

Methylphenidate hydrochloride

Brands

- Concerta XL
- Delmosart
- Equasym XL
- Medikinet
- Matoride
- Xaggitin XL
- Xenidate XL
- Ritalin
- Xenidate XL
- Tranquilyn

see index for additional brand names

Generic?

Yes

Class

- Neuroscience-based nomenclature: pharmacology domain – dopamine, norepinephrine; mode of action – multimodal
- Stimulant; noradrenaline reuptake inhibitor and releaser

Commonly Prescribed for

(bold for BNF indication)

- **Attention deficit hyperactivity disorder (ADHD) in children aged 6–17 years (initiated under specialist supervision)**
- **ADHD in adults (unlicensed use – initiated under specialist supervision)**
- **Narcolepsy (unlicensed use in adults)**

 ## How the Drug Works

* Increases noradrenaline and especially dopamine actions by blocking their reuptake
- Site of action is on cortico-basal ganglia loops
- PET studies have shown decreased binding of the dopamine 2 receptor radioligand [¹¹C]raclopride in the striatum with methylphenidate, suggesting it leads to increased release of dopamine in this brain region
- Increased positive blood-oxygen-level-dependent (BOLD) signal seen in the entorhinal cortex with functional magnetic resonance imaging (fMRI) studies
- Enhancement of dopamine and noradrenaline actions in certain brain regions (e.g. dorsolateral prefrontal cortex) may improve executive function and wakefulness
- Enhancement of dopamine actions in other brain regions (e.g. basal ganglia) may improve hyperactivity
- Enhancement of dopamine and noradrenaline in yet other brain regions (e.g. medial prefrontal cortex, hypothalamus) may improve depression, fatigue, and sleepiness

How Long Until It Works

- Some immediate effects can be seen with first dosing
- Can take several weeks to attain maximum therapeutic benefit

If It Works

- The goal of treatment of ADHD is reduction of symptoms of inattentiveness, motor hyperactivity, and/or impulsiveness that disrupt social, school, and/or occupational functioning
- Continue treatment until all symptoms are under control or improvement is stable and then continue treatment indefinitely as long as improvement persists
- Re-evaluate the need for treatment periodically
- Treatment for ADHD begun in childhood may need to be continued into adolescence and adulthood if continued benefit is documented

If It Doesn't Work

- Inform patient it may take several weeks for full effects to be seen
- Consider adjusting dose or switching to another formulation or another agent. It is important to consider if maximal dose has been achieved before deciding there has not been an effect and switching
- Consider behavioural therapy or cognitive behavioural therapy if appropriate – to address issues such as social skills with peers, problem-solving, self-control, active listening and dealing with and expressing emotions
- Consider the possibility of non-concordance and counsel patients and parents
- Consider evaluation for another diagnosis or for a co-morbid condition (e.g. bipolar disorder, substance abuse, medical illness, etc.)

- In children consider other important factors, such as ongoing conflicts, family psychopathology, adverse environment, for which alternative interventions might be more appropriate (e.g. social care referral, trauma-informed care)
- *Some ADHD patients and some depressed patients may experience lack of consistent efficacy due to activation of latent or underlying bipolar disorder, and require either augmenting with a mood stabiliser or switching to a mood stabiliser

Best Augmenting Combos for Partial Response or Treatment Resistance

- Best to attempt other monotherapies prior to augmenting
- For the expert, can combine immediate-release formulation with a sustained-release formulation for ADHD
- There is no evidence to support using antipsychotics for ADHD symptoms, but risperidone may help in reducing severe co-existent agitation or aggression, especially in patients with moderate learning disability
- There is no clear evidence to support use in combination with atomoxetine

Tests

- Before treatment, assess for presence of cardiac disease (history, family history, physical exam)
- Pulse, BP, appetite, weight, height, psychiatric symptoms should be recorded at initiation of therapy, following every dose change and every 6 months after that
- In children, pulse, BP, height and weight should be recorded on percentile charts; observe growth trajectory by plotting a graph
- Regular FBC and platelet counts may be considered during prolonged therapy (rare leucopenia and/or anaemia can be side effects of treatment)
- Monitor for appearance or worsening of anxiety, depression or tics

SIDE EFFECTS

How Drug Causes Side Effects

- Increases in noradrenaline peripherally can cause autonomic side effects, including tremor, tachycardia, hypertension, and cardiac arrhythmias

- Increases in noradrenaline and dopamine centrally can cause CNS side effects such as insomnia, agitation, psychosis, and substance abuse

Notable Side Effects

- *Insomnia, headache, exacerbation of tics, nervousness, irritability, overstimulation, tremor, dizziness
- Anorexia, nausea, abdominal pain, weight loss
- Can temporarily slow normal growth in children (controversial)
- Blurred vision

Common or very common

- CNS/PNS: abnormal behaviour, altered mood, anxiety, depression, dizziness, drowsiness, headaches, movement disorders, sleep disorders
- CVS: arrhythmias, hypertension, palpitations
- GIT: decreased appetite, decreased weight, diarrhoea, dry mouth, gastrointestinal discomfort, nausea, vomiting
- Other: alopecia, arthralgia, cough, fever, growth retardation (in children), laryngeal pain, nasopharyngitis

Uncommon

- CNS/PNS: hallucinations, psychotic disorder, suicidal tendencies, tic, tremor, vision disorders
- CVS: chest discomfort
- Other: constipation, dyspnoea, fatigue, haematuria, muscle complaint

Rare or very rare

- CNS/PNS: abnormal thinking, cerebrovascular insufficiency, confusion, hyperfocus, seizures
- CVS: angina pectoris, cardiac arrest, myocardial infarction, sudden cardiac death
- GIT: hepatic coma
- Other: anaemia, gynaecomastia, hyperhidrosis, leucopenia, mydriasis, neuroleptic malignant syndrome, peripheral coldness, Raynaud's phenomenon, sexual dysfunction, skin reactions, thrombocytopenia

Frequency not known

- Blood disorders: pancytopenia
- *CNS: delusions, drug dependence, intracranial haemorrhage, logorrhoea
- Other: hyperpyrexia, vasculitis

Life-Threatening or Dangerous Side Effects

∗Rare priapism
- Psychosis
- Seizures
- Rare neuroleptic malignant syndrome
- Sudden death in those with pre-existing cardiac structural abnormalities

What To Do About Side Effects

- Wait
- Can usually be managed by symptomatic management and/or dose reduction
- If lack of appetite and weight is a clinical concern suggest taking medication with or after food and offer high calorie food or snacks early morning or late evening when stimulant effects have worn off
- If child or young person on ADHD medication shows persistent resting heart rate >120 bpm, arrhythmia, or systolic BP (measured on 2 occasions) with clinically significant increase or >95th percentile, then reduce medication dose and refer to specialist physician
- If a person taking stimulants develops tics, consider: are the tics related to the stimulant (tics naturally wax and wane)? Observe tic evolution over 3 months. Consider if the impairment associated with the tics outweighs the benefits of ADHD treatment
- If tics are stimulant-related, reduce the stimulant dose, or consider changing to guanfacine (in children aged 5 years and over and young people only), atomoxetine, clonidine, or stopping medication
- If a person with ADHD presents with seizures (new or worsening), review and stop any ADHD medication that could reduce the seizure threshold. Cautiously reintroduce the ADHD medication after completing necessary tests and confirming it as non-contributory towards the cause of the seizures
- If sleep becomes a problem: assess sleep at baseline. Monitor changes in sleep pattern (for example, with a sleep diary). Adjust medication accordingly. Advise on sleep hygiene as appropriate. Prescription of melatonin may be helpful to promote sleep onset, where behavioural and environmental adjustments have not been effective
- Consider drug holidays to prevent growth retardation in children

- Consider switch to another agent, e.g. atomoxetine or guanfacine

Best Augmenting Agents for Side Effects

- Beta blockers for peripheral autonomic side effects
- Beta blockers or pregabalin for anxiety; do not prescribe benzodiazepines
- SSRIs or SNRIs for depression
- If psychosis develops, stop methylphenidate and add antipsychotics such as olanzapine or quetiapine, consider a switch to atomoxetine
- Consider melatonin for insomnia in children
- Dose reduction or switching to another agent may be more effective

DOSING AND USE

Usual Dosage Range

- ADHD (children 6–17 years): initial minimum dose of 5 mg/day up to 2.1 mg/kg per day; max daily dose of 90 mg/day (max licensed dose 60 mg/day)
- ADHD (adults): 10–100 mg/day
- Narcolepsy: 10–60 mg/day in divided doses

Dosage Forms

- Tablet 5 mg, 10 mg, 20 mg
- Modified-release tablet 18 mg, 20 mg, 27 mg, 36 mg, 54 mg
- Modified-release capsule 5 mg, 10 mg, 20 mg, 30 mg, 40 mg, 50 mg, 60 mg
- For Concerta XL: combined immediate-release (22% of dose) and modified-release (78% of dose) components
- For Equasym XL: combined immediate-release (30% of dose) and modified-release (70% of dose) components
- For Medikinet XL: combined immediate-release (50% of dose) and modified-release (50% of dose) components

How to Dose

∗For immediate-release medicines
- Attention deficit hyperactivity disorder (initiated under specialist supervision)
- Child 6–17 years:
- Initial dose 5 mg 1–2 times per day, can be increased by 5–10 mg/day at weekly intervals, increased if necessary up to 2.1 mg/kg/day in 2–3 divided doses (licensed max dose 60 mg/day in 2–3 doses; higher doses of up to 90 mg/day under specialist

direction), discontinue if no response after one month; if effect wears off in the evening with rebound hyperactivity, a bedtime dose may be used. Treatment may be started using a modified-release preparation
- Adult:
- Initial dose 5 mg 2–3 times per day, can be increased at weekly intervals according to response up to 100 mg/day in 2–3 divided doses; if effect wears off in the evening with rebound hyperactivity a dose at bedtime may be used. Treatment may be started using a modified-release preparation
- Narcolepsy
- Adult:
- 10–60 mg/day in divided doses; usual dose 20–30 mg/day in divided doses taken before meals

＊For Concerta XL
- Attention deficit hyperactivity disorder (initiated under specialist supervision)
- Child 6–17 years:
- Initial dose 18 mg in the morning, increased by 18 mg each week, adjusted according to response; increased as required up to 2.1 mg/kg/day, licensed max dose 54 mg/day, to be increased to higher dose only under specialist direction; discontinue if no response after 1 month; max 108 mg/day
- Adult:
- Initial dose 18 mg in the morning; adjusted at weekly intervals according to response; max 108 mg/day

＊For Delmosart prolonged-release tablet
- Attention deficit hyperactivity disorder (initiated under specialist supervision)
- Child 6–17 years:
- Initial dose 8 mg in the morning, then increased by 18 mg each week as required, discontinue if no response after 1 month; max 54 mg/day
- Adult:
- Initial dose 18 mg in the morning, then increased by 18 mg each week as required, discontinue if no response after 1 month; max 54 mg/day

＊For Equasym XL
- Attention deficit hyperactivity disorder (initiated under specialist supervision)
- Child 6–17 years:
- Initial dose 10 mg in the morning before breakfast; increased gradually at weekly intervals as required; increased as required up to 2.1 mg/kg/day, licensed max dose 60 mg/day, to be increased to higher dose

only under specialist direction; discontinue if no response after 1 month; max 90 mg/day
- Adult:
- Initial dose 10 mg in the morning before breakfast; increased gradually at weekly intervals as required; max 100 mg/day

＊For Medikinet XL
- Attention deficit hyperactivity disorder (initiated under specialist supervision)
- Child 6–17 years:
- Initial dose 10 mg in the morning with breakfast; adjusted at weekly intervals according to response; increased as required up to 2.1 mg/kg/day, licensed max dose 60 mg/day, to be increased to higher dose only under specialist direction; discontinue if no response after 1 month; max 90 mg/day
- Adult:
- Initial dose 10 mg in the morning with breakfast; adjusted at weekly intervals according to response; max 100 mg/day

＊For Xaggitin XL
- Attention deficit hyperactivity disorder (initiated under specialist supervision)
- Child 6–17 years:
- Initial dose 18 mg in the morning, increased by 18 mg each week, adjusted according to response, discontinue if no response after 1 month; max 54 mg/day
- Adult:
- Initial dose 18 mg in the morning, increased by 18 mg each week, adjusted according to response, discontinue if no response after 1 month; max 54 mg/day

 Dosing Tips
- Different versions of modified-release preparations may have a different clinical effect; to avoid confusion prescribers should specify the brand to be dispensed
- Dose equivalence and conversion:
- Total daily dose of 15 mg of standard-release formulation is considered equivalent to Concerta XL 18 mg/day
- Total daily dose of 15 mg of standard-release formulation is considered equivalent to Delmosart prolonged-release tablet 18 mg/day
- Total daily dose of 15 mg of standard-release formulation is considered equivalent to Xaggitin XL 18 mg/day

- Clinical duration of action often differs from pharmacokinetic half-life
- Taking oral formulations with food may delay peak actions for 2–3 hours
- Immediate-release formulations have 2–4 hour duration of clinical action
- Older sustained-release formulations and generic methylphenidate sustained-release all have about 4–6 hour duration of clinical action, which for most patients is generally not long enough for once-daily dosing in the morning and thus generally requires lunchtime dosing at school
- May be possible to dose only during the school week for some ADHD patients
- May be able to give drug holidays over the summer in order to reassess therapeutic utility and effects on growth and to allow catch-up from any growth suppression as well as to assess any other side effects and evaluate whether to continue treatment for the next school term
- Avoid dosing late in day due to risk of insomnia
- Side effects are generally dose-related
- Usually safe to restart methylphenidate at the previous dose after a period of non-concordance

Overdose

- Vomiting, tremor, coma, convulsion, hyperreflexia, euphoria, confusion, hallucination, tachycardia, flushing, palpitations, sweating, hyperpyrexia, hypertension, arrhythmia, mydriasis

Long-Term Use

- Often used long-term for ADHD when ongoing monitoring documents continued efficacy
- Dependence and/or abuse may develop
- Tolerance to therapeutic effects may develop in some patients
- Long-term stimulant use may be associated with growth suppression in children (controversial)
- Periodic monitoring of weight, blood pressure, pulse, height, FBC, platelet count, and liver function may be indicated
- Monitor for insomnia, mood and appetite change, and the development of tics
- Treatment should be stopped immediately if behaviour deteriorates or there are unacceptable adverse effects

Habit Forming

- Yes
- Methylphenidate is a Class B/Schedule 2 drug
- High abuse potential, patients may develop tolerance, psychological dependence

How to Stop

- Taper to avoid withdrawal effects
- Withdrawal following chronic therapeutic use may unmask symptoms of the underlying disorder and may require follow-up and reinstitution of treatment
- Careful supervision is required during withdrawal from abusive use since severe depression may occur

Pharmacokinetics

- Half-life depends on the formulation used: immediate-release – duration of action around 2–4 hours; modified-release – duration of action about 3 to 8 hours or 8 to 12 hours (e.g. Concerta XL)
- Average half-life in adults 3.5 hours (1.3–7.7 hours)
- Average half-life in children 2.5 hours (1.5–5 hours)
- Time to peak action affected if taken with food. On average, the peak plasma time may be achieved at about 2 hours

 Drug Interactions

- Methylphenidate is predicted to increase the risk of a hypertensive crisis when given with selegiline or MAOIs; avoid and for 14 days after stopping the MAOI
- May affect blood pressure and should be used cautiously with agents used to control BP
- May inhibit metabolism of SSRIs, anticonvulsants, TCAs, and coumarin anticoagulants, requiring downward dosage adjustments of these drugs
- Serious adverse effects may occur if combined with clonidine (controversial)
- CNS and cardiovascular actions of methylphenidate could theoretically be enhanced by combination with agents that block noradrenaline reuptake, such as desipramine, venlafaxine, duloxetine, atomoxetine and reboxetine
- Methylphenidate may increase the risk of dyskinesias when given with risperidone or paliperidone

Methylphenidate hydrochloride (Continued)

- Theoretically antipsychotics should inhibit the stimulatory effects of methylphenidate
- Theoretically methylphenidate could inhibit the antipsychotic actions of antipsychotics
- Theoretically methylphenidate could inhibit the mood-stabilising actions of atypical antipsychotics

 Other Warnings/Precautions

- Use carefully in patients with hypertension
- The prevalence of substance misuse and antisocial personality disorder is high in adults with previously undiagnosed ADHD in childhood. Whilst effective in this population, caution with prescribing and monitoring is appropriate
- Children who are not growing or gaining weight should stop treatment, at least temporarily
- May worsen motor and phonic tics
- May worsen anxiety and agitation
- May worsen symptoms of thought disorder and behavioural disturbance in psychotic patients
- Stimulants have a high potential for abuse and must be used with caution in anyone with a history of substance abuse or alcoholism – alcohol potentially decreases methylphenidate metabolism
- Administration for prolonged periods should be avoided when possible or done only with close monitoring, as it may lead to drug tolerance and dependence
- Attention should be paid to the possibility of obtaining stimulants for non-therapeutic use or distribution to others and the drugs should be prescribed sparingly with documentation of appropriate use
- Usual dosing has been associated with sudden death in children with structural cardiac abnormalities
- Not an appropriate first-line treatment for depression or for normal fatigue
- Caution in epilepsy as may lower seizure threshold
- Caution in patients with a family history of Tourette syndrome
- Caution in patients with susceptibility to angle-closure glaucoma
- Emergence or worsening of activation and agitation may represent the induction of a bipolar state, especially a mixed dysphoric bipolar condition associated with suicidal ideation, and require the addition of a

mood stabiliser and/or methylphenidate discontinuation
- If a dose is forgotten, do not give the missed dose, but give the next dose as usual
- Avoid abrupt withdrawal
- Concerta XL: dose form not appropriate in dysphagia or restricted gastrointestinal lumen
- Delmosart prolonged-release tablet: dose form not appropriate in dysphagia or restricted gastrointestinal lumen
- Xaggitin XL: dose form not appropriate in dysphagia

Do Not Use

- In patients with the following:
  - Anorexia nervosa
  - Arrhythmias
  - Cardiomyopathy
  - Cardiovascular disease
  - Cerebrovascular disorders
  - Heart failure
  - Hyperthyroidism
  - Phaeochromocytoma
  - Psychosis
  - Severe depression
  - Severe hypertension
  - Structural cardiac abnormalities
  - Suicidal ideation
  - Uncontrolled bipolar disorder
  - Vasculitis
- If there is a proven allergy to methylphenidate

SPECIAL POPULATIONS

Renal Impairment

- No known additional risk in this population, but use with caution

Hepatic Impairment

- Use with caution
- Rare reports of liver dysfunction and hypersensitivity reactions in this population

Cardiac Impairment

- Contraindicated in cardiovascular disease, cardiomyopathy, heart failure and in patients with structural cardiac abnormalities

Elderly

- Should not be used in the elderly as safety and efficacy have not been established in this group

Children and Adolescents

Before you prescribe:

- Diagnosis of ADHD should only be made by an appropriately qualified healthcare professional, e.g. specialist psychiatrist, paediatrician, and after full clinical and psychosocial assessment in different domains, full developmental and psychiatric history, observer reports across different settings, and opportunity to speak to the child and carer on their own
- Children and adolescents with untreated anxiety, PTSD and mood disorders, or those who do not have a psychiatric diagnosis but social or environmental stressors, may present with anger, irritability, motor agitation, and concentration problems
- Consider undiagnosed learning disability or specific learning difficulties, and sensory impairments that may potentially cause or contribute to inattention and restlessness, especially in school
- ADHD-specific advice on symptom management and environmental adaptations should be offered to all families and teachers, including reducing distractions, seating, shorter periods of focus, movement breaks and teaching assistants
- For children >5 years and young people with moderate ADHD pharmacological treatment should be considered if they continue to show significant impairment in at least one setting after symptom management and environmental adaptations have been implemented
- For severe ADHD, behavioural symptom management may not be effective until pharmacological treatment has been established

Practical notes:

- First-line when a drug is indicated
- Consider using modified-release preparations in children as there is convenience of single-day dosage, improved adherence, reduced stigma, acceptability to schools, or can consider multiple doses of immediate-release, which has benefit of greater flexibility in controlling time-course of action, closer initial titration
- Monitor patients face-to-face regularly, particularly during the first several weeks of treatment

- Monitor for activation of suicidal ideation at the beginning of treatment
- Consider cognitive behavioural therapy (CBT) for those whose ADHD symptoms are still causing significant difficulties in one or more domains, addressing emotion regulation, problem-solving, self-control, and social skills (including active listening skills and interactions with peers)
- Medication for ADHD for a child under 5 years should only be considered on specialist advice from an ADHD service with expertise in managing ADHD in young children (ideally a tertiary service). Use of medicines for treating ADHD is off-label in children aged <5 years
- Same medication choices should be offered to patients with co-morbidities (e.g. anxiety, tic disorders or autism spectrum disorders) as to patients with ADHD alone
- A trial of methylphenidate in children with ADHD and intellectual disability showed that optimal dosing with methylphenidate was effective in some
- NICE conducted a meta-analysis and found clear benefit for methylphenidate in ADHD in the context of learning difficulties
- Insomnia is common
- Methylphenidate has acute effects on growth hormone; long-term effects are unknown, but weight and height should be monitored 6-monthly using a growth chart
- Do not use in children with structural cardiac abnormalities or other serious cardiac problems
- Sudden death in children and adolescents with serious heart problems has been reported
- American Heart Association recommends ECG prior to initiating stimulant treatment in children, but not all experts agree
- Re-evaluate the need for continued treatment regularly
- Provide the Medicines for Children leaflet: Methylphenidate for attention deficit hyperactivity disorder (ADHD)

Pregnancy

- Limited human data on use during pregnancy
- Single study found an increased risk of conotruncal and major arch anomalies following exposure during pregnancy

- Increased risks of spontaneous abortion when used early in pregnancy
- Increased risk of low Apgar score when used in late pregnancy
- Infants whose mothers took methylphenidate during pregnancy may experience withdrawal symptoms
- Use in women of childbearing potential requires weighing potential benefits to the mother against potential risks to the foetus
- *For ADHD patients, methylphenidate should generally be discontinued before anticipated pregnancies

Breastfeeding

- Small amounts found in mother's breast milk
- Infants of women who choose to breastfeed while on methylphenidate should be monitored for possible adverse effects
- If irritability, sleep disturbance, or poor weight gain develop in nursing infant, may need to discontinue drug or bottle feed

THE ART OF PSYCHOPHARMACOLOGY

Potential Advantages

- Established long-term efficacy as a first-line treatment for ADHD
- Multiple options for drug delivery, peak actions, and duration of action, therefore dosing regimes can be adapted to the individual child's needs (e.g. school hours, homework, sleep)
- Effective in ADHD associated with learning difficulties

Potential Disadvantages

- Patients with current or past substance abuse
- Patients with current or past bipolar disorder or psychosis
- Patients where height and weight loss will be an issue
- May exacerbate symptoms in children and adolescents with untreated anxiety and mood disorders, or those who do not have a psychiatric diagnosis, but present with anger, irritability, motor agitation, and concentration problems
- Adverse effects more commonly reported in children with ADHD and intellectual disability than in children with ADHD alone

Primary Target Symptoms

- Concentration, attention span
- Motor hyperactivity
- Impulsiveness
- Physical and mental fatigue
- Daytime sleepiness
- Depression

Pearls

- When switching from immediate-release preparations of methylphenidate to modified-release preparations of methylphenidate – consult product literature
- Many of the modified-release preparations of methylphenidate show a biphasic plasma concentration-time curve
- Duration of action differs between the modified-release preparations of methylphenidate: Medikinet XL (8 hours), Equasym XL (10 hours), Concerta XL (12 hours)
- Stimulant drugs such as methylphenidate are more effective than non-stimulant drugs in the treatment of ADHD
- The number needed to treat (NNT) equals 3 for the effect of methylphenidate in ADHD
- Potential for drug misuse or diversion is lower than with dexamfetamine
- Can be used to potentiate opioid analgesia and reduce sedation, particularly in end-of-life management
- Atypical antipsychotics may be useful in treating stimulant or psychotic consequences of overdose
- Some patients respond to or tolerate methylphenidate better than amfetamine and vice versa
- Taking with food may delay peak actions of oral formulations for 2–3 hours
- Half-life and duration of clinical action tend to be shorter in younger children
- Drug abuse may actually be lower in ADHD adolescents treated with stimulants than in ADHD adolescents who are not treated
- Can consider bupropion in cases with co-morbid substance misuse
- Older modified-release technologies for methylphenidate were not significant advances over immediate-release methylphenidate, because they did not eliminate the need for lunchtime dosing or allow once-daily administration

* Newer modified-release technologies are truly once-a-day dosing
* Concerta has less of an early peak, but a longer duration of action (up to 12 hours)
* Concerta may be preferable for those ADHD patients who work in the evening or do homework up to 12 hours after morning dosing
* Ritalin XL may be preferable for those ADHD patients who lose their appetite for dinner or have insomnia with Concerta
* Some patients may benefit from an occasional addition of 5–10 mg of immediate-release methylphenidate to their daily base of modified-release methylphenidate
* Studies support the efficacy and tolerability of methylphenidate in children with

22q11.2DS; however, ensure cardiovascular assessment prior to and during treatment
* Conflicting and limited data for use in bariatric surgery; one case report of reduced efficacy and other reports of signs of toxicity when used in bariatric surgery
* Although caution advised in epilepsy, some studies at therapeutic doses support safety and efficacy of methylphenidate in children with epilepsy
* There is anecdotal report of successful use of methylphenidate in a patient with psychotic depression non-responsive to therapeutic doses of a combination of an antidepressant and an antipsychotic

 ## Suggested Reading

Azran C, Langguth P, Dahan A. Impaired oral absorption of methylphenidate after Roux-en-Y gastric bypass. Surg Obes Relat Dis 2017;13(7):1245–7.

Huang C-C, Shiah I-S, Chen H-K, et al. Adjunctive use of methylphenidate in the treatment of psychotic unipolar depression. Clin Neuropharmacol 2008;31(4):245–7.

Kanner AM. Management of psychiatric and neurological comorbidities in epilepsy. Nat Rev Neurol 2016;12(2):106–16.

Kimko HC, Cross JT, Abernethy DR. Pharmacokinetics and clinical effectiveness of methylphenidate. Clin Pharmacokinet 1999;37(6):457–70.

Ludvigsson M, Haenni A. Methylphenidate toxicity after Roux-en-Y gastric bypass. Surg Obes Relat Dis 2016;12(5):e55-e57.

Siegel M, Beaulieu AA. Psychotropic medications in children with autism spectrum disorders: a systematic review and synthesis for evidence-based practice. J Autism Dev Disord 2012;42(8):1592–605.

Simonoff E, Taylor E, Baird G, et al. Randomized controlled double-blind trial of optimal dose methylphenidate in children and adolescents with severe attention deficit hyperactivity disorder and intellectual disability. J Child Psychol Psychiatry 2013;54(5):527–35.

Spencer T, Wilens T, Biederman J, et al. A double-blind crossover comparison of methylphenidate and placebo in adults with childhood-onset attention-deficit hyperactivity disorder. Arch Gen Psychiatry 1995;52(6):434–43.

Sung M, Chin CH, Lim CG, et al. What's in the pipeline? Drugs in development for autism spectrum disorder. Neuropsychiatr Dis Treat 2014;10:371–81.

Tang KL, Antshel KM, Fremont WP, et al. Behavioral and psychiatric phenotypes in 22q11.2 deletion syndrome. J Dev Behav Pediatr 2015;36(8):639–50.

Williamson ED, Martin A. Psychotropic medications in autism: practical considerations for parents. J Autism Dev Disord 2012;42(6):1249–55.

Mianserin hydrochloride

Brands
• Non-proprietary

Generic?
Yes

Class
• Neuroscience-based nomenclature: pharmacology domain – norepinephrine; mode of action – multimodal
• Tetracyclic antidepressant
• Noradrenergic agent

Commonly Prescribed for
(bold for BNF indication)
• **Depressive illness (particularly where sedation is required)**
• Anxiety
• Insomnia
• Treatment-resistant depression

 How the Drug Works
• Blocks alpha 2 adrenergic presynaptic receptor, thereby increasing noradrenergic neurotransmission
• This is a novel mechanism independent of noradenergic reuptake blockade
• Blocks alpha 2 adrenergic presynaptic receptors but also alpha 1 adrenergic receptors on serotonin neurons, thereby causing little increase in serotonin neurotransmission
• Blocks 5HT2A, 5HT2C, and 5HT3 serotonin receptors
• Blocks H1 histamine receptors

How Long Until It Works
∗ Actions on insomnia and anxiety can start shortly after initiation of dosing
• Onset of therapeutic actions in depression, however, is usually not immediate, but often delayed 2–4 weeks
• If it is not working within 3–4 weeks for depression, it may require a dosage increase or it may not work at all
• May continue to work for many years to prevent relapse of symptoms

If It Works
• The goal of treatment is complete remission of current symptoms as well as prevention of future relapses
• Treatment most often reduces or even eliminates symptoms, but is not a cure

since symptoms can recur after medicine is stopped
• Continue treatment until all symptoms are gone (remission), especially in depression and whenever possible in anxiety disorders
• Once symptoms are gone, continue treating for at least 6–9 months for the first episode of depression or >12 months if relapse indicators present
• If >5 episodes and/or 2 episodes in the last few years then need to continue for at least 2 years or indefinitely
• Use in anxiety disorders may also need to be indefinite

If It Doesn't Work
• Important to recognise non-response to treatment early on (3–4 weeks)
• Many patients have only a partial response where some symptoms are improved but others persist (especially insomnia, fatigue, and problems concentrating)
• Other patients may be non-responders, sometimes called treatment-resistant or treatment-refractory
• Some patients who have an initial response may relapse even though they continue treatment
• Consider increasing dose, switching to another agent, or adding an appropriate augmenting agent
• Lithium may be added for suicidal patients or those at high risk of relapse
• Consider psychotherapy
• Consider ECT
• Consider evaluation for another diagnosis or for a co-morbid condition (e.g. medical illness, substance abuse, etc.)
• Some patients may experience a switch into mania and so would require antidepressant discontinuation and initiation of a mood stabiliser

⚖ Best Augmenting Combos for Partial Response or Treatment Resistance
• SSRI or SNRI (use combinations of antidepressant with caution as this may activate bipolar disorder and suicidal ideation or lead to the serotonin syndrome)

Mianserin hydrochloride (Continued)

- Lithium or atypical antipsychotics for bipolar depression, psychotic depression, or treatment-resistant depression
- Benzodiazepines if anxiety present

Tests

- Baseline ECG is useful for patients over age 50
- ECGs may be useful for selected patients (e.g. those with personal or family history of QTc prolongation; cardiac arrhythmia; recent myocardial infarction; decompensated heart failure; or taking agents that prolong QTc interval such as pimozide, thioridazine, selected antiarrhythmics, moxifloxacin etc.)
- *Since tricyclic and tetracyclic antidepressants are frequently associated with weight gain, before starting treatment, weigh all patients and determine if the patient is already overweight (BMI 25.0–29.9) or obese (BMI ≥30)
- Before giving a drug that can cause weight gain to an overweight or obese patient, consider determining whether the patient already has:
  - Pre-diabetes – fasting plasma glucose: 5.5 mmol/L to 6.9 mmol/L or HbA1c: 42 to 47 mmol/mol (6.0 to 6.4%)
  - Diabetes – fasting plasma glucose: >7.0 mmol/L or HbA1c: ≥48 mmol/L (≥6.5%)
  - Hypertension (BP >140/90 mm Hg)
  - Dyslipidaemia (increased total cholesterol, LDL cholesterol, and triglycerides; decreased HDL cholesterol)
- Treat or refer such patients for treatment, including nutrition and weight management, physical activity counselling, smoking cessation, and medical management
- *Monitor weight and BMI during treatment
- *While giving a drug to a patient who has gained >5% of initial weight, consider evaluating for the presence of pre-diabetes, diabetes, dyslipidaemia, or consider switching to a different antidepressant
- Patients at risk for electrolyte disturbances (e.g. patients aged >60, patients on diuretic therapy) should have baseline and periodic serum potassium and magnesium measurements
- A full blood count (FBC) is recommended every 4 weeks during the first 3 months
- Patients complaining of sore throat, stomatitis, fever, malaise, flu-like symptoms or other signs of infection should discontinue treatment with mianserin, and FBC obtained

SIDE EFFECTS

How Drug Causes Side Effects

- Most side effects are immediate but often go away with time
- *Histamine 1 receptor antagonism may explain sedative effects
- *Histamine 1 receptor antagonism plus 5HT2C antagonism may explain some aspects of weight gain

Notable Side Effects

- Sedation
- Increased appetite, weight gain

Frequency not known

- Blood disorders: agranulocytosis, bone marrow disorders, granulocytopenia, leucopenia
- CNS/PNS: agitation, altered mood, blurred vision, confusion, dizziness, irritability, neuromuscular irritability, paraesthesia, paranoid delusions, psychosis, sedation, seizure, suicidal behaviours, tremor
- CVS: postural hypotension
- GIT: hepatic disorders, increased appetite, weight gain
- Other: arthritis, breast abnormalities, gynaecomastia, hyperhidrosis, hyponatraemia, joint disorders, lactation in the absence of pregnancy, oedema, rash, sexual dysfunction, withdrawal syndrome

 Life-Threatening or Dangerous Side Effects

- Seizures
- Blood dyscrasias
- Rare induction of mania
- Very rare – neuroleptic malignant syndrome
- Sudden death of patients with cardiac disease
- Rare increase in suicidal ideation and behaviours in adolescents and young adults (up to age 25), hence patients should be warned of this potential adverse event

Weight Gain

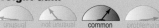

- Many experience and/or can be significant in amount

Sedation

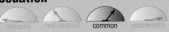

unusual · not unusual · common · problematic

- Many experience and/or can be significant in amount
- Generally transient

What to Do About Side Effects

- Wait
- Wait
- Wait
- Switch to another drug

Best Augmenting Agents for Side Effects

- Often best to try another antidepressant monotherapy prior to resorting to augmentation strategies to treat side effects
- Many side effects are dose-dependent (i.e. they increase as dose increases, or they re-emerge until tolerance redevelops)
- Many side effects are time-dependent (i.e. they start immediately upon dosing and upon each dose increase, but go away with time)
- Many side effects cannot be improved with an augmenting agent
- Increased activation or agitation may represent the induction of a bipolar state, especially a mixed dysphoric bipolar condition sometimes associated with suicidal ideation, and require the addition of lithium, a mood stabiliser or an atypical antipsychotic, and/or discontinuation of mianserin

DOSING AND USE

Usual Dosage Range

- Depressive illness (particularly where sedation is required): 30–90 mg/day

Dosage Forms

- Tablet 10 mg, 30 mg

How to Dose

*Depressive illness (particularly where sedation is required):
- Adult: initial dose 30–40 mg/day at bedtime or in divided doses, increased gradually as needed; usual dose 30–90 mg/day
- Elderly: start at the lower dose of 30 mg

Dosing Tips

- Can be dosed once or twice per day
- If intolerable anxiety, insomnia, agitation, akathisia, or activation occur either upon dosing initiation or discontinuation, consider the possibility of activated bipolar disorder and switch to a mood stabiliser or an atypical antipsychotic

Overdose

- Overdose can lead to sedation, hypertension or hypotension, tachycardia, coma

Long-Term Use

- Safe

Habit Forming

- Not expected

How to Stop

- Taper is prudent to avoid withdrawal effects, but tolerance, dependence, and withdrawal effects not reliably reported

Pharmacokinetics

- 90% protein bound
- Biphasic plasma half-life
- Duration of terminal phase ranges from 6 to 39 hours

 Drug Interactions

- Tramadol increases the risk of seizures in patients taking an antidepressant
- Carbamazepine and phenytoin may reduce mianserin levels
- Theoretically could cause a fatal "serotonin syndrome" when combined with MAOIs, so do not use with MAOIs or for at least 14 days after MAOIs are stopped unless you are an expert and only for treatment-resistant cases that may justify the risk
- Do not start an MAOI for at least 5 half-lives (5 to 7 days for most drugs) after discontinuing mianserin
- Mianserin may affect the metabolism of coumarin derivatives such as warfarin; patients receiving warfarin therapy should receive coagulation monitoring when mianserin is initiated or stopped

Mianserin hydrochloride (Continued)

⚠ Other Warnings/Precautions

- Sudden death of patients with cardiac disease
- Take caution in patients with arrhythmias, cardiovascular disease, heart block, immediate recovery after myocardial infarction, phaeochromocytoma (increased risk of arrhythmias)
- Drug may lower white blood cell count (rare; may not be increased compared to other antidepressants but controlled studies lacking)
- Concomitant alcohol use may increase sedation and cognitive and motor effects
- Use with caution in patients with history of seizures
- Use with caution in patients with diabetes
- Use with caution in the elderly
- Use with caution in patients with prostatic hypertrophy, susceptibility to angle-closure glaucoma
- Use with caution in patients with bipolar disorder (unless treated with concomitant mood-stabilising agent), stop treatment if the patient enters a manic phase
- Warn patients and their caregivers about the possibility of activating side effects and advise them to report such symptoms immediately
- Use with caution in patients with a history of psychosis
- Use with caution in patients with a significant risk of suicide
- Rare increase of suicidal ideation and behaviour in adolescents and young adults (up to age 25), hence patients should be warned of this potential adverse event

Do Not Use

- In acute porphyrias
- During the acute phase of mania
- If patient is taking an MAOI
- If there is a proven allergy to mianserin

SPECIAL POPULATIONS

Renal Impairment

- Use with caution; start with low dose and increase gradually

Hepatic Impairment

- Sedative effects are increased in hepatic impairment; avoid in severe liver disease

Cardiac Impairment

- Baseline ECG is recommended
- Should be used with caution

Elderly

- Baseline ECG is recommended for patients over age 50
- Some patients may tolerate lower doses better
- Blood dyscrasias, though still rare, may be more common in the elderly

Children and Adolescents

- The safety and efficacy of mianserin in children and adolescents have not been satisfactorily established, therefore mianserin should not be used in this population

Pregnancy

- Controlled studies have not been conducted in pregnant women
- Not generally recommended for use during pregnancy, especially during first trimester
- Must weigh the risk of treatment (first trimester foetal development, third trimester newborn delivery) to the child against the risk of no treatment (recurrence of depression, maternal health, infant bonding) to the mother and child
- For many patients this may mean continuing treatment during pregnancy

Breastfeeding

- Small amounts found in mother's breast milk
- Extremely limited evidence of safety
- If child becomes irritable or sedated, breastfeeding or drug may need to be discontinued
- Immediate postpartum period is a high-risk time for depression, especially in women who have had prior depressive episodes, so drug may need to be reinstituted late in the third trimester or shortly after childbirth to prevent a recurrence during the postpartum period
- Must weigh benefits of breastfeeding with risks and benefits of antidepressant treatment versus nontreatment to both the infant and the mother

- For many patients, this may mean continuing treatment during breastfeeding
- Other antidepressants may be preferable, e.g. imipramine or nortriptyline

THE ART OF PSYCHOPHARMACOLOGY

Potential Advantages
- Patients particularly concerned about sexual side effects
- Patients with symptoms of anxiety and insomnia
- As an augmenting agent to boost the efficacy of other antidepressants

Potential Disadvantages
- Patients concerned with weight gain
- Patients with low energy

Primary Target Symptoms
- Depressed mood

- Sleep disturbance
- Anxiety

Pearls
- *Adding alpha 2 antagonism to agents that block serotonin and/or norepinephrine reuptake may be synergistic for severe depression
- Adding mianserin to venlafaxine or SSRIs may reverse drug-induced anxiety and insomnia
- Efficacy of mianserin for depression in cancer patients has been shown in small controlled studies
- *Only causes sexual dysfunction infrequently
- Generally better tolerated than TCAs and safer in overdose
- Mianserin has been used to combat akathisia

 Suggested Reading

Brogden RN, Heel RC, Speight TM, et al. Mianserin: a review of its pharmacological properties and therapeutic efficacy in depressive illness. Drugs 1978;16(4):273–301.

De Ridder JJ. Mianserin: result of a decade of antidepressant research. Pharm Weekbl Sci 1982;4(5):139–45.

Leinonen E, Koponen H, Lepola U. Serum mianserin and ageing. Prog Neuropsychopharmacol Biol Psychiatry 1994;18(5):833–45.

Rotzinger S, Bourin M, Akimoto Y, et al. Metabolism of some "second"- and "fourth"-generation antidepressants: iprindole, viloxazine, bupropion, mianserin, maprotiline, trazodone, nefazodone, and venlafaxine. Cell Mol Neurobiol 1999;19(4):427–42.

Wakeling A. Efficacy and side effects of mianserin, a tetracyclic antidepressant. Postgrad Med J 1983;59(690):229–31

Midazolam

THERAPEUTICS

Brands
- Buccolam
- Epistatus
- Hypnovel

Generic?
Yes

Class
- Neuroscience-based nomenclature: pharmacology domain – GABA; mode of action – positive allosteric modulator (PAM)
- Benzodiazepine (hypnotic)

Commonly Prescribed for
(bold for BNF indication)
- **Seizures: (status epilepticus or febrile convulsions – in children and adults)**
- **Conscious sedation for procedures**
- **Sedation (adjunct to anaesthesia)**
- **Preoperative anxiolytic**
- **Induction of anaesthesia (rarely used)**
- **Sedation of patients receiving intensive care**
- **Palliative care: (confusion and restlessness – adjunct to antipsychotic; convulsions)**

 ### How the Drug Works
- Binds to benzodiazepine receptors at the GABA-A ligand-gated chloride channel complex
- Enhances the inhibitory effects of GABA
- Boosts chloride conductance through GABA-regulated channels
- Inhibitory actions in sleep centres may provide sedative hypnotic effects

How Long Until It Works
- Intravenous injection: onset 1–3 minutes
- IM injection: onset 10–20 minutes, peak 30–60 minutes
- Buccal liquid: onset is 15–30 minutes

If It Works
- Faster onset and shorter duration of action than lorazepam, diazepam or haloperidol
- IV should only be used with extreme caution as a last resort and where resuscitation facilities are available
- Patients generally recover 2–6 hours after awakening

If It Doesn't Work
- Increase the dose
- Repeat after 45–60 minutes if necessary
- Switch to another agent

 ### Best Augmenting Combos for Partial Response or Treatment Resistance
- Combination of IV olanzapine or IV droperidol with IV midazolam seems to be more rapidly effective than IV midazolam alone and results in fewer subsequent doses needed
- IM midazolam is more rapidly sedating than a combination of haloperidol and promethazine

Tests
- None for healthy individuals

SIDE EFFECTS

How Drug Causes Side Effects
- Actions on benzodiazepine receptors that carry over to next day can cause daytime sedation, amnesia, and ataxia

Notable Side Effects
- Oversedation, impaired recall, agitation, involuntary movements, headache
- Nausea, vomiting
- Hicupps, fluctuation of vital signs, pain at site of injection
- Hypotension

Common or very common
- Vomiting

Uncommon
- Skin reactions

Rare or very rare
- CNS: movement disorders
- GIT: dry mouth, hiccups
- Resp: dyspnoea, respiratory disorders

Frequency not known
- Severe disinhibition in children (with sedative and peri-operative use), vertigo

 ### Life-Threatening or Dangerous Side Effects
- Respiratory depression, apnoea, respiratory arrest
- Cardiac arrest

Midazolam (Continued)

Weight Gain

- Reported but not expected

Sedation

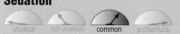

- Frequent and can be significant
- Higher doses prolong sedation and risk of hypoventilation
- Drug accumulates in adipose tissue, which can prolong sedation in obese patients and those with hepatic or renal impairment
- Co-administration with other sedative, hypnotic, or CNS-depressant drugs results in increased sedation

What To Do About Side Effects

- Wait
- Switch to another agent
- Administer flumazenil if side effects are severe or life-threatening

Best Augmenting Agents for Side Effects

- Many side effects cannot be improved with an augmenting agent

DOSING AND USE

Usual Dosage Range

- Status epilepticus and febrile convulsions: adult (buccal; 10 mg, then 10 mg after 10 minutes as required); child (depends on age)
- Conscious sedation for procedures: adult (slow IV, total dose 2.0–7.5 mg per course); elderly (slow IV, 0.5–3.5 mg per course)
- Sedative in combined anaesthesia: adult (IV, 30–100 mcg/kg); elderly (lower doses)
- Premedication: adult (IM, 70–100 mcg/kg or IV, 1–2 mg); elderly and debilitated patients (IM, 25–50 mcg/kg or IV, 0.5 mg)
- Induction of anaesthesia: adult (slow IV, 150–600 mg/kg in divided doses – max per dose 5 mg); elderly and debilitated patients (slow IV, 50–600 mg/kg in divided doses – max per dose 5 mg)
- Sedation of patient receiving intensive care: adult (slow IV, initial dose 30–300 mcg/kg, then 30–200 mcg/kg/hour)
- Adjunct to antipsychotic for confusion and restlessness in palliative care: adult (s/c; initial dose 10–20 mg/24 hours; usual dose 20–60 mg/24 hours)
- Convulsions in palliative care: adult (continuous s/c infusion, 20–40 mg/24 hours)

Dosage Forms

- Oromucosal solution 10 mg/mL, 10 mg/2 mL, 2.5 mg/0.5 mL, 5 mg/mL, 7.5 mg/1.5 mL
- Solution for injection 2 mg/2 mL, 5 mg/5 mL, 10 mg/5 mL, 10 mg/2 mL, 50 mg/10 mL
- Solution for infusion 50 mg/50 mL, 100 mg/50 mL

How to Dose

*Status epilepticus and febrile convulsions:
- Adult: buccal 10 mg, then 10 mg after 10 minutes if required
- Child 1–2 months: 300 mcg/kg; max per dose 2.5 mg, then 300 mcg/kg after 10 minutes; max per dose 2.5 mg if required
- Child 3–11 months: 2.5 mg, then 2.5 mg after 10 minutes if required
- Child 1–4 years: 5 mg, then 5 mg after 10 minutes if required
- Child 5–9 years: 7.5 mg, then 7.5 mg after 10 minutes if required
- Child 10–17 years: 10 mg, then 10 mg after 10 minutes if required
*Conscious sedation for procedures:
- Adult: slow IV, initial dose 2–2.5 mg, to be administered 5–10 minutes before procedure at a rate of about 2 mg/minute, increased by increments of 1 mg if required, usual total dose is 3.5–5 mg; max 7.5 mg per course
- Elderly: slow IV, initial dose 0.5–1 mg, to be administered 5–10 minutes before procedure at a rate of about 2 mg/minute, increased by increments of 0.5–1 mg if required; max 3.5 mg per course
*Sedative in combined anaesthesia:
- Adult: IV, 30–100 mcg/kg, repeated as required, alternatively by continuous IV infusion 30–100 mcg/kg/hour
- Elderly: lower doses
*Premedication:
- Adult: IM, 70–100 mcg/kg, to be administered 20–60 minutes before induction; IV, 1–2 mg, repeated as required, to be administered 5–30 minutes before procedure
- Elderly and debilitated patients: IM, 25–50 mcg/kg, to be administered 20–60 minutes before induction; IV, 0.5 mg, repeated as required, initial dose to be administered

5–30 minutes before procedure, repeat dose slowly as required

* Induction of anaesthesia:
* Adult: slow IV, 150–200 mcg/kg/day in divided doses; max per dose 5 mg, dose to be given at intervals of 2 minutes, max total dose 600 mcg/kg
* Elderly and debilitated patients: slow IV, 50–150 mcg/kg daily in divided doses; max per dose 5 mg, dose to be given at intervals of 2 minutes, max total dose 600 mcg/kg

* Sedation of patient receiving intensive care: 30–300 mcg/kg, dose to be given by increments of 1–2.5 mg every 2 minutes, then by either slow IV injection or continuous IV infusion at a rate of 30–200 mcg/kg/hour; reduce dose or omit initial dose in hypothermia, hypovolaemia, vasoconstriction; lower doses may be enough if opioids also used
* Adult: slow IV, initial dose 30–300 mcg/kg, dose to be given by increments of 1–2.5 mg every 2 minutes, then by either slow IV injection or continuous IV infusion at a rate of 30–200 mcg/kg/hour; reduce dose or omit initial dose in hypothermia, hypovolaemia, vasoconstriction; lower doses may be enough if opioids also used

* Adjunct to antipsychotic for confusion and restlessness in palliative care:
* Adult: s/c; initial dose 10–20 mg/24 hours, adjusted according to response; usual dose 20–60 mg/24 hours

* Convulsions in palliative care:
* Adult: continuous s/c infusion, 20–40 mg/24 hours

 Dosing Tips

* Better to underdose, observe for effects, and then prudently raise dose while monitoring carefully
* For intravenous infusion give continuously in glucose 5% or sodium chloride 0.9%
* For oral use in children solution may be diluted with apple or blackcurrant juice, chocolate sauce, or cola

Overdose

* At high doses (5 mg/mL in 2 mL and 10 mL ampoules or 2 mg/mL in 5 mL ampoules); should only be used in general anaesthesia, intensive care, palliative care, or other situations where the risk has been assessed

* Signs of overdose include ataxia, dysarthria, nystagmus, slurred speech, somnolence, confusion, hypotension, respiratory arrest, vasomotor collapse, impaired motor functions, reflexes, coordination and balance, coma and death
* A midazolam overdose is considered a medical emergency
* Have flumazenil available when midazolam is used

Long-Term Use

* Not generally intended for long-term use
* Avoid prolonged use and abrupt withdrawal thereafter

Habit Forming

* Yes
* Midazolam is a Class C/Schedule 3 controlled drug
* Midazolam infusions may induce tolerance and a withdrawal syndrome in a matter of days

How to Stop

* If administration was prolonged, do not stop abruptly
* Gradual reduction of midazolam after regular use can minimise withdrawal and rebound effects

Pharmacokinetics

* Duration of action 1–6 hours
* Elimination half-life 1.5–2.5 hours in healthy individuals
* Active metabolite
* Recovery may be longer in the elderly, in patients with a low cardiac output, or after repeated dosing
* Excretion via kidneys

 Drug Interactions

* If CNS depressants are used concomitantly, midazolam dose should be reduced by half or more
* Increased depressive effects when taken with other CNS depressants (see Warnings below)
* Drugs that inhibit CYP450 3A4, such as fluvoxamine, may reduce midazolam clearance and raise midazolam levels
* Midazolam decreases the minimum alveolar concentration of halothane needed for general anaesthesia

Other Warnings/Precautions

- Warning regarding the increased risk of CNS-depressant effects (especially alcohol) when benzodiazepines and opioid medications are used together, including specifically the risk of slowed or difficulty breathing and death
- If alternatives to the combined use of benzodiazepines and opioids are not available, clinicians should limit the dosage and duration of each drug to the minimum possible while still achieving therapeutic efficacy
- Patients and their caregivers should be warned to seek medical attention if unusual dizziness, light-headedness, sedation, slowed or difficulty breathing, or unresponsiveness occur
- Dosage changes should be made in collaboration with prescriber
- History of drug or alcohol abuse often creates greater risk for dependency
- Some depressed patients may experience a worsening of suicidal ideation
- Some patients may exhibit abnormal thinking or behavioural changes similar to those caused by other CNS depressants (i.e. either depressant actions or disinhibiting actions)
- Avoid prolonged use and abrupt cessation
- Use lower doses in debilitated patients and the elderly
- Use with caution in patients with myasthenia gravis; respiratory disease
- Use with caution in patients with personality disorder (dependent/avoidant or anankastic types) as may increase risk of dependence
- Use with caution in patients with a history of alcohol or drug dependence/abuse
- Benzodiazepines may cause a range of paradoxical effects including aggression, antisocial behaviours, anxiety, overexcitement, perceptual abnormalities and talkativeness. Adjustment of dose may reduce impulses
- Use with caution in patients with muscle weakness or organic brain changes
- Patients with COPD should receive lower doses
- Use with caution in patients with impaired respiratory function
- Use with caution in adults with cardiac disease, hypothermia, hypovolaemia, and vasoconstriction
- Use with caution in neonates and children especially those with impaired cardiac system
- Sedated paediatric patients should be monitored throughout the procedure
- With intravenous use: concentration of midazolam in children under 15 kg not to exceed 1 mg/mL
- Midazolam should be used only in an environment in which the patient can be closely monitored (e.g. hospital), because of the risk of respiratory depression and respiratory arrest

Do Not Use

- If patient has acute pulmonary insufficiency, respiratory depression, significant neuromuscular respiratory weakness, sleep apnoea syndrome, or unstable myasthenia gravis
- In patients with CNS depression, compromised airway
- Alone in chronic psychosis in adults
- On its own to treat depression, anxiety associated with depression, obsessional states or phobic states
- If patient has angle-closure glaucoma
- If there is a proven allergy to midazolam or any benzodiazepine

SPECIAL POPULATIONS

Renal Impairment

- Longer elimination half-life, prolonging time to recovery
- For all benzodiazepines: increased cerebral sensitivity to benzodiazepines
- For midazolam: use with caution in chronic renal failure

Hepatic Impairment

- Longer elimination half-life; clearance is reduced. Benzodiazepines with shorter half-life are considered safer

- For sedation: use with caution; may precipitate coma
- For febrile convulsions and status epilepticus: use with caution in mild-moderate impairment, avoid in severe impairment
- For parenteral preparations consider dose reduction in all degrees of impairment

Cardiac Impairment

- Longer elimination half-life; clearance is reduced

Elderly

- Longer elimination half-life; clearance is reduced
  Intravenous:
- Sedation: initial dose 0.5–1 mg, administered 5–10 minutes before procedure at a rate of 2 mg/minute, increased by increments of 0.5–1 mg as required; max 3.5 mg per course
- Premedication: 0.5 mg, repeated if needed, initial dose to be administered 5–30 minutes before procedure, repeat dose slowly as required
- Induction of anaesthesia: 50–150 mcg/kg daily in divided doses (max per dose 5 mg), dose to be given at intervals of 2 minutes, max total dose 600 mcg/kg
  IM injection:
- Premedication: 25–50 mcg/kg, to be administered 20–60 minutes before induction

Children and Adolescents

- In most paediatric populations, pharmacokinetic properties are similar to those in adults
- Caution if cardiovascular impairment
- Concentration in children under 15 kg should not exceed 1 mg/mL
- Seriously ill neonates have reduced clearance and longer elimination half-life, so reduce dose
- Risk of airway obstruction and hypoventilation in children under 6 months (monitor respiratory rate and oxygen saturation)
- Hypotension has occurred in neonates given midazolam and fentanyl
- Intravenous dose: dependent on age, weight, route, procedure
- Buccal administration: dependent on age

- 1–2 months: 300 mcg/kg (max per dose 2.5 mg), then 300 mcg/kg after 10 minutes (max per dose 2.5 mg) if required
- 3–11 months: 2.5 mg, then 2.5 mg after 10 minutes if required
- 1–4 years: 5 mg, then 5 mg after 10 minutes if required
- 5–9 years: 7.5 mg, then 7.5 mg after 10 minutes if required
- 10–17 years: 10 mg, then 10 mg after 10 minutes if required

Pregnancy

- Possible increased risk of birth defects when benzodiazepines taken during pregnancy
- Use during pregnancy may be justified if the benefit to the mother exceeds any associated risk
- Drug should be tapered if discontinued
- Infants whose mothers received a benzodiazepine late in pregnancy may experience withdrawal effects
- Neonatal flaccidity has been reported in infants whose mothers took a benzodiazepine during pregnancy
- Seizures, even mild seizures, may cause harm to the embryo/foetus

Breastfeeding

- Small amounts found in mother's breast milk
- Effects of benzodiazepines on infant have been observed and include feeding difficulties, sedation, and weight loss
- Caution should be taken with the use of benzodiazepines in breastfeeding mothers, seek to use low doses for short periods to reduce infant exposure
- Considered not to pose a risk to the infant when given as a single dose (e.g. for pre-medication)
- Avoid breastfeeding for 24 hours after midazolam administration

THE ART OF PSYCHOPHARMACOLOGY

Potential Advantages
- Fast onset
- Parenteral dosage forms

Potential Disadvantages
- Can be oversedating

Primary Target Symptoms
- Anxiety

Midazolam (Continued)

Pearls

- Recovery (e.g. ability to stand/walk) generally takes 2–6 hours after wakening
- Half-life may be longer in obese patients
- Patients with premenstrual syndrome may be less sensitive to midazolam than healthy women throughout the cycle
- Midazolam clearance may be reduced in postmenopausal women compared to premenopausal women

- Though not systematically studied, benzodiazepines have been used effectively to treat catatonia and are the initial recommended treatment
- People experiencing amnesia as a side effect of midazolam are generally unaware their memory is impaired
- In USA, midazolam in combination with an antipsychotic drug is indicated for the acute management of agitation in schizophrenia

 Suggested Reading

Blumer JL. Clinical pharmacology of midazolam in infants and children. Clin Pharmacokinet 1998;35(1):37–47.

Chan EW, Taylor DM, Knott JC, et al. Intravenous droperidol or olanzapine as an adjunct to midazolam for the acutely agitated patient: a multicenter, randomized, double-blind, placebo-controlled clinical trial. Ann Emerg Med 2013;61(1):72–81.

Fountain NB, Adams RE. Midazolam treatment of acute and refractory status epilepticus. Clin Neuropharmacol 1999;22(5):261–7.

Patel MX, Sethi FN, Barnes TR, et al. Joint BAP NAPICU evidence-based consensus guidelines for the clinical management of acute disturbance: de-escalation and rapid tranquillisation. J Psychopharmacol 2018;32(6):601–40.

Shafer A. Complications of sedation with midazolam in the intensive care unit and a comparison with other sedative regimens. Crit Care Med 1998;26(5):947–56.

TREC Collaborative Group. Rapid tranquillisation for agitated patients in emergency psychiatric rooms: a randomised trial of midazolam versus haloperidol plus promethazine. BMJ 2003;327(7417):708–13.

Yuan R, Flockhart DA, Balian JD. Pharmacokinetic and pharmacodynamic consequences of metabolism-based drug interactions with alprazolam, midazolam, and triazolam. J Clin Pharmacol 1999;39(11):1109–25.

Zaman H, Sampson SJ, Beck AL, et al. Benzodiazepines for psychosis-induced aggression or agitation. Cochrane Database Syst Rev 2017;12:CD003079.

Mirtazapine

Brands
• Non-proprietary

Generic?
Yes

Class
• Neuroscience-based nomenclature: low-dose mirtazapine: pharmacology domain – histamine; mode of action – antagonist; upper-dose mirtazapine: pharmacology domain – norepinephrine, serotonin; mode of action – antagonist
• Alpha 2 antagonist; NaSSA (noradrenaline and specific serotonergic agent); dual serotonin and norepinephrine agent: serotonin (5HT2, 5HT3) and norepinephrine receptor antagonist (SN-RAn); antidepressant

Commonly Prescribed for
(bold for BNF indication)
• **Major depression**
• Panic disorder
• Generalised anxiety disorder
• Post-traumatic stress disorder

 How the Drug Works
• Boost neurotransmitters serotonin and noradrenaline
• Blocks alpha 2 adrenergic presynaptic receptor, thereby increasing noradrenaline neurotransmission
• Blocks alpha 2 adrenergic presynaptic receptor on serotonin neurons (heteroreceptors), thereby increasing serotonin neurotransmission
• This is a novel mechanism independent of noradrenaline and serotonin reuptake blockade
• Blocks 5HT2A, 5HT2C, and 5HT3 serotonin receptors
• Blocks H1 histamine receptors

How Long Until It Works
∗Actions on insomnia and anxiety can start shortly after initiation
• Onset of therapeutic actions with some antidepressants can be seen within 1–2 weeks, but often delayed 2–4 weeks

• If it is not working within 3–4 weeks for depression, it may require a dosage increase or it may not work at all
• By contrast, for generalised anxiety, onset of response and increases in remission rates may still occur after 8 weeks, and for up to 6 months after initiating dosing
• May continue to work for many years to prevent relapse of symptoms

If It Works
• The goal of treatment is complete remission of current symptoms as well as prevention of future relapses
• Treatment most often reduces or even eliminates symptoms, but is not a cure since symptoms can recur after medicine is stopped
• Continue treatment until all symptoms are gone (remission), especially in depression and whenever possible in anxiety disorders
• Once symptoms are gone, continue treating for at least 6–9 months for the first episode of depression or >12 months if relapse indicators present
• If >5 episodes and/or 2 episodes in the last few years then need to continue for at least 2 years or indefinitely
• Use in anxiety disorders may also need to be indefinite

If It Doesn't Work
• Important to recognise non-response to treatment early on (3–4 weeks)
• Many patients have only a partial response where some symptoms are improved but others persist (especially insomnia, fatigue, and problems concentrating)
• Other patients may be non-responders, sometimes called treatment-resistant or treatment-refractory
• Some patients who have an initial response may relapse even though they continue treatment
• Consider increasing dose, switching to another agent, or adding an appropriate augmenting agent
• Lithium may be added for suicidal patients or those at high risk of relapse
• Consider psychotherapy
• Consider ECT
• Consider evaluation for another diagnosis or for a co-morbid condition (e.g. medical illness, substance abuse, etc.)

Mirtazapine (Continued)

- Some patients may experience a switch into mania and so would require antidepressant discontinuation and initiation of a mood stabiliser

 Best Augmenting Combos for Partial Response or Treatment Resistance

- Mood stabilisers or atypical antipsychotics for bipolar depression
- Atypical antipsychotics for psychotic depression
- Atypical antipsychotics as first-line augmenting agents (quetiapine MR 300 mg/day or aripiprazole at 2.5–10 mg/day) for treatment-resistant depression
- Atypical antipsychotics as second-line augmenting agents (risperidone 0.5–2 mg/day or olanzapine 2.5–10 mg/day) for treatment-resistant depression
- *Add SSRI or SNRI (observe for switch into mania, increase in suicidal ideation or serotonin syndrome)
- Although T3 (20–50 mcg/day) is another second-line augmenting agent the evidence suggests that it works best with tricyclic antidepressants
- Other augmenting agents but with less evidence include bupropion (up to 400 mg/day), buspirone (up to 60 mg/day) and lamotrigine (up to 400 mg/day)
- Benzodiazepines if agitation present
- Hypnotics or trazodone for insomnia (but beware of serotonin syndrome with trazodone)
- Augmenting agents reserved for specialist use include: modafinil for sleepiness, fatigue and lack of concentration; stimulants, oestrogens, testosterone
- Lithium is particularly useful for suicidal patients and those at high risk of relapse including with factors such as severe depression, psychomotor retardation, repeated episodes (>3), significant weight loss, or a family history of major depression (aim for lithium plasma levels 0.6–1.0 mmol/L)
- For elderly patients lithium is a very effective augmenting agent
- For severely ill patients other combinations may be tried especially in specialist centres
- Augmenting agents that may be tried include omega-3, SAM-e, L-methylfolate

- Additional non-pharmacological treatments such as exercise, mindfulness, CBT, and IPT can also be helpful
- If present after treatment response (4–8 weeks) or remission (6–12 weeks), the most common residual symptoms of depression include cognitive impairments, reduced energy and problems with sleep

Tests

- None for healthy individuals
- May need liver function tests for those with hepatic abnormalities before initiating treatment
- May need to monitor blood count during treatment for those with blood dyscrasias, leucopenia, or granulocytopenia
- Since some antidepressants such as mirtazapine can be associated with significant weight gain, before starting treatment, weigh all patients and determine if the patient is already overweight (BMI >25.0–29.9) or obese (BMI ≥30)
- Before giving a drug that can cause weight gain to an overweight or obese patient, consider determining whether the patient already has pre-diabetes (fasting plasma glucose 5.5–6.9 mmol/L), diabetes (fasting plasma glucose >7.0 mmol/L), or dyslipidaemia (increased total cholesterol, LDL cholesterol, and triglycerides; decreased HDL cholesterol), and treat or refer such patients for treatment, including nutrition and weight management, physical activity counselling, smoking cessation, and medical management
- *Monitor weight and BMI during treatment
- *While giving a drug to a patient who has gained >5% of initial weight, consider evaluating for the presence of pre-diabetes, diabetes, or dyslipidaemia, or consider switching to a different antidepressant

SIDE EFFECTS

How Drug Causes Side Effects

- Most side effects are immediate but often go away with time
- *Histamine 1 receptor antagonism may explain sedative effects
- *Histamine 1 receptor antagonism plus 5HT2C antagonism may explain some aspects of weight gain

Notable Side Effects

- Dry mouth, constipation, increased appetite, weight gain
- Sedation, dizziness, abnormal dreams, confusion
- Flu-like symptoms (may indicate low white blood cell or granulocyte count)
- Change in urinary function
- Hypotension

Common or very common

- CNS/PNS: anxiety, confusion, dizziness, drowsiness, headache (on discontinuation), sleep disorders, tremor
- CVS: postural hypotension
- GIT: decreased appetite, constipation, diarrhoea, dry mouth, increased weight, nausea, vomiting
- Other: arthralgia, back pain, fatigue, myalgia, oedema

Uncommon

- Hallucination, mania, movement disorders, oral disorders, syncope

Rare or very rare

- Aggression, pancreatitis

Frequency not known

- Blood disorders: agranulocytosis, bone marrow disorders, eosinophilia, granulocytopenia, thrombocytopenia
- CNS/PNS: dysarthria, seizure, suicidal tendencies
- CVS: arrhythmias, QT interval prolongation
- Other: hyponatraemia, jaundice (discontinue), rhabdomyolysis, serotonin syndrome, severe cutaneous adverse reactions (SCARs), SIADH, skin reactions, sudden death, urinary retention, withdrawal syndrome

 Life-Threatening or Dangerous Side Effects

- Seizures
- Induction of mania (uncommon)
- Rare increase in suicidal ideation and behaviours in adolescents and young adults (up to age 25), hence patients should be warned of this potential adverse event
- Blood dyscrasias have been reported

Weight Gain

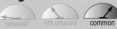

- Many experience and can be significant in amount

Sedation

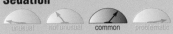

- Many experience and/or can be significant

What to Do About Side Effects

- Warn in advance about sedation and weight gain
- Wait
- Wait
- Switch to another drug

Best Augmenting Agents for Side Effects

- Often best to try another antidepressant monotherapy prior to resorting to augmentation strategies to treat side effects
- Many side effects are dose-dependent (i.e. they increase as dose increases, or they re-emerge until tolerance redevelops)
- Many side effects are time-dependent (i.e. they start immediately upon dosing and upon each dose increase, but go away with time)
- Many side effects cannot be improved with an augmenting agent
- Increased activation or agitation may represent the induction of a bipolar state, especially a mixed dysphoric bipolar condition sometimes associated with suicidal ideation, and requires the addition of lithium, a mood stabiliser or an atypical antipsychotic, and/or discontinuation of mirtazapine

DOSING AND USE

Usual Dosage Range

- 15–45 mg at night

Dosage Forms

- Tablet 15 mg, 30 mg, 45 mg
- Orodispersible tablet 15 mg, 30 mg, 45 mg
- Oral solution 15 mg/mL

How to Dose

- Initial dose 15 mg at bedtime; increase every 1–2 weeks until desired efficacy is reached; max generally 45 mg/day (at bedtime or in 2 divided doses)

 Dosing Tips

- Sedation may not worsen as dose increases when using doses of 15 mg and higher, but it is not likely that it decreases

* Breaking a 15 mg tablet in half and administering 7.5 mg dose may actually increase sedation, though this dose is below the dose needed for antidepressant effect
* Some patients require more than 45 mg daily, including up to 90 mg in difficult cases and in patients that can tolerate such doses (off-label)
* If intolerable anxiety, insomnia, agitation, akathisia, or activation occur either upon dosing initiation or discontinuation, consider the possibility of activated bipolar disorder and switch to a mood stabiliser or an atypical antipsychotic

Overdose
* Associated with tachycardia, mild hypertension and mild CNS depression not requiring intervention. Rarely lethal; all fatalities have involved other medications; symptoms include sedation, disorientation, memory impairment, rapid heartbeat

Long-Term Use
* Safe

Habit Forming
* Not expected

How to Stop
* Taper over several weeks is prudent to avoid withdrawal effects including nausea, vomiting, dizziness, agitation, anxiety, and headache

Pharmacokinetics
* Half-life 20–40 hours
* Substrate for CYP450 2D6, 3A4, and 1A2 (smoking reduces levels by 30%)
* Food does not affect absorption

 Drug Interactions

* Tramadol increases the risk of seizures in patients taking an antidepressant
* No significant pharmacokinetic drug interactions
* Can cause a fatal "serotonin syndrome" when combined with MAOIs, so do not use with MAOIs or for at least 14 days after MAOIs are stopped
* Do not start an MAOI for at least 5 half-lives (5 to 7 days for most drugs) after discontinuing mirtazapine

 Other Warnings/Precautions

* Drug may lower white blood cell count (rare; may not be increased compared to other antidepressants but controlled studies lacking; not a common problem reported in postmarketing surveillance)
* Drug may increase cholesterol
* May cause photosensitivity
* Avoid alcohol, which may increase sedation and cognitive and motor effects
* Use with caution in patients with cardiac disorders and hypotension, diabetes mellitus, history of seizures, history of urinary retention and susceptibility to angle-closure glaucoma
* Use with caution in patients with bipolar disorder unless treated with concomitant mood-stabiliser
* Use with caution in patients with psychoses (may aggravate psychotic symptoms)
* Warn patients and their caregivers about the possibility of activating side effects and advise them to report such symptoms immediately
* Monitor all patients for activation of suicidal ideation, especially those below the age of 25

Do Not Use
* If patient is taking an MAOI
* If there is a proven allergy to mirtazapine

SPECIAL POPULATIONS

Renal Impairment
* Drug should be used with caution as clearance is reduced

Hepatic Impairment
* Drug should be used with caution
* May require lower dose

Cardiac Impairment
* Drug should be used with caution
* The potential risk of hypotension should be considered

Elderly
* Some patients may tolerate lower doses better
* Reduction in the risk of suicidality with antidepressants compared to placebo in adults age 65 and older

Children and Adolescents

- Safety and efficacy in children and adolescents have not been established
- Mirtazapine is not licensed in the UK for use in children and adolescents
- Prescribing is reserved for the specialist, after first- or second-line options have been tried

Before you prescribe:
- Carefully weigh the risks and benefits of pharmacological treatment against the risks and benefits of nontreatment with antidepressants and make sure to document this in the patient's chart
- For mild to moderate depression psychotherapy (individual or systemic) should be the first-line treatment.
  For moderate to severe depression, pharmacological treatment may be offered when the young person is unresponsive after 4–6 sessions of psychological therapy. Combined initial therapy (SSRI and psychological therapy) may be considered
- For anxiety disorders evidence-based psychological treatments should be offered as first-line treatment including psychoeducation and skills training for parents, to support development of the child's or adolescent's coping skills, cognitive reframing and exposure to feared or avoided situations
- For both severe depression and anxiety disorders, pharmacological interventions may have to commence prior to psychological treatments to enable the child/young person to engage in psychological therapy
- Where a child or young person presents with self-harm and suicidal thoughts the immediate risk management may take first priority
- All children and young people presenting with depression/anxiety should be supported with sleep management, anxiety management, exercise and activation schedules, and healthy diet
- Mirtazapine may be considered as third-line option

Practical notes:
- Inform parents and child/young person that improvements may take several weeks to emerge
- The earliest effects may only be apparent to outsiders
- A risk management plan should be discussed prior to start of medication because of the possible increase in suicidal ideation and behaviours in adolescents and young adults
- Monitor patients face-to-face regularly, and weekly during the first 2–3 weeks of treatment or after increase
- Monitor for activation of suicidal ideation at the beginning of treatment
- Use with caution, observing for activation of known or unknown bipolar disorder and/or suicidal ideation; and inform parents or guardians of this risk so they can help observe child or adolescent patients

If it does not work:
- Review child's/young person's profile, consider new/changing contributing individual or systemic factors such as peer or family conflict. Consider physical health problems
- Consider non-concordance, especially in adolescents. In all children consider non-concordance by parent or child, address underlying reasons for non-concordance
- Consider dose adjustment before switching or augmentation. Be vigilant of polypharmacy especially in complex and highly vulnerable children/adolescents
- Re-evaluate the need for continued treatment regularly

Pregnancy

- Very limited data for the use of mirtazapine in pregnancy
- Limited evidence does not suggest increased risk of congenital malformation, preterm delivery or low birth weight
- Evidence suggests no association with intrauterine death, neurodevelopmental delay or neonatal complications but data too limited to exclude increased risk
- Not generally recommended for use during pregnancy, especially during first trimester
- Although there is no data to substantiate, there is a theoretical risk that as with SSRIs when used beyond the 20th week of pregnancy there is increased risk of persistent pulmonary hypertension (PPHN) in newborns

- Must weigh the risk of treatment (first trimester foetal development, third trimester newborn delivery) to the child against the risk of no treatment (recurrence of depression, maternal health, infant bonding) to the mother and child
- For many patients this may mean continuing treatment during pregnancy

Breastfeeding

- Small amounts found in human breast milk
- If child becomes irritable or sedated, breastfeeding or drug may need to be discontinued
- Immediate postpartum period is a high-risk time for depression, especially in women who have had prior depressive episodes, so drug may need to be reinstituted late in the third trimester or shortly after childbirth to prevent a recurrence during the postpartum period
- Must weigh benefits of breastfeeding with risks and benefits of antidepressant treatment versus nontreatment to both the infant and the mother
- For many patients, this may mean continuing treatment during breastfeeding
- Other antidepressants may be preferable, e.g. paroxetine, sertraline, imipramine, or nortriptyline

THE ART OF PSYCHOPHARMACOLOGY

Potential Advantages

- Patients particularly concerned about sexual side effects
- Patients with symptoms of anxiety and agitation
- Patients on concomitant medications
- As an augmenting agent to boost the efficacy of other antidepressants

Potential Disadvantages

- Patients particularly concerned about gaining weight
- Patients with low energy

Primary Target Symptoms

- Depressed mood
- Sleep disturbance
- Anxiety

 Pearls

* Adding alpha 2 antagonism to agents that block serotonin and/or norepinephrine reuptake may be synergistic for severe depression
- Adding mirtazapine to venlafaxine or SSRIs may reverse drug-induced anxiety and insomnia and improve sexual function
- Adding mirtazapine's 5HT3 antagonism to venlafaxine or SSRIs may reverse drug-induced nausea, diarrhoea, stomach cramps, and gastrointestinal side effects
- SSRIs, venlafaxine, bupropion or stimulants may mitigate mirtazapine-induced weight gain
- If weight gain has not occurred by week 6 of treatment, it is less likely for there to be significant weight gain
- Has been demonstrated to have an earlier onset of action than SSRIs
* Fewer effects on CYP450 system, and so may be preferable in patients requiring concomitant medications
- Preliminary evidence suggests efficacy as an augmenting agent to haloperidol in treating negative symptoms of schizophrenia
- Anecdotal reports of efficacy in recurrent brief depression
- Weight gain as a result of mirtazapine treatment is more likely in women than in men, and before menopause rather than after
* May cause sexual dysfunction only infrequently
- Patients can have carryover sedation and intoxicated-like feeling if particularly sensitive to sedative side effects when initiating dosing
- Rarely, patients may complain of visual "trails" or after-images on mirtazapine

Suggested Reading

Anttila SA, Leinonen EV. A review of the pharmacological and clinical profile of mirtazapine. CNS Drug Rev 2001;7(3):249–64.

Benkert O, Muller M, Szegedi A. An overview of the clinical efficacy of mirtazapine. Hum Psychopharmacol 2002;17(Suppl 1):S23–6.

Cipriani A, Furukawa TA, Salanti G, et al. Comparative efficacy and acceptability of 21 antidepressant drugs for the acute treatment of adults with major depressive disorder: a systematic review and network meta-analysis. Lancet 2018;391(10128):1357–66.

Falkai P. Mirtazapine: other indications. J Clin Psychiatry 1999;60(Suppl 17):36–40; discussion 46–8.

Fawcett J, Barkin RL. A meta-analysis of eight randomized, double-blind, controlled clinical trials of mirtazapine for the treatment of patients with major depression and symptoms of anxiety. J Clin Psychiatry 1998;59(3):123–7.

Masand PS, Gupta S. Long-term side effects of newer-generation antidepressants: SSRIS, venlafaxine, nefazodone, bupropion, and mirtazapine. Ann Clin Psychiatry 2002;14(3):175–82.

Shuman M, Chukwu A, Van Veldhuizen N, et al. Relationship between mirtazapine dose and incidence of adrenergic side effects: an exploratory analysis. Ment Health Clin 2019;9(1):41–7.

Watanabe N, Omori IM, Nakagawa A, et al. Mirtazapine versus other antidepressive agents for depression. Cochrane Database Syst Rev 2011;7(12):CD006528.

Moclobemide

THERAPEUTICS

Brands
• Manerix

Generic?
Yes

Class
• Neuroscience-based nomenclature: pharmacology domain – serotonin, norepinephrine, dopamine; mode of action – enzyme inhibitor
• Reversible inhibitor of monoamine oxidase A (MAO-A) (RIMA)

Commonly Prescribed for
(bold for BNF indication)
• **Depressive illness**
• **Social anxiety disorder**

How the Drug Works
• Reversibly blocks MAO-A from breaking down noradrenaline, dopamine, and serotonin
• This presumably boosts noradrenergic, serotonergic, and dopaminergic neurotransmission
• MAO-A inhibition predominates unless significant concentrations of monoamines build up (e.g. due to dietary tyramine), in which case MAO-A inhibition is theoretically reversed

How Long Until It Works
• Onset of therapeutic actions with some antidepressants can be seen within 1–2 weeks, but often delayed 2–4 weeks
• If it is not working within 3–4 weeks for depression, it may require a dosage increase or it may not work at all
• For anxiety, onset of response and increases in remission rates may still occur after 8 weeks, and for up to 6 months after initiating dosing
• May continue to work for many years to prevent relapse of symptoms

If It Works
• The goal of treatment is complete remission of current symptoms as well as prevention of future relapses
• Treatment most often reduces or even eliminates symptoms, but is not a cure since symptoms can recur after medicine is stopped
• Continue treatment until all symptoms are gone (remission), especially in depression and whenever possible in anxiety disorders
• Once symptoms are gone, continue treating for at least 6–9 months for the first episode of depression or >12 months if relapse indicators present
• If >5 episodes and/or 2 episodes in the last few years then need to continue for at least 2 years or indefinitely
• Use in anxiety disorders may also need to be indefinite

If It Doesn't Work
• Important to recognise non-response to treatment early on (3–4 weeks)
• Many patients have only a partial response where some symptoms are improved but others persist (especially insomnia, fatigue, and problems concentrating)
• Other patients may be non-responders, sometimes called treatment-resistant or treatment-refractory
• Some patients who have an initial response may relapse even though they continue treatment
• Consider increasing dose, switching to another agent, or adding an appropriate augmenting agent
• Lithium may be added for suicidal patients or those at high risk of relapse
• Consider psychotherapy
• Consider ECT
• Consider evaluation for another diagnosis or for a co-morbid condition (e.g. medical illness, substance abuse, etc.)
• Some patients may experience a switch into mania and so would require antidepressant discontinuation and initiation of a mood stabiliser

Best Augmenting Combos for Partial Response or Treatment Resistance
* Augmentation of MAOIs has not been systematically studied, and this is something for the expert, to be done with caution and with careful monitoring
• Lithium is particularly useful for suicidal patients and those at high risk of relapse including with factors such as severe depression, psychomotor retardation,

repeated episodes (>3), significant weight loss, or a family history of major depression (aim for lithium plasma levels 0.6–1.0 mmol/L)
- Atypical antipsychotics (with special caution for those agents with monoamine reuptake blocking properties)
- Mood-stabilising anticonvulsants
* A stimulant such as dexamfetaime or methylphenidate (with caution; may activate bipolar disorder and suicidal ideation; may elevate blood pressure)

Tests
- Patients should be monitored for changes in blood pressure

SIDE EFFECTS

How Drug Causes Side Effects
- Theoretically due to increases in monoamines in parts of the brain and body and at receptors other than those that cause therapeutic actions (e.g. unwanted actions of serotonin in sleep centres causing insomnia, unwanted actions of norepinephrine on vascular smooth muscle causing changes in blood pressure)
- Side effects are generally immediate, but immediate side effects often subside in time

Notable Side Effects
- Insomnia, dizziness, agitation, anxiety, restlessness
- Dry mouth, diarrhoea, constipation, nausea, vomiting
- Galactorrhoea
- Rare hypertension

Common or very common
- CNS/PNS: anxiety, dizziness, headache, irritability, paraesthesia, sleep disorder
- CVS: hypotension
- GIT: constipation, diarrhoea, dry mouth, nausea, vomiting
- Other: skin reactions

Uncommon
- Altered taste, asthenia, confusion, flushing, oedema, suicidal tendencies, visual impairment

Rare or very rare
- Decreased appetite, delusions, hyponatraemia, serotonin syndrome

 ### Life-Threatening or Dangerous Side Effects
- Hypertensive crisis (especially when MAOIs are used with certain tyramine-containing foods – reduced risk compared to irreversible MAOIs)
- Induction of mania
- Rare increase in suicidal ideation and behaviours in adolescents and young adults (up to age 25), hence patients should be warned of this potential adverse event
- Seizures

Weight Gain

unusual   not unusual   common   problematic

- Reported but not expected

Sedation

unusual   not unusual   common   problematic

- Occurs in significant minority

What to Do About Side Effects
- Wait
- Wait
- Wait
- Lower the dose
- Switch to an SSRI or newer antidepressant

Best Augmenting Agents for Side Effects
- Trazodone (with caution) for insomnia
- Benzodiazepines for insomnia
- Many side effects cannot be improved with an augmenting agent

---

DOSING AND USE

Usual Dosage Range
- 150–600 mg/day

Dosage Forms
- Tablet 150 mg, 300 mg
- Oral suspension is available on special order

How to Dose
* Depressive illness:
- Initial dose 300 mg/day in divided doses, adjusted according to response; usual dose 150–600 mg/day, dose to be taken after food

*For social anxiety disorder:
• Initial dose 300 mg/day for 3 days, increased to 600 mg/day in 2 divided doses; assess efficacy after 8–12 weeks of treatment

 Dosing Tips

*At higher doses, moclobemide also inhibits MAO-B and thereby loses its selectivity for MAO-A, with uncertain clinical consequences
*Taking moclobemide after meals as opposed to before may minimise the chances of interactions with tyramine
• May be less toxic in overdose than TCAs and older MAOIs
• Clinical duration of action may be longer than biological half-life and allow twice-daily dosing in some patients, or even once-daily dosing, especially at lower doses

Overdose
• Agitation, aggression, behavioural disturbances, gastrointestinal irritation

Long-Term Use
• MAOIs may lose efficacy long-term

Habit Forming
• Some patients have developed dependence to MAOIs

How to Stop
• Taper not generally necessary

Pharmacokinetics
• Partially metabolised by CYP450 2C19 and 2D6
• Inactive metabolites
• Elimination half-life about 2–4 hours
• Clinical duration of action at least 24 hours

 Drug Interactions

• Moclobemide is claimed to cause less potentiation of the pressor effect of tyramine than the traditional (irreversible) MAOIs, but patients should avoid consuming large amounts of tyramine-rich foods (such as mature cheese, salami, pickled herring, Bovril®, Oxo®, Marmite® or any similar meat or yeast extract or fermented soya bean extract, and some beers, lagers or wines)

• Tramadol may increase the risk of seizures in patients taking an MAOI
• Can cause a fatal "serotonin syndrome" when combined with drugs that block serotonin reuptake, so do not use with a serotonin reuptake inhibitor or for 5 half-lives after stopping the serotonin reuptake inhibitor (see Table 1 after Pearls)
• Hypertensive crisis with headache, intracranial bleeding, and death may result from combining MAOIs with sympathomimetic drugs (e.g. amfetamines, methylphenidate, cocaine, dopamine, epinephrine, norepinephrine, and related compounds methyldopa, levodopa, L-tryptophan, L-tyrosine, and phenylalanine)
• Do not combine with another MAOI, alcohol, or guanethidine
• Adverse drug reactions can result from combining MAOIs with tricyclic/tetracyclic antidepressants and related compounds, including carbamazepine and mirtazapine, and should be avoided except by experts to treat difficult cases
• MAOIs in combination with spinal anaesthesia may cause combined hypotensive effects
• Combination of MAOIs and CNS depressants may enhance sedation and hypotension
• Cimetidine may increase plasma concentrations of moclobemide
• Moclobemide is a potent inhibitor of CYP450 2C19 substrates (warfarin, omeprazole, phenytoin)
• Moclobemide may enhance the effects of NSAIDs such as ibuprofen

 Other Warnings/Precautions

• Use still requires low-tyramine diet, although more tyramine may be tolerated with moclobemide than with other MAOIs before eliciting a hypertensive reaction (see Table 2 after Pearls)
• Patient and prescriber must be vigilant to potential interactions with any drug, including antihypertensives and over-the-counter cough/cold preparations
• Over-the-counter medications to avoid include cough and cold preparations, including those containing dextromethorphan, nasal decongestants

(tablets, drops, or spray), hay-fever medications, sinus medications, asthma inhalant medications, anti-appetite medications, weight-reducing preparations, "pep" pills (see Table 3 after Pearls)
• Use cautiously in hypertensive or thyrotoxic patients
• Moclobemide is not recommended for use in patients who cannot be monitored closely
• Ensure patients read the leaflets provided with the medication
• Warn patients and their caregivers about the possibility of activating side effects and advise them to report such symptoms immediately
• Monitor patients for activation of suicidal ideation, especially young adults

Do Not Use
• In agitated patients or in the manic phase
• If patient is taking pethidine
• If patient is taking a sympathomimetic agent or taking guanethidine
• If patient is taking another MAOI
• If patient is taking any agent that can inhibit serotonin reuptake (e.g. SSRIs, sibutramine, tramadol, duloxetine, venlafaxine, clomipramine, etc.)
• If patient is in an acute confusional state
• If patient has phaeochromocytoma
• If patient has frequent or severe headaches
• If patient is undergoing elective surgery and requires general anaesthesia
• If there is a proven allergy to moclobemide

Elderly
• Elderly patients may have greater sensitivity to adverse effects
• Reduction in the risk of suicidality with antidepressants compared to placebo in adults age 65 and older

 Children and Adolescents
• Not recommended for use in children and adolescents

Pregnancy
• Controlled studies have not been conducted in pregnant women
• Not generally recommended for use during pregnancy, especially during first trimester
• Use in pregnancy may be justified if the benefit of continued treatment exceeds any associated risk

Breastfeeding
• Small amounts found in mother's breast milk
• Effects on infant are unknown
• Immediate postpartum period is a high-risk time for depression, especially in women who have had prior depressive episodes, so drug may need to be reinstituted late in the third trimester or shortly after childbirth to prevent a recurrence during the postpartum period
• The benefits of continuing treatment during breastfeeding should be weighed against possible risks to the infant

SPECIAL POPULATIONS

Renal Impairment
• Use with caution

Hepatic Impairment
• Plasma concentrations are increased
• May require one-half to one-third of usual adult dose

Cardiac Impairment
• Cardiac impairment may require lower than usual adult dose
• Patients with angina pectoris or coronary artery disease should limit their exertion

THE ART OF PSYCHOPHARMACOLOGY

Potential Advantages
• Atypical depression
• Severe depression
• Treatment-resistant depression or anxiety disorders

Potential Disadvantages
• Patients non-concordant with dietary restrictions, concomitant drug restrictions, and twice-daily dosing after meals

Primary Target Symptoms
• Depressed mood

Pearls

- MAOIs are generally reserved for use after SSRIs, SNRIs, TCAs and combinations of newer antidepressants have failed
- Patient should be advised not to take any prescription or over-the-counter drugs without consulting his/her doctor because of possible drug interactions with the MAOI
- Headache is often the first symptom of hypertensive crisis
- Moclobemide has a much reduced risk of interactions with tyramine than non-selective MAOIs
- Foods with high tyramine need to be avoided, especially at higher doses of moclobemide (see Table 2)
- The rigid dietary restrictions may reduce adherence
- *May be a safer alternative to classical irreversible non-selective MAO-A and MAO-B inhibitors with less propensity for tyramine and drug interactions and hepatotoxicity (although not entirely free of interactions)
- May not be as effective at low doses, and may have more side effects at higher doses
- Moclobemide's profile at higher doses may be more similar to classical MAOIs
- MAOIs are a viable treatment option in depression, but are not frequently used
- *Myths about the danger of dietary tyramine can be exaggerated, but prohibitions against concomitant drugs often not followed closely enough
- Orthostatic hypotension, insomnia, and sexual dysfunction are some of the most troublesome side effects
- *MAOIs should be for the specialist, and particular caution needed if combining with agents of potential risk (e.g. stimulants, trazodone, TCAs)
- *MAOIs should not be neglected as therapeutic agents for the treatment-resistant
- Although generally prohibited, a heroic but potentially dangerous treatment for severely treatment-resistant patients is for an expert to give a tricyclic/tetracyclic antidepressant other than clomipramine simultaneously with an MAOI for patients who fail to respond to numerous other antidepressants
- Use of MAOIs with clomipramine is always prohibited because of the risk of serotonin syndrome and death
- Although very strict dietary and concomitant drug restrictions must be observed to prevent hypertensive crises and serotonin syndrome, the most common side effects of MAOI and tricyclic/tetracyclic combinations may be weight gain and orthostatic hypotension

Table 1. Drugs contraindicated due to risk of serotonin syndrome/toxicity

Do Not Use:			
Antidepressants	Drugs of Abuse	Opioids	Other
SSRIs	MDMA (ecstasy)	Pethidine	Non-subcutaneous sumatriptan
SNRIs	Cocaine	Tramadol	Chlorphenamine
Clomipramine	Metamfetamine	Methadone	Brompheniramine
St. John's wort	High-dose or injected amfetamine	Fentanyl	Dextromethorphan
			Procarbazine?

Moclobemide (Continued)

Table 2. Dietary guidelines for patients taking MAOIs

Foods to avoid*	Foods allowed
Dried, aged, smoked, fermented, spoiled, or improperly stored meat, poultry, and fish	Fresh or processed meat, poultry, and fish; properly stored pickled or smoked fish
Broad bean pods	All other vegetables
Aged cheeses	Processed cheese slices, cottage cheese, ricotta cheese, yoghurt, cream cheese
Keg and unpasteurised beer	Canned or bottled beer and alcohol
Marmite	Brewer's and baker's yeast
Sauerkraut, kimchee	
Soy products/tofu	Peanuts
Banana peel	Bananas, avocados, raspberries
Tyramine-containing nutritional supplement	

*Not necessary for 6-mg transdermal or low-dose oral selegiline

Table 3. Drugs that boost norepinephrine: should only be used with caution with MAOIs

Use With Caution:			
Decongestants	Stimulants	Antidepressants with norepinephrine reuptake inhibition	Other
Phenylephrine	Amfetamines	Most tricyclics	Phentermine
Pseudoephedrine	Methylphenidate	NRIs	Local anaesthetics containing vasoconstrictors
	Cocaine	NDRIs	
	Metamfetamine		
	Modafinil		Tapentadol
	Armodafinil		

 Suggested Reading

Bandelow B. Current and novel psychopharmacological drugs for anxiety disorders. Adv Exp Med Biol 2020;1191:347–65.

Fulton B, Benfield P. Moclobemide. An update of its pharmacological properties and therapeutic use. Drugs 1996;52(3):450–74. Erratum in Drugs 1996;52(6):869.

Gillman PK. A reassessment of the safety profile of monoamine oxidase inhibitors: elucidating tired old tyramine myths. J Neural Transm (Vienna) 2018;125(11):1707–17.

Kennedy SH. Continuation and maintenance treatments in major depression: the neglected role of monoamine oxidase inhibitors. J Psychiatry Neurosci 1997;22(2):127–31.

Lippman SB, Nash K. Monoamine oxidase inhibitor update. Potential adverse food and drug interactions. Drug Saf 1990;5(3):195–204.

Nutt D, Montgomery SA. Moclobemide in the treatment of social phobia. Int Clin Psychopharmacol 1996;11(Suppl 3):77–82.

Modafinil

Brands
• Provigil

Generic?
Yes

Class
• Neuroscience-based nomenclature: pharmacology domain – dopamine; mode of action – reuptake inhibitor
• Wake-promoting

Commonly Prescribed for
(bold for BNF indication)
• **Excessive sleepiness associated with narcolepsy with or without cataplexy**
• Fatigue and sleepiness in depression or bipolar depression
• Attention deficit hyperactivity disorder

How the Drug Works
• Unknown, but clearly different from classical stimulants such as methylphenidate and amfetamine
• Binds to and requires the presence of the dopamine transporter; also requires the presence of alpha-adrenergic receptors
• Can inhibit reuptake of dopamine via the dopamine transporter
• Increases neuronal activity selectively in the hypothalamus
∗ Presumably enhances activity in hypothalamic wakefulness centre (tuberomammillary nucleus – TMN) within the hypothalamic sleep-wake switch by an unknown mechanism
∗ Activates TMN neurons that release histamine
∗ Activates other hypothalamic neurons that release orexin/hypocretin

How Long Until It Works
• Can immediately reduce daytime sleepiness and improve cognitive task performance within 2 hours of first dosing
• Can take several days to optimise dosing and clinical improvement

If It Works
∗ Improves daytime sleepiness and may improve attention as well as fatigue
∗ Does not generally prevent one from falling asleep when needed

• May not completely normalise wakefulness
• Treat until improvement stabilises and then continue treatment indefinitely as long as improvement persists (studies support at least 12 weeks of treatment)

If It Doesn't Work
∗ Change dose; some patients do better with an increased dose, but some actually do better with a decreased dose
• Augment or consider an alternative treatment for daytime sleepiness, fatigue, or ADHD

Best Augmenting Combos for Partial Response or Treatment Resistance
∗ Modafinil is itself an augmenting therapy to antidepressants for residual sleepiness and fatigue in major depressive disorder
∗ Best to attempt another monotherapy prior to augmenting with other drugs in the treatment of sleepiness associated with sleep disorders or problems concentrating in ADHD
• Combination of modafinil with stimulants such as methylphenidate or amfetamine or with atomoxetine for ADHD has not been systematically studied and safety is not established
• However, such combinations may be useful options for experts, with close monitoring, when numerous monotherapies for sleepiness or ADHD have failed

Tests
• ECG required before initiation
• Monitor blood pressure and heart rate in hypertensive patients

How Drug Causes Side Effects
• Unknown
• CNS side effects presumably due to excessive CNS actions on various neurotransmitter systems

Notable Side Effects
∗ Headache (dose-dependent)
• Anxiety, nervousness, insomnia
• Dry mouth, diarrhoea, nausea, anorexia
• Pharyngitis, rhinitis, infection

- Hypertension
- Palpitations

Common or very common

- CNS/PNS: abnormal sensation, abnormal thinking, altered mood, anxiety, confusion, depression, dizziness, drowsiness, headaches, sleep disorders, vision disorders
- CVS: arrhythmias, chest pain, palpitations, vasodilation
- GIT: abnormal appetite, constipation, diarrhoea, dry mouth, gastrointestinal discomfort, nausea
- Other: asthenia

Uncommon

- Blood disorders: eosinophilia, leucopenia
- CNS/PNS: abnormal behaviour, CNS stimulation, memory loss, movement disorders, psychiatric disorders, speech disorder, suicidal ideation, tremor, vertigo
- CVS: hypertension, hypotension
- Endocrine/metabolic: diabetes, hypercholesterolaemia, hyperglycaemia
- GIT: altered taste, dysphagia, gastrointestinal disorders, oral disorders, thirst, vomiting, weight changes
- Other: abnormal urine, allergic rhinitis, arthralgia, asthma, decreased libido, dry eye, dyspnoea, epistaxis, hyperhidrosis, increased muscle tone, increased risk of infection, menstrual disorder, muscle complaints, muscle weakness, pain, peripheral oedema, skin reactions, urinary frequency, worsening cough

Rare or very rare

- Hallucination, psychosis

Frequency not known

- Delusions, fever, hypersensitivity, lymphadenopathy, severe cutaneous adverse reactions (SCARs)

 Life-Threatening or Dangerous Side Effects

- Transient ECG ischaemic changes in patients with mitral valve prolapse or left ventricular hypertrophy
- Activation of hypomania/mania, anxiety, hallucinations and suicidal ideation
- Severe dermatological reactions (Stevens-Johnsons syndrome and others)
- Angioedema, anaphylactoid reactions and multi-organ hypersensitivity reactions

Weight Gain

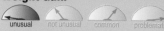

- Reported but not expected
- Uncommon

Sedation

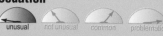

- Reported but not expected
- Patients are usually awakened and some may be activated

What To Do About Side Effects

- Wait
- Lower the dose
- Give only once daily
- Give smaller split doses 2 or more times daily
- For activation or insomnia, do not give in the evening
- If unacceptable side effects persist, discontinue use
- For life-threatening or dangerous side effects, discontinue immediately (e.g. at first sign of a drug-related rash)

Best Augmenting Agents for Side Effects

- Many side effects cannot be improved with an augmenting agent

DOSING AND USE

Usual Dosage Range

- Adults: 200–400 mg/day in 1 or 2 divided doses

Dosage Forms

- Tablet 100 mg, 200 mg

How to Dose

- Adults: initial dose 200 mg/day in 2 doses (morning and noon) or 200 mg/day once daily (morning); can be adjusted according to response to 200–400 mg in 2 divided doses or 1 dose
- Elderly: initial dose 100 mg/day
- Titration up or down only necessary if not optimally efficacious at the standard starting dose

Dosing Tips

- Higher doses may be better than lower doses in patients with daytime sleepiness in sleep disorders
- For problems concentrating and fatigue: lower doses (50–200 mg/day) may be paradoxically better than higher doses (200–400 mg/day) in some patients
- At high doses, may slightly induce its own metabolism, possibly by actions of inducing CYP450 3A4
- Dose may creep upward in some patients with long-term treatment due to auto-induction: drug holiday may restore efficacy at original dose

Overdose

- Can be fatal alone or in combination; CNS: agitation, anxiety, confusion, disorientation, excitation, hallucinations, insomnia, restlessness; GIT: diarrhoea, nausea; CVS: bradycardia, chest pain, hypertension, tachycardia

Long-Term Use

- Efficacy in reducing excessive sleepiness in sleep disorders has been demonstrated in 9- to 12-week trials
- Unpublished data show safety for up to 136 weeks
- The need for continued treatment should be re-evaluated periodically

Habit Forming

- May have potential for abuse

How to Stop

- Taper not necessary, but patients may have sleepiness on discontinuation

Pharmacokinetics

- Metabolised by the liver
- Excreted renally
- Composed of 2 enantiomers: 'R' and 'S'
- Elimination half-life of 'R' enantiomer after multiple doses is about 15 hours
- Half-life for 'S' enantiomer is about 4 hours
- Inhibits CYP450 2C19 (and perhaps 2C9)
- Induces CYP450 3A4 – especially 'R' enantiomer (and slightly 1A2 and 2B6)

Drug Interactions

- May increase plasma levels of drugs metabolised by CYP450 2C19 (e.g. diazepam, phenytoin, propranolol)
- Modafinil may increase plasma levels of CYP450 2D6 substrates such as TCAs and SSRIs, perhaps requiring downward dose adjustments of these agents
- Modafinil may decrease plasma levels of CYP450 3A4 substrates such as ethinylestradiol and cyclosporine
- Due to induction of CYP450 3A4, effectiveness of steroidal contraceptives may be reduced by modafinil, including 1 month after discontinuation (additional or alternative methods of contraception required and women should be warned of the risk of congenital malformations)
- Inducers or inhibitors of CYP450 3A4 may affect levels of modafinil (e.g. carbamazepine may lower modafinil plasma levels; fluvoxamine and fluoxetine may raise modafinil plasma levels)
- Modafinil may slightly reduce its own levels by auto-induction of CYP450 3A4
- Modafinil may increase clearance of drugs dependent on CYP450 1A2 and reduce their plasma levels
- Patients on modafinil and warfarin should have prothrombin times monitored
- Methylphenidate may delay absorption of modafinil by an hour
- *However, co-administration with methylphenidate does not significantly change the pharmacokinetics of either modafinil or methylphenidate
- *Co-administration with dexamfetamine also does not significantly change the pharmacokinetics of either modafinil or dexamfetamine
- Interaction studies with MAOIs have not been performed, but MAOIs can be given with modafinil by experts with cautious monitoring

Other Warnings/Precautions

- Use with caution in patients with a history of alcohol or drug abuse
- Use with caution in patients with a history of depression, mania or psychosis
- Possibility of dependence

Modafinil (Continued)

Do Not Use

- In patients with arrhythmias
- In patients with a history of clinically significant signs of CNS stimulant-induced mitral valve prolapse including ischaemic ECG changes, chest pain and arrhythmias
- In patients with a history of cor-pulmonale, left ventricular hypertrophy or moderate/ severe uncontrolled hypertension
- If there is a proven allergy to modafinil

SPECIAL POPULATIONS

Renal Impairment

- Use with caution; end-stage renal disease start at 50% dose and increase gradually according to response

Hepatic Impairment

- Dose adjustment – halve the dose in severe impairment

Cardiac Impairment

- Monitor blood pressure and heart rate in hypertensive patients

Elderly

- Initial dose 100 mg/day
- Limited experience in people >65 years old
- Clearance may be reduced in older people

Children and Adolescents

- For ADHD: modafinil [unlicensed] has been used in the management of ADHD, but due to limited evidence its use is not recommended without specialist advice

Pregnancy

- Controlled studies have not been conducted in pregnant women
- Limited data suggest a three-fold increase in risk of congenital malformation
- Intrauterine growth restriction and spontaneous abortion have been reported with armodafinil and modafinil
- In animal studies, developmental toxicity was observed at clinically relevant plasma exposures of armodafinil and modafinil
- Use in women of childbearing potential requires weighing potential benefits to the mother against potential risks to the foetus

* Generally, modafinil should be discontinued prior to anticipated pregnancies

Breastfeeding

- Unknown if modafinil is secreted in human breast milk, but all psychotropics assumed to be secreted in breast milk
- Extremely limited evidence of safety
- Monitor the infant for side effects seen in adults
- For narcolepsy dexamfetamine may be preferable

THE ART OF PSYCHOPHARMACOLOGY

Potential Advantages

- Selective for areas of brain involved in sleep/wake promotion
- Less activating and less abuse potential than stimulants

Potential Disadvantages

- May not work as well as stimulants in some patients with ADHD

Primary Target Symptoms

- Sleepiness
- Concentration
- Physical and mental fatigue

Pearls

* Modafinil is not a replacement for sleep
* The treatment for sleep deprivation is sleep, not modafinil
* May be useful to treat fatigue in younger patients with depression. Experience in older people >65 years is limited
- Use in other CNS disorders, such as multiple sclerosis, is not recommended by NICE and all such use is off-label as the evidence base is equivocal and risks may outweigh benefits
- In depression, modafinil's actions on sleepiness also appear to be independent of actions (if any) on mood, but may be linked to actions on fatigue or on global functioning
- Several controlled studies in depression show improvement in sleepiness or global functioning, especially for depressed patients with sleepiness and fatigue

- May be useful adjunct to mood stabilisers for bipolar depression, but should be used with caution
- Subjective sensation associated with modafinil is usually one of normal wakefulness, not of stimulation, although jitteriness can rarely occur
- Anecdotally, some patients may experience wearing off of efficacy over time, especially for off-label uses, with restoration of efficacy after a drug holiday; such wearing off is less likely with intermittent dosing
- *Compared to stimulants, modafinil has a novel mechanism of action, novel therapeutic uses, and less abuse potential, but is often inaccurately classified as a stimulant
- Alpha 1 antagonists such as prazosin may block the therapeutic actions of modafinil

 Suggested Reading

Goss AJ, Kaser M, Costafreda SG, et al. Modafinil augmentation therapy in unipolar and bipolar depression: a systematic review and meta-analysis of randomized controlled trials. J Clin Psychiatry 2013;74(11):1101–7.

Jasinski DR, Koyacevic-Ristanovic R. Evaluation of the abuse liability of modafinil and other drugs for excessive daytime sleepiness associated with narcolepsy. Clin Neuropharmacol 2000;23(3):149–56.

Kumar R. Approved and investigational uses of modafinil: an evidence-based review. Drugs 2008;68(13):1803–39.

Wesensten NJ, Belenky G, Kautz MA, et al. Maintaining alertness and performance during sleep deprivation: modafinil versus caffeine. Psychopharmacology (Berl) 2002;159(3):238–47.

Nalmefene

THERAPEUTICS

Brands
• Selincro

Generic?
No, not in UK

Class
• Neuroscience-based nomenclature: pharmacology domain – opioid; mode of action – antagonist
• Alcohol dependence treatment: mu and delta receptor antagonist and kappa opioid receptor partial agonist

Commonly Prescribed for
(bold for BNF indication)
• **Reduction of alcohol consumption in patients with alcohol dependence who have high drinking risk level (without physical withdrawal symptoms and who do not require immediate detoxification)**
• Pathological gambling
• Management of opiate overdose

 ### How the Drug Works
• Reduces alcohol consumption through modulation of opioid systems, thereby reducing the reinforcing effects of alcohol
• Blockade of mu opioid receptors prevents the pleasurable effects of alcohol, whereas modulation of the kappa opioid receptors may reduce dysphoria associated with alcohol withdrawal
• Blocks human brain mu receptors for 24 hours as seen on PET

How Long Until It Works
• Can begin working immediately and used as needed

If It Works
• Reduces alcohol consumption by diminishing reinforcing properties of alcohol (rewarding effects, cravings)
• Reduced number of heavy and very heavy drinking days and total alcohol consumption

If It Doesn't Work
• Evaluate and address contributing factors
• Consider switching to another agent

 ### Best Augmenting Combos for Partial Response or Treatment Resistance
• Should be prescribed alongside psychosocial support in groups or as an individual for successful treatment
• Limited evidence for augmentation with other drugs

Tests
• None for healthy individuals, but baseline liver function testing useful as they may be altered by treatment

SIDE EFFECTS

How Drug Causes Side Effects
• Blockade of mu opioid receptors

Notable Side Effects
• Nausea, vomiting
• Dizziness, insomnia, headaches
• Decreased appetite

Common or very common
• CNS/PNS: abnormal sensation, confusion, dizziness, drowsiness, feeling abnormal, headache, impaired concentration, restlessness, sleep disorders, tremor
• CVS: palpitations, tachycardia
• GIT: decreased appetite, decreased weight, diarrhoea, dry mouth, nausea, vomiting
• Other: asthenia, decreased libido, hyperhidrosis, malaise, muscle spasms

Frequency not known
• Dissociation, hallucinations

 ### Life-Threatening or Dangerous Side Effects
• Confusion, dissociation and hallucinations

Weight Gain
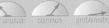
unusual   not unusual   common   problematic
• Weight loss and reduced appetite are common

Sedation

unusual   not unusual   common   problematic
• Drowsiness is common
• Sedation occurs in significant minority

What To Do About Side Effects
• Wait or switch to another agent

Best Augmenting Agents for Side Effects
• Switching to another agent may be more effective since most side effects cannot be improved with an augmenting agent

DOSING AND USE

Usual Dosage Range
• 18 mg/day as needed

Dosage Forms
• Tablet 18 mg

How to Dose
• Before initiating treatment, evaluate the patient's clinical status, alcohol dependence, and level of alcohol consumption. After an initial visit, the patient should keep a record of alcohol consumption for 2 weeks. Those who continue to have a high drinking risk level (more than 7.5 units/day for men and 5 units/day for women) during those 2 weeks can be initiated on nalmefene
• Patient should be opioid-free for 7–10 days before initiating treatment
• Nalmefene is taken as needed: 18 mg to be taken on each day there is a risk of drinking alcohol, 1–2 hours before the anticipated time of drinking
• If a dose has not been taken before starting to drink alcohol, 1 dose should be taken as soon as possible
• Max dose 18 mg/day

Dosing Tips
• Tablet should be swallowed whole, not chewed or crushed as nalmefene can cause skin irritation
• Can be taken with or without food
• Nalmefene should only be prescribed in conjunction with continuous psychosocial support focused on treatment adherence and reduced alcohol consumption

Overdose
• Limited experience

Long-Term Use
• Caution with use over 1 year (trial evaluation only up to 1 year – greatest effect in first 4 weeks); patients should be monitored regularly and the need for continued treatment should be assessed

Habit Forming
• No

How to Stop
• Taper not necessary

Pharmacokinetics
• Extensively metabolised by the liver
• Terminal half-life about 10.8 +/– 5.3 hours
• Excretion mainly via kidneys

 Drug Interactions
• Increased depressive effects, particularly respiratory depression, have occurred when taken with other CNS depressants; consider dose reduction of either or both when taken concomitantly
• UGT2B7 inhibitors (e.g. diclofenac, fluconazole, medroxyprogesterone acetate, meclofenamic acid) may increase nalmefene levels
• UGT2B7 inducers (e.g. dexamethasone, phenobarbital, rifampicin, omeprazole) may decrease nalmefene levels
• Decreased efficacy of opioid-based drugs with nalmefene

 Other Warnings/Precautions
• To prevent withdrawal in patients dependent on opioids, patients must be opioid-free for 7–10 days before initiating treatment
• Individuals receiving nalmefene who require pain management with opioid analgesia may need a higher dose than usual and may experience deeper and more prolonged respiratory depression; pain management with non-opioid or rapid-acting opioid analgesics recommended if possible
• Nalmefene should be temporarily discontinued 1 week prior to anticipated use of opioids, e.g. analgesia during elective surgery
• Caution when using products containing opioids, e.g. cough medicines
• Risk of respiratory depression is increased with concomitant use of CNS depressants
• Use with caution in patients with psychiatric illness

- Use with caution in patients with a history of seizure disorders including alcohol withdrawal seizures
- Caution when continuing treatment for more than 1 year

Do Not Use
- If patient is taking opioid analgesics, is dependent on opioids or is in acute opioid withdrawal
- If patient has a recent history of acute alcohol withdrawal syndrome
- If patient has severe hepatic or renal impairment
- If patient has galactose intolerance, lactase deficiency, or glucose-galactose malabsorption
- If there is a proven allergy to nalmefene

SPECIAL POPULATIONS

Renal Impairment
- No dose adjustment recommended in mild or moderate impairment, but use with caution
- Avoid in severe impairment

Hepatic Impairment
- No dose adjustment recommended in mild or moderate impairment, but use with caution
- Avoid in severe impairment

Cardiac Impairment
- Not studied

Elderly
- Limited data

Children and Adolescents
- Safety/efficacy not established – no data available

Pregnancy
- Controlled studies have not been conducted in pregnant women
- Some animal studies have shown adverse effects
- Pregnant women needing to stop drinking may consider behavioural therapy before pharmacotherapy

- Not generally recommended for use during pregnancy, especially during first trimester

Breastfeeding
- Unknown if nalmefene is secreted in human breast milk, but all psychotropics assumed to be secreted in breast milk
- * Recommended either to discontinue drug or bottle feed

THE ART OF PSYCHOPHARMACOLOGY

Potential Advantages
- Individuals who are not ready to abstain completely from alcohol

Potential Disadvantages
- Individuals whose goal is immediate abstinence

Primary Target Symptoms
- Alcohol dependence

Pearls
- Nalmefene was originally used as a parenteral agent to reverse the opioid agonist effects of opioid anaesthesia or in opioid overdose
- Nalmefene is intended for patients with the goal of reduced-risk drinking; it has been shown to reduce alcohol consumption on average by 60%
- Reduction in alcohol consumption has been shown to be maintained at 13 months
- Nalmefene can be used for patients who do not need detoxification, i.e. in "less severe" dependence
- Alcohol withdrawal-related dysphoria is reduced by nalmefene's partial agonist action on kappa opioid receptors
- Nalmefene is unique in that it is taken as needed when the patient perceives a risk of drinking alcohol
- Nalmefene does not provide any therapeutic opioid analgesia
- The common side effects of nausea and insomnia are likely to go away after a few days of use
- Nalmefene may have a better safety profile than naltrexone with less risk of liver toxicity

Nalmefene (Continued)

- An indirect meta-analysis showed nalmefene to be superior to naltrexone in reducing the quantity and frequency of heavy drinking
- However, controversy exists as another meta-analysis showed nalmefene to have

only limited efficacy in reducing alcohol consumption
- Intravenous doses of nalmefene have been shown effective at counteracting the respiratory depression produced by opioid overdose

 ## Suggested Reading

Keating GM. Nalmefene: a review of its use in the treatment of alcohol dependence. CNS Drugs 2013;27(9):761–72.

Lingford-Hughes AR, Welch S, Peters L, et al. BAP updated guidelines: evidence-based guidelines for the pharmacological management of substance abuse, harmful use, addiction and comorbidity: recommendations from BAP. J Psychopharmacol 2012;26(7):899–952.

Mann K, Torup L, Sorensen P, et al. Nalmefene for the management of alcohol dependence: review on its pharmacology, mechanism of action and meta-analysis on its clinical efficacy. Eur Neuropsychopharmacol 2016;26(12):1941–9.

van den Brink W, Sørensen P, Torup L, et al. Long-term efficacy, tolerability and safety of nalmefene as-needed in patients with alcohol dependence: a 1-year, randomised controlled study. J Psychopharmacol 2014;28(8):733–44.

Naltrexone hydrochloride

Brands
• Adepend

Generic?
Yes

Class
• Neuroscience-based nomenclature: pharmacology domain – opioid; mode of action – antagonist
• Alcohol or opioid dependence treatment; mu receptor antagonist

Commonly Prescribed for
(bold for BNF indication)
• **Adjunct to prevent relapse in formerly opioid-dependent patients who have remained opioid-free for at least 7–10 days (initiated under specialist supervision)**
• **Adjunct to prevent relapse in formerly alcohol-dependent patients (initiated under specialist supervision)**

 How the Drug Works

• Blocks mu opioid receptors, preventing exogenous opioids from binding there and thus preventing the pleasurable effects of opioid consumption
• Reduces alcohol consumption through modulation of opioid systems, thereby reducing the reinforcing effects of alcohol
• Human PET studies show that it blocks most of the mu and some of the delta receptors after 4 days of treatment in abstinent patients with alcohol dependence

How Long Until It Works
• Maximum effect may take a few weeks, but begins working within a few days
• Continue treatment for 6 months

If It Works
• Reduces alcohol and opioid consumption by diminishing their reinforcing properties (cravings and feelings of euphoria); can decrease impulsivity and can moderate the stress response
• Reduces quantity, frequency and severity of relapse to drinking in alcohol dependence
• Blocks the effects of opiates in opiate dependence

If It Doesn't Work
• If still drinking after 4–6 weeks, discontinue
• Evaluate and address contributing factors
• Consider switching to another agent or augmenting with acamprosate

 Best Augmenting Combos for Partial Response or Treatment Resistance

• Should augment with psychosocial support for increased success
• Can be combined with acamprosate (combination better than with acamprosate alone, but not with naltrexone alone)
• Some evidence for increased response when combined with disulfiram for concurrent alcohol and cocaine addiction
• Possible use with alpha 2 adrenergic agonists in managing opioid withdrawal, but close monitoring needed with initial naltrexone administration due to vomiting, diarrhoea or delirium

Tests
• Ask about use of opioid-containing agents, possibly taken unknowingly, e.g. over-the-counter analgesia
• Urine screen for opioids
• Naloxone challenge – test dose 0.2–0.8 mg given IM prior to starting naltrexone treatment, will precipitate withdrawal symptoms but for shorter duration than if precipitated by naltrexone
• Check and monitor renal and liver function

How Drug Causes Side Effects
• Blockade of mu opioid receptors

Notable Side Effects
• Nausea, vomiting, decreased appetite
• Dizziness, dysphoria, anxiety

Common or very common
• CNS/PNS: altered mood, anxiety, dizziness, eye disorders, headache, sleep disorders
• CVS: chest pain, palpitations, tachycardia
• GIT: abdominal pain, abnormal appetite, constipation, diarrhoea, nausea, thirst, vomiting
• Other: arthralgia, asthenia, chills, hyperhidrosis, myalgia, sexual dysfunction, skin reactions

Naltrexone hydrochloride (Continued)

Uncommon
- CNS/PNS: confusion, depression, drowsiness, hallucination, paranoia, tinnitus, tremor, vertigo, vision disorders
- GIT: dry mouth, flatulence, hepatic disorders, oropharyngeal pain, weight changes
- Other: alopecia, cough, dysphonia, dyspnoea, ear discomfort, eye discomfort, eye swelling, feeling hot, fever, flushing, increased sputum, lymphadenopathy, nasal complaints, pain, peripheral coldness, seborrhoea, sinus disorder, ulcer, urinary disorders, yawning

Rare or very rare
- Immune thrombocytopenic purpura, rhabdomyolysis, suicidal behaviours

Frequency not known
- Withdrawal syndrome

 Life-Threatening or Dangerous Side Effects
- Eosinophilic pneumonia
- Hepatocellular injury at excessive doses

Weight Gain

unusual   not unusual   common   problematic
- Reported but not expected

Sedation

unusual   not unusual   common   problematic
- Occurs in significant minority
- Some increase in daytime sleepiness

What To Do About Side Effects
- Wait
- Adjust dose, or discontinue if side effects persist or not tolerated
- Possible reduction in nausea if taken with food
- GI problems and sedative effects are the main issues reported

Best Augmenting Agents for Side Effects
- Dose reduction or switching to another agent may be more effective since most side effects cannot be improved with an augmenting agent
- Increase in diarrhoea and nausea when naltrexone combined with acamprosate compared with naltrexone alone

DOSING AND USE

Usual Dosage Range
- 50 mg/day
- Maximum 350 mg/week, can be divided into 3 doses (e.g. 100 mg on Monday and Wednesday and 150 mg on Friday) to increase concordance

Dosage Forms
- Tablet 50 mg
- Oral solution, oral suspension or capsule available on special order from manufacturer
- Prolonged-release tablet: 8 mg naltrexone hydrochloride + 90 mg bupropion hydrochloride (Mysimba)

How to Dose
- 25 mg/day on day 1–2, monitor for 4 hours for signs of withdrawal especially if using for opioid dependence, then if tolerated increase to 50 mg/day from day 2–3
- Total weekly dose can be divided and given 3 times per week to improve concordance (e.g. 100 mg/day on Monday and Wednesday, then 150 mg on Friday)
- Maximum 350 mg/week
- Patient should be opioid-free for 7–10 days prior to initiating treatment, confirmed by negative urine screen and/or naloxone challenge test
- Patients initiated on naltrexone for alcohol dependence can begin while still drinking or during medically assisted alcohol withdrawal but discontinue naltrexone if still drinking after 4–6 weeks or feel unwell taking it

 Dosing Tips
- Adjunct use at 25 mg dose is unlicensed dose
- Combine with psychosocial support for increased chance of success
- Individuals who abstain from alcohol for several day prior to initiating treatment with naltrexone may have greater reductions in the number of drinking days as well as heavy drinking days and may also be more likely to abstain completely throughout treatment
- Prescribe for 6 months, or longer if perceived benefit

- Unlicensed use for self-injurious behaviour in those with learning disabilities – very limited evidence, specialist use only)

Overdose

- Limited experience, possible nausea, abdominal pain, sedation, dizziness

Long-Term Use

- Has been studied in trials up to 1 year

Habit Forming

- No

How to Stop

- Taper not necessary

Pharmacokinetics

- Plasma half-life of naltrexone hydrochloride is about 4 hours
- Plasma half-life of metabolite 6-beta-naltrexol is 13 hours

 Drug Interactions

- Hepatically metabolised by dihydrodiol dehydrogenase and not by the CYP450 enzyme system so unlikely to be affected by drugs that induce or inhibit CYP450 enzymes
- Can block the effects of opioid-containing medications, e.g. some cough/cold remedies, anti-diarrhoeal preparations, opioid analgesics)
- Concomitant administration with acamprosate may increase plasma levels of acamprosate, but this does not seem clinically significant and dose adjustment is not recommended
- Avoid concurrent use of opioids if possible

 Other Warnings/Precautions

- Increased risk of fatal opioid overdose as individual's tolerance decreases markedly following detoxification and at any period of abstinence, including after discontinuation of naltrexone treatment
- Attempts by patients to overcome blockade of opioid receptors by taking large amounts of exogenous opioids could lead to opioid intoxication or fatal overdose

- Those using naltrexone who require pain management with opioid analgesia may need higher dose than usual or experience deeper/more prolonged respiratory depression – manage with non-opioid or rapid-acting opioid analgesia where possible

Do Not Use

- If patient is currently dependent on opioids or in acute opioid withdrawal
- If patient has failed the naloxone challenge or has positive opioid urine screen
- If patient has acute hepatitis, hepatic failure or severe impairment (risk of hepatocellular injury with high doses of naltrexone)
- If there is a proven allergy to naltrexone

SPECIAL POPULATIONS

Renal Impairment

- Dose adjustment not necessary in mild impairment
- Avoid in severe impairment

Hepatic Impairment

- Dose adjustment not necessary in mild impairment
- Avoid in severe impairment
- Contraindicated in acute hepatitis or hepatic failure

Cardiac Impairment

- Limited data available

Elderly

- Limited evidence, some patients may tolerate lower doses better

 Children and Adolescents

- Not licensed for use in children
- However, evidence base for naltrexone is evolving and better supported than for acamprosate or disulfiram

Pregnancy

- Controlled studies have not been conducted in pregnant women
- Toxicity reported in animal studies

- Pregnant women needing to stop drinking may consider behavioural therapy before pharmacotherapy
- Not generally recommended for use during pregnancy, especially during first trimester
- Risk of acute withdrawal syndrome with serious consequences to mother and foetus if mother also using opiates

Breastfeeding

- Very limited evidence of safety
- Negligible amounts in mother's breast milk, but potential toxicity, so recommend to either discontinue drug or bottle feed

Potential Advantages

- Individuals who are not ready to abstain completely from alcohol
- For binge drinkers
- Individuals who want to abstain from opioid use

Potential Disadvantages

- Cannot be used in those currently using or withdrawing from opioids
- Less effective in those still drinking at time of treatment initiation
- World Health Organization guidelines suggest that most patients should be advised to use agonists rather than antagonists like naltrexone, due to their superiority in reducing mortality and retaining patients in care
- Increased risk of fatal opioid overdose

Primary Target Symptoms

- Alcohol or opioid dependence

Pearls

- Not only increases total abstinence, but also can reduce days of heavy drinking
- May be a preferred treatment if the goal is reduced-risk drinking (i.e. 3–4 drinks per day in men, maximum 16 drinks per week; 2–3 drinks per day in women, maximum 12 drinks per week)
- Less effective in patients who are not abstinent at the time of treatment initiation, therefore best started after detox if possible
- Some patients complain of apathy or loss of pleasure with chronic treatment
- Decreased rates of relapse to heavy drinking from a lapse
- No need for routine LFTs, but would need to follow-up if impaired
- For alcohol dependence and co-morbid mental health disorders: depressed patients (naltrexone 100 mg/day with sertraline 200 mg superior outcome than each drug alone and placebo; no benefit with citalopram); bipolar patients (first-line agent); PTSD patients (naltrexone alone or combination with disulfiram improved drinking outcomes compared with placebo); schizophrenia (naltrexone or acamprosate can be used); borderline personality disorder (limited evidence for efficacy of naltrexone in reducing self-harm and dissociative symptoms); tardive dyskinesia (some evidence to support use at a 200 mg dose with a benzodiazepine to treat tardive dyskinesia)
- Mysimba (naltrexone/bupropion combination) used as an adjunct to a reduced-calorie diet and increased physical activity, for the management of weight in obese adult patients or overweight (BMI>27) patients with co-morbid diabetes, dyslipidaemia or controlled hypertension

 **Switching**

- From buprenorphine – washout period of up to 7 days if final dose >2 mg, used for >2 weeks (naltrexone can sometimes be started in 2–3 days if buprenorphine dose <2 mg, used for <2 weeks)
- If opioid analgesia is necessary and anticipated, it can be initiated 48–72 hours after cessation of naltrexone

Suggested Reading

Anton RF, O'Malley SS, Ciraulo DA, et al. Combined pharmacotherapies and behavioral interventions for alcohol dependence: the COMBINE study: a randomized controlled trial. JAMA 2006;295(17):2003–17.

Johansson BA, Berglund M, Lindgren A. Efficacy of maintenance treatment with naltrexone for opioid dependence: a meta-analytical review. Addiction 2006;101(4):491–503.

Mason BJ, Heyser CJ. Alcohol use disorder: the role of medication in recovery. Alcohol Res 2021;41(1):07.

Rosner S, Leucht S, Lehert P, et al. Acamprosate supports abstinence, naltrexone prevents excessive drinking: evidence from a meta-analysis with unreported outcomes. J Psychopharmacol 2008;22(1):11–23.

Schmitz JM, Stotts AL, Sayre SL, et al. Treatment of cocaine-alcohol dependence with naltrexone and relapse prevention therapy. Am J Addict 2004;13(4):333–41.

Nitrazepam

THERAPEUTICS

Brands
• Mogadon

Generic?
Yes

Class
• Neuroscience-based nomenclature: pharmacology domain – GABA; mode of action – positive allosteric modulator (PAM)
• Benzodiazepine; hypnotic

Commonly Prescribed for
(bold for BNF indication)
• **Insomnia (short-term use)**

 How the Drug Works
• Binds to benzodiazepine receptors at the GABA-A ligand-gated chloride channel complex
• Enhances the inhibitory effects of GABA
• Boosts chloride conductance through GABA-regulated channels
• Inhibitory actions in sleep centres may provide sedative hypnotic effects

How Long Until It Works
• Reaches peak plasma concentrations following oral administration in 2 hours (range 0.5–5 hours)

If It Works
• Most patients contraindication would respond positively in the management of insomnia

If It Doesn't Work
• Adjust dose to reach maximum level, if no other contra-indication
• Use alternative hypnotics
• Where possible behavioural therapies (e.g. CBT for insomnia) should be offered before prescribing hypnotics

 Best Augmenting Combos for Partial Response or Treatment Resistance
• Generally best to switch to another agent
• RCTs support the effectiveness of Z-hypnotics over a period of at least 6 months
• Trazodone

• Agents with antihistamine actions (e.g. promethazine, TCAs)
• Use melatonin and melatonin-related drugs (adults over the age of 55)

Tests
• No routine tests recommended
• When known renal or hepatic impairment then periodic LFTs and FBC recommended

SIDE EFFECTS

How Drug Causes Side Effects
• Same mechanism for side effects as for therapeutic effects – namely due to excessive actions at benzodiazepine receptors
• Actions at benzodiazepine receptors that carry over to the next day can cause daytime sedation, amnesia, and ataxia
• Long-term adaptations in benzodiazepine receptors may explain the development of dependence, tolerance, and withdrawal

Notable Side Effects
• Amnesia, ataxia, confusion, hangover effect, aggression
• Muscle weakness
• Tolerance and drug dependence

Common or very common
• Movement disorders

Uncommon
• Impaired concentration

Rare or very rare
• Abdominal distress, muscle cramps, psychiatric disorder, skin reactions, Stevens-Johnson syndrome

Frequency not known
• Drug abuse

 Life-Threatening or Dangerous Side Effects
• Sedation
• Coma

Weight Gain

unusual   not unusual   common   problematic
• Not reported

Sedation

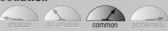

unusual   not unusual   **common**   problematic

- Frequent and can be significant in amount
- Some patients may not tolerate it
- Can wear off over time

What To Do About Side Effects

- Wait
- To avoid problems with memory, only take nitrazepam if planning to have a full night's sleep
- Lower the dose
- Switch to a shorter-acting sedative hypnotic
- Switch to a non-benzodiazepine hypnotic
- Administer flumazenil if side effects are severe or life-threatening

Best Augmenting Agents for Side Effects

- Many side effects cannot be improved with an augmenting agent

DOSING AND USE

Usual Dosage Range

- 2.5–10 mg at bedtime (depends on age of patient, and degree of debilitation)

Dosage Forms

- Tablet 5 mg
- Oral suspension 2.5 mg/5 mL

How to Dose

- For adult: 5–10 mg at bedtime
- For elderly or debilitated patient: 2.5–5 mg at bedtime

 Dosing Tips

- Reduce dose for elderly or the debilitated patient
- Caution in acute porphyria, hypoalbuminaemia, muscle weakness

Overdose

- Drowsiness, ataxia, dysarthria, nystagmus, occasionally respiratory depression, and coma

Long-Term Use

- Avoid prolonged use (and abrupt withdrawal thereafter)
- Should not be routinely used for more than 1 month

- Those with panic disorder may benefit from CBT during the taper period

Habit Forming

- Yes
- Nitrazepam is a Class C/Schedule 4 drug
- Tolerance and dependence can occur in as little as 4 weeks

How to Stop

- Systematic reduction strategies are twice as likely to lead to abstinence than simply advising patient to stop, especially after prolonged use
- Rapid discontinuation may lead to withdrawal symptoms
- Reduce by 1 mg/day every 1–2 weeks until stopped

Pharmacokinetics

- Average half-life 24 hours (range 16.5–48.3 hours: lower in young people and longer in elderly)
- Cerebrospinal fluid half-life 68 hours
- Concomitant food intake has no influence on the rate of absorption or on its bioavailability
- Hepatic metabolism
- Excretion via kidneys

 Drug Interactions

- Caution with other CNS-depressant drugs – may affect ability to perform skilled tasks
- Caution with rifampicin, as it increases the clearance of nitrazepam, thus reducing the therapeutic effect
- Metabolised by CYP450 3A4, which is inhibited by erythromycin, several SSRIs and ketoconazole, thus co-administration of these drugs would result in higher serum levels
- Important interaction with methadone
- Use with caution in patients prescribed clozapine – increased risk of cardio-pulmonary depression

 Other Warnings/Precautions

- Warning regarding the increased risk of CNS-depressant effects (especially alcohol) when benzodiazepines and opioid medications are used together, including specifically the risk of slowed or difficulty breathing and death

- If alternatives to the combined use of benzodiazepines and opioids are not available, clinicians should limit the dosage and duration of each drug to the minimum possible while still achieving therapeutic efficacy
- Patients and their caregivers should be warned to seek medical attention if unusual dizziness, light-headedness, sedation, slowed or difficulty breathing, or unresponsiveness occur
- Dosage changes should be made in collaboration with prescriber
- History of drug or alcohol abuse often creates greater risk for dependency
- Some depressed patients may experience a worsening of suicidal ideation
- Some patients may exhibit abnormal thinking or behavioural changes similar to those caused by other CNS depressants (i.e. either depressant actions or disinhibiting actions)
- Avoid prolonged use and abrupt cessation
- Use lower doses in debilitated patients and the elderly
- Use with caution in patients with myasthenia gravis; respiratory disease
- Use with caution in patients with acute porphyrias; hypoalbuminaemia
- Use with caution in patients with personality disorder (dependent/avoidant or anankastic types) as may increase risk of dependence
- Use with caution in patients with a history of alcohol or drug dependence/abuse
- Benzodiazepines may cause a range of paradoxical effects including aggression, antisocial behaviours, anxiety, overexcitement, perceptual abnormalities and talkativeness. Adjustment of dose may reduce impulses
- Use with caution as nitrazepam can cause muscle weakness
- Insomnia may be a symptom of a primary disorder, rather than a primary disorder itself
- Nitrazepam should be administered only at bedtime

Do Not Use

- If patient has acute pulmonary insufficiency, respiratory depression, significant neuromuscular respiratory weakness, sleep apnoea syndrome or unstable myasthenia gravis
- Alone in chronic psychosis in adults
- On its own to treat depression, anxiety associated with depression, obsessional states or phobic states
- If patient has angle-closure glaucoma
- If there is a proven allergy to nitrazepam or any benzodiazepine

SPECIAL POPULATIONS

Renal Impairment

- Less than 5% excreted unchanged in urine
- Use with caution; start with lower doses in end-stage renal failure
- Monitor patient for increased cerebral sensitivity

Hepatic Impairment

- Caution in mild to moderate impairment: reduce dose and adjust according to response
- Avoid in severe impairment
- Shorter half-life drugs are safer

Cardiac Impairment

- Dosage adjustment may not be necessary
- Benzodiazepines have been used to treat insomnia associated with acute myocardial infarction

Elderly

- Reduce dose

Children and Adolescents

- Greater risk of anxiety, agitation, and aggression
- Tablets not licensed for use in children

Pregnancy

- Possible increased risk of birth defects when benzodiazepines taken during pregnancy
- Because of the potential risks, nitrazepam is not generally recommended as treatment for insomnia during pregnancy, especially during the first trimester

Nitrazepam (Continued)

- Drug should be tapered if discontinued
- Infants whose mothers received a benzodiazepine late in pregnancy may experience withdrawal effects
- Neonatal flaccidity has been reported in infants whose mothers took a benzodiazepine during pregnancy
- Seizures, even mild seizures, may cause harm to the embryo/foetus

Breastfeeding

- Some drug is found in mother's breast milk
- Effects on infant have been observed and include feeding difficulties, sedation, and weight loss
- Caution should be taken with the use of benzodiazepines in breastfeeding mothers; seek to use low doses for short periods to reduce infant exposure
- Use of shorter-acting 'Z' drugs zopiclone or zolpidem preferred
- Mothers taking hypnotics should be warned about the risks of co-sleeping

Pearls

- NICE Guidelines recommend medication for insomnia only as a second-line treatment after non-pharmacological treatment options have been tried (e.g. cognitive behavioural therapy for insomnia)
- Psychiatric symptoms and paradoxical reactions may be quite severe and more frequent compared to other benzodiazepines
- Paradoxical reactions include restlessness, agitation, irritability, aggression, delusions, rage, nightmares, hallucinations, psychosis, inappropriate behaviour, and other adverse behavioural effects
- In combination with alcohol affects judgement and inhibitions and can reduce recall of events
- Since 2000, calorimetric compound added that turns the drug blue when added to a liquid
- Best for short-term use up to 10 days

THE ART OF PSYCHOPHARMACOLOGY

Potential Advantages

- Reduces pathological anxiety, agitation, and tension
- Can augment SSRIs

Potential Disadvantages

- Dependence potential

Primary Target Symptoms

- Anxiety
- Insomnia

THE ART OF SWITCHING

 **Switching**

- Patients on nitrazepam should be offered an equivalent dose of diazepam – has a longer half-life and thus less severe withdrawal
- Nitrazepam 10 mg is approximately equivalent to diazepam 10 mg
- Precautions apply in patients with hepatic dysfunction, as diazepam can accumulate to toxic levels

 Suggested Reading

Mason M, Cates CJ, Smith I. Effects of opioid, hypnotic and sedating medications on sleep-disordered breathing in adults with obstructive sleep apnoea. Cochrane Database Syst Rev 2015;(7):CD011090.

Riemann D, Baglioni C, Bassetti C, et al. European guideline for the diagnosis and treatment of insomnia. J Sleep Res 2017;26(6):675–700.

Schweizer E, Rickels K. Benzodiazepine dependence and withdrawal: a review of the syndrome and its clinical management. Acta Psychiatr Scand Suppl 1998;393:95–101.

Soyka M. Treatment of benzodiazepine dependence. N Engl J Med 2017;376(12):1147–57.

Voshaar RCO, Couvée JE, van Balkom AJLM, et al. Strategies for discontinuing long-term benzodiazepine use: meta-analysis. Br J Psychiatry 2006;189:213–20.

Winkler A, Auer C, Doering BK, et al. Drug treatment of primary insomnia: a meta-analysis of polysomnographic randomized controlled trials. CNS drugs 2014;28(9):799–816.

Nortriptyline

Brands
• Non-proprietary

Generic?
Yes

Class
• Neuroscience-based nomenclature: pharmacology domain – norepinephrine; mode of action – reuptake inhibitor
• Tricyclic antidepressant (TCA); serotonin, noradrenaline reuptake inhibitor (predominantly a noradrenaline reuptake inhibitor)

Commonly Prescribed for
(bold for BNF indication)
• **Depressive illness**
• **Neuropathic pain (not licensed)**
• Anxiety
• Insomnia
• Treatment-resistant depression

How the Drug Works
• Boosts neurotransmitter noradrenaline
• Blocks noradrenaline reuptake pump (noradrenaline transporter), presumably increasing noradrenergic neurotransmission
• Since dopamine is deactivated by noradrenaline reuptake in frontal cortex, which largely lacks dopamine transporters, nortriptyline can increase dopamine neurotransmission in this part of the brain
• A more potent inhibitor of noradrenaline reuptake pump than serotonin reuptake pump (serotonin transporter)
• At high doses may also boost neurotransmitter serotonin and presumably increase serotonergic neurotransmission

How Long Until It Works
• May have immediate effects in treating insomnia or anxiety
• Onset of therapeutic actions with some antidepressants can be seen within 1–2 weeks, but often delayed up to 2–4 weeks
• If it is not working within 3–4 weeks for depression, it may require a dosage increase or it may not work at all
• By contrast, for generalised anxiety, onset of response and increases in remission rates may still occur after 8 weeks, and for up to 6 months after initiating dosing

If It Works
• The goal of treatment is complete remission of current symptoms as well as prevention of future relapses
• Treatment often reduces or even eliminates symptoms, but it is not a cure since symptoms can recur after medicine stopped
• Continue treatment until all symptoms are gone (remission)
• Once symptoms are gone, continue treating for at least 6–9 months for the first episode of depression or >12 months if relapse indicators present
• If >5 episodes and/or 2 episodes in the last few years then need to continue for at least 2 years or indefinitely
• The goal of treatment of chronic neuropathic pain is to reduce symptoms as much as possible, especially in combination with other treatments
• Treatment of chronic neuropathic pain may reduce symptoms, but rarely eliminates them completely, and is not a cure since symptoms can recur after medicine is stopped
• Use in anxiety disorders and chronic pain may also need to be indefinite, but long-term treatment is not well studied in these conditions

If It Doesn't Work
• Many depressed patients have only a partial response where some symptoms are improved but others persist (especially insomnia, fatigue, and problems concentrating)
• Other depressed patients may be non-responders
• It is important to recognise non-response to treatment early on (3–4 weeks)
• Consider increasing dose, switching to another agent, or adding an appropriate augmenting agent
• Lithium may be added for suicidal patients or those at high risk of relapse
• Consider psychotherapy
• Consider ECT
• Consider evaluation for another diagnosis or for a co-morbid condition (e.g. medical illness, substance abuse, etc.)
• Some patients may experience a switch into mania and so would require antidepressant discontinuation and initiation of a mood stabiliser

⚖ Best Augmenting Combos for Partial Response or Treatment Resistance

- Mood stabilisers or atypical antipsychotics for bipolar depression
- Atypical antipsychotics for psychotic depression
- Atypical antipsychotics as first-line augmenting agents (quetiapine MR 300 mg/day or aripiprazole at 2.5–10 mg/day) for treatment-resistant depression
- Atypical antipsychotics as second-line augmenting agents (risperidone 0.5–2 mg/day or olanzapine 2.5–10 mg/day) for treatment-resistant depression
- Mirtazapine at 30–45 mg/day as another second-line augmenting agent (a dual serotonin and noradrenaline combination, but observe for switch into mania, increase in suicidal ideation or serotonin syndrome)
- T3 (20–50 mcg/day) is another second-line augmenting agent that works best with tricyclic antidepressants
- Other augmenting agents but with less evidence include bupropion (up to 400 mg/day), buspirone (up to 60 mg/day) and lamotrigine (up to 400 mg/day)
- Benzodiazepines if agitation present
- Hypnotics or trazodone for insomnia (but beware of serotonin syndrome with trazodone)
- Augmenting agents reserved for specialist use include: modafinil for sleepiness, fatigue and lack of concentration; stimulants, oestrogens, testosterone
- Lithium is particularly useful for suicidal patients and those at high risk of relapse including with factors such as severe depression, psychomotor retardation, repeated episodes (>3), significant weight loss, or a family history of major depression (aim for lithium plasma levels 0.6–1.0 mmol/L)
- For elderly patients lithium is a very effective augmenting agent
- For severely ill patients other combinations may be tried especially in specialist centres
- Augmenting agents that may be tried include omega-3, SAM-e, L-methylfolate
- Additional non-pharmacological treatments such as exercise, mindfulness, CBT, and IPT can also be helpful

- If present after treatment response (4–8 weeks) or remission (6–12 weeks), the most common residual symptoms of depression include cognitive impairments, reduced energy and problems with sleep
- For chronic pain: gabapentin, tiagabine, opioids – requires careful monitoring and specialist input advised

Tests

- Baseline ECG is useful for patients over age 50
- ECGs may be useful for selected patients (e.g. those with personal or family history of QTc prolongation; cardiac arrhythmia; recent myocardial infarction; decompensated heart failure; or taking agents that prolong QTc interval such as pimozide, thioridazine, selected antiarrhythmics, moxifloxacin etc.)
- *Since tricyclic and tetracyclic antidepressants are frequently associated with weight gain, before starting treatment, weigh all patients and determine if the patient is already overweight (BMI 25.0–29.9) or obese (BMI ≥30)
- Before giving a drug that can cause weight gain to an overweight or obese patient, consider determining whether the patient already has:
- Pre-diabetes – fasting plasma glucose: 5.5 mmol/L to 6.9 mmol/L or HbA1c: 42 to 47 mmol/mol (6.0 to 6.4%)
- Diabetes – fasting plasma glucose: >7.0 mmol/L or HbA1c: ≥48 mmol/L (≥6.5%)
- Hypertension (BP >140/90 mm Hg)
- Dyslipidaemia (increased total cholesterol, LDL cholesterol, and triglycerides; decreased HDL cholesterol)
- Treat or refer such patients for treatment, including nutrition and weight management, physical activity counselling, smoking cessation, and medical management
- *Monitor weight and BMI during treatment
- *While giving a drug to a patient who has gained >5% of initial weight, consider evaluating for the presence of pre-diabetes, diabetes, dyslipidaemia, or consider switching to a different antidepressant
- Patients at risk for electrolyte disturbances (e.g. patients aged >60, patients on diuretic therapy) should have baseline and periodic serum potassium and magnesium measurements

• Monitoring of plasma levels is available, however there is little evidence that this is beneficial. Target range for trough levels is 50–150 mcg/L

• Other: alopecia, asthenia, bone marrow disorders, drug cross-reactivity, drug fever, fever, flushing, hyperhidrosis, increased risk of fracture, increased risk of infection, malaise, mydriasis, oedema, photosensitivity, sexual dysfunction, SIADH, skin reactions, testicular swelling, urinary disorders, urinary tract dilation

SIDE EFFECTS

How Drug Causes Side Effects

• Anticholinergic activity may explain sedative effects, dry mouth, constipation, and blurred vision
• Sedative effects and weight gain may be due to antihistamine properties
• Blockade of alpha adrenergic 1 receptors may explain dizziness, sedation, and hypotension
• Cardiac arrhythmias and seizures, especially in overdose, may be caused by blockade of ion channels

Notable Side Effects

• Blurred vision, constipation, urinary retention, dry mouth, increased appetite, weight gain
• Fatigue, weakness, dizziness, hypotension, sedation, headache, anxiety, restlessness, agitation
• Sexual dysfunction (impotence, change in libido)
• Sweating, rash, itching

Frequency not known

• Blood disorders: agranulocytosis, eosinophilia, thrombocytopenia
• CNS/PNS: abnormal sensation, anxiety, confusion, delusions, dizziness, drowsiness, hallucination, headache, hypomania, movement disorders, peripheral neuropathy, psychosis exacerbated, seizure, sleep disorders, stroke, suicidal behaviours, tinnitus, tremor, vision disorders
• CVS: arrhythmias, atrioventricular block, hypertension, hypotension, myocardial infarction, palpitations
• Endocrine: breast enlargement, galactorrhoea, gynaecomastia
• GIT: altered taste, decreased appetite, constipation, diarrhoea, dry mouth, gastrointestinal discomfort, hepatic disorders, nausea, oral disorders, paralytic ileus, vomiting, weight changes

 ### Life-Threatening or Dangerous Side Effects

• Agranulocytosis, bone marrow disorders
• Paralytic ileus, hepatic failure
• Lowered seizure threshold and rare seizures
• Orthostatic hypotension, sudden death, arrhythmias, tachycardia
• QTc prolongation
• Increased intraocular pressure
• Rare induction of mania and paranoid delusions
• Rare increase in suicidal ideation and behaviours in adolescents and young adults (up to age 25), hence patients should be warned of this potential adverse event

Weight Gain

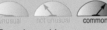

• Experienced by many and/or can be significant in amount
• Can increase appetite and carbohydrate craving

Sedation

• Experienced by many and/or can be significant in amount
• Tolerance to sedative effect may develop with long-term use

What To Do About Side Effects

• Wait
• Wait
• Wait
• The risk of side effects is reduced by titrating slowly to the minimum effective dose (every 2–3 days)
• Consider using a lower starting dose in elderly patients
• Manage side effects that are likely to be transient (e.g. drowsiness) by explanation, reassurance and, if necessary, dose reduction and re-titration

- Giving patients simple strategies for managing mild side effects (e.g. dry mouth) may be useful
- For persistent, severe or distressing side effects the options are:
- Dose reduction and re-titration if possible
- Switching to an antidepressant with a lower propensity to cause that side effect
- Non-drug management of the side effect (e.g. diet and exercise for weight gain)

Best Augmenting Agents for Side Effects

- Many side effects cannot be improved with an augmenting agent

DOSING AND USE

Usual Dosage Range

- Depressive illness: 75–150 mg/day in divided doses; 30–50 mg/day in divided doses (elderly)
- Neuropathic pain: 10–75 mg/day (higher doses to be given under specialist supervision)

Dosage Forms

- Tablet 10 mg, 25 mg, 50 mg
- Capsule 10 mg, 25 mg
- Oral suspension 10 mg/5 mL, or 25 mg/5 mL

How to Dose

*Depressive illness:
- Adult: initiate at low dose, then increased as needed to 75–100 mg/day at night or in divided doses, max 150 mg/day
- Elderly: initiate at low dose, then increased as needed to 30–50 mg/day in divided doses

*Neuropathic pain:
- Initial dose 10 mg at night, increased gradually as needed to 75 mg/day; higher doses under specialist supervision

 Dosing Tips

- If given in a single dose, should generally be administered at bedtime because of its sedative properties
- If given in split doses, largest dose should generally be given at bedtime because of its sedative properties

- If patients experience nightmares, split dose and do not give large dose at bedtime
- Risk of seizure increases with dose
- Some formulations of nortriptyline contain sodium bisulphate, which may cause allergic reactions in some patients, perhaps more frequently in asthmatics
- If intolerable anxiety, insomnia, agitation, akathisia, or activation occur either upon dosing initiation or discontinuation, consider the possibility of activated bipolar disorder, and switch to a mood stabiliser or an atypical antipsychotic

Overdose

- Symptoms of overdose include arrhythmias, cardiac conduction defects, coma, dilated pupils, dry mouth, extensor plantar responses, hyperreflexia, hypotension, hypothermia, respiratory failure, seizures, tachycardia and urinary retention
- Assessment in hospital is strongly advised in case of overdose
- Supportive measures to ensure a clear airway and adequate ventilation during transfer are mandatory
- Activated charcoal given within 1 hour of the overdose reduces absorption of the drug

Long-Term Use

- Safe
- The risk of withdrawal symptoms is increased if the antidepressant is stopped suddenly after regular administration for 8 weeks or more

Habit Forming

- No

How to Stop

- Taper gradually to avoid withdrawal effects
- Even with gradual dose reduction some withdrawal symptoms may appear within the first 2 weeks
- It is best to reduce the dose gradually over 4 weeks or longer if withdrawal symptoms emerge
- If severe withdrawal symptoms emerge during discontinuation, raise dose to stop symptoms and then restart withdrawal much more slowly (over at least 6 months in patients on long-term maintenance treatment)

Pharmacokinetics

- Substrate for CYP450 2D6 and 3A4
- Nortriptyline is the active metabolite of amitriptyline, formed by demethylation via CYP450 1A2
- Half-life about 25–38 hours
- Food does not affect absorption

Drug Interactions

- Tramadol increases the risk of seizures in patients taking TCAs
- Use of TCAs with anticholinergic drugs may result in paralytic ileus or hyperthermia
- Fluoxetine, paroxetine, bupropion, duloxetine, terbinafine and other CYP450 2D6 inhibitors may increase TCA concentrations
- Cimetidine may increase plasma concentrations of TCAs and cause anticholinergic symptoms
- Phenothiazines or haloperidol may raise TCA blood concentrations
- May alter effects of antihypertensive drugs; may inhibit hypotensive effects of clonidine
- Use with sympathomimetic agents may increase sympathetic activity
- Methylphenidate may inhibit metabolism of TCAs
- Nortriptyline can increase the effects of adrenaline/epinephrine
- Carbamazepine decreases the exposure to nortriptyline
- Both nortriptyline and carbamazepine can increase the risk of hyponatraemia
- Nortriptyline is predicted to increase the risk of severe toxic reaction when given with MAOIs; avoid and for 14 days after stopping the MAOI
- Both nortriptyline and MAOIs can increase the risk of hypotension
- Do not start an MAOI for at least 5 half-lives (5 to 7 days for most drugs) after discontinuing nortriptyline
- Activation and agitation, especially following switching or adding antidepressants, may represent the induction of a bipolar state, especially a mixed dysphoric bipolar condition sometimes associated with suicidal ideation, and require the addition of lithium, a mood stabiliser or an atypical antipsychotic, and/or discontinuation of nortriptyline

 Other Warnings/Precautions

- Use with caution in patients with cardiovascular disease
- Can potentially prolong QTc interval at higher doses
- Arrhythmias may occur at higher doses, but are rare
- Increased risk of arrhythmias in patients with hyperthyroidism or phaeochromocytoma
- Caution if patient is taking agents capable of significantly prolonging QTc interval or if there is a history of QTc prolongation
- Caution if the patient is taking drugs that inhibit TCA metabolism, including CYP450 2D6 inhibitors
- Because TCAs can prolong QTc interval, use with caution in patients who have bradycardia or who are taking drugs that can induce bradycardia (e.g. beta blockers, calcium channel blockers, clonidine, digitalis)
- Because TCAs can prolong QTc interval, use with caution in patients who have hypokalaemia and/or hypomagnesaemia or who are taking drugs that can induce hypokalaemia and/or hypo-magnesaemia (e.g. diuretics, stimulant laxatives, intravenous amphotericin B, glucocorticoids, tetracosactide)
- Caution if there is reduced CYP450 2D6 function, such as patients who are poor 2D6 metabolisers
- Can exacerbate chronic constipation
- Use caution when treating patients with epilepsy
- Use caution in patients with diabetes
- Use with caution in patients with a history of bipolar disorder, psychosis or significant risk of suicide
- Use with caution in patients with increased intra-ocular pressure or susceptibility to angle-closure glaucoma
- Use with caution in patients with prostatic hypertrophy or urinary retention

Do Not Use

- In patients during a manic phase
- If there is a history of cardiac arrhythmia, recent acute myocardial infarction, heart block
- In patients with acute porphyrias
- If there is a proven allergy to nortriptyline or amitriptyline

SPECIAL POPULATIONS

Renal Impairment

- No need for adjustment if eGFR >10 mL/minute/1.73m²
- If eGFR <10 mL/minute/1.73m² start at a low dose
- Plasma concentrations of active metabolites are raised in renal impairment, so plasma level monitoring recommended

Hepatic Impairment

- Sedative effects are increased in hepatic impairment
- Avoid in severe liver disease

Cardiac Impairment

- Baseline ECG is recommended
- TCAs have been reported to cause arrhythmias, prolongation of conduction time, postural hypotension, sinus tachycardia, and heart failure, especially in the diseased heart
- Myocardial infarction and stroke have been reported with TCAs
- TCAs produce QTc prolongation, which may be enhanced by the existence of bradycardia, hypokalaemia, congenital or acquired long QTc interval, which should be evaluated prior to administering nortriptyline
- Use with caution if treating concomitantly with a medication likely to produce prolonged bradycardia, hypokalaemia, heart block, or prolongation of the QTc interval
- Avoid TCAs in patients with a known history of QTc prolongation, recent acute myocardial infarction, and decompensated heart failure
- TCAs may cause a sustained increase in heart rate in patients with ischaemic heart disease and may worsen (decrease) heart rate variability, an independent risk of mortality in cardiac populations
- Since SSRIs may improve (increase) heart rate variability in patients following a myocardial infarct and may improve survival as well as mood in patients with acute angina or following a myocardial infarction, these are more appropriate agents for cardiac populations than tricyclic/ tetracyclic antidepressants
- *Risk/benefit ratio may not justify use of TCAs in cardiac impairment

Elderly

- Baseline ECG is recommended for patients over age 50
- May be more sensitive to anticholinergic, cardiovascular, hypotensive, and sedative effects
- To be initiated at a low dose, then increased if necessary to 30–50 mg daily in divided doses
- Initial dose should be increased with caution and under close supervision
- Reduction in the risk of suicidality with antidepressants compared to placebo in adults age 65 and older

Children and Adolescents

- Depressive illness (child 12–17 years): to be initiated at a low dose, then increased as needed to 30–50 mg/day in divided doses, alternatively increased as needed to 30–50 mg at bedtime; max 150 mg/day

Pregnancy

- No strong evidence of TCA maternal use during pregnancy being associated with an increased risk of congenital malformations
- Risk of malformations cannot be ruled out due to limited information on specific TCAs
- Poor neonatal adaptation syndrome and/or withdrawal have been reported in infants whose mothers took a TCA during pregnancy or near delivery
- Maternal use of more than one CNS-acting medication is likely to lead to more severe symptoms in the neonate
- Must weigh the risk of treatment (first trimester foetal development, third trimester newborn delivery) to the child against the risk of no treatment (recurrence of depression, maternal health, infant bonding) to the mother and child
- For many patients this may mean continuing treatment during pregnancy

Breastfeeding

- Small amounts found in mother's breast milk
- Infant should be monitored for sedation and poor feeding
- Immediate postpartum period is a high-risk time for depression, especially in women who have had prior depressive episodes;

antidepressants may need to be reinstituted late in the third trimester or shortly after childbirth to prevent a recurrence during the postpartum period
- Must weigh benefits of breastfeeding with risks and benefits of antidepressant treatment versus nontreatment to both the infant and the mother
- For many patients this may mean continuing treatment during breastfeeding
- Imipramine and nortriptyline are preferred TCAs for depression in breastfeeding mothers

THE ART OF PSYCHOPHARMACOLOGY

Potential Advantages
- Patients with insomnia
- Severe or treatment-resistant depression
- Patients for whom therapeutic drug monitoring is desirable

Potential Disadvantages
- Paediatric and geriatric patients
- Patients concerned with weight gain
- Cardiac patients

Primary Target Symptoms
- Depressed mood
- Chronic pain

Pearls
- TCAs are often a first-line treatment option for chronic pain
- TCAs are no longer generally considered a first-line option for depression because of their side-effect profile
- TCAs continue to be useful for severe or treatment-resistant depression
- Noradrenergic reuptake inhibitors such as nortriptyline can be used as a second-line treatment for smoking cessation, cocaine dependence, and attention deficit disorder
- TCAs may aggravate psychotic symptoms, nevertheless nortriptyline is an effective treatment for psychotic depression when combined with an antipsychotic

- Useful when a more noradrenergic agent is required
- Less likely to cause anticholinergic side effects when compared to other TCAs
- Dosage range more limited when compared to other TCAs; doses above 150 mg/day not recommended
- Alcohol should be avoided because of additive CNS effects
- Underweight patients may be more susceptible to adverse cardiovascular effects
- Children, patients with inadequate hydration, and patients with cardiac disease may be more susceptible to TCA-induced cardiotoxicity than healthy adults
- Patients on TCAs should be aware that they may experience symptoms such as photosensitivity or blue-green urine
- SSRIs may be more effective than TCAs in women, and TCAs may be more effective than SSRIs in men
- Not recommended for first-line use in children with ADHD because of the availability of safer treatments with better documented efficacy and because of nortriptyline's potential for sudden death in children
- *Nortriptyline is one of the few TCAs where monitoring of plasma drug levels has been well studied especially with doses above 100 mg/day; the therapeutic window falls between 50–150 mcg/L, but in recent years it has been uncertain whether checking levels is of any real practical value
- Since tricyclic/tetracyclic antidepressants are substrates for CYP450 2D6, and 7% of the population (especially Whites) may have a genetic variant leading to reduced activity of 2D6, such patients may not safely tolerate normal doses of tricyclic/-tetracyclic antidepressants and may require dose reduction
- Patients who seem to have extraordinarily severe side effects at normal or low doses may have this phenotypic CYP450 2D6 variant and require low doses or switching to another antidepressant not metabolised by 2D6

Nortriptyline (Continued)

 Suggested Reading

Anderson IM. Selective serotonin reuptake inhibitors versus tricyclic antidepressants: a meta-analysis of efficacy and tolerability. J Affect Disord 2000;58(1):19–36.

Anderson IM. Meta-analytical studies on new antidepressants. Br Med Bull 2001;57:161–78.

Hughes JR, Stead LF, Hartmann-Boyce J, et al. Antidepressants for smoking cessation. Cochrane Database Syst Rev 2014;(1):CD000031.

Wilens TE, Biederman J, Baldessarini RJ, et al. Cardiovascular effects of therapeutic doses of tricyclic antidepressants in children and adolescents. J Am Acad Child Adolesc Psychiatry 1996;35(11):1491–501.

Olanzapine

Brands
- Zypadhera (olanzapine embonate)
- Zalasta
- Zyprexa

Generic?
Yes

Class
- Neuroscience-based nomenclature: pharmacology domain – dopamine, serotonin; mode of action – antagonist
- Atypical antipsychotic (serotonin-dopamine antagonist; second-generation antipsychotic; also a mood stabiliser)

Commonly Prescribed for
(bold for BNF indication)
- **Schizophrenia (ages 12 and older)**
- **Mania (as monotherapy or as part of combination therapy) (ages 12 and older)**
- **Preventing recurrence in bipolar disorder**
- **Control of agitation and disturbed behaviour in schizophrenia or mania (intramuscular)**

 How the Drug Works
- Blocks dopamine 2 receptors, reducing positive symptoms of psychosis and stabilising affective symptoms
- Blocks serotonin 2A receptors, causing enhancement of dopamine release in certain brain regions and thus reducing motor side effects and possibly improving cognitive and affective symptoms
- Interactions at a myriad of other neurotransmitter receptors may contribute to olanzapine's efficacy
- * Specifically, antagonist actions at 5HT2C receptors may contribute to efficacy for cognitive and affective symptoms in some patients

How Long Until It Works
- Psychotic and manic symptoms can improve within 1 week, but it may take several weeks for full effect on behaviour as well as on cognition and affective stabilisation
- Classically recommended to wait at least 4–6 weeks to determine efficacy of drug, but in practice some patients require up to 16–20 weeks to show a good response, especially on cognitive symptoms
- IM formulation for rapid tranquillisation can reduce agitation in 15–30 minutes

If It Works
- Most often reduces positive symptoms in schizophrenia but does not eliminate them
- Can improve negative symptoms, as well as aggressive, cognitive, and affective symptoms in schizophrenia
- Most schizophrenic patients do not have a total remission of symptoms but rather a reduction of symptoms by about a third
- Perhaps 5–15% of schizophrenic patients can experience an overall improvement of >50–60%, especially when receiving stable treatment for >1 year
- Such patients are considered super-responders or "awakeners" since they may be well enough to be employed, live independently, and sustain long-term relationships
- Many bipolar patients may experience a reduction of symptoms by half or more
- Continue treatment until reaching a plateau of improvement
- After reaching a satisfactory plateau, continue treatment for at least 1 year after first episode of psychosis, but it may be preferable to continue treatment indefinitely to avoid subsequent episodes
- After any subsequent episodes of psychosis, treatment may need to be indefinite
- Treatment may not only reduce mania but also prevent recurrences of mania in bipolar disorder

If It Doesn't Work
- Try one of the other atypical antipsychotics (risperidone should be considered first before considering other agents such as quetiapine, aripiprazole, amisulpride, or lurasidone)
- If 2 or more antipsychotic monotherapies do not work, consider clozapine
- Some patients may require treatment with a conventional antipsychotic
- If no first-line atypical antipsychotic is effective, consider higher doses or augmentation with valproate or lamotrigine
- Consider non-concordance and switch to another antipsychotic with fewer side

effects or to an antipsychotic that can be given by depot injection
- Consider initiating rehabilitation and psychotherapy such as cognitive remediation
- Consider presence of concomitant drug abuse

Best Augmenting Combos for Partial Response or Treatment Resistance

- Valproic acid (Depakote or Epilim)
- Other mood-stabilising anticonvulsants (carbamazepine, oxcarbazepine, lamotrigine)
- Lithium
- Benzodiazepines
- Fluoxetine and other antidepressants may be effective augmenting agents to olanzapine for bipolar depression, psychotic depression, and for unipolar depression not responsive to antidepressants alone (e.g. olanzapine-fluoxetine combination)

Tests

Before starting an atypical antipsychotic

*Measure weight, BMI, and waist circumference
- Get baseline personal and family history of diabetes, obesity, dyslipidaemia, hypertension, and cardiovascular disease
*Check pulse and blood pressure, fasting plasma glucose or glycosylated haemoglobin (HbA1c), fasting lipid profile, and prolactin level
- Full blood count (FBC), urea and electrolytes (including creatinine and eGFR), liver function tests (LFTs)
- Assessment of nutritional status, diet, and level of physical activity
- Determine if the patient:
- is overweight (BMI 25.0–29.9)
- is obese (BMI ≥30)
- has pre-diabetes – fasting plasma glucose: 5.5 mmol/L to 6.9 mmol/L or HbA1c: 42 to 47 mmol/mol (6.0 to 6.4%)
- has diabetes – fasting plasma glucose: >7.0 mmol/L or HbA1c: ≥48 mmol/L (≥6.5%)
- has hypertension (BP >140/90 mm Hg)
- has dyslipidaemia (increased total cholesterol, LDL cholesterol, and triglycerides; decreased HDL cholesterol)

- Treat or refer such patients for treatment, including nutrition and weight management, physical activity counselling, smoking cessation, and medical management
- Baseline ECG for: inpatients; those with a personal history or risk factor for cardiac disease

Children and adolescents:
- As for adults
- Also check for history of congenital heart problems, history of dizziness when stressed or on exertion, history of long-QT syndrome, family history of long-QT syndrome, bradycardia, myocarditis, family history of cardiac myopathies, low K/low Mg/low Ca
- Measure weight, BMI, and waist circumference plotted on a growth chart
- Pulse, BP plotted on a percentile chart
- ECG. Note for QTc interval: machine-generated may be incorrect in children as different formula needed if HR <60 or >100
- Baseline prolactin levels

Monitoring after starting an atypical antipsychotic

- FBC annually to detect chronic bone marrow suppression, stop treatment if neutrophils fall below 1.5×10^9/L and refer to specialist care if neutrophils fall below 0.5×10^9/L
- Urea and electrolytes (including creatinine and eGFR) annually
- LFTs annually
- Prolactin levels at 6 months and then annually (olanzapine may increase prolactin levels)
*Weight/BMI/waist circumference, weekly for the first 6 weeks, then at 12 weeks, at 1 year, and then annually
*Pulse and blood pressure at 12 weeks, 1 year, and then annually
*Fasting blood glucose, HbA1c, and blood lipids at 12 weeks, at 1 year, and then annually
*For patients with type 2 diabetes, measure HbA1c at 3–6 month intervals until stable, then every 6 months
*Even in patients without known diabetes, be vigilant for the rare but life-threatening onset of diabetic ketoacidosis, which always requires immediate treatment, by monitoring for the rapid onset of polyuria, polydipsia, weight loss, nausea, vomiting, dehydration, rapid respiration, weakness and clouding of sensorium, even coma

✱If HbA1c remains ≥48 mmol/mol (6.5%) then drug therapy should be offered, e.g. metformin

- Treat or refer for treatment or consider switching to another atypical antipsychotic for patients who become overweight, obese, pre-diabetic, diabetic, hypertensive, or dyslipidaemic while receiving an atypical antipsychotic

Children and adolescents:
- As for adults
- Weight/BMI/waist circumference, weekly for the first 6 weeks, then at 12 weeks, and then every 6 months, plotted on a growth/ percentile chart
- Pulse and blood pressure at 12 weeks, then every 6 months plotted on a percentile chart
- ECG prior to starting and 2 weeks after dose increase for monitoring of QTc interval. Machine-generated may be incorrect in children as different formula needed if HR <60 or >100
- Prolactin levels: prior to starting and after 12 weeks, 24 weeks, and 6-monthly thereafter. Consider additional monitoring in young adults (under 25) who have not yet reached peak bone mass
- In prepubertal children monitor sexual maturation
- Post-pubertal children and young person monitor sexual side effects (both sexes: loss of libido, sexual dysfunction, galactorrhoea, infertility; male: diminished ejaculate, gynaecomastia; female: oligorrhoea/amenorrhoea, reduced vaginal lubrication, dyspareunia, acne, hirsutism)

SIDE EFFECTS
How Drug Causes Side Effects
- By blocking histamine 1 receptors in the brain, it can cause sedation and possibly weight gain
- By blocking alpha 1 adrenergic receptors, it can cause dizziness, sedation, and hypotension
- By blocking muscarinic 1 receptors, it can cause dry mouth, constipation, and sedation
- By blocking dopamine 2 receptors in the striatum, it can cause motor side effects (unusual)

- Mechanism of weight gain and increased incidence of diabetes and dyslipidaemia with atypical antipsychotics is unknown but insulin regulation may be impaired by blocking pancreatic M3 muscarinic receptors

Notable Side Effects
✱Increased risk for diabetes and dyslipidaemia
- Appetite increased and weight gain
- Dizziness, sedation
- Dry mouth, constipation, dyspepsia
- Arthralgia
- Oedema
- For long-acting injection (LAI) side effects may persist until the drug has been cleared from the injection site; also post-injection reactions have been reported leading to signs and symptoms of overdose

Common or very common
- Blood disorders: eosinophilia
- Other: anticholinergic effects, arthralgia, fatigue, fever, glycosuria, increased appetite, oedema, sexual dysfunction
- IM use: dyslipidaemia
- Oral use: hypersomnia

Uncommon
- CNS: dysarthria, memory loss
- GIT: abdominal distension
- Other: alopecia, breast enlargement, diabetes mellitus, epistaxis, photosensitivity, urinary disorder
- IM use: hypoventilation
- Oral use: diabetes mellitus (coma, ketoacidosis), oculogyric crisis

Rare or very rare
- Blood disorders: thrombocytopenia
- GIT: hepatic disorders, pancreatitis
- Other: hypothermia, rhabdomyolysis
- IM use: withdrawal syndrome
- Long-acting injection use: DRESS (Drug Reaction with Eosinophilia and Systemic Symptoms)

Frequency not known
- IM use: abnormal gait, cardiovascular event, falls, hallucinations, pneumonia
- Long-acting injection use: abnormal gait, erythema, falls, hallucinations (visual), pneumonia

Life-Threatening or Dangerous Side Effects

- Hyperglycaemia, in some cases extreme and associated with ketoacidosis or diabetic coma
- Drug reaction with eosinophilia and systemic symptoms (DRESS) syndrome
- Rare neuroleptic malignant syndrome (much reduced risk compared to conventional antipsychotics but still reported)
- Increased risk of death and cerebrovascular events in elderly patients with dementia-related psychosis

Weight Gain

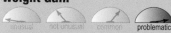

- Weight gain can be a common side effect due to increased appetite; this can become a health problem in some but not all patients experience this

Sedation

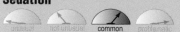

- Hypersomnia (increased tiredness) is a common side effect of olanzapine, particularly associated with oral use. The level of tiredness can be quite significant, but is usually transient

What To Do About Side Effects

- Wait
- Wait
- Wait
- Reduce the dose
- Low-dose benzodiazepine or beta blocker may reduce akathisia
- Take more of the dose at bedtime to help reduce daytime sedation
- Weight loss, exercise programmes, and medical management for high BMIs, diabetes, and dyslipidaemia
- Switch to another antipsychotic (atypical) – quetiapine or clozapine are best in cases of tardive dyskinesia

Best Augmenting Agents for Side Effects

- Dystonia: antimuscarinic drugs (e.g. procyclidine) as oral or IM depending on the severity; botulinum toxin if antimuscarinics not effective
- Parkinsonism: antimuscarinic drugs (e.g. procyclidine)
- Akathisia: beta blocker propranolol (30–80 mg/day) or low-dose benzodiazepine (e.g. 0.5–3.0 mg/day of clonazepam) may help; other agents that may be tried include the 5HT2 antagonists such as cyproheptadine (16 mg/day) or mirtazapine (15 mg at night – caution in bipolar disorder); clonidine (0.2–0.8 mg/day) may be tried if the above ineffective
- Tardive dyskinesia: stop any antimuscarinic, consider tetrabenazine
- Addition of low doses (2.5–5 mg) of aripiprazole can reverse the hyperprolactinaemia/galactorrhoea caused by other antipsychotics
- Addition of aripiprazole (5–15 mg/day) or metformin (500–2000 mg/day) to weight-inducing atypical antipsychotics such as olanzapine and clozapine can help mitigate against weight gain

DOSING AND USE

Usual Dosage Range

- Schizophrenia, or combination therapy or monotherapy therapy for mania, or preventing recurrence in bipolar disorder: 5–20 mg/day
- Long-acting injection maintenance in schizophrenia in patients tolerant to olanzapine by mouth: 210 mg every 2 weeks (or 405 mg every 4 weeks) to 300 mg every 2 weeks
- Control of agitation and disturbed behaviour in schizophrenia or mania: IM injection 5–10 mg per dose (max 20 mg in 24 hours)

Dosage Forms

- Tablet 2.5 mg, 5 mg, 7.5 mg, 10 mg, 15 mg, 20 mg
- Oral lyophilisate 5 mg, 10 mg, 15 mg, 20 mg
- Orodispersible tablet 5 mg, 10 mg, 15 mg, 20 mg
- Intramuscular formulation 5 mg/mL
- Long-acting injection 210 mg, 300 mg, 405 mg

How to Dose
Oral
- Schizophrenia, or combination therapy for mania, or preventing recurrence in bipolar disorder: 10 mg/day, adjusted according

to response, usual dose range 5–20 mg/day, doses above 10 mg/day only after reassessment, consider lower starting dose and more gradual increase in dose in those likely to have a slower metabolism (e.g. older adults, women, non-smokers); max 20 mg/day
- Monotherapy for mania: 15 mg/day, adjusted according to response, usual dose range 5–20 mg/day, doses above 5 mg/day only after reassessment, consider lower starting dose and more gradual increase in dose in those likely to have a slower metabolism (e.g. older adults, women, non-smokers); max 20 mg/day

Intramuscular
- Control of agitation and disturbed behaviour in schizophrenia or mania: initial dose 5–10 mg (usually 10 mg for 1 dose), followed by 5–10 mg after 2 hours as needed, max 3 injections per day for 3 days; max combined oral and parenteral dose 20 mg/day, consider lower starting dose and more gradual increase in dose in those likely to have a slower metabolism (e.g. older adults, women, non-smokers)

 ### Dosing Tips
- Minimum effective dose is 5 mg/day for first episode of psychosis in schizophrenia and 10 mg/day for relapses
- Monitoring blood concentration of olanzapine may be helpful in certain circumstances, such as patients presenting symptoms suggestive of toxicity, or when concomitant medicines may interact to increase blood concentration of olanzapine

Overdose
- Rarely lethal in monotherapy overdose
- Sedation and slurred speech may occur

Long-Term Use
- Approved to maintain response in long-term treatment of schizophrenia
- Approved for long-term maintenance in bipolar disorder
- Often used for long-term maintenance in various behavioural disorders

Habit Forming
- No

How to Stop
- The risk of relapse is high if medication is stopped after 1–2 years
- Withdrawal of antipsychotic drugs after long-term therapy should be gradual and closely monitored to avoid the risk of withdrawal symptoms or rapid relapse
- After withdrawal of an antipsychotic, patients should be monitored for signs and symptoms of relapse for 2 years
- See Switching section of individual agents for how to stop olanzapine

Pharmacokinetics
- Metabolites are inactive
- Parent drug has a half-life of about 21–54 hours
- Olanzapine is a substrate for CYP450 1A2 and 2D6
- Food does not affect absorption

 ### Drug Interactions
- May increase effect of antihypertensive agents
- May antagonise levodopa, dopamine agonists
- Dose may need to be lowered if given with CYP450 1A2 inhibitors (e.g. fluvoxamine) and raised if given in conjunction with CYP450 1A2 inducers (e.g. tobacco, carbamazepine)

 ### Other Warnings/Precautions
- All antipsychotics should be used with caution in patients with angle-closure glaucoma, blood disorders, cardiovascular disease, depression, diabetes, epilepsy and susceptibility to seizures, history of jaundice, myasthenia gravis, Parkinson's disease, photosensitivity, prostatic hypertrophy, severe respiratory disorders
- Olanzapine long-acting injection may be associated with DRESS. This may begin as a rash but can progress to other parts of the body and can include symptoms such as fever, swollen lymph nodes, swollen face, inflammation of organs, and an increase in white blood cells known as eosinophilia. In some cases, DRESS can lead to death. Clinicians should inform patients about the risk of DRESS; patients who develop a fever with rash and swollen lymph nodes

Olanzapine (Continued)

or swollen face should seek medical care. However, patients are not advised to stop their medication without consulting their prescribing clinician
- With long-acting injection: caution in bone-marrow depression; hypereosinophilia; low leucocyte and neutrophil count; myeloproliferative disease; paralytic ileus; during a switch from oral to depot, the oral dose should be reduced gradually
- Use with caution in patients with conditions that predispose to hypotension (dehydration, overheating)
- Use with caution in patients with prostatic hypertrophy, angle-closure glaucoma, paralytic ileus
- Patients receiving the intramuscular formulation of olanzapine should be observed closely for hypotension
- Intramuscular formulation is not generally recommended to be administered with parenteral benzodiazepines; if patient requires a parenteral benzodiazepine it should be given at least 1 hour after intramuscular olanzapine
- Olanzapine should be used cautiously in patients at risk for aspiration pneumonia, as dysphagia has been reported

Do Not Use
- Intramuscular olanzapine in patients with cardiovascular conditions including acute myocardial infarction, bradycardia, hypotension (severe), recent heart surgery, sick sinus syndrome, unstable angina
- Olanzapine long-acting injection in children
- In any form if there is a proven allergy to olanzapine

SPECIAL POPULATIONS

Renal Impairment
- Consider lower initial dose of 5 mg/day
- Long-acting injection: initial dose 150 mg every 4 weeks

Hepatic Impairment
- Consider lower initial dose of 5 mg/day
- Long-acting injection: manufacturer advises caution
- Liver function should be tested a few times a year

Cardiac Impairment
- Contraindicated in acute myocardial infarction, bradycardia, recent heart surgery, severe hypotension, sick sinus syndrome, unstable angina
- Use with caution in these circumstances due to the risk of orthostatic hypotension

Elderly
- Olanzapine increases the risk of cerebrovascular events in elderly patients with dementia-related psychosis
- Consider lower starting dose and more gradual increase in dose
- IM in elderly: initial dose 2.5–5 mg, followed by 2.5–5 mg after 2 hours as needed, max 3 injections per day for 3 days; max combined oral and parenteral dose 20 mg/day, consider lower starting dose and more gradual increase in dose in those likely to have a slower metabolism (e.g. older adults, women, non-smokers)

Children and Adolescents
- Approved for schizophrenia and for combination therapy or monotherapy in mania for children aged 12–17 years under expert supervision

Before you prescribe:
- Do not offer antipsychotic medication when transient or attenuated psychotic symptoms or other mental state changes associated with distress, impairment, or help-seeking behaviour are not sufficient for a diagnosis of psychosis or schizophrenia. Consider individual CBT with or without family therapy and other treatments recommended for anxiety, depression, substance use, or emerging personality disorder
- For first-episode psychosis (FEP) antipsychotic medication should only be started by a specialist following a comprehensive multidisciplinary assessment and in conjunction with recommended psychological interventions (CBT, family therapy)
- As first-line treatment: allow patient to choose from aripiprazole, olanzapine or risperidone. As second-line treatment switch to alternative from list
- For bipolar disorder: if bipolar disorder is suspected in primary care in children or adolescents refer them to a specialist service
- Choice of antipsychotic medication should be an informed choice depending on individual factors and side-effect profile (metabolic, cardiovascular, extrapyramidal, hormonal, other)

- All children and young people with FEP/bipolar should be supported with sleep management, anxiety management, exercise and activation schedules, and healthy diet
- Where a child or young person presents with self-harm and suicidal thoughts the immediate risk management may take first priority
- A risk management plan is important prior to start of medication because of the possible increase in suicidal ideation and behaviours in adolescents and young adults

Practical notes:

- Carefully weigh the risks and benefits of pharmacological treatment against the risks and benefits of non-treatment and make sure to document this in the patient's chart
- Monitor weight, weekly for the first 6 weeks, then at 12 weeks, and then every 6 months (plotted on a growth chart)
- Monitor height every 6 months (plotted on a growth chart)
- Monitor waist circumference every 6 months (plotted on a percentile chart)
- Monitor pulse and blood pressure (plotted on a percentile chart) at 12 weeks and then every 6 months
- Monitor fasting blood glucose, HbA1c, blood lipid and prolactin levels at 12 weeks and then every 6 months
- Monitor for activation of suicidal ideation at the beginning of treatment. Inform parents or guardians of this risk so they can help observe child or adolescent patients
- If it does not work: review child's/young person's profile, consider new/changing contributing individual or systemic factors such as peer or family conflict. Consider drug/substance misuse. Consider dose adjustment before switching or augmentation. Be vigilant of polypharmacy especially in complex and highly vulnerable children/adolescents
- Consider non-concordance by parent or child, consider non-concordance in adolescents, address underlying reasons for non-concordance
- Children are more sensitive to most side effects
  - There is an inverse relationship between age and incidence of EPS
  - Exposure to antipsychotics during childhood and young age is associated with a three-fold increase of diabetes mellitus

- Treatment with all second-generation antipsychotics (SGAs) has been associated with changes in most lipid parameters
  - Olanzapine is strongly associated with weight gain, changes in lipid parameters, sedation
  - Weight gain correlates with time on treatment. Any childhood obesity is associated with obesity in adults
  - Aripiprazole is least associated with weight gain, changes in lipid parameters, sedation, and prolactin increase amongst SGAs
- Dose adjustments may be necessary in the presence of interacting drugs
- Re-evaluate the need for continued treatment regularly
- Provide Medicines for Children leaflet for olanzapine for schizophrenia-bipolar-disorder-and-agitation
- Monitoring of endocrine function (weight, height, sexual maturation and menses) is required when a child is taking an antipsychotic drug that is known to cause hyperprolactinaemia

Pregnancy

- Controlled studies have not been conducted in pregnant women
- Increased risks to baby have been reported for antipsychotics as a group although evidence is limited
- There is a risk of abnormal muscle movements and withdrawal symptoms in newborns whose mothers took an antipsychotic during the third trimester; symptoms may include agitation, abnormally increased or decreased muscle tone, tremor, sleepiness, severe difficulty breathing, and difficulty feeding
- Psychotic symptoms may worsen during pregnancy, and some form of treatment may be necessary
- Use in pregnancy may be justified if the benefit of continued treatment exceeds any associated risk
- Switching antipsychotics may increase the risk of relapse
- Olanzapine has been associated with maternal hyperglycaemia which may lead to developmental toxicity; blood glucose levels should be monitored

• Olanzapine may be preferable to anticonvulsant mood stabilisers if treatment or prophylaxis are required during pregnancy

• Depot antipsychotics should only be used when there is a good response to the depot and a history of non-concordance with oral medication

Breastfeeding

• Small amounts expected in mother's breast milk

• Risk of accumulation in infant due to long half-life

• Haloperidol is considered to be the preferred first-generation antipsychotic, and quetiapine the preferred second-generation antipsychotic

• Sedation reported in breastfed infants

• Infants of women who choose to breastfeed should be monitored for possible adverse effects

THE ART OF PSYCHOPHARMACOLOGY

Potential Advantages

• Some cases of psychosis and bipolar disorder refractory to treatment with other antipsychotics

∗ Often a preferred augmenting agent in bipolar depression or treatment-resistant unipolar depression

∗ Patients needing rapid onset of antipsychotic action without drug titration

• Patients switching from intramuscular olanzapine to an oral preparation

Potential Disadvantages

• Patients concerned about gaining weight

∗ Patients with diabetes mellitus, obesity, and/or dyslipidaemia

Primary Target Symptoms

• Positive symptoms of psychosis
• Negative symptoms of psychosis
• Cognitive symptoms
• Unstable mood (both depressed mood and mania)
• Aggressive symptoms

 Pearls

• Olanzapine may show greater efficacy in schizophrenia versus some other atypical or conventional antipsychotics

• Olanzapine may show greater propensity for metabolic side effects in schizophrenia versus some other atypical or conventional antipsychotics

• Well accepted for use in schizophrenia and bipolar disorder, including more complex cases especially at higher doses

• Effective at lower doses as an augmenting agent when added to SSRI antidepressants in non-psychotic depression

• Effective in treating bipolar depression when combined with fluoxetine

• Although may cause more weight gain than many other antipsychotics, this does not occur in all patients

• Motor side effects unlikely at low-moderate doses

• Smoking can reduce plasma levels and so smokers tend to need higher doses

• Some patients who do not respond to regular doses of olanzapine may respond to high dosing guided by plasma drug levels

• Short-acting IM injection effective for rapid tranquillisation, but cannot be given together at the same time as lorazepam

• Long-acting injection effective, but due to potential side effects in the first few hours after administration, each monthly dose must be given in an environment with access to medical care. The patient must show capacity in deciding to accept this regimen

OLANZAPINE LONG-ACTING INJECTION

Zypadhera Properties

Vehicle	Water
Duration of action	1 day–4 weeks
Tmax	2–4 days
T1/2 with multiple dosing	30 days
Time to steady state	About 12 weeks
Able to be loaded	Yes
Dosing schedule (maintenance)	Every 2 weeks or 4 weeks
Injection site	Intramuscular gluteal
Needle gauge	19
Dosage forms	210 mg, 300 mg, 405 mg (powder and solvent for prolonged-release suspension for injection)
Injection volume	210 mg/mL, 300 mg/mL, 405 mg/mL

Usual Dosage Range
- 300 mg every 2 weeks or 405 mg every 4 weeks

How to Dose
- Not recommended for patients who have not first demonstrated tolerability to oral olanzapine
- Maintenance in schizophrenia in patients tolerant to oral olanzapine (10 mg/day) – adult 18–75 years: initial dose 210 mg every 2 weeks, otherwise initial dose 405 mg every 4 weeks, then maintenance 150 mg every 2 weeks, alternatively maintenance 300 mg every 4 weeks, maintenance dose to start after 2 months of initial treatment
- Maintenance in schizophrenia in patients tolerant to oral olanzapine (15 mg/day) – adult 18–75 years: initial dose 300 mg every 2 weeks, then maintenance 210 mg every 2 weeks, alternatively maintenance 405 mg every 4 weeks, maintenance dose to start after 2 months of initial treatment
- Maintenance in schizophrenia in patients tolerant to oral olanzapine (20 mg/day) – adult: initial dose 300 mg every 2 weeks, then maintenance 300 mg every 2 weeks (max per dose 300 mg every 2 weeks), adjusted according to response
- Oral supplementation may be required if adequate loading dose not used

 Dosing Tips
- With long-acting injections, the absorption rate constant is slower than the elimination rate constant, thus resulting in "flip-flop" kinetics – i.e. time to steady state is a function of absorption rate, while concentration at steady state is a function of elimination rate

- The rate-limiting step for plasma drug levels for long-acting injections is not drug metabolism, but rather slow absorption from the injection site
- In general, 5 half-lives of any medication are needed to achieve 97% of steady-state levels
- The long half-life of depot/long-acting injection antipsychotics means that one must either adequately load the dose (if possible) or provide oral supplementation
- The failure to adequately load the dose leads either to prolonged cross-titration from oral antipsychotic or to sub-therapeutic antipsychotic plasma levels for weeks or months in patients who are not receiving (or adhering to) oral supplementation
- Because plasma antipsychotic levels increase gradually over time, dose requirements may ultimately decrease; if possible obtaining periodic plasma levels can be beneficial to prevent unnecessary plasma level creep
- The time to get a blood level for patients receiving long-acting injection is the morning of the day they will receive their next injection
- Advantages: efficacy advantage of oral olanzapine
- Disadvantages: 3-hour post-injection monitoring required due to risk (about 0.1%) of post-injection syndrome from vascular breach
- Typical symptoms of post-injection syndrome: agitation, anxiety, ataxia, confusion, delirium, dysarthria, sedation
- Olanzapine assay can be useful to check adherence, assess for adequacy of dosage, and investigate any suspected acute poisoning. A steady-state reference range of 20–40 mcg/L suggested

THE ART OF SWITCHING

 **Switching from Oral Antipsychotic to Olanzapine Long-Acting Injection**

- Discontinuation of oral antipsychotic can begin immediately if adequate loading is pursued
- How to discontinue oral formulations:
  - Down-titration is not required for: amisulpride, aripiprazole, cariprazine, olanzapine, paliperidone
  - 1-week down-titration is required for: lurasidone, risperidone, asenapine, quetiapine
  - 4+-week down-titration may be required for: clozapine

Switching from Oral Antipsychotics to Oral Olanzapine

- With aripiprazole, amisulpride, and paliperidone, immediate stop is possible; begin olanzapine at middle dose
- With risperidone and lurasidone, begin olanzapine gradually, titrating over at least 2 weeks to allow patients to become tolerant to the sedating effect

*May need to taper clozapine slowly over 4 weeks or longer

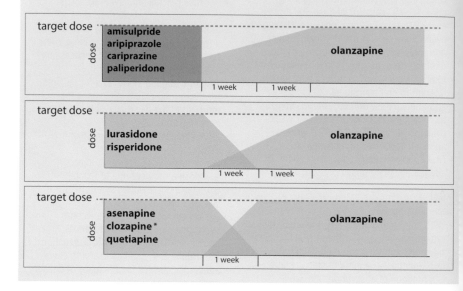

📖 Suggested Reading

Bahji A, Ermacora D, Stephenson C, et al. Comparative efficacy and tolerability of pharmacological treatments for the treatment of acute bipolar depression: a systematic review and network meta-analysis. J Affect Disord 2020;269:154–84.

Baldessarini RJ, Vazquez GH, Tondo L. Bipolar depression: a major unsolved challenge. Int J Bipolar Disord 2020;8(1):1.

Detke HC, Zhao F, Garhyan P, et al. Dose correspondence between olanzapine long-acting injection and oral olanzapine: recommendations for switching. Int Clin Psychopharmacol 2011;26(1):35–42.

Hirsch L, Yang J, Bresee L, et al. Second-generation antipsychotics and metabolic side effects: a systematic review of population-based studies. Drug Saf 2017;40(9):771–81.

Huhn M, Nikolakopoulou A, Schneider-Thoma J, et al. Comparative efficacy and tolerability of 32 oral antipsychotics for the acute treatment of adults with multi-episode schizophrenia: a systematic review and network meta-analysis. Lancet 2019;394(10202):939–51.

Komossa K, Rummel-Kluge C, Hunger H, et al. Olanzapine versus other atypical antipsychotics for schizophrenia. Cochrane Database Syst Rev 2010;(3):CD006654.

Meyer JM, Stahl SM. The Clinical Use of Antipsychotic Plasma Levels. Cambridge University Press, Cambridge, 2021.

Nasrallah HA. Atypical antipsychotic-induced metabolic side effects: insights from receptor-binding profiles. Mol Psychiatry 2008;13(1):27–35.

Pillinger T, McCutcheon RA, Vano L, et al. Comparative effects of 18 antipsychotics on metabolic function in patients with schizophrenia, predictors of metabolic dysregulation, and association with psychopathology: a systematic review and network meta-analysis. Lancet Psychiatry 2020;7(1):64–77.

Takeshima M. Treating mixed mania/hypomania: a review and synthesis of the evidence. CNS Spectr 2017;22(2):177–85.

Oxazepam

Brands
• Non-proprietary

Generic?
Yes

Class
• Neuroscience-based nomenclature: pharmacology domain – GABA; mode of action – positive allosteric modulator (PAM)
• Benzodiazepine (anxiolytic); hypnotic

Commonly Prescribed for
(bold for BNF indication)
• **Anxiety (short-term use)**
• **Insomnia associated with anxiety**
• Anxiety associated with depression
• Alcohol withdrawal
• Catatonia

 How the Drug Works
• Binds to benzodiazepine receptors at the GABA-A ligand-gated chloride channel complex
• Enhances the inhibitory effects of GABA
• Boosts chloride conductance through GABA-regulated channels
• Inhibits neuronal activity presumably in amygdala-centred fear circuits to provide therapeutic benefits in anxiety disorders

How Long Until It Works
• Some immediate relief with first dosing is common; can take several weeks for maximal therapeutic benefit with daily dosing

If It Works
• For short-term symptoms of anxiety – after a few weeks, discontinue use or use on an "as-needed" basis
• For chronic anxiety disorders, the goal of treatment is complete remission of symptoms as well as prevention of future relapses
• For chronic anxiety disorders, treatment most often reduces or even eliminates symptoms, but is not a cure since symptoms can recur after medicine stopped
• For long-term symptoms of anxiety, consider switching to an SSRI or SNRI for long-term maintenance
• Avoid long-term maintenance with a benzodiazepine

• If symptoms re-emerge after stopping a benzodiazepine, consider treatment with an SSRI or SNRI, or consider restarting the benzodiazepine; sometimes benzodiazepines have to be used in combination with SSRIs or SNRIs at the start of treatment for best results

If It Doesn't Work
• Consider switching to another agent or adding an appropriate augmenting agent
• Consider psychotherapy, especially cognitive behavioural psychotherapy
• Consider presence of concomitant substance abuse
• Consider presence of oxazepam abuse
• Consider another diagnosis such as a co-morbid medical condition

 Best Augmenting Combos for Partial Response or Treatment Resistance
• Benzodiazepines are frequently used as augmenting agents for antipsychotics and mood stabilisers in the treatment of psychotic and bipolar disorders
• Benzodiazepines are frequently used as augmenting agents for SSRIs and SNRIs in the treatment of anxiety disorders
• Not generally rational to combine with other benzodiazepines
• Caution if using as an anxiolytic concomitantly with other sedative hypnotics for sleep

Tests
• In patients with seizure disorders, concomitant medical illness, and/or those with multiple concomitant long-term medications, periodic liver tests and blood counts may be prudent

How Drug Causes Side Effects
• Same mechanism for side effects as for therapeutic effects – namely due to excessive actions at benzodiazepine receptors
• Long-term adaptations in benzodiazepine receptors may explain the development of dependence, tolerance, and withdrawal
• Side effects are generally immediate, but immediate side effects often disappear in time

Notable Side Effects

* ✳Sedation, fatigue, depression
* ✳Dizziness, ataxia, slurred speech, weakness
* ✳Forgetfulness, confusion
* ✳Hyperexcitability, nervousness
* Rare hallucinations, mania
* Rare hypotension
* Hypersalivation, dry mouth

Frequency not known

* Altered saliva, fever, leucopenia, memory loss, oedema, slurred speech, syncope, urticaria

 Life-Threatening or Dangerous Side Effects

* Respiratory depression, especially when taken with CNS depressants in overdose
* Rare hepatic dysfunction, renal dysfunction, blood dyscrasias

Weight Gain

unusual   not unusual   common   problematic

* Reported but not expected

Sedation

unusual   not unusual   common   problematic

* Many experience and/or can be significant in amount
* Especially at initiation of treatment or when dose increases
* Tolerance often develops over time

What to Do About Side Effects

* Wait
* Wait
* Wait
* Lower the dose
* Take largest dose at bedtime to avoid sedative effects during the day
* Switch to another agent
* Administer flumazenil if side effects are severe or life-threatening

Best Augmenting Agents for Side Effects

* Many side effects cannot be improved with an augmenting agent

---

DOSING AND USE

Usual Dosage Range

* Short-term use in anxiety (adults): 15–30 mg 3–4 times per day
* Short-term use in anxiety (elderly/debilitated): 10–20 mg 3–4 times per day
* Insomnia associated with anxiety (adults): 15–50 mg at bedtime

Dosage Forms

* Tablet 10 mg, 15 mg

How to Dose

* ✳Short-term use in anxiety:
* Adults: 15–30 mg 3–4 times per day
* Elderly or debilitated patients: 10–20 mg 3–4 times per day
* ✳Insomnia associated with anxiety:
* Adults: 15–25 mg at bedtime (max per dose 50 mg)

 Dosing Tips

* Use lowest possible effective dose for the shortest possible period of time (a benzodiazepine-sparing strategy)
* Some forms of tablet contain tartrazine dye, which may cause allergic reactions in certain patients, particularly those who are sensitive to aspirin
* For inter-dose symptoms of anxiety, can either increase dose or maintain same total daily dose but divide into more frequent doses
* Can also use an as-required occasional "top up" dose for inter-dose anxiety
* Because anxiety disorders can require higher doses, the risk of dependence may be greater in these patients
* Some severely ill patients may require doses higher than the generally recommended maximum dose
* Frequency of dosing in practice is often greater than predicted from half-life, as duration of biological activity is often shorter than pharmacokinetic terminal half-life
* Oxazepam 2 mg = diazepam 1 mg

Overdose

* Fatalities can occur; ataxia, confusion, excessive somnolence, hypotension, respiratory depression, coma

- Oxazepam is generally less toxic in overdose than other benzodiazepines

Long-Term Use

- Evidence of efficacy up to 16 weeks
- Risk of dependence, particularly for treatment periods longer than 12 weeks and especially in patients with past or current polysubstance abuse

Habit Forming

- Oxazepam is a Class C/Schedule 4 drug
- Patients may develop dependence and/or tolerance with long-term use

How to Stop

- Patients with history of seizure may experience seizures upon withdrawal, especially if withdrawal is abrupt
- Taper by 0.5 mg every 3 days to reduce chances of withdrawal effects
- For difficult to taper cases, consider reducing dose much more slowly once reaching 3 mg/day, perhaps by as little as 0.25 mg per week or less
- For other patients with severe problems discontinuing a benzodiazepine, dosing may need to be tapered over many months (i.e. reduce dose by 1% every 3 days by crushing tablet and suspending or dissolving in 100 mL of fruit juice and then disposing of 1 mL while drinking the rest; 3–7 days later, dispose of 2 mL, and so on). This is both a form of very slow biological tapering and a form of behavioural desensitisation
- Be sure to differentiale re-emergence of symptoms requiring reinstitution of treatment from withdrawal symptoms
- Benzodiazepine-dependent anxiety patients are not addicted to their medications. When benzodiazepine-dependent patients stop their medication, disease symptoms can re-emerge, disease symptoms can worsen (rebound), and/or withdrawal symptoms can emerge

Pharmacokinetics

- Half-life of about 3–21 hours
- Metabolism via hepatic glucuronidation
- No active metabolites
- Excretion via kidneys

 Drug Interactions

- Increased depressive effects when taken with other CNS depressants (see Warnings below)

 Other Warnings/Precautions

- Warning regarding the increased risk of CNS-depressant effects (especially alcohol) when benzodiazepines and opioid medications are used together, including specifically the risk of slowed or difficulty breathing and death
- If alternatives to the combined use of benzodiazepines and opioids are not available, clinicians should limit the dosage and duration of each drug to the minimum possible while still achieving therapeutic efficacy
- Patients and their caregivers should be warned to seek medical attention if unusual dizziness, lightheadedness, sedation, slowed or difficulty breathing, or unresponsiveness occur
- Dosage changes should be made in collaboration with prescriber
- History of drug or alcohol abuse often creates greater risk for dependency
- Some depressed patients may experience a worsening of suicidal ideation
- Some patients may exhibit abnormal thinking or behavioural changes similar to those caused by other CNS depressants (i.e. either depressant actions or disinhibiting actions)
- Avoid prolonged use and abrupt cessation
- Use lower doses in debilitated patients and the elderly
- Use with caution in patients with myasthenia gravis; respiratory disease
- Use with caution in patients with personality disorder (dependent/avoidant or anankastic types) as may increase risk of dependence
- Use with caution in patients with a history of alcohol or drug dependence/abuse
- Benzodiazepines may cause a range of paradoxical effects including aggression, antisocial behaviours, anxiety, overexcitement, perceptual abnormalities and talkativeness. Adjustment of dose may reduce impulses

Oxazepam (Continued)

- Use with caution as oxazepam can cause muscle weakness and organic brain changes
- Insomnia may be a symptom of a primary disorder, rather than a primary disorder itself

Do Not Use

- If patient has acute pulmonary insufficiency, respiratory depression, significant neuromuscular respiratory weakness, sleep apnoea syndrome or unstable myasthenia gravis
- Alone in chronic psychosis in adults
- On its own to try to treat depression, anxiety associated with depression, obsessional states or phobic states
- If patient has angle-closure glaucoma
- If there is a proven allergy to oxazepam or any benzodiazepine

SPECIAL POPULATIONS

Renal Impairment

- Start with small doses in severe impairment

Hepatic Impairment

- Can precipitate coma
- If treatment is necessary, benzodiazepines with a shorter half-life are safer
- Avoid in severe impairment
- Dose adjustments: start with smaller initial doses or reduce dose

Cardiac Impairment

- Benzodiazepines have been used to treat anxiety associated with acute myocardial infarction

Elderly

- For short-term use in anxiety, 10–20 mg 3–4 times per day

Children and Adolescents

- Not recommended in children and adolescents

Pregnancy

- Possible increased risk of birth defects when benzodiazepines taken during pregnancy

- Because of the potential risks, oxazepam is not generally recommended as treatment for anxiety during pregnancy, especially during the first trimester
- Drug should be tapered if discontinued
- Infants whose mothers received a benzodiazepine late in pregnancy may experience withdrawal effects
- Neonatal flaccidity has been reported in infants whose mothers took a benzodiazepine during pregnancy
- Seizures, even mild seizures, may cause harm to the embryo/foetus

Breastfeeding

- Some drug is found in mother's breast milk
- Effects of benzodiazepines on infant have been observed and include feeding difficulties, sedation, and weight loss
- Caution should be taken with the use of benzodiazepines in breastfeeding mothers; seek to use low doses for short periods to reduce infant exposure
- Use of short-acting agents, e.g. oxazepam or lorazepam, preferred

THE ART OF PSYCHOPHARMACOLOGY

Potential Advantages

- Rapid onset of action

Potential Disadvantages

- Euphoria may lead to abuse
- Abuse especially risky in past or present substance abusers

Primary Target Symptoms

- Panic attacks
- Anxiety
- Agitation

Pearls

- NICE Guidelines recommend medication for insomnia only as a second-line treatment after non-pharmacological treatment options have been tried (e.g. cognitive behavioural therapy for insomnia)
- Can be a very useful adjunct to SSRIs and SNRIs in the treatment of numerous anxiety disorders
- Not effective for treating psychosis as a monotherapy, but can be used as an adjunct to antipsychotics

- Not effective for treating bipolar disorder as a monotherapy, but can be used as an adjunct to mood stabilisers and antipsychotics
* Because of its short half-life and inactive metabolites, oxazepam may be preferred over some benzodiazepines for patients with liver disease
- Oxazepam may be preferred over some other benzodiazepines for the treatment of delirium
- Can both cause and treat depression in different patients
- When using to treat insomnia, remember that insomnia may be a symptom of some other primary disorder itself, and thus warrant evaluation for co-morbid psychiatric and/or medical conditions
- Though not systematically studied, benzodiazepines have been used effectively to treat catatonia and are the initial recommended treatment
- Oxazepam has been shown to suppress cortisol levels
- Studies suggest that oxazepam is the most slowly absorbed and has the slowest onset of action of all the common benzodiazepines

 ## Suggested Reading

Ayd Jr FJ. Oxazepam: update 1989. Int Clin Psychopharmacol 1990;5(1):1–15.

Buckley NA, Dawson AH, Whyte IM, et al. Relative toxicity of benzodiazepines in overdose. BMJ 1995;310(6974):219–21.

Christensen P, Lolk A, Gram LF, et al. Benzodiazepine-induced sedation and cortisol suppression. A placebo-controlled comparison of oxazepam and nitrazepam in healthy male volunteers. Psychopharmacology (Berl) 1992;106(4):511–16.

Garattini S. Biochemical and pharmacological properties of oxazepam. Acta Psychiatr Scand Suppl 1978;(274):9–18.

Greenblatt DJ. Clinical pharmacokinetics of oxazepam and lorazepam. Clin Pharmacokinet 1981;6(2):89–105.

Paliperidone

Brands

- Invega (modified-release tablets)
- Xeplion (suspension for injecting)
- Trevicta (prolonged-release suspension for injection)

Generic?

No, not in UK

Class

- Neuroscience-based nomenclature: pharmacology domain – dopamine, serotonin, norepinephrine; mode of action – antagonist
- Atypical antipsychotic (serotonin dopamine antagonist; second-generation antipsychotics; also a mood stabiliser)

Commonly Prescribed for

(bold for BNF indication)

- **Schizophrenia**
- **Psychotic or manic symptoms of schizoaffective disorder**
- **Maintenance of schizophrenia in patients who are clinically stable on once-monthly intramuscular paliperidone**
- **Maintenance in schizophrenia in patients previously responsive to paliperidone or risperidone**

 How the Drug Works

- Paliperidone (9-hydroxy risperidone) is a metabolite of risperidone via CYP450 2D6 metabolism
- Blocks dopamine 2 receptors, reducing positive symptoms of psychosis and stabilising affective symptoms
- Blocks serotonin 2A receptors, causing enhancement of dopamine release in certain brain regions and thus reducing motor side effects and possibly improving cognitive and affective symptoms
- *Serotonin 7 antagonist properties may contribute to antidepressant actions

How Long Until It Works

- Psychotic symptoms can improve within 1 week, but it may take several weeks for full effect on behaviour as well as on cognition
- Classically recommended to wait at least 4–6 weeks to determine efficacy of drug, but in practice some patients may require up to 16–20 weeks to show a good response, especially on cognitive symptoms

If It Works

- Most often reduces positive symptoms in schizophrenia but does not eliminate them
- Can improve negative symptoms, as well as aggressive, cognitive, and affective symptoms in schizophrenia
- Most patients with schizophrenia do not have a total remission of symptoms but rather a reduction of symptoms by about a third
- Perhaps 5–15% of patients with schizophrenia can experience an overall improvement of >50–60%, especially when receiving stable treatment for >1 year
- Such patients are considered super-responders or "awakeners" since they may be well enough to work, live independently, and sustain long-term relationships
- Many bipolar patients may experience a reduction of symptoms by half or more
- Continue treatment until reaching a plateau of improvement
- After reaching a satisfactory plateau, continue treatment for at least 1 year after first episode of psychosis, but it may be preferable to continue treatment indefinitely to avoid subsequent episodes
- After any subsequent episodes of psychosis, treatment may need to be indefinite

If It Doesn't Work

- Try one of the other atypical antipsychotics (olanzapine should be considered first before considering other agents such as quetiapine, aripiprazole, amisulpride or lurasidone)
- If 2 or more antipsychotic monotherapies do not work, consider clozapine
- Some patients may require treatment with a conventional antipsychotic
- If no first-line atypical antipsychotic is effective, consider higher doses or augmentation with valproate or lamotrigine
- Consider non-concordance and switch to another antipsychotic with fewer side effects or to an antipsychotic that can be given by depot injection (a depot formulation of paliperidone is available)
- Consider initiating rehabilitation and psychotherapy such as cognitive remediation
- Consider presence of concomitant drug abuse

Best Augmenting Combos for Partial Response or Treatment Resistance

- Valproic acid (Depakote or Epilim)
- Other mood-stabilising anticonvulsants (carbamazepine, oxcarbazepine, lamotrigine)
- Lithium
- Benzodiazepines

Tests

Before starting an atypical antipsychotic

* Measure weight, BMI, and waist circumference
- Get baseline personal and family history of diabetes, obesity, dyslipidaemia, hypertension, and cardiovascular disease
* Check pulse and blood pressure, fasting plasma glucose or glycosylated haemoglobin (HbA1c), fasting lipid profile, and prolactin level
- Full blood count (FBC), urea and electrolytes (including creatinine and eGFR), liver function tests (LFTs)
- Assessment of nutritional status, diet, and level of physical activity
- Determine if the patient:
  - is overweight (BMI 25.0–29.9)
  - is obese (BMI ≥30)
  - has pre-diabetes – fasting plasma glucose: 5.5 mmol/L to 6.9 mmol/L or HbA1c: 42 to 47 mmol/mol (6.0 to 6.4%)
  - has diabetes – fasting plasma glucose: >7.0 mmol/L or HbA1c: ≥48 mmol/L (≥6.5%)
  - has hypertension (BP >140/90 mm Hg)
  - has dyslipidaemia (increased total cholesterol, LDL cholesterol, and triglycerides; decreased HDL cholesterol)
- Treat or refer such patients for treatment, including nutrition and weight management, physical activity counselling, smoking cessation, and medical management
- Baseline ECG for: inpatients; those with a personal history or risk factor for cardiac disease

Monitoring after starting an atypical antipsychotic

- FBC annually to detect chronic bone marrow suppression, stop treatment if neutrophils fall below 1.5x10⁹/L, and refer to specialist care if neutrophils fall below 0.5x10⁹/L

- Urea and electrolytes (including creatinine and eGFR) annually
- LFTs annually
- Prolactin levels at 6 months and then annually (paliperidone is likely to increase prolactin levels)
* Weight/BMI/waist circumference, weekly for the first 6 weeks, then at 12 weeks, at 1 year, and then annually
* Pulse and blood pressure at 12 weeks, 1 year, and then annually
* Fasting blood glucose, HbA1c, and blood lipids at 12 weeks, at 1 year, and then annually
* For patients with type 2 diabetes, measure HbA1c at 3–6 month intervals until stable, then every 6 months
* Even in patients without known diabetes, be vigilant for the rare but life-threatening onset of diabetic ketoacidosis, which always requires immediate treatment, by monitoring for the rapid onset of polyuria, polydipsia, weight loss, nausea, vomiting, dehydration, rapid respiration, weakness and clouding of sensorium, even coma
- If HbA1c remains ≥48 mmol/mol (6.5%) then drug therapy should be offered, e.g. metformin
- Treat or refer for treatment or consider switching to another atypical antipsychotic for patients who become overweight, obese, pre-diabetic, diabetic, hypertensive, or dyslipidaemic while receiving an atypical antipsychotic

SIDE EFFECTS

How Drug Causes Side Effects

- By blocking alpha 1 adrenergic receptors, it can cause dizziness, sedation, and hypotension
- By blocking dopamine 2 receptors in the striatum, it can cause motor side effects, especially at high doses
- By blocking dopamine 2 receptors in the pituitary, it can cause elevations in prolactin
- Mechanism of weight gain and increased incidence of diabetes and dyslipidaemia with atypical antipsychotics is unknown

Notable Side Effects

* Dose-dependent extrapyramidal side effects
* Hyperprolactinaemia
* May increase risk for diabetes and dyslipidaemia

Common or very common

- CNS/PNS: altered mood, anxiety, depression, headache, vision disorders
- CVS: cardiac conduction disorders, hypertension
- GIT: abnormal appetite, diarrhoea, gastrointestinal discomfort, nausea, oral disorders
- Other: asthenia, cough, fever, hyperglycaemia, increased risk of infection, joint disorders, laryngeal pain, nasal congestion, pain, skin reactions
- With oral use: decreased weight

Uncommon

- Blood disorders: anaemia, thrombocytopenia
- CNS/PNS: abnormal gait, abnormal sensation, dysarthria, fall, seizure, sleep disorders, tinnitus, vertigo
- CVS: palpitations, syncope
- GIT: altered taste, dysphagia, gastrointestinal disorders, thirst
- Other: alopecia, breast abnormalities, chest discomfort, chills, conjunctivitis, cystitis, dry eye, dyspnoea, ear pain, epistaxis, hypoglycaemia, induration, malaise, menstrual cycle irregularities, muscle spasms, muscle weakness, oedema, respiratory disorders, sexual dysfunction, urinary disorders
- With oral use: confusion, diabetes mellitus, impaired concentration

Rare or very rare

- CNS/PNS: abnormal posture, cerebrovascular insufficiency, coma, dysphonia, eye disorders, impaired consciousness, sleep apnoea
- GIT: jaundice, pancreatitis
- Other: angioedema, dandruff, diabetic ketoacidosis, flushing, glaucoma, hypothermia, ischaemia, polydipsia, rhabdomyolysis, SIADH, vaginal discharge, water intoxication, withdrawal syndrome

Frequency not known

- With IM use: injection site necrosis

☠ Life-Threatening or Dangerous Side Effects

- Hyperglycaemia, in some cases extreme and associated with ketoacidosis or hyperosmolar coma or death, has been reported in patients taking atypical antipsychotics
- Increased risk of death and cerebrovascular events in elderly patients with dementia-related psychosis
- Rare neuroleptic malignant syndrome (much reduced risk compared to conventional antipsychotics but still reported)
- Seizures

Weight Gain

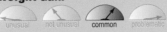

- Many patients experience and/or can be significant in amount
- May be dose-dependent
- May be less than for some antipsychotics, more than for others

Sedation

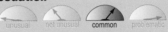

- Many patients experience and/or can be significant in amount
- May be dose-dependent
- May be less than for some antipsychotics, more than for others

What To Do About Side Effects

- Wait
- Wait
- Wait
- Reduce the dose
- Low-dose benzodiazepine or beta blocker may reduce akathisia
- Take more of the dose at bedtime to help reduce daytime sedation
- Weight loss, exercise programmes, and medical management for high BMIs, diabetes, and dyslipidaemia
- Switch to another antipsychotic (atypical) – quetiapine or clozapine are best in cases of tardive dyskinesia

Best Augmenting Agents for Side Effects

- Dystonia: antimuscarinic drugs (e.g. procyclidine) as oral or IM depending on the severity; botulinum toxin if antimuscarinics not effective
- Parkinsonism: antimuscarinic drugs (e.g. procyclidine)
- Akathisia: beta blocker propranolol (30–80 mg/day) or low-dose benzodiazepine

(e.g. 0.5–3.0 mg/day of clonazepam) may help; other agents that may be tried include the 5HT2 antagonists such as cyproheptadine (16 mg/day) or mirtazapine (15 mg at night – caution in bipolar disorder); clonidine (0.2–0.8 mg/day) may be tried if the above ineffective
- Tardive dyskinesia: stop any antimuscarinic, consider tetrabenazine
- Addition of low doses (2.5–5 mg) of aripiprazole can reverse the hyperprolactinaemia/galactorrhoea caused by other antipsychotics
- Addition of aripiprazole (5–15 mg/day) or metformin (500–2000 mg/day) to weight-inducing atypical antipsychotics such as olanzapine and clozapine can help mitigate against weight gain

DOSING AND USE

Usual Dosage Range
- Schizophrenia; psychotic or manic symptoms of schizoaffective disorder: 3–12 mg/day
- Maintenance in schizophrenia in patients previously responsive to paliperidone or risperidone: deep IM injection 25–150 mg every month
- Maintenance of schizophrenia in patients who are clinically stable on once-monthly intramuscular paliperidone: deep IM injection 175–525 mg every 3 months

Dosage Forms
- Modified-release tablet (prolonged-release) 3 mg, 6 mg, 9 mg
- Suspension for injection Xeplion 50 mg in 0.5 mL, 75 mg in 0.75 mL, 100 mg in 1 mL, 150 mg in 1.5 mL
- Prolonged-release suspension for injection Trevicta 175 mg in 0.875 mL, 263 mg in 1.315 mL, 350 mg in 1.75 mL, 525 mg in 2.265 mL

How to Dose
＊Schizophrenia; psychotic or manic symptoms of schizoaffective disorder:
- Initial dose 6 mg in the morning, then adjust dose by increments of 3 mg/day every 5 days as needed; usual dose 3–12 mg/day

＊Maintenance in schizophrenia in patients who have previously responded to paliperidone or risperidone:
- Initial dose 150 mg on day 1, then 100 mg on day 8, injection into deltoid muscle. After this adjust dose at monthly intervals according to response; maintenance dose 75 mg once/month (range 25–150 mg once/month). Maintenance doses can be injected into deltoid or gluteal muscle
＊Maintenance of schizophrenia in patients who are clinically stable on once-monthly IM paliperidone:
- Initial dose 175–525 mg every 3 months, adjusted according to response, administered into deltoid or gluteal muscle. Dose based on previous once-monthly IM paliperidone and initiated in place of next scheduled dose
- Long-acting injected paliperidone is not recommended for patients who have not first demonstrated tolerability to oral paliperidone or risperidone

Dosing Tips
- Tablet should not be divided or chewed, but rather should only be swallowed whole
- Tablet does not change shape in the gastrointestinal tract and generally should not be used in patients with gastrointestinal narrowing because of the risk of intestinal obstruction
- Some patients may benefit from doses above 6 mg/day; alternatively, for some patients 3 mg/day may be sufficient
- A common dosage error is to assume the paliperidone prolonged-release oral dose is the same as the risperidone oral dose in mg, and that paliperidone should be titrated. However, many patients can do well starting at a dose of 6 mg orally of paliperidone prolonged-release without titration
- There is a dose-dependent increase in some side effects, including extrapyramidal symptoms and weight gain, above 6 mg/day
- Rather than raise the dose above these levels in acutely agitated patients requiring acute antipsychotic actions, consider augmentation with a benzodiazepine or conventional antipsychotic, either orally or intramuscularly
- Rather than raise the dose above these levels in partial responders, consider augmentation

with a mood-stabilising anticonvulsant, such as valproate or lamotrigine
- Children and elderly should generally be dosed at the lower end of the dosage spectrum
- Treatment should be suspended if absolute neutrophil count falls below less than 1.5×10^9/L

Overdose
- Extrapyramidal symptoms, gait unsteadiness, sedation, tachycardia, hypotension, QT prolongation

Long-Term Use
- Approved for maintenance in schizophrenia

Habit Forming
- No

How to Stop
- There is a high risk of relapse if medication is stopped after 1–2 years
- Rapid oral discontinuation may lead to rebound psychosis and worsening of symptoms
- Withdrawal of antipsychotic drugs after long-term therapy should always be gradual and closely monitored to avoid the risk of acute withdrawal syndromes or rapid relapse
- Patients should be monitored for 2 years after withdrawal of antipsychotic medication for signs and symptoms of relapse
- See Switching section of individual agents for how to stop paliperidone

Pharmacokinetics
- Absorption is reduced if taken on an empty stomach
- Oral paliperidone has a much lower bioavailability than risperidone (doses 2–2.5 times greater are required to achieve comparable plasma levels and antipsychotic effect)
- Paliperidone is the major active metabolite of risperidone
- Half-life about 23 hours (paliperidone has a longer half-life than risperidone)
- Paliperidone is largely excreted unchanged

 Drug Interactions
- May increase effects of antihypertensive agents
- May antagonise levodopa, dopamine agonists

- May enhance QTc prolongation of other drugs capable of prolonging QTc interval
- CYP450 3A4 inducers (e.g. carbamazepine, phenytoin, rifampicin) can reduce plasma levels of paliperidone and increase them on their withdrawal
- Precautions required with CYP450 3A4 inhibitors (fluvoxamine, fluoxetine, paroxetine, ciprofloxacin, cimetidine, ketaconazole) – may require lower doses
- Precautions required with CYP450 2D6 inhibitors (bupropion, duloxetine, paroxetine, fluoxetine) – may require lower doses

 Other Warnings/Precautions
- All antipsychotics should be used with caution in patients with angle-closure glaucoma, blood disorders, cardiovascular disease, depression, diabetes, epilepsy and susceptibility to seizures, history of jaundice, myasthenia gravis, Parkinson's disease, photosensitivity, prostatic hypertrophy, severe respiratory disorders
- Patients with schizoaffective disorder treated with paliperidone should be carefully monitored for a potential switch from manic to depressive symptoms
- Use with caution in patients with conditions that predispose to hypotension (dehydration, overheating)
- Dysphagia has been associated with antipsychotic use, and paliperidone should be used cautiously in patients at risk for aspiration pneumonia
- Paliperidone prolongs QTc interval more than some other antipsychotics
- Use with caution in cataract surgery (risk of intraoperative floppy iris syndrome)
- Use with caution if at all in Parkinson's disease or dementia with Lewy bodies
- Use with caution in elderly patients with dementia or elderly patients with risk factors for stroke
- Use caution in patients with a predisposition to gastrointestinal obstruction
- Use with caution in patients with possible prolactin-dependent tumours

Do Not Use
- Intramuscular paliperidone injections in children
- If there is a proven allergy to paliperidone or risperidone

Paliperidone (Continued)

Renal Impairment

- With oral use: avoid if creatinine clearance less than 10 mL/minute
- With intramuscular use: avoid if creatinine clearance less than 50 mL/minute

Hepatic Impairment

- Caution in severe impairment

Cardiac Impairment

- In cardiac impairment, use with caution due to risk of orthostatic hypotension
- An ECG may be required, particularly if physical examination identifies cardiovascular risk factors, personal history of cardiovascular disease, or if the patient is being admitted as an inpatient

Elderly

- Use with caution in elderly with dementia or elderly with risk factors for stroke

Children and Adolescents

- Do not administer intramuscular paliperidone injections in children
- Oral paliperidone is also not licensed for children. It is occasionally used, but is not recommended for children under the age of 15
- If used, regular monitoring of endocrine function is suggested including height, weight, menstruation and sexual maturation

Pregnancy

- Controlled studies have not been conducted in pregnant women
- There is a risk of abnormal muscle movements and withdrawal symptoms in newborns whose mothers took an antipsychotic during the third trimester; symptoms may include agitation, abnormally increased or decreased muscle tone, tremor, sleepiness, severe difficulty breathing, and difficulty feeding
- Psychotic symptoms may worsen during pregnancy and some form of treatment may be necessary
- Use in pregnancy may be justified if the benefit of continued treatment exceeds any associated risk

- Switching antipsychotics may increase the risk of relapse
- Antipsychotics may be preferable to anticonvulsant mood stabilisers if treatment is required for mania during pregnancy
- Effects of hyperprolactinaemia on the foetus are unknown
- Olanzapine and clozapine have been associated with maternal hyperglycaemia which may lead to developmental toxicity; risk may also apply for other atypical antipsychotics
- Depot antipsychotics should only be used when there is a good response to the depot and a history of non-concordance with oral medication

Breastfeeding

- Some drug is found in mother's breast milk
- Risk of accumulation in infant due to long half-life
- Haloperidol is considered to be the preferred first-generation antipsychotic, and quetiapine the preferred second-generation antipsychotic
- Infants of women who choose to breastfeed should be monitored for possible adverse effects

Potential Advantages

- Some cases of psychosis and schizoaffective disorder refractory to treatment with other antipsychotics
- Patients requiring rapid onset of antipsychotic action without dosage titration

Potential Disadvantages

- Patients for whom elevated prolactin may not be desired (e.g. possibly pregnant patients; pubescent girls with amenorrhoea; postmenopausal women with low oestrogen who do not take oestrogen replacement therapy)

Primary Target Symptoms

- Positive symptoms of psychosis
- Negative symptoms of psychosis
- Cognitive symptoms
- Unstable mood (both depression and mania)
- Aggressive symptoms

Pearls

- Paliperidone may cause less weight gain than some antipsychotics (e.g. clozapine, olanzapine) and more than others
- Some patients may respond better to paliperidone than risperidone
- Some patients respond to or tolerate paliperdone better than the parent drug risperidone
- Paliperidone may cause more motor side effects especially at higher doses and in patients with Lewy body disease
- Hyperprolactinaemia in women with low oestrogen may accelerate osteoporosis
- Paliperidone long-acting injection does not require simultaneous oral medication
- Paliperidone long-acting injection may be well tolerated
- Paliperidone long-acting injection may be combined with a second antipsychotic in complex cases
- Therapeutic drug monitoring may be helpful
- Paliperidone long-acting injection paliperidone is absorbed more slowly after gluteal injection versus deltoid injection

PALIPERDONE LONG-ACTING INJECTIONS

Xeplion Properties

Vehicle	Water
Tmax	13 days
T1/2 with multiple dosing	25–49 days
Time to steady state	About 20 weeks
Able to be loaded	Yes
Dosing schedule (maintenance)	Every month
Injection site	IM (deltoid for 2 first loading doses, then either deltoid or gluteal)
Needle gauge	22 or 23
Dosage forms	Suspension for injection (50 mg, 75 mg, 100 mg, 150 mg)
Injection volume	50 mg in 0.5 mL, 75 mg in 0.75 mL, 100 mg in 1 mL, 150 mg in 1.5 mL; range 0.5–1.5 mL

Trevicta Properties

Vehicle	Water
Tmax	30–33 days
T1/2 with multiple dosing	84–95 days (deltoid), 118–139 days (gluteal)
Time to steady state	
Able to be loaded	N/A
Dosing schedule (maintenance)	Every 3 months
Injection site	IM (gluteal region/ deltoid muscle)
Needle gauge	22
Dosage forms	Prolonged-release suspension for injection pre-filled syringes (175 mg, 263 mg, 350 mg, 525 mg)
Injection volume	175 mg/0.875 mL, 263 mg/1.315 mL, 350 mg/1.75 mL, 525 mg/2.265 mL; range 0.875–2.265 mL

Usual Dosage Range

- 1-month injectable maintenance dose: usually between 75–150 mg
- 3-month injectable maintenance dose: usually between 175–525 mg every 3 months, adjusted according to response

How to Dose

- Not recommended for patients who have not first demonstrated tolerability to oral risperidone
- There is no need to use oral paliperidone instead of oral risperidone before starting long-acting injection
- 1-month injectable maintenance dose: first loading dose of 150 mg on day 1 followed by second loading dose of 100 mg on day 8, followed by a maintenance dose of between 75–150 mg after 1 month and repeated each calendar month (patients who are overweight or obese may require doses in the upper range)
- 3-month injectable maintenance dose: initial dose 175–525 mg every 3 months, adjusted according to response, to be administered into the deltoid or gluteal muscle. Dose is based on previous once-monthly IM paliperidone and should be initiated in place of the next scheduled dose

Paliperidone (Continued)

Dosing Tips

- With long-acting injections, the absorption rate constant is slower than the elimination rate constant, thus resulting in "flip-flop" kinetics – i.e. time to steady state is a function of absorption rate, while concentration at steady state is a function of elimination rate
- The rate-limiting step for plasma drug levels for long-acting injections is not drug metabolism, but rather slow absorption from the injection site
- In general, 5 half-lives of any medication are needed to achieve 97% of steady-state levels
- The long half-life of depot/long-acting injection antipsychotics means that one must either adequately load the dose (if possible) or provide oral supplementation
- The failure to adequately load the dose leads either to prolonged cross-titration from oral antipsychotic or to sub-therapeutic antipsychotic plasma levels for weeks or months in patients who are not receiving (or adhering to) oral supplementation
- Because plasma antipsychotic levels increase gradually over time, dose requirements may ultimately decrease; if possible obtaining periodic plasma levels can be beneficial to prevent unnecessary plasma level creep
- The time to get a blood level for patients receiving long-acting injection is the morning of the day they will receive their next injection
- The therapeutic threshold for paliperidone is 20 ng/mL; initial target range: 28–112 ng/mL (aim for the upper half of the therapeutic range in treatment-resistant cases)
- Kinetics of paliperidone long-acting injection are determined by particle size: smaller particles (1 month) vs larger particles (3 months)
- Advantages: no need for oral coverage; 3-month injection schedule with Trevicta
- Disadvantages: must not be stored above 30°C

THE ART OF SWITCHING

Switching from Oral Antipsychotics to Paliperidone Monthly Injections

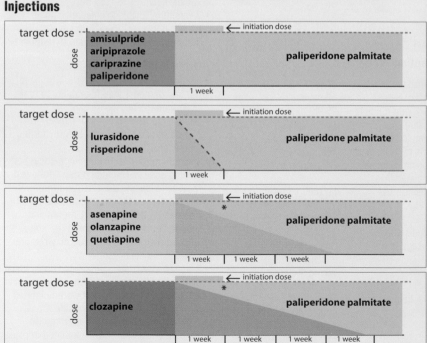

- Discontinuation of oral antipsychotic can begin immediately if adequate loading is pursued
- How to discontinue oral formulations:
  - Down-titration is not required for: amisulpride, aripiprazole, cariprazine, paliperidone
  - 1-week down-titration is required for: lurasidone, risperidone
  - 3–4-week down-titration is required for: asenapine, olanzapine, quetiapine
  - 4+-week down-titration is required for: clozapine
  ∗For patients taking benzodiazepine or anticholinergic medication, this can be continued during cross-titration to help alleviate side effects such as insomnia, agitation, and/or psychosis. Once the patient is stable on long-acting injections, these can be tapered one at a time as appropriate

Switching from Oral Antipsychotics to Oral Paliperidone

- Paliperidone can be initiated at full desired dose; however, titration over 1–2 weeks may be appropriate for some patients
- With aripiprazole and amisulpride, immediate stop is possible; begin paliperidone prolonged-release at an intermediate, or if needed, effective dose
- Risperidone and lurasidone can be tapered off over a period of 1 week due to the risk of withdrawal symptoms such as insomnia
- Clinical experience has shown that quetiapine, olanzapine, and asenapine should be tapered off slowly over a period of 3–4 weeks, to allow patients to readapt to the withdrawal of blocking cholinergic, histaminergic, and alpha 1 receptors
- Clozapine should always be tapered off slowly, over a period of 4 weeks or more
∗Benzodiazepine or anticholinergic medication can be administered during cross-titration to help alleviate side effects such as insomnia, agitation, and/or psychosis

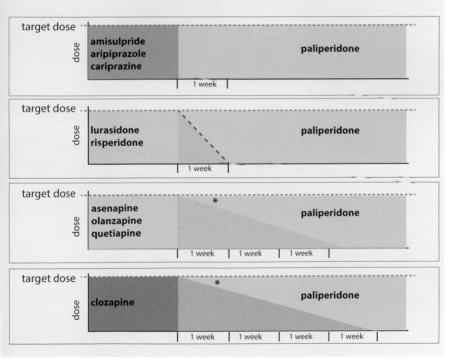

Paliperidone (Continued)

 Suggested Reading

Bernardo M, Bioque M. Three-month paliperidone palmitate – a new treatment option for schizophrenia. Expert Rev Clin Pharmacol 2016;9(7):899–904.

Harrington CA, English C. Tolerability of paliperidone: a meta-analysis of randomized, controlled trials. Int Clin Psychopharmacol 2010;25(6):334–41.

Huhn M, Nikolakopoulou A, Schneider-Thoma J, et al. Comparative efficacy and tolerability of 32 oral antipsychotics for the acute treatment of adults with multi-episode schizophrenia: a systematic review and network meta-analysis. Lancet 2019;394(10202):939–51.

Morris MT, Tarpada SP. Long-acting injectable paliperidone palmitate: a review of efficacy and safety. Psychopharmacol Bull 2017;47(2):42–52.

Nussbaum AM, Stroup TS. Paliperidone for treatment of schizophrenia. Schizophr Bull 2008;34(3):419–22.

Nussbaum AM, Stroup TS. Paliperidone palmitate for schizophrenia. Cochrane Database Syst Rev 2012;(6):CD008296.

Nussbaum AM, Stroup TS. Paliperidone palmitate for schizophrenia. Schizophr Bull 2012;38(6):1124–7.

Patel C, Emond B, Lafeuille MH, et al. Real-world analysis of switching patients with schizophrenia from oral risperidone or oral paliperidone to once-monthly paliperidone palmitate. Drugs Real World Outcomes 2020 Mar;7(1):19–29.

Pillinger T, McCutcheon RA, Vano L, et al. Comparative effects of 18 antipsychotics on metabolic function in patients with schizophrenia, predictors of metabolic dysregulation, and association with psychopathology: a systematic review and network meta-analysis. Lancet Psychiatry 2020;7(1):64–77.

Paroxetine

Brands
• Seroxat

Generic?
Yes

Class
• Neuroscience-based nomenclature: pharmacology domain – serotonin; mode of action – reuptake inhibitor
• SSRI (selective serotonin reuptake inhibitor); often classified as an antidepressant, but it is not just an antidepressant

Commonly Prescribed for
(bold for BNF indication)
• **Major depression**
• **Social anxiety disorder**
• **Post-traumatic stress disorder**
• **Generalised anxiety disorder**
• **Obsessive-compulsive disorder**
• **Panic disorder**
• **Menopausal symptoms, particularly hot flushes, in women with breast cancer (except those taking tamoxifen) – unlicensed use**

How the Drug Works
• Boosts neurotransmitter serotonin
• Blocks serotonin reuptake pump (serotonin transporter)
• Desensitises serotonin receptors, especially serotonin 1A autoreceptors
• Presumably increases serotonergic neurotransmission
• Paroxetine also has mild anticholinergic actions
• Paroxetine may have mild noradrenergic reuptake blocking actions

How Long Until It Works
∗Some patients may experience relief of insomnia or anxiety early after initiation of treatment
• Onset of therapeutic actions with some antidepressants can be seen within 1–2 weeks, but often delayed 2–4 weeks
• If it is not working within 3–4 weeks for depression, it may require a dosage increase or it may not work at all

• By contrast, for generalised anxiety, onset of response and increases in remission rates may still occur after 8 weeks, and for up to 6 months after initiating dosing
• May continue to work for many years to prevent relapse of symptoms

If It Works
• The goal of treatment is complete remission of current symptoms as well as prevention of future relapses
• Treatment most often reduces or even eliminates symptoms, but is not a cure since symptoms can recur after medicine is stopped
• Continue treatment until all symptoms are gone (remission), especially in depression and whenever possible in anxiety disorders
• Once symptoms are gone, continue treating for at least 6–9 months for the first episode of depression or >12 months if relapse indicators present
• If >5 episodes and/or 2 episodes in the last few years then need to continue for at least 2 years or indefinitely
• Use in anxiety disorders may need to be indefinite

If It Doesn't Work
• Important to recognise non-response to treatment early on (3–4 weeks)
• Many patients have only a partial response where some symptoms are improved but others persist (especially insomnia, fatigue, and problems concentrating)
• Other patients may be non-responders, sometimes called treatment-resistant or treatment-refractory
• Some patients who have an initial response may relapse even though they continue treatment
• Consider increasing dose, switching to another agent, or adding an appropriate augmenting agent
• Lithium may be added for suicidal patients or those at high risk of relapse
• Consider psychotherapy
• Consider ECT
• Consider evaluation for another diagnosis or for a co-morbid condition (e.g. medical illness, substance abuse, etc.)
• Some patients may experience a switch into mania and so would require antidepressant discontinuation and initiation of a mood stabiliser

Best Augmenting Combos for Partial Response or Treatment Resistance

- Mood stabilisers or atypical antipsychotics for bipolar depression
- Atypical antipsychotics for psychotic depression
- Atypical antipsychotics as first-line augmenting agents (quetiapine MR 300 mg/day or aripiprazole at 2.5–10 mg/day) for treatment-resistant depression
- Atypical antipsychotics as second-line augmenting agents (risperidone 0.5–2 mg/day or olanzapine 2.5–10 mg/day) for treatment-resistant depression
- Mirtazapine at 30–45 mg/day as another second-line augmenting agent (a dual serotonin and noradrenaline combination, but observe for switch into mania, increase in suicidal ideation or rare risk of non-fatal serotonin syndrome)
- Although T3 (20–50 mcg/day) is another second-line augmenting agent the evidence suggests that it works best with tricyclic antidepressants
- Other augmenting agents but with less evidence include bupropion (up to 400 mg/day), buspirone (up to 60 mg/day) and lamotrigine (up to 400 mg/day)
- Benzodiazepines if agitation present
- Hypnotics or trazodone for insomnia (but there is a rare risk of non-fatal serotonin syndrome with trazodone)
- Augmenting agents reserved for specialist use include: modafinil for sleepiness, fatigue and lack of concentration; stimulants, oestrogens, testosterone
- Lithium is particularly useful for suicidal patients and those at high risk of relapse including with factors such as severe depression, psychomotor retardation, repeated episodes (>3), significant weight loss, or a family history of major depression (aim for lithium plasma levels 0.6–1.0 mmol/L)
- For elderly patients lithium is a very effective augmenting agent
- For severely ill patients other combinations may be tried especially in specialist centres
- Augmenting agents that may be tried include omega-3, SAM-e, L-methylfolate

- Additional non-pharmacological treatments such as exercise, mindfulness, CBT, and IPT can also be helpful
- If present after treatment response (4–8 weeks) or remission (6–12 weeks), the most common residual symptoms of depression include cognitive impairments, reduced energy and problems with sleep

Tests

- None for healthy individuals

SIDE EFFECTS

How Drug Causes Side Effects

- Theoretically due to increases in serotonin concentrations at serotonin receptors in parts of the brain and body other than those that cause therapeutic actions (e.g. unwanted actions of serotonin in sleep centres causing insomnia, unwanted actions of serotonin in the gut causing diarrhoea, etc.)
- Increasing serotonin can cause diminished dopamine release and might contribute to emotional flattening, cognitive slowing, and apathy in some patients
- Most side effects are immediate but often go away with time, in contrast to most therapeutic effects, which are delayed and are enhanced over time
- *Paroxetine's weak antimuscarinic properties can cause constipation, dry mouth, sedation

Notable Side Effects

- CNS: insomnia but also sedation, agitation, tremors, headache, dizziness
- GIT: decreased appetite, nausea, diarrhoea, constipation, dry mouth
- Sexual dysfunction (men: delayed ejaculation, erectile dysfunction; men and women: decreased sexual desire, anorgasmia)
- SIADH (syndrome of inappropriate antidiuretic hormone secretion)
- Mood elevation in diagnosed or undiagnosed bipolar disorder
- Sweating (dose-dependent)
- Bruising and rare bleeding
- Weight gain

Common or very common

- Blurred vision

Uncommon
- Impaired diabetic control

Rare or very rare
- Acute glaucoma, hepatic disorders, peripheral oedema

 Life-Threatening or Dangerous Side Effects
- Rare seizures
- Rare induction of mania
- Rare increase in suicidal ideation and behaviours in adolescents and young adults (up to age 25), hence patients should be warned of this potential adverse event

Weight Gain

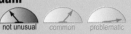

- Occurs in significant minority

Sedation

- Many experience and/or can be significant in amount
- Generally transient

What To Do About Side Effects
- Wait
- Wait
- Wait
- If paroxetine is sedating, take at night to reduce daytime drowsiness
- Reduce dose to 5–10 mg until side effects abate, then increase as tolerated, usually to at least 20 mg
- In a few weeks, switch or add other drugs

Best Augmenting Agents for Side Effects
- Many side effects are dose-dependent (i.e. they increase as dose increases, or they re-emerge until tolerance redevelops)
- Many side effects are time-dependent (i.e. they start immediately upon dosing and upon each dose increase, but go away with time)
- Often best to try another antidepressant monotherapy prior to resorting to augmentation strategies to treat side effects
- Trazodone, mirtazapine or hypnotic for insomnia

- Mirtazapine for agitation and gastrointestinal side effects
- Bupropion for emotional flattening, cognitive slowing, or apathy
- For sexual dysfunction: can augment with bupropion for women, sildenafil for men; or otherwise switch to another antidepressant
- Benzodiazepines for jitteriness and anxiety, especially at initiation of treatment and especially for anxious patients
- Increased activation or agitation may represent the induction of a bipolar state, especially a mixed dysphoric bipolar condition sometimes associated with suicidal ideation, and requires the addition of lithium, a mood stabiliser or an atypical antipsychotic, and/or discontinuation of the SSRI

DOSING AND USE

Usual Dosage Range
- Major depression: adult (20–50 mg/day); elderly (20–40 mg/day)
- Social anxiety disorder: adult (20–50 mg/day); elderly (20–40 mg/day)
- Post-traumatic stress disorder: adult (20–50 mg/day); elderly (20–40 mg/day)
- Generalised anxiety disorder: adult (20–50 mg/day); elderly (20–40 mg/day)
- Obsessive-compulsive disorder: adult (20–60 mg/day); elderly (20–40 mg/day)
- Panic disorder: adult (10–60 mg/day); elderly (10–40 mg/day)
- Menopausal symptoms, particularly hot flushes, in women with breast cancer (except those taking tamoxifen): adult (10 mg/day)

Dosage Forms
- Tablet 10 mg, 20 mg, 30 mg, 40 mg
- Oral suspension 20 mg/10 mL (150 mL bottle)

How to Dose
- Major depression
- Social anxiety disorder
- Post-traumatic stress disorder
- Generalised anxiety disorder
  - Adult: 20 mg in the morning, no evidence of greater efficacy at higher doses; max 50 mg/day

- Elderly: 20 mg in the morning, no evidence of greater efficacy at higher doses; max 40 mg/day
- Obsessive-compulsive disorder
  - Adult: initial dose 20 mg in the morning, increased gradually by 10 mg increments up to to 40 mg/day, no evidence of greater efficacy at higher doses; max 60 mg/day
  - Elderly: initial dose 20 mg in the morning, increased gradually by 10 mg increments up to max 40 mg/day
- Panic disorder
  - Adult: initial dose 10 mg in the morning, increased gradually by 10 mg increments to 40 mg/day, no evidence of greater efficacy at higher doses; max 60 mg/day
  - Elderly: initial dose 10 mg in the morning, increased gradually by 10 mg increments; max 40 mg/day
- Menopausal symptoms, particularly hot flushes, in women with breast cancer (except those taking tamoxifen)
  - Adult: 10 mg/day

Dosing Tips

- Given once daily, often at bedtime, but any time of day tolerated
- 20 mg/day is often sufficient for patients with social anxiety disorder and depression
- Other anxiety disorders, as well as difficult cases in general, may require higher dosing
- Occasional patients are dosed above 60 mg/ day, but this is for experts and requires caution
- If intolerable anxiety, insomnia, agitation, akathisia, or activation occur either upon dosing initiation or discontinuation, consider the possibility of activated bipolar disorder and switch to a mood stabiliser or an atypical antipsychotic
- Liquid formulation easiest for doses below 10 mg when used for cases that are very intolerant to paroxetine or especially for very slow down-titration during discontinuation for patients with withdrawal symptoms
- Unlike other SSRIs and antidepressants where dosage increments can be double and triple the starting dose, paroxetine's dosing increments are by 10 mg increments (i.e. 20, 30, 40)
- Paroxetine inhibits its own metabolism and thus plasma concentrations can double

when oral doses increase by 50%; plasma concentrations can increase 2–7-fold when oral doses are doubled
* For patients with severe problems discontinuing paroxetine, dosing may need to be tapered over many months (i.e. reduce dose by 1% every 3 days by crushing tablet and suspending or dissolving in 100 mL of fruit juice and then disposing of 1 mL while drinking the rest; 3–7 days later, dispose of 2 mL, and so on). This is both a form of very slow biological tapering and a form of behavioural desensitisation
- For some patients with severe problems discontinuing paroxetine, it may be useful to add an SSRI with a long half-life, especially fluoxetine, prior to taper of paroxetine; while maintaining fluoxetine dosing, first slowly taper paroxetine and then taper fluoxetine
- Be sure to differentiate between re-emergence of symptoms requiring reinstitution of treatment and withdrawal symptoms

Overdose

- Rarely lethal in monotherapy overdose: vomiting, sedation, heart rhythm disturbances, dilated pupils, dry mouth
- Management of SSRI poisoning is supportive; activated charcoal given within 1 hour of the overdose reduces absorption of the drug
- Convulsions can be treated with lorazepam, diazepam, or buccal midazolam

Long-Term Use
- Safe

Habit Forming
- No

How to Stop

- If taking SSRIs for more than 6–8 weeks, it is not recommended to stop them suddenly due to the risk of withdrawal effects (dizziness, nausea, stomach cramps, sweating, tingling, dysaesthesias)
- Taper dose gradually over 4 weeks, or longer if withdrawal symptoms emerge
- Inform all patients of the risk of withdrawal symptoms
- If withdrawal symptoms emerge during discontinuation, raise dose to stop

symptoms and then restart withdrawal much more slowly

∗Withdrawal effects can be more common or more severe with paroxetine than with some other SSRIs

• Paroxetine's withdrawal effects may be related in part to the fact that it inhibits its own metabolism

• Thus, when paroxetine is withdrawn, the rate of its decline can be faster as it stops inhibiting its metabolism

• Re-adaptation of cholinergic receptors after prolonged blockade may contribute to withdrawal effects of paroxetine

Pharmacokinetics

• Inactive metabolites
• Half-life about 24 hours
• Inhibits CYP450 2D6

 Drug Interactions

• Tramadol increases the risk of seizures in patients taking an antidepressant

• Can increase TCA levels; use with caution with TCAs or when switching from a TCA to paroxetine

• Can cause a fatal "serotonin syndrome" when combined with MAOIs, so do not use with MAOIs or for at least 14 days after MAOIs are stopped

• Do not start an MAOI for at least 5 half-lives (5 to 7 days for most drugs) after discontinuing paroxetine

• Can rarely cause weakness, hyperreflexia, and incoordination when combined with sumatriptan or possibly with other triptans, requiring careful monitoring of patient

• Increased risk of bleeding when used in combination with NSAIDs, aspirin, alteplase, anti-platelets, and anticoagulants

• NSAIDs may impair effectiveness of SSRIs

• Increased risk of hyponatraemia when paroxetine is used in combination with other agents that cause hyponatraemia, e.g. thiazides

• May increase anticholinergic effects of procyclidine and other drugs with anticholinergic properties

• Via CYP450 2D6 inhibition, paroxetine could theoretically interfere with the therapeutic actions of codeine and tamoxifen, and increase the plasma levels of some beta blockers and of atomoxetine

• Via CYP450 3A4 inhibition, paroxetine could theoretically increase the concentrations of pimozide, and cause QTc prolongation and dangerous cardiac arrhythmias

 Other Warnings/Precautions

• Add or initiate other antidepressants with caution for up to 2 weeks after discontinuing paroxetine

• Use with caution in patients with diabetes

• Use with caution in patients with susceptibility to angle-closure glaucoma

• Use with caution in patients receiving ECT or with a history of seizures

• Use with caution in patients with a history of bleeding disorders

• Use with caution in patients with bipolar disorder unless treated with concomitant mood-stabiliser

• When treating children, carefully weigh the risks and benefits of pharmacological treatment against the risks and benefits of nontreatment with antidepressants and make sure to document this in the patient's chart

• Warn patients and their caregivers about the possibility of activating side effects and advise them to report such symptoms immediately

• Monitor patients for activation of suicidal ideation, especially children and adolescents

• Achlorhydria and high gastric pH can reduce the absorption of the oral suspension formulation of paroxetine

Do Not Use

• If patient has poorly controlled epilepsy
• If patient enters a manic phase
• If patient is already taking an MAOI (risk of serotonin syndrome)
• If patient is taking pimozide or tamoxifen
• If there is a proven allergy to paroxetine

Paroxetine (Continued)

Renal Impairment
- Reduce dose if eGFR less than 30 mL/minute/1.73 m^2

Hepatic Impairment
- Caution due to prolonged half-life; use doses at lower end of the range

Cardiac Impairment
- Preliminary research suggests paroxetine is safe
- Treating depression with SSRIs in patients with acute angina or following an MI may reduce cardiac events and improve survival as well as mood

Elderly
- Lower dose (initial dose 10 mg/day, max 40 mg/day)
- Risk of SIADH with SSRIs is higher in the elderly
- Reduction in the risk of suicidality with antidepressants compared to placebo in adults age 65 and older

Children and Adolescents
- Not licensed for use in those under the age of 18
- Not specifically approved, but preliminary evidence suggests efficacy in children and adolescents with OCD, social phobia, or depression
- Carefully weigh the risks and benefits of pharmacological treatment against the risks and benefits of nontreatment with antidepressants and make sure to document this in the patient's chart
- Monitor patients face-to-face regularly, particularly during the first several weeks of treatment
- Use with caution, observing for activation of known or unknown bipolar disorder and/or suicidal ideation, and inform parents or guardians of this risk so they can help observe child or adolescent patients

Pregnancy
- Not generally recommended for use during pregnancy, especially during first trimester
- Nonetheless, continuous treatment during pregnancy may be necessary and has not been proven to be harmful to the foetus
- Must weigh the risk of treatment (first trimester foetal development, third trimester newborn delivery) to the child against the risk of no treatment (recurrence of depression, maternal health, infant bonding) to the mother and child
- For many patients, this may mean continuing treatment during pregnancy
- Exposure to SSRIs in pregnancy has been associated with cardiac malformations, however recent studies have suggested that these findings may be due to other patient factors
- Exposure to SSRIs in pregnancy has been associated with an increased risk of spontaneous abortion, low birth weight and preterm delivery. Data is conflicting and the effects of depression cannot be ruled out from some studies
- SSRI use beyond the 20th week of pregnancy may be associated with increased risk of persistent pulmonary hypertension (PPHN) in newborns. Whilst the risk of PPHN remains low it presents potentially serious complications
- SSRI/SNRI antidepressant use in the month before delivery may result in a small increased risk of postpartum haemorrhage
- Neonates exposed to SSRIs or SNRIs late in the third trimester have developed complications requiring prolonged hospitalisation, respiratory support, and tube feeding; reported symptoms are consistent with either a direct toxic effect of SSRIs and SNRIs or, possibly, a drug discontinuation syndrome, and include respiratory distress, cyanosis, apnoea, seizures, temperature instability, feeding difficulty, vomiting, hypoglycaemia, hypotonia, hypertonia, hyperreflexia, tremor, jitteriness, irritability, and constant crying

Breastfeeding
- Small amounts found in mother's breast milk
- Trace amounts may be present in nursing children whose mothers are taking paroxetine
- If child becomes irritable or sedated, breastfeeding or drug may need to be discontinued
- Immediate postpartum period is a high-risk time for depression, especially in women

who have had prior depressive episodes, so drug may need to be reinstituted late in the third trimester or shortly after childbirth to prevent a recurrence during the postpartum period

- Must weigh benefits of breastfeeding with risks and benefits of antidepressant treatment versus nontreatment to both the infant and the mother
- For many patients, this may mean continuing treatment during breastfeeding
- Sertraline or paroxetine are the preferred SSRIs for breastfeeding mothers

THE ART OF PSYCHOPHARMACOLOGY

Potential Advantages
- Patients with anxiety disorders and insomnia
- Patients with mixed anxiety/depression

Potential Disadvantages
- Patients with hypersomnia
- Alzheimer's disease/cognitive disorders
- Patients with psychomotor retardation, fatigue, and low energy

Primary Target Symptoms
- Depressed mood
- Anxiety
- Sleep disturbance, especially insomnia
- Panic attacks, avoidant behaviour, re-experiencing, hyperarousal

Pearls
- Often a preferred treatment of anxious depression as well as major depressive disorder co-morbid with anxiety disorders

* Withdrawal effects may be more likely than for some other SSRIs when discontinued (especially akathisia, restlessness, gastrointestinal symptoms, dizziness, tingling, dysaesthesias, nausea, stomach cramps, restlessness)
- Inhibits own metabolism, so dosing is not linear
* Paroxetine has mild anticholinergic actions that can enhance the rapid onset of anxiolytic and hypnotic effects, but also cause mild anticholinergic side effects
- Can cause cognitive and affective "flattening"
- May be less activating than other SSRIs
- Paroxetine is a potent CYP450 2D6 inhibitor
- SSRIs may be less effective in women over 50, especially if they are not taking oestrogen
- SSRIs may be useful for hot flushes in perimenopausal women
- Some anecdotal reports suggest greater weight gain and sexual dysfunction than some other SSRIs, but the clinical significance of this is unknown
- For sexual dysfunction, can augment with bupropion or sildenafil or switch to a non-SSRI such as mirtazapine
- Some postmenopausal depression will respond better to paroxetine plus oestrogen augmentation than to paroxetine alone
- Non-response to paroxetine in elderly may require consideration of mild cognitive impairment or Alzheimer's disease
- Can be better tolerated than some SSRIs for patients with anxiety and insomnia and can reduce these symptoms early in dosing

Suggested Reading

Bourin M, Chue P, Guillon Y. Paroxetine: a review. CNS Drug Rev 2001;7(1):25–47.

Cipriani A, Furukawa TA, Salanti G, et al. Comparative efficacy and acceptability of 21 antidepressant drugs for the acute treatment of adults with major depressive disorder: a systematic review and network meta-analysis. Lancet 2018;391(10128):1357–66.

Gibiino S, Serretti A. Paroxetine for the treatment of depression: a critical update. Expert Opin Pharmacother 2012;13(3):421–31.

Green B. Focus on paroxetine. Curr Med Res Opin 2003;19(1):13–21.

Wagstaff AJ, Cheer SM, Matheson AJ, et al. Paroxetine: an update of its use in psychiatric disorders in adults. Drugs 2002;62(4):655–703. Erratum in Drugs 2002;62(10):1461.

Phenelzine

THERAPEUTICS

Brands
• Nardil

Generic?
No, not in UK

Class
• Neuroscience-based nomenclature: pharmacology domain – serotonin, norepinephrine, dopamine; mode of action – enzyme inhibitor
• Monoamine oxidase inhibitor (MAOI)

Commonly Prescribed for
(bold for BNF indication)
• **Depressive illness**
• Depressed patients with atypical, hypochondriacal, "non-endogenous" or hysterical features
• Treatment-refractory depression
• Treatment-resistant phobic or panic disorder
• Treatment-resistant social anxiety disorder

How the Drug Works
• Irreversibly blocks monoamine oxidase (MAO) from breaking down noradrenaline, serotonin, and dopamine
• This presumably boosts noradrenergic, serotonergic, and dopaminergic neurotransmission

How Long Until It Works
• Onset of therapeutic actions usually not immediate, but often delayed 2–4 weeks
• If it is not working within 3–4 weeks, it may require a dosage increase or it may not work at all
• May continue to work for many years to prevent relapse of symptoms

If It Works
• The goal of treatment is complete remission of current symptoms as well as prevention of future relapses
• Treatment most often reduces or even eliminates symptoms, but is not a cure since symptoms can recur after medicine stopped
• Continue treatment until all symptoms are gone (remission)
• Once symptoms are gone, continue treating for at least 6–9 months for the first episode of depression or >12 months if relapse indicators present
• If >5 episodes and/or 2 episodes in the last few years then need to continue for at least 2 years or indefinitely
• Use in anxiety disorders may also need to be indefinite

If It Doesn't Work
• Important to recognise non-response to treatment early on (3–4 weeks)
• Many patients have only a partial response where some symptoms are improved but others persist (especially insomnia, fatigue, and problems concentrating)
• Other patients may be non-responders, sometimes called treatment-resistant or treatment-refractory
• Some patients who have an initial response may relapse even though they continue treatment
• Consider increasing dose, switching to another agent, or adding an appropriate augmenting agent
• Lithium may be added for suicidal patients or those at high risk of relapse
• Consider psychotherapy
• Consider ECT
• Consider evaluation for another diagnosis or for a co-morbid condition (e.g. medical illness, substance abuse, etc.)
• Some patients may experience a switch into mania and so would require antidepressant discontinuation and initiation of a mood stabiliser

Best Augmenting Combos for Partial Response or Treatment Resistance
* Augmentation of MAOIs has not been systematically studied, and this is something for the expert, to be done with caution and with careful monitoring
• Lithium is particularly useful for suicidal patients and those at high risk of relapse including with factors such as severe depression, psychomotor retardation, repeated episodes (>3), significant weight loss, or a family history of major depression (aim for lithium plasma levels 0.6–1.0 mmol/L)
• Atypical antipsychotics (with special caution for those agents with monoamine reuptake blocking properties)

- Mood-stabilising anticonvulsants
*A stimulant such as dexamfetamine or methylphenidate (with caution; may activate bipolar disorder and suicidal ideation; may elevate blood pressure)

Tests

- Patients should be monitored for changes in blood pressure
- Patients receiving high doses or long-term treatment should have hepatic function evaluated periodically
*Since MAOIs are frequently associated with weight gain, before starting treatment, weigh all patients and determine if the patient is already overweight (BMI 25.0–29.9) or obese (BMI ≥30)
- Before giving a drug that can cause weight gain to an overweight or obese patient, consider determining whether the patient already has pre-diabetes (fasting plasma glucose 5.5–6.9 mmol/L), diabetes (fasting plasma glucose >7 mmol/L), or dyslipidaemia (increased total cholesterol, LDL cholesterol, and triglycerides; decreased HDL cholesterol), and treat or refer such patients for treatment, including nutrition and weight management, physical activity counselling, smoking cessation, and medical management
*Monitor weight and BMI during treatment
*While giving a drug to a patient who has gained >5% of initial weight, consider evaluating for the presence of pre-diabetes, diabetes, or dyslipidaemia, or consider switching to a different antidepressant

SIDE EFFECTS

How Drug Causes Side Effects

- Theoretically due to increases in monoamines in parts of the brain and body and at receptors other than those that cause therapeutic actions (e.g. unwanted actions of serotonin in sleep centres causing insomnia, unwanted actions of norepinephrine on vascular smooth muscle causing changes in blood pressure, etc.)
- Side effects are generally immediate, but immediate side effects often disappear with time

Notable Side Effects

- Dizziness, agitation, sedation, headache, sleep disturbances, fatigue, weakness,

tremor, movement problems, blurred vision, increased sweating
- Orthostatic hypotension (dose-related); syncope may develop at high doses
- Constipation, dry mouth, nausea, change in appetite, weight gain
- Sexual dysfunction

Frequency not known

- CNS/PNS: altered mood, coma, delirium, feeling jittery, impaired driving ability, intracranial haemorrhage, movement disorders, nystagmus, repetitive speech, schizophrenia, seizure
- CVS: cardiovascular insufficiency, hypertensive crisis
- GIT: fatal progressive hepatocellular necrosis, gastrointestinal disorder
- Other: electrolyte imbalance, fever, glaucoma, hypermetabolism, increased muscle tone, lupus-like syndrome, malaise, muscle twitching, neuroleptic malignant syndrome, oedema, respiratory disorders, sexual dysfunction

Life-Threatening or Dangerous Side Effects

- Hypertensive crisis (especially when MAOIs are used with certain tyramine-containing foods or prohibited drugs)
- Induction of mania
- Rare increase in suicidal ideation and behaviours in adolescents and young adults (up to age 25), hence patients should be warned of this potential adverse event
- Seizures
- Hepatotoxicity
- Phenelzine is probably the safest of the MAOIs

Weight Gain

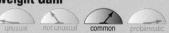

- Some experience and/or can be significant in amount

Sedation

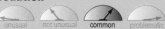

- Many experience and/or can be significant in amount
- Can also cause activation

What to Do About Side Effects

- Wait
- Wait
- Wait
- Lower the dose
- Take at night if daytime sedation
- Switch after appropriate washout to an SSRI or newer antidepressant

Best Augmenting Agents for Side Effects

- Trazodone (with caution) for insomnia
- Benzodiazepines for insomnia
- Many side effects cannot be improved with an augmenting agent

DOSING AND USE

Usual Dosage Range

- 45–60 mg/day (up to 90 mg/day in hospitalised patients)

Dosage Forms

- Tablet 15 mg

How to Dose

- Initial dose 45 mg/day in 3 divided doses; increase to 60–90 mg/day; after desired therapeutic effect is achieved lower the dose as far as possible (15 mg on alternate days may be adequate)

 Dosing Tips

- Once dosing is stabilised, some patients may tolerate once- or twice-daily dosing rather than 3-times-a-day dosing
- Orthostatic hypotension, especially at high doses, may require splitting into 4 daily doses
- Patients receiving high doses may need to be evaluated periodically for effects on the liver
- Little evidence to support efficacy of phenelzine below doses of 45 mg/day in treating acute depression

Overdose

- Can be fatal; dizziness, ataxia, sedation, headache, insomnia, restlessness, anxiety, irritability, cardiovascular effects, confusion, respiratory depression, coma

Long-Term Use

- May require periodic evaluation of hepatic function
- MAOIs may lose efficacy long-term

Habit Forming

- Some patients have developed dependence on MAOIs

How to Stop

- Generally no need to taper, as the drug wears off slowly over 2–3 weeks as new MAO is produced; however there can be withdrawal effects and risk of relapse

Pharmacokinetics

- Clinical duration of action may be up to 14 days due to irreversible enzyme inhibition
- Half-life about 1.2 hours

 Drug Interactions

- Fentanyl, pethidine and tramadol may increase the risk of seizures in patients taking an MAOI
- Can cause a fatal "serotonin syndrome" when combined with drugs that block serotonin reuptake, so do not use with a serotonin reuptake inhibitor or for 5 half-lives of the SSRI after stopping the serotonin reuptake inhibitor (see Table 1 after Pearls)
- Hypertensive crisis with headache, intracranial bleeding, and death may result from combining MAOIs with sympathomimetic drugs (e.g. amfetamines, methylphenidate, cocaine, dopamine, epinephrine, norepinephrine, and related compounds methyldopa, levodopa, L-tryptophan, L-tyrosine, and phenylalanine)
- Do not combine with another MAOI, alcohol, or guanethidine
- Adverse drug reactions can result from combining MAOIs with tricyclic/tetracyclic antidepressants and related compounds, including carbamazepine and mirtazapine, and should be avoided except by experts to treat difficult cases
- MAOIs in combination with spinal anaesthesia may cause combined hypotensive effects
- Combination of MAOIs and CNS depressants may enhance sedation and hypotension

Other Warnings/Precautions

- Use requires low-tyramine diet (see Table 2 after Pearls)
- Patient and prescriber must be vigilant to potential interactions with any drug, including antihypertensives and over-the-counter cough/cold preparations
- Over-the-counter medications to avoid include cough and cold preparations, including those containing dextromethorphan, nasal decongestants (tablets, drops, or spray), hay-fever medications, sinus medications, asthma inhalant medications, anti-appetite medications, weight-reducing preparations, "pep" pills (see Table 3 after Pearls)
- Hypoglycaemia may occur in diabetic patients receiving insulin or oral antidiabetic agents
- Use cautiously in patients receiving reserpine, anaesthetics, disulfiram, anticholinergic agents
- Phenelzine is not recommended for use in patients who cannot be monitored closely
- Use with caution in acute porphyrias, blood disorders, cardiovascular disease, diabetes, epilepsy
- Use with caution in patients undergoing ECT
- Use with great caution in the elderly
- Use with caution in patients undergoing surgery
- When treating children, carefully weigh the risks and benefits of pharmacological treatment against the risks and benefits of nontreatment with antidepressants and make sure to document this in the patient's chart
- Distribute leaflet provided by the drug companies concerning dietary restrictions
- Warn patients and their caregivers about the possibility of activating side effects and advise them to report such symptoms immediately
- Monitor patients for activation of suicidal ideation, especially those up to the age of 25

Do Not Use

- In agitated patients or in the manic phase
- If patient is taking pethidine
- If patient is taking a sympathomimetic agent or taking guanethidine
- If patient is taking another MAOI
- If patient is taking any agent that can inhibit serotonin reuptake (e.g. SSRIs, sibutramine, tramadol, duloxetine, venlafaxine, clomipramine, etc.)
- If patient is taking diuretics
- If patient has pheochromocytoma
- If patient has severe cardiovascular disease or cerebrovascular disease
- If patient has frequent or severe headaches
- If patient is undergoing elective surgery and requires general anaesthesia
- If patient has a history of liver disease or abnormal liver function tests
- If patient is taking a prohibited drug
- If patient is not compliant with a low-tyramine diet
- If there is a proven allergy to phenelzine

SPECIAL POPULATIONS

Renal Impairment

- Use with caution – drug may accumulate in plasma
- May require lower than usual adult dose

Hepatic Impairment

- Phenelzine should not be used

Cardiac Impairment

- Contraindicated in patients with congestive heart failure or hypertension
- Any other cardiac impairment may require lower than usual adult dose
- Patients with angina pectoris or coronary artery disease should limit their exertion

Elderly

- Only use with great caution (increased risk of postural hypotension)
- Initial dose 7.5 mg/day; increase every few days by 7.5–15 mg/day
- Elderly patients may have greater sensitivity to adverse effects
- Reduction in the risk of suicidality with antidepressants compared to placebo in adults age 65 and older

Children and Adolescents

- Not recommended for use for those under the age of 18

Pregnancy

- Controlled studies have not been conducted in pregnant women
- Not generally recommended for use during pregnancy, especially during first and third trimesters
- Possible increased incidence of foetal malformations if phenelzine is taken during the first trimester
- Should evaluate patient for treatment with an antidepressant with a better risk/benefit ratio

Breastfeeding

- Some drug is found in mother's breast milk
- Effects on infant unknown
- Immediate postpartum period is a high-risk time for depression, especially in women who have had prior depressive episodes, so drug may need to be reinstituted shortly after childbirth to prevent a recurrence during the postpartum period
- Should evaluate patient for treatment with an antidepressant with a better risk/benefit ratio

THE ART OF PSYCHOPHARMACOLOGY

Potential Advantages

- Atypical depression
- Severe depression
- Treatment-resistant depression or anxiety disorders

Potential Disadvantages

- Requires compliance to dietary restrictions, concomitant drug restrictions
- Patients with cardiac problems or hypertension
- Multiple daily doses

Primary Target Symptoms

- Depressed mood
- Somatic symptoms
- Anxiety
- Sleep and eating disturbances
- Psychomotor retardation
- Morbid preoccupation

Pearls

- MAOIs are generally reserved for use after SSRIs, SNRIs, TCAs or combinations of newer antidepressants have failed
- Patient should be advised not to take any prescription or over-the-counter drugs without consulting their doctor because of possible drug interactions with the MAOI
- Headache is often the first symptom of hypertensive crisis
- The rigid dietary restrictions may reduce compliance (see Table 2 after Pearls)
- Response can be delayed and usually only when side effects are apparent
- Can be a dramatic response when other treatments have failed
- Patients who have remained well for long periods can relapse on withdrawal and may need to accept long-term treatment
- It is vital that patients inform other doctors because of interactions including prior to surgery
- Mood disorders can be associated with eating disorders (especially in adolescent females), and phenelzine can be used to treat both depression and bulimia
- MAOIs are viable treatment options in depression when other classes of antidepressants have not worked, but they are not frequently used

*Myths about the danger of dietary tyramine can be exaggerated, but prohibitions against concomitant drugs often not followed closely enough

• Orthostatic hypotension, insomnia, and sexual dysfunction are often the most troublesome common side effects

*MAOIs should be for the expert, especially if combining with agents of potential risk (e.g. stimulants, trazodone, TCAs)

*MAOIs should not be neglected as therapeutic agents for the treatment-resistant

• Although generally prohibited, a heroic but potentially dangerous treatment for severely treatment-resistant patients is for an expert to give a tricyclic/tetracyclic antidepressant other than clomipramine simultaneously with an MAOI for patients who fail to respond to numerous other antidepressants

• Use of MAOIs with clomipramine is always prohibited because of the risk of serotonin syndrome and death

• Start the MAOI with the tricyclic/tetracyclic antidepressant simultaneously at low doses after appropriate drug washout, then alternately increase doses of these agents every few days to a week as tolerated

• Although very strict dietary and concomitant drug restrictions must be observed to prevent hypertensive crises and serotonin syndrome, the most common side effects of MAOI and tricyclic/ tetracyclic combinations may be weight gain and orthostatic hypotension

Table 1. Drugs contraindicated due to risk of serotonin syndrome/toxicity

Do Not Use			
Antidepressants	Drugs of Abuse	Opioids	Other
SSRIs	MDMA (ecstasy)	Pethidine	Non-subcutaneous sumatriptan
SNRIs	Cocaine	Tramadol	Chlorphenamine
Clomipramine	Metamfetamine	Methadone	Procarbazine?
St. John's wort	High-dose or injected amfetamine	Fentanyl	Morphinan-containing compounds

Table 2. Dietary guidelines for patients taking MAOIs

Foods to avoid*	Foods allowed
Dried, aged, smoked, fermented, spoiled, or improperly stored meat, poultry, and fish	Fresh or processed meat, poultry, and fish; properly stored pickled or smoked fish
Broad bean pods	All other vegetables
Aged cheeses	Processed cheese slices, cottage cheese, ricotta cheese, yoghurt, cream cheese
Tap and unpasteurised beer	Canned or bottled beer and alcohol
Marmite	Brewer's and baker's yeast
Sauerkraut, kimchee	
Soy products/tofu esp soy sauce	Peanuts
Banana peel	Bananas, avocados, raspberries
Tyramine-containing nutritional supplement	

*Not necessary for 6-mg transdermal or low-dose oral selegiline

Table 3. Drugs that boost norepinephrine: should only be used with caution with MAOIs

Use With Caution:			
Decongestants	**Stimulants**	**Antidepressants with norepinephrine reuptake inhibition**	**Other**
Phenylephrine	Amfetamines	Most tricyclics	Local anaesthetics containing vasoconstrictors
Pseudoephedrine	Methylphenidate	NRIs	Tapentadol
	Cocaine	NDRIs	
	Metamfetamine		
	Modafinil		

Suggested Reading

Amsterdam JD, Kim TT. Relative effectiveness of monoamine oxidase inhibitor and tricyclic antidepressant combination therapy for treatment-resistant depression. J Clin Psychopharmacol 2019;39(6):649–52.

Gillman PK. A reassessment of the safety profile of monoamine oxidase inhibitors: elucidating tired old tyramine myths. J Neural Transm (Vienna) 2018;125(11):1707–17.

Kennedy SH. Continuation and maintenance treatments in major depression: the neglected role of monoamine oxidase inhibitors. J Psychiatry Neurosci 1997;22(2):127–31.

Kim T, Xu C, Amsterdam JD. Relative effectiveness of tricyclic antidepressant versus monoamine oxidase inhibitor monotherapy for treatment-resistant depression. J Affect Disord 2019;250:199–203.

Lippman SB, Nash K. Monoamine oxidase inhibitor update. Potential adverse food and drug interactions. Drug Saf 1990;5(3):195–204.

Parsons B, Quitkin FM, McGrath PJ, et al. Phenelzine, imipramine, and placebo in borderline patients meeting criteria for atypical depression. Psychopharmacol Bull 1989;25(4):524–34.

Pimozide

Brands
• Orap

Generic?
No, not in UK

Class
• Neuroscience-based nomenclature: pharmacology domain – dopamine; mode of action – antagonist
• Tourette syndrome/tic suppressant; conventional antipsychotic (neuroleptic, dopamine 2 antagonist); dopamine receptor antagonist (D-RAn)

Commonly Prescribed for
(bold for BNF indication)
• **Schizophrenia**
• **Monosymptomatic hypochondriacal psychosis**
• **Paranoid psychosis**
• **Tourette syndrome in children (unlicensed use – under expert supervision)**

 ## How the Drug Works
• Blocks dopamine 2 receptors in the nigrostriatal dopamine pathway, reducing tics in Tourette syndrome
• When used for psychosis, can block dopamine 2 receptors in the mesolimbic dopamine pathway, reducing positive symptoms of psychosis

How Long Until It Works
• Relief from tics may occur more rapidly than antipsychotic actions
• Psychotic symptoms can improve within 1 week, but it may take several weeks for full effect on behaviour

If It Works
*Is not a first-line treatment option for Tourette syndrome
*Is not a first-line treatment option for schizophrenia or paranoid psychosis
*Has been shown historically to be effective in the treatment of monosymptomatic hypochondriacal psychosis

If It Doesn't Work
• Consider trying one of the first-line atypical antipsychotics (risperidone, olanzapine, quetiapine, aripiprazole, amisulpride)
• Consider trying another conventional antipsychotic
• If 2 or more antipsychotic monotherapies do not work, consider clozapine

 ## Best Augmenting Combos for Partial Response or Treatment Resistance
*Augmentation of pimozide has not been systematically studied and can be dangerous, especially with drugs that can either prolong QTc interval or raise pimozide plasma levels
• Addition of a mood-stabilising anticonvulsant such as valproate or lamotrigine may be considered in schizophrenia and psychosis
• Addition of a benzodiazepine, especially short term for agitation

Tests

Baseline for typical antipsycotic
*Measure weight, BMI, and waist circumference
• Get baseline personal and family history of diabetes, obesity, dyslipidaemia, hypertension, and cardiovascular disease
• Check for personal history of drug-induced leucopenia/neutropenia
*Check pulse and blood pressure, fasting plasma glucose or glycosylated haemoglobin (HbA1c), fasting lipid profile, and prolactin levels
• Full blood count (FBC)
• Assessment of nutritional status, diet, and level of physical activity
• Determine if the patient:
  • is overweight (BMI 25.0–29.9)
  • is obese (BMI ≥30)
  • has pre-diabetes – fasting plasma glucose: 5.5 mmol/L to 6.9 mmol/L or HbA1c: 42 to 47 mmol/mol (6.0 to 6.4%)
  • has diabetes – fasting plasma glucose: >7.0 mmol/L or HbA1c: ≥48 mmol/L (≥6.5%)
  • has hypertension (BP >140/90 mm Hg)

Pimozide (Continued)

- has dyslipidaemia (increased total cholesterol, LDL cholesterol, and triglycerides; decreased HDL cholesterol)
- Treat or refer such patients for treatment, including nutrition and weight management, physical activity counselling, smoking cessation, and medical management
- Baseline ECG for: inpatients; those with a personal history or risk factor for cardiac disease

Children and adolescents:
- As for adults
- Also check history of congenital heart problems, history of dizziness when stressed or on exertion, history of long-QT syndrome, family history of long-QT syndrome, bradycardia, myocarditis, family history of cardiac myopathies, low K+/low Mg++/low Ca++
- Measure weight, BMI, and waist circumference plotted on a growth chart
- Pulse, BP plotted on a percentile chart
- ECG: note for QTc interval – machine-generated may be incorrect in children as different formula needed if HR <60 or >100
- Baseline prolactin levels

Monitoring for typical antipsychotic

- Monitor weight and BMI during treatment
- Consider monitoring fasting triglycerides monthly for several months in patients at high risk for metabolic complications and when initiating or switching antipsychotics
- While giving a drug to a patient who has gained >5% of initial weight, consider evaluating for the presence of pre-diabetes, diabetes, or dyslipidaemia, or consider switching to a different antipsychotic
- Patients with low white blood cell count (WBC) or history of drug-induced leucopenia/neutropenia should have full blood count (FBC) monitored frequently during the first few months and pimozide should be discontinued at the first sign of decline of WBC in the absence of other causative factors
- Monitor prolactin levels and for signs and symptoms of hyperprolactinaemia

Children and adolescents:
- As for adults
- Weight/BMI/waist circumference, weekly for the first 6 weeks, then at 12 weeks, and then every 6 months, plotted on a growth/percentile chart
- Height every 6 months, plotted on a growth chart

- Pulse and blood pressure at 12 weeks, then every 6 months plotted on a percentile chart
- ECG prior to starting and after 2 weeks after dose increase for monitoring of QTc interval. Machine-generated may be incorrect in children as different formula needed if HR <60 or >100
- Prolactin levels: prior to starting and after 12 weeks, 24 weeks, and 6-monthly thereafter. Consider additional monitoring in young adults (under 25) who have not yet reached peak bone mass. In comparison quetiapine is only associated with marginal increase of prolactin
- In prepubertal children monitor sexual maturation
- In post-pubertal children and YP monitor sexual side effects (both sexes: loss of libido, sexual dysfunction, galactorrhoea, infertility; male: diminished ejaculate, gynaecomastia; female: oligorrhoea/amenorrhoea, reduced vaginal lubrication, dyspareunia, acne, hirsutism)

Additional tests for pimozide

- Baseline ECG and serum potassium levels for all patients
- *Periodic evaluation of ECG and serum potassium levels, especially during dose titration. If repolarisation changes (prolongation of QTc interval, T-wave changes or U-wave development) appear or arrhythmias develop, the need for treatment with pimozide should be reviewed and the dose reduced or the drug discontinued
- Serum Mg levels may also need to be monitored
- Check blood pressure in the elderly before starting and for the first few weeks of treatment

SIDE EFFECTS

How Drug Causes Side Effects

- By blocking dopamine 2 receptors in the striatum, it can cause motor side effects
- By blocking dopamine 2 receptors in the pituitary, it can cause elevations in prolactin
- By blocking dopamine 2 receptors excessively in the mesocortical and mesolimbic dopamine pathways, especially at high doses, it can cause worsening of negative and cognitive

symptoms (neuroleptic-induced deficit syndrome)
• Anticholinergic actions may cause sedation, blurred vision, constipation, dry mouth
• Antihistaminergic actions may cause sedation, weight gain
• By blocking alpha 1 adrenergic receptors, it can cause dizziness, sedation, and hypotension
• Mechanism of weight gain and any possible increased incidence of diabetes or dyslipidaemia with conventional antipsychotics is unknown
∗ Mechanism of potentially dangerous QTc prolongation may be related to actions at ion channels

Notable Side Effects

∗ Neuroleptic malignant syndrome (uncommon)
∗ Akathisia
∗ Extrapyramidal symptoms, parkinsonism, tardive dyskinesia
∗ Hypotension
• Sedation, akinesia
• Galactorrhoea, amenorrhoea
• Dry mouth, constipation, blurred vision
• Sexual dysfunction
∗ Weight gain

Common or very common
• CNS: blurred vision, depression, headache, restlessness
• GIT: decreased appetite, hypersalivation
• Other: hyperhidrosis, sebaceous gland overactivity, urinary disorders

Uncommon
• CNS: dysarthria, oculogyric crisis
• Other: facial oedema, muscle spasms, skin reactions

Frequency not known
• CNS: seizure
• CVS: cardiac arrest
• Other: decreased libido, glycosuria, hyponatraemia, neck stiffness, temperature dysregulation

Life-Threatening or Dangerous Side Effects

• Neuroleptic malignant syndrome (discontinue as potentially fatal)
• Seizures
∗ Dose-dependent QTc prolongation
• Ventricular arrhythmias and sudden death

• Increased risk of death and cerebrovascular events in elderly patients with dementia-related psychosis

Weight Gain

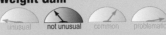

• Occurs in significant minority

Sedation

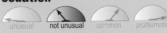

• Occurs in significant minority

What To Do About Side Effects

• Wait
• Wait
• Wait
• Reduce the dose
• Low-dose benzodiazepine or beta blocker may reduce akathisia
• Take more of the dose at bedtime to help reduce daytime sedation
• Weight loss, exercise programmes, and medical management for high BMIs, diabetes, and dyslipidaemia
• Switch to another antipsychotic (atypical) – quetiapine or clozapine are best in cases of tardive dyskinesia

Best Augmenting Agents for Side Effects

• Dystonia: antimuscarinic drugs (e.g. procyclidine) as oral or IM depending on the severity; botulinum toxin if antimuscarinics not effective
• Parkinsonism: antimuscarinic drugs (e.g. procyclidine)
• Akathisia: beta blocker propranolol (30–80 mg/day) or low-dose benzodiazepine (e.g. 0.5–3.0 mg/day of clonazepam) may help; other agents that may be tried include the 5HT2 antagonists such as cyproheptadine (16 mg/day) or mirtazapine (15 mg at night – caution in bipolar disorder); clonidine (0.2–0.8 mg/day) may be tried if the above ineffective
• Tardive dyskinesia: stop any antimuscarinic, consider tetrabenazine (caution – risk of QTc interval prolongation)
∗ Augmentation of pimozide has not been systematically studied and can be dangerous, especially with drugs that can either prolong QTc interval or raise pimozide plasma levels

DOSING AND USE

Usual Dosage Range

- Schizophrenia: 2–20 mg/day (elderly: 1–20 mg/day; child 12–17 years: 1–20 mg/day)
- Psychosis: 4–16 mg/day (elderly: 2–16 mg/day)
- Tourette syndrome: 1–4 mg/day (child 2–12 years); 2–10 mg/day (child 12–17 years)

Dosage Forms

- Tablet 1 mg, 4 mg

How to Dose

*Schizophrenia:
- Adult: initial dose 2 mg/day, adjusted according to response, increased by increments of 2–4 mg at weekly intervals; usual dose 2–20 mg/day
- Elderly: initial dose 1 mg/day, adjusted according to response, increased by increments of 2–4 mg at weekly intervals; usual dose 2–20 mg/day
- Child 12–17 years (under expert supervision): initial dose 1 mg/day, adjusted according to response, increased by increments of 2–4 mg at weekly intervals; usual dose 2–20 mg/day

*Psychosis:
- Adult: initial dose 4 mg/day, adjusted according to response, increased by increments of 2–4 mg at weekly intervals; max 16 mg/day
- Elderly: initial dose 2 mg/day, adjusted according to response, increased by increments of 2–4 mg at weekly intervals; max 16 mg/day

*Tourette syndrome:
- Child 2–11 years (under expert supervision): 1–4 mg/day
- Child 12–17 years (under expert supervision): 2–10 mg/day

 Dosing Tips

- The effects of pimozide on the QTc interval are dose-dependent, so start low and go slow while carefully monitoring QTc interval
- Sudden unexpected deaths have occurred in patients taking high doses of pimozide for conditions other than Tourette syndrome; thus patients should be instructed not to exceed the prescribed dose

- Do not exceed the maximum dose in acutely agitated patients, instead consider adding a benzodiazepine for the short term, or another antipsychotic especially IM
- If QTc exceeds 500 msec, pimozide should be discontinued
- Treatment should be suspended if absolute neutrophil count falls below 1.5 x 10^9/L

Overdose

- Patients who have taken an overdose of pimozide should be observed for at least 4 days as pimozide has a long half-life
- Deaths have occurred; extrapyramidal symptoms, ECG changes, hypotension, respiratory depression, coma

Long-Term Use

- Should periodically re-evaluate long-term usefulness in individual patients, but treatment may need to continue for many years for some patients
- Some side effects may be irreversible (e.g. tardive dyskinesia)

Habit Forming

- No

How to Stop

- Slow down-titration (over 6 to 8 weeks), especially when simultaneously beginning a new antipsychotic while switching (i.e. cross-titration)
- Rapid discontinuation may lead to acute withdrawal symptoms, rebound psychosis and worsening of symptoms
- If antiparkinsonian agents are being used, they should be continued for a few weeks after pimozide is discontinued

Pharmacokinetics

- Metabolised by CYP450 3A and to a lesser extent 1A2
- Mean elimination half-life about 55 hours

 Drug Interactions

- May decrease the effects of levodopa, dopamine agonists
- May enhance QTc prolongation of other drugs capable of prolonging QTc interval
- May increase the effects of antihypertensive drugs

*Use with CYP450 3A4 inhibitors (e.g. drugs such as fluoxetine, sertraline, fluvoxamine; foods such as grapefruit juice) can raise pimozide levels and increase the risks of dangerous arrhythmias
- Use of pimozide and fluoxetine may lead to bradycardia
- Additive effects may occur if used with CNS depressants
- Additive effects may occur if used with anticholinergic drugs
- Some patients taking a neuroleptic and lithium have developed an encephalopathic syndrome similar to neuroleptic malignant syndrome
- Combined use with adrenaline may lower blood pressure

 Other Warnings/Precautions

- All antipsychotics should be used with caution in patients with angle-closure glaucoma, blood disorders, cardiovascular disease, depression, diabetes, epilepsy and susceptibility to seizures, history of jaundice, myasthenia gravis, Parkinson's disease, photosensitivity, prostatic hypertrophy, severe respiratory disorders
- If signs of neuroleptic malignant syndrome develop, treatment should be immediately discontinued
- Use cautiously in patients with alcohol withdrawal or convulsive disorders because of possible lowering of seizure threshold
- Use cautiously in patients consuming alcohol as increased risk of CNS depression and hypotension
- Antiemetic effect can mask signs of other disorders or overdose
- Do not use adrenaline in event of overdose as interaction with some pressor agents may lower blood pressure
- Because pimozide may dose-dependently prolong QTc interval, use with caution in patients who have bradycardia or who are taking drugs that can induce bradycardia (e.g. beta blockers, calcium channel blockers, clonidine, digitalis)
- Because pimozide may dose-dependently prolong QTc interval, use with caution in patients who have hypokalaemia and/or hypomagnesaemia or who are taking drugs that can induce hypokalaemia and/or hypomagnesaemia (e.g. diuretics, stimulant laxatives, intravenous amphotericin

B, glucocorticoids, beta agonists, tetracosactide, theoretical risk with aminophylline)
*Pimozide can increase the QTc interval and potentially cause arrhythmia or sudden death, especially in combination with drugs that raise its levels
- Use only with caution if at all in a patient with a recent acute myocardial infarction or decompensated heart failure
- Use only with caution if at all in a patient taking drugs that can cause tics
- Use only with caution if at all in Lewy body disease
- Pimozide has been shown to increase tumours in mice (dose-related effect)

Do Not Use
- If patient has phaeochromocytoma
- If patient is in a comatose state or has CNS depression
- If patient has a personal history or family history of congenital QT prolongation
*If there is a history of QTc prolongation or cardiac arrhythmia
*If patient is taking an agent capable of significantly prolonging QTc interval (e.g. selected antiarrhythmics, citalopram, selected antipsychotics, moxifloxacin)
*If patient is taking drugs that inhibit pimozide metabolism, such as macrolide antibiotics, azole antifungal agents (ketoconazole, itraconazole), protease inhibitors, antiretroviral agents, fluvoxamine, fluoxetine, sertraline, etc.
- If there is a proven allergy to pimozide
- If there is a known sensitivity to other antipsychotics

Renal Impairment
- Use with caution in renal failure

Hepatic Impairment
- Use with caution

Cardiac Impairment
- A baseline ECG is required, this is particularly important if physical examination identifies cardiovascular risk factors, personal history of cardiovascular disease, or if the patient has been admitted to hospital

- Pimozide produces a dose-dependent prolongation of QTc interval, which may be enhanced by the existence of bradycardia, hypokalaemia, congenital or acquired long QTc interval, which should be evaluated prior to administering pimozide
- Caution if treating concomitantly with a medication likely to produce prolonged bradycardia, hypokalaemia, slowing of intracardiac conduction, or prolongation of QTc interval
- Use only with caution if at all in a patient with a recent acute myocardial infarction or decompensated heart failure
- Avoid if patient has a personal history or family history of congenital QT prolongation
* Avoid if there is a history of QTc prolongation or cardiac arrhythmia
* Avoid if patient is taking an agent capable of significantly prolonging QTc interval (e.g. selected antiarrhythmics, citalopram, selected antipsychotics, moxifloxacin)

Elderly

- Some patients may tolerate lower doses better
- Although conventional antipsychotics are commonly used for behavioural disturbances in dementia, no agent has been approved for treatment of elderly patients with dementia-related psychosis
- Elderly patients with dementia-related psychosis treated with antipsychotics are at an increased risk of death compared to placebo, and also have an increased risk of cerebrovascular events

Children and Adolescents

- Use in Tourette syndrome is not licensed
- May be used to treat schizophrenia in children aged 12–17 years
- Should only be prescribed under expert supervision

Before you prescribe:

- Do not offer antipsychotic medication when transient or attenuated psychotic symptoms or other mental state changes associated with distress, impairment, or help-seeking behaviour are not sufficient for a diagnosis of psychosis or schizophrenia. Consider individual CBT with or without family therapy and other treatments recommended for anxiety, depression, substance use, or emerging personality disorder
- For first-episode psychosis (FEP) antipsychotic medication should only be started by a specialist following a comprehensive multidisciplinary assessment and in conjunction with recommended psychological interventions (CBT, family therapy)
- As first-line treatment: allow patient to choose from aripiprazole, olanzapine or risperidone. As second-line treatment switch to alternative from list. Consider quetiapine depending on desired profile. Pimozide to be considered as third- or fourth-line option depending on response and/or patient profile
- Choice of antipsychotic medication should be an informed choice depending on individual factors and side-effect profile (metabolic, cardiovascular, extrapyramidal, hormonal, other)
- All children and young people with FEP/ bipolar should be supported with sleep management, anxiety management, exercise and activation schedules, and healthy diet
- Where a child or young person presents with self-harm and suicidal thoughts the immediate risk management may take first priority
- Persistent severe aggression in children with autism or pervasive developmental disorders, when other treatments are ineffective or not tolerated. There are many reasons for challenging behaviours in autism spectrum disorder (ASD) and consideration should be given to possible physical, psychosocial, environmental or ASD-specific causes (e.g. sensory processing difficulties, communication). These should be addressed first. Consider behavioural interventions and family support. Pharmacological treatment can be offered alongside the above. It may be prudent to periodically discontinue prescriptions if symptoms are well controlled, and as irritability may lessen as the patient is going through neurodevelopmental changes
- Severe tic disorder including Tourette syndrome under expert supervision, when educational, psychological and other pharmacological treatments are ineffective or not tolerated: transient tics occur in up to 20% of children. Tourette syndrome occurs in 1% of children. Tics

wax and wane over time and are variably exacerbated by external factors such as stress, inactivity, fatigue. Tics are a lifelong disorder, but often get better over time. As many as 65% of young people with Tourette syndrome have only mild tics in adult life. Psychoeducation and evidence-based psychological interventions such as habit reversal therapy (HRT) or exposure and response prevention (ERP) should be offered first. Pharmacological treatment may be considered in conjunction with psychological interventions where tics result in significant impairment or psychosocial consequences, and/or where psychological interventions have been ineffective. If co-morbid with ADHD other choices (clonidine/guanfacine) may be better options to avoid polypharmacy

- A risk management plan is important prior to start of medication because of the possible increase in suicidal ideation and behaviours in adolescents and young adults
Practical notes:
- Carefully weigh the risks and benefits of pharmacological treatment against the risks and benefits of non-treatment and make sure to document this in the patient's chart
- Monitor weight, weekly for the first 6 weeks, then at 12 weeks, and then every 6 months (plotted on a growth chart)
- Monitor height every 6 months (plotted on a growth chart)
- Monitor waist circumference every 6 months (plotted on a percentile chart)
- Monitor pulse and blood pressure (plotted on a percentile chart) at 12 weeks and then every 6 months
- Monitor fasting blood glucose, HbA1c, blood lipid and prolactin levels at 12 weeks and then every 6 months
- Monitor for activation of suicidal ideation at the beginning of treatment. Inform parents or guardians of this risk so they can help observe child or adolescent patients
If it does not work:
- Review child's/young person's profile, consider new/changing contributing individual or systemic factors such as peer or family conflict. Consider drug/substance misuse. Consider dose adjustment before switching or augmentation. Be vigilant of polypharmacy especially in complex and highly vulnerable children/adolescents

- Consider non-concordance by parent or child, consider non-concordance in adolescents, address underlying reasons for non-concordance
- Children are more sensitive to most side effects
  - There is an inverse relationship between age and incidence of EPS
  - Exposure to antipsychotics during childhood and young age is associated with a three-fold increase of diabetes mellitus
  - Treatment with all second-generation antipsychotics has been associated with changes in most lipid parameters
  - Weight gain correlates with time on treatment. Any childhood obesity is associated with obesity in adults
- Dose adjustments may be necessary in the presence of interacting drugs
- Re-evaluate the need for continued treatment regularly
- Monitoring of endocrine function (weight, height, sexual maturation and menses) is required when a child is taking an antipsychotic drug that is known to cause hyperprolactinaemia

Pregnancy

- Controlled studies have not been conducted in pregnant women
- Very limited evidence of safety in pregnancy
- There is a risk of abnormal muscle movements and withdrawal symptoms in newborns whose mothers took an antipsychotic during the third trimester; symptoms may include agitation, abnormally increased or decreased muscle tone, tremor, sleepiness, severe difficulty breathing, and difficulty feeding
- Reports of extrapyramidal symptoms, jaundice, hyperreflexia, hyporeflexia in infants whose mothers took a phenothiazine during pregnancy
- Psychotic symptoms may worsen during pregnancy and some form of treatment may be necessary
- Use in pregnancy may be justified if the benefit of continued treatment exceeds any associated risk
- Switching antipsychotics may increase the risk of relapse
- Effects of hyperprolactinaemia on the foetus are unknown

Pimozide (Continued)

Breastfeeding

- Unknown if pimozide is secreted in human breast milk, but all psychotropics assumed to be secreted in breast milk
- Not recommended for use because of potential for tumorigenicity or cardiovascular effects on infant
- Haloperidol is considered to be the preferred first-generation antipsychotic, and quetiapine the preferred second-generation antipsychotic
- Infants of women who choose to breastfeed should be monitored for possible adverse effects

THE ART OF PSYCHOPHARMACOLOGY

Potential Advantages

- Only for patients who respond to this agent and not to other antipsychotics
- Useful in monosymptomatic hypochondriacal psychosis

Potential Disadvantages

- Vulnerable populations such as children and elderly
- Patients on other drugs

Primary Target Symptoms

- Vocal and motor tics in patients who fail to respond to treatment with other antipsychotics
- Monosymptomatic hypochondriacal psychosis
- Psychotic symptoms in patients who fail to respond to treatment with other antipsychotics

Pearls

* Although indicated in the BNF for Tourette syndrome, schizophrenia and other psychoses such as monosymptomatic hypochondriacal psychosis, it is now recognised that the benefits of pimozide generally do not outweigh its risks in most patients
* Because of its effects on QTc interval, pimozide is not intended for use unless other options for tic disorders (or psychotic disorders) have failed

 Suggested Reading

Huhn M, Nikolakopoulou A, Schneider-Thoma J, et al. Comparative efficacy and tolerability of 32 oral antipsychotics for the acute treatment of adults with multi-episode schizophrenia: a systematic review and network meta-analysis. Lancet 2019;394(10202):939–51.

McPhie ML, Kirchhof MG. A systematic review of antipsychotic agents for primary delusional infestation. J Dermatolog Treat 2022;33(2):709–21.

Mothi M, Sampson S. Pimozide for schizophrenia or related psychoses. Cochrane Database Syst Rev 2013;(11):CD001949.

Pringsheim T, Marras C. Pimozide for tics in Tourette's syndrome. Cochrane Database Syst Rev 2009;(2):CD006996.

Rathbone J, McMonagle T. Pimozide for schizophrenia or related psychoses. Cochrane Database Syst Rev 2007;(3):CD001949.

Prazosin

THERAPEUTICS

Brands
- Hypovase
- Minipress

Generic?
No, not in UK

Class
- Neuroscience-based nomenclature: pharmacology domain – norepinephrine; mode of action – antagonist
- Alpha 1 adrenergic receptor blocker

Commonly Prescribed for
(bold for BNF indication)
- **Hypertension (includes children)**
- **Congestive heart failure (includes children)**
- **Raynaud's syndrome**
- **Benign prostatic hyperplasia**
- Nightmares in post-traumatic stress disorder (PTSD)
- Blood circulation disorders
- Passing of kidney stones

 ### How the Drug Works
- Blocks alpha 1 adrenergic receptors to reduce noradrenergic hyperactivation
- Stimulation of central noradrenergic receptors during sleep may activate traumatic memories, so blocking this activation may reduce nightmares

How Long Until It Works
- Within a few days to a few weeks

If It Works
- Reduces the frequency and severity of nightmares associated with PTSD

If It Doesn't Work
- Increase dose
- Switch to another agent

 ### Best Augmenting Combos for Partial Response or Treatment Resistance
- Prazosin is itself an adjunct for the treatment of nightmares in PTSD

Tests
- None for healthy individuals
- False-positive results may occur in screening tests for phaeochromocytoma in patients who are being treated with prazosin; if an elevated urinary vanillylmandelic acid (VMA) is found, prazosin should be discontinued and the patient retested after a month

SIDE EFFECTS

How Drug Causes Side Effects
- Excessive blockade of alpha 1 peripheral noradrenergic receptors

Notable Side Effects
- Dizziness, lightheadedness, headache, fatigue, blurred vision
- Nausea

Common or very common
- CNS/PNS: blurred vision, depression, dizziness, drowsiness, headache, nervousness, vertigo
- CVS: palpitations, postural hypotension, syncope
- GIT: constipation, dry mouth, nausea, vomiting
- Other: asthenia, dyspnoea, nasal congestion, oedema, sexual dysfunction, skin reactions, urinary disorders

Uncommon
- CNS/PNS: paraesthesia, sleep disorders, tinnitus
- CVS: angina pectoris, arrhythmias
- GIT: gastrointestinal discomfort
- Other: arthralgia, epistaxis, eye pain, eye redness, hyperhidrosis

Rare or very rare
- GIT: hepatic dysfunction, pancreatitis
- Other: alopecia, fever, flushing, gynaecomastia, hallucination, pain, vasculitis

 ### Life-Threatening or Dangerous Side Effects
- Syncope with sudden loss of consciousness

Weight Gain

unusual   not unusual   common   problematic

- Reported but not expected

Sedation

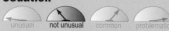

unusual | not unusual | common | problematic

- Occurs in significant minority

What To Do About Side Effects

- Lower the dose
- Wait
- Wait
- Wait
- In a few weeks switch to another agent

Best Augmenting Agents for Side Effects

- Often best to try another treatment prior to resorting to augmentation strategies to treat side effects

DOSING AND USE

Usual Dosage Range

Adult:

Hypertension
- 1–20 mg/day in divided doses

Congestive heart failure (rarely used)
- 1–20 mg/day in divided doses

Raynaud's syndrome (but efficacy not established)
- 1–4 mg/day in divided doses

Benign prostatic hyperplasia
- 1–4 mg/day in divided doses

Nightmares in PTSD
- 1–16 mg/day, generally in divided doses

Children and adolescents:

Hypertension
- Range from 10 mcg/kg twice per day to a max of 20 mg/day in divided doses

Congestive heart failure (rarely used)
- Range from 5 mcg/kg twice per day to a max of 20 mg/day in divided doses

Nightmares in PTSD
- 1–4 mg/day, generally in divided doses

Dosage Forms

- Tablet 500 mcg, 2 mg, 5 mg

How to Dose

Adult:

Hypertension
- Initial dose 500 mcg 2–3 times per day for 3–7 days, first dose at bedtime, increased to 1 mg 2–3 times per day for another 3–7 days, then increased if needed up to 20 mg/day in divided doses

Congestive heart failure (rarely used)
- 500 mcg 2–4 times per day, first dose at bedtime, increased to 4 mg/day in divided doses; maintenance 4–20 mg/day in divided doses

Raynaud's syndrome (but efficacy not established)
- Initial dose 500 mcg twice per day, first dose at bedtime, dose may be increased after 3–7 days if needed to 1–2 mg twice per day

Benign prostatic hyperplasia
- Initial dose 500 mcg twice per day for 3–7 days, adjusted according to response, maintenance 2 mg twice per day; start with lowest possible dose in the elderly

Nightmares in PTSD
- Formal dosing recommendation not established
- Initial dose 1 mg at bedtime, increase dose (divided) until the nightmares resolve or until the drug is not tolerated due to side effects

Children and adolescents:

Hypertension
- Child 1 month–11 years: initial dose 10–15 mcg/kg 2–4 times per day, first dose at bedtime, then increased gradually to 500 mcg/kg/day in divided doses, max 20 mg/day
- Child 12–17 years: initial dose 500 mcg 2–3 times per day for 3–7 days, first dose at bedtime, increased to 1 mg 2–3 times per day for a further 3–7 days, then increased as needed gradually up to 20 mg/day in divided doses

Congestive heart failure (rarely used)
- Child 1 month–11 years: 5 mcg/kg twice per day, first dose at bedtime, then increased gradually to 100 mcg/kg/day in divided doses
- Child 12–17 years: 500 mcg 2–4 times per day, first dose at bedtime, then increased to 4 mg/day in divided doses; maintenance 4–20 mg/day in divided doses

Nightmares in PTSD
- Formal dosing recommendation not established
- Initial dose 1 mg at bedtime, increase dose to a maximum of 2–4 mg nocte

Dosing Tips
- In PTSD dosing may be extremely individualised with as little as 2 mg/day being helpful for some patients, whilst others need doses as high as 40 mg/day
- Therapeutic dose does not correlate with blood levels
- Divided dosing may be preferable; in particular giving a small dose during the day may be beneficial if the patient has persistent hyperarousal and is re-experiencing symptoms during the day
- Risk of syncope can be decreased by limiting the initial dose to 1 mg and using slow dose titration
- In PTSD for children and adolescents titrate the dose slowly, e.g. 1 mg per week

Overdose
- Sedation, depressed reflexes and hypotension in overdose

Long-Term Use
- Prazosin has not been evaluated against placebo in long-term trials
- Nightmares may return if prazosin is stopped

Habit Forming
- No

How to Stop
- Taper to avoid hypertension

Pharmacokinetics
- Elimination half-life about 2–3 hours

Drug Interactions
- Concomitant use with a phosphodiesterase-5 inhibitor (PDE-5) such as sildenafil can have additive effects on blood pressure, potentially leading to hypotension; thus, a PDE-5 inhibitor should be initiated at the lowest possible dose
- Concomitant use with a beta blocker (e.g. propranolol) can have additive effects on blood pressure

- Concomitant use with other alpha 1 blockers, which include many psychotropic agents, can have additive effects leading to hypotension

Other Warnings/Precautions
- Beware of first dose hypotension
- Use with caution in the elderly
- Prazosin can cause syncope with sudden loss of consciousness, most often in association with rapid dose increases or the introduction of another antihypertensive drug
- Intraoperative floppy iris syndrome (IFIS) has been observed during cataract surgery in some patients treated with alpha 1 adrenergic blockers, which may require modifications to the surgical technique; however, there does not appear to be a benefit of stopping the alpha 1 adrenergic blocker prior to cataract surgery
- Avoid situations that can cause orthostatic hypotension, such as extensive periods of standing, prolonged or intense exercise, and exposure to heat

Do Not Use
- In a patient with benign prostatic hypertrophy who has a history of micturition syncope
- If patient has a history of postural hypotension
- If patient has congestive heart failure due to a mechanical obstruction (e.g. aortic stenosis)
- If there is proven allergy to quinazolines or prazosin

SPECIAL POPULATIONS

Renal Impairment
- Moderate-severe impairment: initial dose reduction to 500 mcg/day; increase dose with caution

Hepatic Impairment
- Use with caution
- Initial dose reduction to 500 mcg/day advised
- Increase dose with caution

Cardiac Impairment
- Do not use if patient has congestive heart failure due to a mechanical obstruction (e.g. aortic stenosis)

Prazosin (Continued)

- Use with caution in patients who are predisposed to hypotensive or syncopal episodes

Elderly

- Use with caution in the elderly due to higher risk of orthostatic hypotension and syncope
- Some patients may tolerate lower doses better
- Prescription potentially inappropriate in those with symptomatic orthostatic hypotension, micturition syncope or persistent postural hypotension

 Children and Adolescents

- BNF indications for use in children and adolescents include hypertension and congestive heart failure
- Not licensed for use in children under 12 years of age
- Evidence for use in PTSD in children and adolescents limited
- Slow titration recommended, e.g. 1 mg per week
- Risk of orthostatic hypotension
- Monitor blood pressure especially early in treatment

 Pregnancy

- No evidence of teratogenicity
- Limited data of safety in humans
- Animal studies indicate low risk
- Only use when potential benefit outweighs risk

Breastfeeding

- Present in milk, but in amounts too small to be likely to be harmful
- No published evidence of safety
- Manufacturer advises use with caution
- If drug is continued while breastfeeding, infant should be monitored for hypotension

THE ART OF PSYCHOPHARMACOLOGY

Potential Advantages

- For patients with PTSD who do not respond to SSRIs/SNRIs or exposure therapy
- Specifically for nightmares and other symptoms of autonomic arousal

Potential Disadvantages

- Patients with cardiovascular disease
- Patients taking concomitant psychotropic drugs with alpha 1 antagonist properties

Primary Target Symptoms

- Nightmares

 Pearls

- The evidence base for using prazosin to treat nightmares associated with PTSD is limited but generally positive, and prazosin is recommended in USA by the Department of Veterans Affairs as an adjunctive treatment for this purpose
- Initiate treatment early in the onset of nightmares following exposure to trauma
- May also be useful for nightmares and symptoms of autonomic arousal in other trauma and stress-related disorders in addition to PTSD

Suggested Reading

Hudson N, Burghart S, Reynoldson J, et al. Evaluation of low dose prazosin for PTSD-associated nightmares in children and adolescents. Ment Health Clin 2021;11(2):45–9.

Kung S, Espinel Z, Lapid MI. Treatment of nightmares with prazosin: a systematic review. Mayo Clin Proc 2012;87(9):890–900.

Reist C, Streja E, Tang CC, et al. Prazosin for treatment of post-traumatic stress disorder: a systematic review and meta-analysis. CNS Spectr 2021;26(4):338–44.

Schoenfeld FB, Deviva JC, Manber R. Treatment of sleep disturbances in posttraumatic stress disorder: a review. J Rehabil Res Dev 2012;49(5):729–52.

van Berkel VM, Bevelander SE, Mommersteeg PM. Placebo-controlled comparison of prazosin and cognitive-behavioral treatments for sleep disturbances in US military veterans. J Psychosom Res 2012;73(2):153; author reply 154–5.

Pregabalin

THERAPEUTICS

Brands
- Lyrica
- Alzain
- Axalid

Generic?
Yes

Class
- Neuroscience-based nomenclature: pharmacology domain – glutamate; mode of action – channel blocker
- Anticonvulsant, antineuralgic for chronic pain, alpha 2 delta ligand at voltage-sensitive calcium channels

Commonly Prescribed for
(bold for BNF indication)
- **Peripheral and central neuropathic pain**
- **Adjunctive therapy for focal seizures with or without secondary generalisation**
- **Generalised anxiety disorder (GAD)**
- Diabetic peripheral neuropathy
- Postherpetic neuralgia
- Fibromyalgia
- Neuropathic pain associated with spinal cord injury
- Partial seizures in adults (adjunctive)
- Panic disorder
- Social anxiety disorder

How the Drug Works
- Is a leucine analogue and is transported both into the blood from the gut and also across the blood–brain barrier into the brain from the blood by the system L transport system (a sodium-independent transporter) as well as by additional sodium-dependent amino acid transporter systems
- *Binds to the alpha 2 delta subunit of voltage-sensitive calcium channels
- This closes N and P/Q presynaptic calcium channels, diminishing excessive neuronal activity and neurotransmitter release
- Although structurally related to gamma-aminobutyric acid (GABA), no known direct actions on GABA or its receptors

How Long Until It Works
- Can reduce neuropathic pain and anxiety within a week
- Should reduce seizures by 2 weeks

- If it is not producing clinical benefits within 6–8 weeks, it may require a dosage increase or it may not work at all

If It Works
- The goal of treatment of neuropathic pain, seizures, and anxiety disorders is to reduce symptoms as much as possible, and if necessary in combination with other treatments
- Treatment of neuropathic pain most often reduces, but does not eliminate all symptoms and is not a cure since symptoms usually recur after medicine stopped
- Continue treatment until all symptoms are gone or until improvement is stable and then continue treating indefinitely as long as improvement persists

If It Doesn't Work
- Many patients have only a partial response where some symptoms are improved, but others persist
- Other patients may be non-responders, sometimes called treatment-resistant or treatment-refractory
- Consider increasing dose, switching to another agent, or adding an appropriate augmenting agent
- Consider biofeedback or hypnosis for pain
- Consider psychotherapy for anxiety
- Consider the presence of non-concordance and counsel patient
- Consider evaluation for another diagnosis or for a co-morbid condition (e.g. medical illness, substance abuse, etc.)

Best Augmenting Combos for Partial Response or Treatment Resistance
- *Pregabalin can itself act as an augmenting agent to other anticonvulsants in treating epilepsy
- For postherpetic neuralgia, pregabalin can decrease concomitant opiate use
- *For neuropathic pain, TCAs and SNRIs as well as tiagabine, other anticonvulsants, and even opiates can augment pregabalin if done by experts while carefully monitoring in difficult cases
- For anxiety, SSRIs, SNRIs, or benzodiazepines can augment pregabalin

Tests
- None for healthy individuals

SIDE EFFECTS

How Drug Causes Side Effects

- CNS side effects may be due to excessive blockade of voltage-sensitive calcium channels

Notable Side Effects

- *Sedation, dizziness
- Ataxia, fatigue, tremor, dysarthria, paraesthesia, memory impairment, coordination abnormal, impaired attention, confusion, euphoric mood, irritability
- Vomiting, dry mouth, constipation, increased appetite, weight gain, flatulence
- Blurred vision, diplopia
- Peripheral oedema
- Libido decreased, erectile dysfunction

Common or very common

- CNS/PNS: abnormal gait, abnormal sensation, altered mood, confusion, dizziness, drowsiness, feeling abnormal, headache, impaired concentration, memory loss, movement disorders, sleep disorders, speech impairment, vertigo, vision disorders
- GIT: abdominal distension, abnormal appetite, constipation, diarrhoea, dry mouth, gastrointestinal disorders, nausea, vomiting, weight changes
- Other: asthenia, cervical spasm, increased risk of infection, joint disorders, muscle complaints, oedema, pain, sexual dysfunction

Uncommon

- CNS/PNS: aggression, anxiety, decreased reflexes, depression, hallucination, impaired consciousness, hyperacusia, psychiatric disorders
- CVS: arrhythmias, atrioventricular block, hypertension, hypotension, syncope, vasodilation
- GIT: oral disorders, taste loss, thirst
- Other: breast abnormalities, chest tightness, chills, cough, dry eye, dyspnoea, epistaxis, eye discomfort, eye disorders, eye inflammation, fever, hypoglycaemia, malaise, menstrual cycle irregularities, nasal complaints, neutropenia, peripheral coldness, skin reactions, snoring, sweat changes, urinary disorders

Rare or very rare

- CNS: altered smell sensation, dysgraphia
- CVS: QT interval prolongation
- GIT: ascites, dysphagia, gynaecomastia, hepatic disorders, pancreatitis, throat tightness
- Other: renal impairment, rhabdomyolysis, Stevens-Johnson syndrome

 Life-Threatening or Dangerous Side Effects

- Rare activation of suicidal ideation and behaviour (suicidality)

Weight Gain

- Occurs in significant minority

Sedation

- Many experience and/or can be significant in amount
- Dose-related
- Can wear off with time

What to Do About Side Effects

- Wait
- Wait
- Wait
- Take more of the dose at night to reduce daytime sedation
- Lower the dose
- Switch to another agent

Best Augmenting Agents for Side Effects

- Many side effects cannot be improved with an augmenting agent

DOSING AND USE

Usual Dosage Range

- Peripheral and central neuropathic pain: adult (150–600 mg/day)
- Adjunctive therapy for focal seizures with or without secondary generalisation: adult (50–600 mg/day)
- Generalised anxiety disorder: adult (150–600 mg/day)

Dosage Forms

- Oral solution 20 mg/mL
- Capsule 25 mg, 50 mg, 75 mg, 100 mg, 150 mg, 200 mg, 225 mg, 300 mg

How to Dose

* Peripheral and central neuropathic pain:
- Initial dose 150 mg/day in 2–3 divided doses, increased as needed after 3–7 days to 300 mg/day in 2–3 divided doses, then increased after 1 week up to 600 mg/day in 2–3 divided doses if required

* Adjunctive therapy for focal seizures with or without secondary generalisation:
- Initial dose 25 mg twice per day, increased by increments of 50 mg/day each week to 300 mg/day in 2–3 divided for 1 week, then increased up to 600 mg/day in 2–3 divided doses if required

* Generalised anxiety disorder:
- Initial dose 150 mg/day in 2–3 divided doses, increased by increments of 150 mg/day each week as needed, then increased up to 600 mg/day in 2–3 divided doses if required

 Dosing Tips

- Because of its short elimination half-life, pregabalin is administered 2 to 3 times per day to maintain therapeutic levels
* Generally given in one-third to one-sixth the dose of gabapentin
- If pregabalin is added to a second sedating agent, such as another anticonvulsant, a benzodiazepine, or an opiate, the titration period should be at least a week to improve tolerance to sedation
- Most patients need to take pregabalin only twice per day
- At the high end of the dosing range, tolerability may be enhanced by splitting dose into 3 or more divided doses
- For intolerable sedation, can give most of the dose at night and less during the day
- To improve slow-wave sleep, may only need to take pregabalin at bedtime
- May be taken with or without food

Overdose

- Not likely to be fatal; agitation, confusion, restlessness, somnolence, seizures and coma may be seen

Long-Term Use
- Safe

Habit Forming
- Yes

- Following concerns about abuse, pregabalin has been reclassified as a Class C controlled substance and is now a Schedule 3 drug, but is exempt from safe custody requirements. Healthcare professionals should evaluate patients carefully for a history of drug abuse before prescribing pregabalin, and observe patients for signs of abuse and dependence. Patients should be informed of the potentially fatal risks of interactions between pregabalin and alcohol, and with other medicines that cause CNS depression, particularly opioids

How to Stop
- Taper over a minimum of 1 week
- Epilepsy patients may seize upon withdrawal, especially if withdrawal is abrupt
- Discontinuation symptoms uncommon

Pharmacokinetics
- Peak plasma within 1 hour (fasted) and 2 to 3 hours (with food)
- Pregabalin is not metabolised much but mostly excreted intact renally
- Elimination half-life about 6.3 hours (5 to 7 hours)

 Drug Interactions
- Pregabalin has not been shown to have significant pharmacokinetic drug interactions
- Because pregabalin is excreted unchanged, it is unlikely to have significant pharmacokinetic drug interactions
- May add to or potentiate the sedative effects of opioids, benzodiazepines, and alcohol

 Other Warnings/Precautions
- Dizziness and sedation could increase the chances of accidental injury (falls) in the elderly
- Increased incidence of haemangiosarcoma at high doses in mice involves platelet changes and associated endothelial cell proliferation not present in rats or humans; no evidence to suggest an associated risk for humans
- Warn patients and their caregivers about the possibility of activation of suicidal ideation and advise them to report such side effects immediately

Pregabalin (Continued)

- Caution in patients with a history of substance misuse, and in conditions that may precipitate encephalopathy or severe congestive heart failure
- Dose adjustments may be necessary in patients at higher risk of respiratory depression including those with compromised respiratory function, respiratory or neurological disease
- Dose adjustments may be necessary in the elderly, in patients with renal impairment, and in patients taking other CNS depressants (e.g. opioid-containing medicines)
- Caution in patient with seizures as these may be exacerbated

Do Not Use

- If patient has a problem of galactose intolerance, the Lapp lactase deficiency, or glucose-galactose malabsorption
- If there is a proven allergy to pregabalin or gabapentin

Pregnancy

- Controlled studies have not been conducted in pregnant women
- In animal studies, pregabalin was teratogenic in rats and rabbits
- Use in women of childbearing potential requires weighing potential benefits to the mother against the risks to the foetus
- Taper drug if discontinuing
- Seizures, even mild seizures, may cause harm to the embryo/foetus

Breastfeeding

- Small amounts found in mother's breast milk
- If drug is continued while breastfeeding, infant should be monitored for possible adverse effects
- If infant becomes irritable or sedated, breastfeeding or drug may need to be discontinued

SPECIAL POPULATIONS

Renal Impairment

- Initial dose 75 mg/day and max dose 300 mg/day if eGFR 30–60 mL/minute/1.73 m^2
- Initial dose 25–50 mg/day and max dose 150 mg/day in 1–2 divided doses if eGFR 15–30 mL/minute/1.73 m^2
- Initial dose 25 mg/day and max dose 75 mg/day if eGFR less than 15 mL/minute/1.73 m^2

Hepatic Impairment

- Dose adjustment not necessary

Cardiac Impairment

- Caution in severe congestive heart failure

Elderly

- Some patients may tolerate lower doses better
- Elderly patients may be more susceptible to adverse effects

Children and Adolescents

- Safety and efficacy have not been established

THE ART OF PSYCHOPHARMACOLOGY

Potential Advantages

- Generalised anxiety disorder
- Improves sleep architecture
- Diabetic peripheral neuropathy
- Fibromyalgia
- Has relatively mild side-effect profile
- Has few pharmacokinetic drug interactions
- More potent and probably better tolerated than gabapentin

Potential Disadvantages

- Requires 2–3 times a day dosing
- Abuse potential

Primary Target Symptoms

- Seizures
- Pain
- Anxiety

Pearls

- Licensed for use in generalised anxiety disorder
- *Should observe patients for signs of abuse and dependence
- Useful for fibromyalgia

- Useful for neuropathic pain associated with diabetic peripheral neuropathy
- Useful in postherpetic neuralgia
- Improves sleep disruption as well as pain in patients with painful diabetic peripheral neuropathy, fibromyalgia, or postherpetic neuralgia
- Well studied in epilepsy, peripheral neuropathic pain, and GAD
- Off-label use for panic disorder and social anxiety disorder may be justified
- May have uniquely robust therapeutic actions for both the somatic and the psychic symptoms of GAD
* Off-label use as an adjunct for bipolar disorder may not be justified

* One of the few agents that enhances slow-wave delta sleep, which may be helpful in chronic neuropathic pain syndromes
- Pregabalin is generally well tolerated, with only mild adverse effects
* Although no head-to-head studies, appears to be better tolerated and more consistently efficacious at high doses than gabapentin
* Drug absorption and clinical efficacy may be more consistent at high doses for pregabalin compared to gabapentin, because of the higher potency of pregabalin and the fact that, unlike gabapentin, it is transported by more than one transport system

 ## Suggested Reading

Bandelow B. Current and novel psychopharmacological drugs for anxiety disorders. Adv Exp Med Biol 2020;1191:347–65.

Bockbrader HN, Radulovic LL, Posvar EL, et al. Clinical pharmacokinetics of pregabalin in healthy volunteers. J Clin Pharmacol 2010;50(8):941–50.

Derry S, Bell RF, Straube S, et al. Pregabalin for neuropathic pain in adults. Cochrane Database Syst Rev 2019;1(1):CD007076.

Lauria-Horner BA, Pohl RB. Pregabalin: a new anxiolytic. Expert Opin Investig Drugs 2003;12(4):663–72.

Stahl SM. Anticonvulsants and the relief of chronic pain: pregabalin and gabapentin as alpha(2) delta ligands at voltage-gated calcium channels. J Clin Psychiatry 2004;65(5):596–7.

Stahl SM. Anticonvulsants as anxiolytics, part 2: pregabalin and gabapentin as alpha(2)delta ligands at voltage-gated calcium channels. J Clin Psychiatry 2004;65(4):460–1.

Stahl SM, Porreca F, Taylor CP, et al. The diverse therapeutic actions of pregabalin: is a single mechanism responsible for several pharmacologic activities? Trends Pharmacol Sci 2013;34(6):332–9.

Prochlorperazine

Brands

- Buccastem
- Stemetil

Generic?

Yes

Class

- Conventional antipsychotic (neuroleptic, phenothiazine, dopamine 2 antagonist, antiemetic)

Commonly Prescribed for

(bold for BNF indication)

- **Schizophrenia and other psychoses**
- **Mania**
- **Short-term adjunctive management of severe anxiety**
- **Nausea and vomiting (acute attack; prevention; in previously diagnosed migraine)**
- **Labyrinthine disorders**
- **Acute migraine**

 How the Drug Works

- Blocks dopamine 2 receptors, reducing positive symptoms of psychosis and improving other behaviours
- Blocks alpha-adrenergic receptors
- Weak anti-muscarinic properties
- Interacts with a range of other receptors producing antiemetic, antipruritic, serotonin-blocking, weak antihistamine and ganglion-blocking activity
- Inhibits the heat-regulating centre
- Can relax smooth muscle
- Membrane-stabilising properties that produce local anaesthetic properties
- Acts on the autonomic system to produce vasodilatation, hypotension and tachycardia
- Reduces salivary and gastric secretions

How Long Until It Works

- Psychotic and manic symptoms can improve within 1 week, but may take several weeks for full effect on behaviour as well as on cognition and affective stabilisation
- Actions on nausea and vomiting are immediate
- Onset time of 30–40 minutes following oral administration
- Onset time of 10–20 minutes following intramuscular administration

- Duration of action is 3–4 hours for all routes of administration

If It Works

- Most often reduces positive symptoms in schizophrenia but does not eliminate them
- Most patients with schizophrenia do not have a total remission of symptoms but rather a reduction of symptoms by about a third
- Continue treatment in schizophrenia until reaching a plateau of improvement
- After reaching a satisfactory plateau, continue treatment for at least a year after the first episode of psychosis
- For second and subsequent episodes of psychosis in schizophrenia, treatment may need to be indefinite
- Reduces symptoms of acute psychotic mania but not proven as a mood stabiliser or as an effective maintenance treatment in bipolar disorder
- After reducing acute psychotic symptoms in mania, switch to a mood stabiliser and/ or an atypical antipsychotic for mood stabilisation and maintenance

If It Doesn't Work

- Consider trying one of the first-line atypical antipsychotics (risperidone, olanzapine, quetiapine, aripiprazole, paliperidone, amisulpride)
- Consider trying another conventional antipsychotic
- If two or more antipsychotic monotherapies do not work, consider clozapine
- In the case of treatment of nausea and vomiting, use ondansetron if ineffective after 30–60 minutes. If symptoms return and it is more than 6–8 hours since the last dose, repeat the dose

Best Augmenting Combos for Partial Response or Treatment Resistance

- Augmentation of conventional antipsychotics has not been systematically studied
- Addition of a mood-stabilising anticonvulsant such as valproate, carbamazepine, or lamotrigine may be helpful in both schizophrenia and bipolar mania

- Augmentation with lithium in bipolar mania may be helpful
- Addition of a benzodiazepine, especially short-term for agitation
- Alternative long-term treatments (pharmacological or psychological) for anxiety will likely provide the best response as prochlorperazine is an adjunct therapy used when anxiety is not controlled by other medications

Tests
Baseline
＊Measure weight, BMI, and waist circumference
- Get baseline personal and family history of diabetes, obesity, dyslipidaemia, hypertension, and cardiovascular disease
- Check for personal history of drug-induced leucopenia/neutropenia
＊Check pulse and blood pressure, fasting plasma glucose or glycosylated haemoglobin (HbA1c), fasting lipid profile, and prolactin levels
- Full blood count (FBC)
- Assessment of nutritional status, diet, and level of physical activity
- Determine if the patient:
  - is overweight (BMI 25.0–29.9)
  - is obese (BMI ≥30)
  - has pre-diabetes – fasting plasma glucose: 5.5 mmol/L to 6.9 mmol/L or HbA1c: 42 to 47 mmol/mol (6.0 to 6.4%)
  - has diabetes – fasting plasma glucose: >7.0 mmol/L or HbA1c: ≥48 mmol/L (≥6.5%)
  - has hypertension (BP >140/90 mm Hg)
  - has dyslipidaemia (increased total cholesterol, LDL cholesterol, and triglycerides; decreased HDL cholesterol)
- Treat or refer such patients for treatment, including nutrition and weight management, physical activity counselling, smoking cessation, and medical management
- Baseline ECG for: inpatients; those with a personal history or risk factor for cardiac disease

Monitoring
- Monitor weight and BMI during treatment
- Consider monitoring fasting triglycerides monthly for several months in patients at high risk for metabolic complications and when initiating or switching antipsychotics
- While giving a drug to a patient who has gained >5% of initial weight, consider evaluating for the presence of pre-diabetes, diabetes, or dyslipidaemia, or consider switching to a different antipsychotic
- Patients with low white blood cell count (WBC) or history of drug-induced leucopenia/neutropenia should have full blood count (FBC) monitored frequently during the first few months and prochlorperazine should be discontinued at the first sign of decline of WBC in the absence of other causative factors
- Monitor prolactin levels and for signs and symptoms of hyperprolactinaemia

SIDE EFFECTS
How Drug Causes Side Effects
- By blocking dopamine 2 receptors in the striatum, it can cause motor side effects
- By blocking dopamine 2 receptors in the pituitary, it can cause elevations in prolactin
- By blocking dopamine 2 receptors excessively in the mesocortical and mesolimbic dopamine pathways, especially at high doses, it can cause worsening of negative and cognitive symptoms (neuroleptic-induced deficit syndrome)
- Anticholinergic actions may cause sedation, blurred vision, constipation, dry mouth
- Antihistaminergic actions may cause sedation, weight gain
- By blocking alpha 1 adrenergic receptors, it can cause dizziness, sedation, and hypotension
- Mechanism of weight gain and any possible increased incidence of diabetes or dyslipidaemia with conventional antipsychotics is unknown, but insulin regulation may be impaired by blocking pancreatic M3 muscarinic receptors

Notable Side Effects
- Agitation
- Hyperprolactinaemia which may result in: amenorrhoea, galactorrhoea, gynaecomastia, erectile dysfunction
- Cardiovascular effects: hypotension (dose-related, usually postural), QT interval prolongation, arrhythmias
- Constipation, dry mouth, urinary retention
- Dizziness
- Drowsiness

- Leucopenia, neutropenia
- Movement disorders, parkinsonism, tremor
- Acute dystonia (risk is increased in men, young adults, children, antipsychotic-naive patients, rapid dose escalation, and abrupt treatment discontinuation)
- Rash

Rare or very rare
- Impaired glucose tolerance and hyperglycaemia, hyponatraemia, SIADH
- With buccal use: blood disorder, hepatic disorders

Frequency not known
- Photosensitivity
- With buccal use: oral disorders, skin eruption
- With IM use: atrioventricular block, cardiac arrest, eye disorders, jaundice, muscle rigidity, nasal congestion, respiratory depression, skin reactions
- With oral use: atrioventricular block, autonomic dysfunction, cardiac arrest, hyperthermia, impaired consciousness, jaundice, muscle rigidity, nasal congestion, oculogyric crisis, respiratory depression, skin reactions

 Life-Threatening or Dangerous Side Effects
- QT interval prolongation and arrhythmias
- Seizures
- Neuroleptic malignant syndrome

Weight Gain

unusual   not unusual   common   problematic

- Many patients experience and/or can be significant in amount

Sedation

unusual   not unusual   common   problematic

- Many patients experience and/or can be significant in amount
- Drowsiness is common
- Tolerance to sedation occurs quickly

What To Do About Side Effects
- Wait
- Wait
- Wait
- Reduce the dose

- Low-dose benzodiazepine or beta blocker may reduce akathisia
- Take more of the dose at bedtime to help reduce daytime sedation
- Weight loss, exercise programmes, and medical management for high BMIs, diabetes, and dyslipidaemia
- Switch to another antipsychotic (atypical) – quetiapine or clozapine are best in cases of tardive dyskinesia

Best Augmenting Agents for Side Effects
- Dystonia: antimuscarinic drugs (e.g. procyclidine) as oral or IM depending on the severity; botulinum toxin if antimuscarinics not effective
- Parkinsonism: antimuscarinic drugs (e.g. procyclidine)
- Akathisia: beta blocker propranolol (30–80 mg/day) or low-dose benzodiazepine (e.g. 0.5–3.0 mg/day of clonazepam) may help; other agents that may be tried include the 5HT2 antagonists such as cyproheptadine (16 mg/day) or mirtazapine (15 mg at night – caution in bipolar disorder); clonidine (0.2–0.8 mg/day) may be tried if the above ineffective
- Tardive dyskinesia: stop any antimuscarinic, consider tetrabenazine

DOSING AND USE

Usual Dosage Range
- Schizophrenia, other psychoses and mania: 25–100 mg/day (oral); 25–75 mg/day (injection)
- Adjunct for severe anxiety: 15–40 mg/day (oral)
- Nausea and vomiting (acute attack): 20–30 mg/day (oral); 12.5 mg as required (injection)
- Nausea and vomiting (prevention): 10–30 mg/day (oral); 12.5 mg as required (injection)
- Labyrinthine disorders: 15–30 mg/day
- Nausea and vomiting in previously diagnosed migraine: 6–12 mg/day (buccal)
- Acute migraine: 10 mg (oral)

Dosage Forms
- Tablet 5 mg
- Buccal tablet 3 mg

- Solution for injection 12.5 mg/mL
- Oral solution 5 mg/5 mL syrup

How to Dose

For schizophrenia, other psychoses and mania
Oral:
- 12.5 mg twice per day for 7 days
- Dose to be adjusted at intervals of 4–7 days according to response
- Usual dose 75–100 mg/day
- Dose varies widely depending on patient
IM injection:
- 12.5–25 mg 2–3 times per day

Adjunct for severe anxiety
Oral:
- 15–20 mg/day in divided doses
- Max 40 mg/day
- Duration of treatment should be less than 12 weeks

Nausea and vomiting (adults)
Oral:
- Acute attacks: initial dose 20 mg, then 10 mg after 2 hours
- Prevention: 5–10 mg 2–3 times per day; 5 mg 4–6 times per day can be used for nausea associated with alcohol withdrawal
IM injection:
- Acute and prevention: 12.5 mg as required, to be followed if necessary after 6 hours by an oral dose

Nausea and vomiting, attacks and prevention (children)
Oral:
- 1–11 years (body weight >10 kg): 250 mcg/kg 2–3 times per day
- 12–17 years: 5–10 mg up to 3 times per day if required
- IM injection:
- 2–4 years: 1.25–2.5 mg up to 3 times per day if required
- 5–11 years: 5–6.25 mg up to 3 times per day if required
- 12–17 years: 12.5 mg up to 3 times per day if required

Labyrinthine disorders
Oral:
- 5 mg 3 times per day
- Increase if necessary to 30 mg/day in divided doses
- Dose to be increased gradually, then reduced to 5–10 mg/day
- Dose is reduced after several weeks

Migraine (nausea and vomiting symptoms)
- 3–6 mg twice per day using buccal tablet
- Tablets to be placed high between upper lip and gum and left to dissolve
- 10 mg oral tablet for 1 dose in acute migraine. Taken as soon as symptoms develop

 Dosing Tips
- Prochlorperazine is available as prochlorperazine maleate or mesilate. 1 mg maleate = 1 mg mesilate

Overdose
- Signs and symptoms of overdose are predominantly extrapyramidal and may be accompanied by agitation, restlessness or CNS depression
- Poisoning can be complicated by hypotension, hypothermia, sinus tachycardia and arrhythmias
- However, phenothiazines cause less depression of consciousness and respiration than other sedatives
- Treatment is symptomatic and supportive
- Pharmacological emesis is unlikely to be of any use
- Do not use adrenaline

Long-Term Use
- Due to the likelihood that some patients with chronic use of antipsychotics will develop tardive dyskinesia, they should be informed of this risk
- Patients with a history of long-term therapy should be evaluated periodically to decide whether the maintenance dose could be lowered or drug therapy discontinued
- Balance disorders can be exacerbated, in part, by the use of labyrinthine sedatives and so prochlorperazine should only be given for a maximum of 2 weeks when used for acute vertigo

Habit Forming
- No

How to Stop
- High risk of relapse if medication is stopped after 1–2 years
- Withdrawal after long-term therapy should be gradual and closely monitored to avoid the risk of acute withdrawal syndromes or rapid relapse

- Acute withdrawal symptoms include nausea, vomiting and insomnia
- Monitor patients for 2 years after withdrawal for relapse
- In schizophrenia, the response to treatment may be delayed and recurrence of symptoms may not become apparent for some time after withdrawal
- Prochlorperazine may continue to be excreted in the urine for up to 3 weeks after cessation of long-term therapy

Pharmacokinetics

- Elimination half-life for oral tablets about 9 hours
- Plasma concentrations following oral administration are much lower than those following IM injection
- Rate of metabolism and excretion decreases in old age

 Drug Interactions

- CNS-depressant actions may be intensified by alcohol, barbiturates and other sedatives
- Anticholinergic agents may reduce antipsychotic effect
- Mild anticholinergic effects may be enhanced by other anticholinergic drugs
- Antacids, anti-Parkinson drugs and lithium can interfere with absorption
- Concurrent use of lithium may increase extrapyramidal side effects and/or neurotoxicity
- Opposes the action of amfetamine, levodopa, clonidine, guanethidine, and adrenaline
- Exaggerates hypotensive effect of most antihypertensives, especially alpha adrenoceptor blocking agents
- Simultaneous administration of dexferrioxamine and prochlorperazine has been observed to induce transient metabolic encephalopathy characterised by loss of consciousness for 48–72 hours

 Other Warnings/Precautions

- All antipsychotics should be used with caution in patients with angle-closure glaucoma, blood disorders, cardiovascular disease, depression, diabetes, epilepsy and susceptibility to seizures, history of jaundice, myasthenia gravis, Parkinson's disease, photosensitivity, prostatic hypertrophy, severe respiratory disorders
- Skin photosensitivity may occur at higher doses. Advise to avoid undue exposure to sunlight and use sun screen if necessary
- Prescription potentially inappropriate in patients with parkinsonism (risk of exacerbating parkinsonian symptoms)
- Increased risk of arrhythmias when used with concomitant QT prolonging drugs and drugs causing electrolyte imbalance
- Discontinue in the event of unexplained fever as this may be a sign of neuroleptic malignant syndrome (pallor, hyperthermia, autonomic dysfunction, altered consciousness, muscle rigidity)
- Monitor risk factors for venous thromboembolism. Cases have been reported with antipsychotic drugs
- Increased risk of agranulocytosis when used concurrently with drugs with myelosuppressive potential
- May lower seizure threshold. Close monitoring is required in patients with epilepsy or a history of seizures
- Hyperglycaemia or intolerance to glucose has been reported. Appropriate glycaemic monitoring during treatment should be present in patients with diabetes mellitus or risk factors
- Do not use alone where depression is predominant but may be combined with antidepressant therapy
- Drowsiness may affect performance of skilled tasks
- Caution in lactose intolerance. Oral tablet (5 mg) contains 61 mg lactose monohydrate
- Caution in prostatic hypertrophy, history of narrow-angle glaucoma, and history of agranulocytosis
- Caution in patients with hypothyroidism

Do Not Use

- Avoid oral route in children under 10 kg
- Avoid concomitant treatment with other antipsychotics
- If there is CNS depression
- If there is hepatic impairment
- If the patient is in a comatose state
- If the patient has phaeochromocytoma
- In myasthenia gravis (buccal tablets)

- If there is a proven allergy to prochlorperazine
- If there is a known sensitivity to any phenothiazine

SPECIAL POPULATIONS

Renal Impairment

- Initiate with small doses in severe renal impairment due to increased cerebral sensitivity

Hepatic Impairment

- Avoid

Cardiac Impairment

- Avoid in cardiac failure

Elderly

- Use with caution
- Lower initial dose is recommended
- Risk of postural hypotension is greater in elderly patients (especially after IM injection)
- Increased risk of drug-induced parkinsonism, particularly after prolonged use

Children and Adolescents

- Indicated for use in the treatment and prevention of nausea and vomiting: oral – child 1–17 years; IM – child 2–17 years
- Indicated for use in the treatment of nausea and vomiting in previously diagnosed migraine: buccal – child 12–17 years
- Associated with dystonic reactions particularly after a cumulative dosage of 0.5 mg/kg
- Use with caution

Pregnancy

- Controlled studies have not been conducted in pregnant women
- Some animal studies have shown reproductive toxicity
- Considered low risk if used occasionally at low doses
- There is a risk of abnormal muscle movements and withdrawal symptoms in newborns whose mothers took an antipsychotic during the third trimester; symptoms may include agitation, abnormally increased or decreased muscle tone, tremor, sleepiness, severe difficulty breathing, and difficulty feeding
- Reports of extrapyramidal symptoms, jaundice, hyperreflexia, hyporeflexia in infants whose mothers took a phenothiazine during pregnancy
- Psychotic symptoms may worsen during pregnancy and some form of treatment may be necessary
- Use in pregnancy may be justified if the benefit of continued treatment exceeds any associated risk
- Switching antipsychotics may increase the risk of relapse

Breastfeeding

- Unknown if prochlorperazine is secreted in human breast milk, but all psychotropics assumed to be secreted in breast milk
- Haloperidol is considered to be the preferred first-generation antipsychotic, and quetiapine the preferred second-generation antipsychotic
- Infants of women who choose to breastfeed should be monitored for possible adverse effects

THE ART OF PSYCHOPHARMACOLOGY

Potential Advantages

- Less sedating than chlorpromazine
- Available over the counter for patients who have nausea and vomiting with previously diagnosed migraine
- Risk of nausea is low when used as pre-treatment for emesis associated with chemotherapy
- Effective early option for reducing uncomplicated nausea and vomiting
- Lower risk of tissue damage when administered intravenously compared to promethazine

Potential Disadvantages

- Risk of tardive dyskinesia
- Risk of drug-induced parkinsonism/ extrapyramidal side effects
- Limited formulations licensed in children

Primary Target Symptoms

- Nausea and vomiting
- Positive symptoms of psychosis

Pearls

- Prochlorperazine has a licence for the treatment of psychoses such as schizophrenia or mania, but in practice it is prescribed more for other disorders such as nausea and vomiting
- Prochlorperazine is associated with an increased risk of tardive dyskinesia and the availability of alternative treatments make its use limited
- Prochlorperazine is less potent in its actions on adrenergic, histaminergic, and muscarinic receptors in comparison to chlorpromazine
- Patients have very similar antipsychotic responses when treated with any of the conventional antipsychotics, which is different from atypical antipsychotics where antipsychotic responses of individual patients can occasionally vary greatly from one atypical to another
- Patients with inadequate responses to atypical antipsychotics may benefit from a trial of augmentation with a conventional antipsychotic such as prochlorperazine or from switching to a conventional antipsychotic such as prochlorperazine
- However, long-term polypharmacy with a combination of a conventional antipsychotic such as prochlorperazine with an atypical antipsychotic may combine their side effects without clearly augmenting the efficacy of either
- For treatment-resistant patients, especially those with impulsivity, aggression, violence, and self-harm, long-term polypharmacy with 2 atypical antipsychotics and 1 conventional antipsychotic may be useful or even necessary while closely monitoring
- In such cases, it may be beneficial to combine 1 depot antipsychotic with 1 oral antipsychotic

Suggested Reading

Casey JF, Lasky JJ, Klett CJ, et al. Treatment of schizophrenic reactions with phenothiazine derivatives. A comparative study of chlorpromazine, triflupromazine, mepazine, prochlorperazine, perphenazine, and phenobarbital. Am J Psychiatry 1960;117:97–105.

Fenton WS, Wyatt RJ, McGlashan TH. Risk factors for spontaneous dyskinesia in schizophrenia. Arch Gen Psychiatry 1994;51(8):643–50.

Nigam P, Rastogi CK, Kapoor KK, et al. Prochlorperazine in anxiety. Indian J Psychiatry 1985;27(3):227–32.

Procyclidine hydrochloride

Brands
• Kemadrin

Generic?
Yes

Class
• Antimuscarinic agent

Commonly Prescribed for
(bold for BNF indication)
• **Parkinsonism**
• **Extrapyramidal symptoms (excluding tardive dyskinesia)**
• **Acute dystonia**

How the Drug Works
• Blocks excitatory effects of acetylcholine at M1, M2 and M4 central muscarinic receptor in corpus striatum, thereby reducing effects of relative central cholinergic excess resulting from dopamine deficiency

How Long Until It Works
• For extrapyramidal disorders and parkinsonism, onset of action of the oral tablet can be within minutes or hours
• Intramuscular or intravenous injection usually effective in 5–10 minutes

If It Works
• Reduces motor side effects
• Does not lessen the ability of antipsychotics to cause tardive dyskinesia
• Periodic cessation of treatment recommended in patients who require long-term therapy

If It Doesn't Work
• Increase dose
• Consider switching to another anticholinergic
• Disorders that develop after prolonged antipsychotic use may not respond to treatment
• Consider discontinuing the agent that precipitated the extrapyramidal symptoms

 Best Augmenting Combos for Partial Response or Treatment Resistance
• If ineffective, switch to another agent rather than augment

Tests
• None for healthy adults

How Drug Causes Side Effects
• Prevents the action of acetylcholine on muscarinic receptors

Notable Side Effects
• Dry mouth, blurred vision, diplopia
• Confusion, hallucinations
• Constipation, nausea, vomiting
• Dilation of colon/paralytic ileus/bowel obstruction
• Erectile dysfunction

Common or very common
• Blurred vision, constipation, dry mouth, urinary retention

Uncommon
• CNS: anxiety, cognitive impairment, confusion, dizziness, hallucination, memory loss
• GIT: gingivitis, nausea, vomiting
• Other: rash

Rare or very rare
• Psychosis

 Life-Threatening or Dangerous Side Effects
• Precipitation of psychotic episode when procyclidine is administered for extrapyramidal side effects may occur in patients with mental health conditions
• May affect performance of skilled tasks, e.g. driving

Weight Gain

unusual   not unusual   common   problematic

• Reported but not expected

Procyclidine hydrochloride (Continued)

Sedation

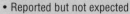

- Reported but not expected
- Patients are usually awakened and some may be activated

What To Do About Side Effects

- For confusion or hallucinations discontinue use
- For dry mouth: chew gum/drink water/ice chips
- For urinary retention: may need to discontinue use

Best Augmenting Agents for Side Effects

- Many side effects cannot be improved with an augmenting agent

---

DOSING AND USE

Usual Dosage Range

- Parkinsonism: adult (7.5–60 mg/day); elderly (lower end of range)
- Extrapyramidal side effects of neuroleptic drugs:(7.5–60 mg/day); elderly (lower end of range)
- Acute dystonia: adult (5–10 mg/day); elderly (lower end of range)

Dosage Forms

- Tablet 5 mg
- Oral solution 2.5 mg/5 mL, 5 mg/5 mL
- Solution for injection 10 mg/2 mL

How to Dose

Adults:

Parkinsonism

- Oral: 2.5 mg 3 times per day, then increased by increments of 2.5–5 mg/day as needed, increased if necessary up to 30 mg/day in 2–4 divided doses, to be increased at 2–3-day intervals. Max daily dose only to be used in exceptional circumstances; max 60 mg/day

Extrapyramidal symptoms

- Oral: starting dose 2.5 mg 3 times per day; increase by 2.5 mg/day increments until symptoms relieved; max 60 mg/day

Acute dystonia

- By IM injection, or by intravenous injection: 5–10 mg, occasionally more than 10 mg,

dose usually effective in 5–10 minutes but may need 30 minutes for relief

Children and adolescents:

Acute dystonia

By IM injection, or by intravenous injection
- Child 1 month–1 year: 0.5–2 mg for 1 dose, dose usually effective in 5–10 minutes but may need 30 minutes for relief
- Child 2–9 years: 2–5 mg for 1 dose, dose usually effective in 5–10 minutes but may need 30 minutes for relief
- Child 10–17 years: 5–10 mg, occasionally more than 10 mg, dose usually effective in 5–10 minutes but may need 30 minutes for relief

Dystonia

Oral
- Child 7–11 years: 1.25 mg 3 times per day
- Child 12–17 years: 2.5 mg 3 times per day

Dosing Tips

- Usual maintenance dose to achieve optimal response is 15–30 mg/day
- Twice-daily dosing may be adequate
- In rare cases 60 mg/day doses may be required
- Younger patients may require higher doses for therapeutic response than older patients

Overdose

- Symptoms and signs: agitation, restlessness, confusion, severe sleeplessness, visual and auditory hallucinations, euphoria, dilated non-reactive pupils. CNS depression has been reported following very large overdoses
- Treatment: activated charcoal within 1–2 hours, gastric lavage if clinically appropriate. Administration of cholinergic agents or haemodialysis unlikely to have clinical effect. Diazepam if convulsions occur

Long-Term Use

- Withdraw after 3–4 months and observe patient for returning signs of extrapyramidal symptoms. Reintroduce if symptoms return

Habit Forming

- Yes – rare but has been observed in a minority of patients

How to Stop
- Avoid abrupt discontinuation due to risk of rebound parkinsonism

Pharmacokinetics
- Gastrointestinal absorption with bioavailability of 75%
- 20% oral intake is metabolised hepatically by CYP450 and then conjugates with glucuronic acid
- Almost 100% bound to albumin
- Urinary excretion of conjugated form
- Plasma elimination half-life after oral administration is about 12 hours

 Drug Interactions
- Daily administration of paroxetine increases the levels of plasma procyclidine significantly: monitor dose and adjust where required
- Monoamine oxidase inhibitors may increase anticholinergic effect of procyclidine
- Use of drugs with cholinergic properties may reduce therapeutic response to procyclidine
- Procyclidine may reduce the efficacy of levodopa by increasing gastric emptying time, resulting in enhanced gastric degradation. The basis for this interaction is theoretical
- May reduce absorption of ketoconazole
- Procyclidine may antagonise the gastrointestinal effects of cisapride, domperidone and metoclopramide

⚠ **Other Warnings/Precautions**
- Use with caution in patients with cardiovascular disease or hypertension
- Use with caution in the elderly
- Use with caution in psychotic disorders
- Use with caution in patients liable to abuse substances
- Use with caution in patients with pyrexia
- Use with caution in patients with prostatic hypertrophy or susceptible to angle-closure glaucoma

Do Not Use
- In patients with gastrointestinal obstruction
- In patients with untreated urinary retention
- In patients with angle-closure glaucoma
- In hereditary galactose intolerance
- In Lapp lactase deficiency
- In glucose-galactose malabsorption
- If there is a proven allergy to procyclidine

Renal Impairment
- Use with caution

Hepatic Impairment
- Use with caution

Cardiac Impairment
- Use with caution

Elderly
- Lower end of dose range preferable
- Older people may be more sensitive to the anticholinergic effects of procyclidine; a reduced dose may be required

 Children and Adolescents
- Used for treatment of dystonias (unlicensed use)

 Pregnancy
- Controlled studies have not been conducted in pregnant women
- Where clinically indicated, procyclidine should be offered providing the woman is carefully counselled regarding limited human pregnancy safety data or the prescriber considers risk of not treating greater than the undetermined foetal risk
- Use of centrally acting drugs throughout pregnancy or around time of delivery is associated with an increased risk of poor neonatal adaptation syndrome
- Maternal exposure prior to delivery may cause anticholinergic side effects in the newborn

Breastfeeding
- Unknown if procyclidine is secreted in human breast milk, but all psychotropics assumed to be secreted in breast milk
- *Recommended either to discontinue drug or bottle feed unless the potential benefit to the mother justifies the potential risk to the child
- Infants of women who choose to breastfeed while on procyclidine should be monitored for possible adverse effects

Procyclidine hydrochloride (Continued)

THE ART OF PSYCHOPHARMACOLOGY

Potential Advantages
- Extrapyramidal disorders related to antipsychotic use
- Generalised dystonias (well tolerated in younger age groups)

Potential Disadvantages
- May worsen tardive dyskinesia if used in combination with neuroleptics, or may reduce threshold at which dyskinesias occur in patients predisposed to dyskinesia
- Procyclidine generally unhelpful for relief of akathisia, effect mainly seen if parkinsonism also present

Primary Target Symptoms
- Rigidity, akinesia, tremor, speech and writing difficulties, gait, sialorrhoea and drooling, sweating, oculogyric crises and depressed mood in Parkinson's disease respond well to procyclidine therapy
- Pseudo-parkinsonism, acute dystonia and akathisia secondary to neuroleptic drugs

Pearls
- First-line agent for extrapyramidal disorders related to antipsychotic disorders, but not for tardive dyskinesia (which it may worsen)
- Not first-line treatment for akathisia
- As required procyclidine should always be prescribed when IM haloperidol is prescribed
- Use with great caution in elderly as may cause confusion, memory loss, disorientation. Monitor also for constipation and urinary retention
- Patients with cognitive impairment may do poorly
- Can cause cognitive side effects with chronic use, so periodic trials of discontinuation should be undertaken, especially to justify chronic use
- Can be abused in institutional or prison settings (as may induce euphoria or hallucinations)
- May be used in Parkinson's disease with tremor/post encephalitic Parkinson's disease

 Suggested Reading

Bergman H, Soares-Weiser K. Anticholinergic medication for antipsychotic-induced tardive dyskinesia. Cochrane Database Syst Rev 2018;1(1):CD000204.

Brocks DR. Anticholinergic drugs used in Parkinson's disease: An overlooked class of drugs from a pharmacokinetic perspective. J Pharm Pharm Sci 1999;2(2):39–46.

Van Harten PN, Hoek HW, Kahn RS. Acute dystonia induced by drug treatment. BMJ 1999;319(7210):623–6.

Promethazine hydrochloride

Brands
- Phenergan
- Sominex

Generic?
Yes

Class
- Neuroscience-based nomenclature: pharmacology domain – histamine, dopamine; mode of action – antagonist
- Anti-histamine (anxiolytic, hypnotic, anti-emetic); dopamine antagonist

Commonly Prescribed for
(bold for BNF indication)
- **Sedation (short-term use)**
- **Symptomatic relief of allergy such as hay fever and urticaria**
- **Insomnia associated with urticaria and pruritis**
- **Nausea; vomiting**
- **Vertigo; labyrinthine disorders; motion sickness**
- **Emergency treatment of anaphylactic reactions**
- Insomnia
- Anxiety and tension associated with psychoneurosis

 How the Drug Works
- Promethazine hydrochloride is a phenothiazine derivative with H1 antagonist, anticholinergic (antagonist at muscarinic M1–M4 receptors) and sedative properties
- It is used as an anti-allergic, an anti-emetic, in pruritus, for sedation and in the treatment of insomnia
- Promethazine hydrochloride competes with free histamine for binding at H1 receptors in the gastrointestinal tract, uterus, blood vessels and bronchial muscle. This is how it mediates its anti-allergic effects
- It is also a moderate antagonist at muscarinic receptors and a weak/moderate antagonist at serotonin 5HT2A/5HT2C, D2 receptors, and alpha-7-nicotinic acetylcholine receptor
- Inhibits NMDA-mediated membrane currents

- Readily penetrates the blood–brain barrier leading to cognitive effects such as drowsiness, confusion, dizziness, CNS depression and lowering of seizure threshold
- The relief of nausea is related to its central anticholinergic actions in the medullary chemoreceptor trigger zone

How Long Until It Works
- Onset of clinical effect ranges from 20–30 minutes
- Some immediate relief with first dosing is common; can take several weeks with daily dosing for maximal therapeutic benefit in chronic conditions

If It Works
- Promethazine hydrochloride should only be used in the short-term
- Consider replacing with an antipsychotic or switching to another hypnotic if further sedation is required
- For short-term symptoms of anxiety – after a few weeks, discontinue use or use on an "as needed" basis
- For chronic anxiety disorders, the goal of treatment is complete remission of symptoms as well as prevention of future relapses
- For chronic anxiety disorders, treatment most often reduces or even eliminates symptoms, but is not a cure since symptoms can recur after medicine stopped
- For long-term symptoms of anxiety, consider switching to an SSRI or SNRI for long-term maintenance

If It Doesn't Work
- Consider switching to another agent or adding an appropriate augmenting agent such as an antipsychotic or another hypnotic
- Consider SSRI or SNRI for longer treatment in anxiety

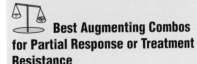 Best Augmenting Combos for Partial Response or Treatment Resistance
- Promethazine hydrochloride can be used off-licence in combination with haloperidol in adults for better-tolerated rapid tranquillisation

Promethazine hydrochloride (Continued)

Tests

- ECG monitoring for patients given an antipsychotic and promethazine
- Physical monitoring post rapid tranquillisation – every 15 minutes in the first hour then hourly: temperature, pulse, blood pressure, respiratory rate

SIDE EFFECTS

How Drug Causes Side Effects

- Blocking histamine 1 receptors can cause sedation
- Moderate antagonist at muscarinic receptors, it can cross the blood–brain barrier, and cause anticholinergic side effects
- Anticholinergic effects include drowsiness, sedation, blurred vision, dizziness, urinary retention, delirium, hallucinations, agitation, tachycardia, dry mouth, constipation, reduced sweating and hyperthermia
- Weak dopamine antagonist with rare reports of neuroleptic malignant syndrome

Notable Side Effects

- Drowsiness, dizziness, fatigue
- Dry mouth, constipation
- Movement disorders
- Palpitations

Frequency not known

- CNS: blurred vision, confusion, dizziness, headache, movement disorders
- CVS: arrhythmia, hypotension, palpitations
- GIT: constipation, dry mouth, jaundice
- Other: blood disorder, photosensitivity, urinary retention

With oral use

- Blood disorders: agranulocytosis, leucopenia, thrombocytopenia
- CNS: anxiety, insomnia, seizure, tinnitus, tremor
- GIT: nausea, vomiting
- Other: blood disorders, photosensitivity, urinary retention

With parenteral use

- Blood disorders: haemolytic anaemia
- CNS: nightmares, restlessness
- GIT: decreased appetite, epigastric discomfort
- Other: fatigue, hypersensitivity, muscle spasms, skin reactions

 Life-Threatening or Dangerous Side Effects

- Should be avoided in neonates due to significant antimuscarinic activity
- Patients should take care when driving or operating heavy machinery as promethazine hydrochloride can increase drowsiness during the day
- Studies have reported that promethazine may occasionally elicit acute dystonia in some individuals, especially in young children and pregnant women
- Elderly patients are more susceptible to anticholinergic side effects as well as movement disorders – case of orofacial dystonia reported

Weight Gain

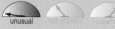

- Reported but not expected

Sedation

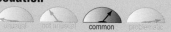

- Frequent and can be significant in amount

What To Do About Side Effects

- Patients should take care when driving and operating heavy machinery
- If side effects are clinically significant discontinue use of promethazine hydrochloride
- Switch to another agent

Best Augmenting Agents for Side Effects

- Many side effects cannot be improved with an augmenting agent
- If using promethazine hydrochloride for anti-allergic effects, switch to a selective antihistamine
- If using promethazine hydrochloride for sedative effects, switch to another hypnotic or sedating agent

DOSING AND USE

Usual Dosage Range

- 5–100 mg/day in divided doses

Dosage Forms

- Solution for injection 25 mg/mL ampoule

- Oral solution 5 mg/5 mL
- Tablet 10 mg, 20 mg, 25 mg

How to Dose

For Sedation (short-term use)
Oral dose:
- Child 2–4 years, 15–20 mg
- Child 5–9 years, 20–25 mg
- Child 10–17 years, 25–50 mg
- Adult 25–50 mg
Deep IM injection:
- Adult 25–50 mg

Symptomatic relief of allergy such as hay fever and urticaria; insomnia associated with urticaria and pruritis
Oral dose:
- Child 2–4 years, 5 mg twice per day OR 5–15 mg at night
- Child 5–9 years, 5–10 mg twice per day OR 10–25 mg at night
- Child 10–17 years, 10–20 mg 2–3 times per day OR 25 mg at night, increased if necessary, to 25 mg twice per day
- Adult 10–20 mg, 2–3 times per day
IM injection:
- Adult 25–50 mg (max per dose 100 mg)

Nausea; vomiting; vertigo; labyrinthine disorders; motion sickness
Oral dose:
- Child 2–4 years, 5 mg at bedtime on night before travel, repeat on the next morning if needed
- Child 5–9 years, 10 mg at bedtime on night before travel, repeat on the next morning if needed
- Child 10–17 years, 20–25 mg at bedtime on night before travel, repeat on the next morning if needed
- Adult, 20–25 mg at bedtime on night before travel, repeat on the next morning if needed

Emergency treatment of anaphylactic reactions
Slow intravenous injection:
- Adult: 25–50 mg, to be administered as a solution containing 2.5 mg/mL in water for injections; max 100 mg per course

 Dosing Tips

- In addition to a coordinated care plan, 25–50 mg of promethazine hydrochloride can be given in the short term to manage crisis in borderline personality disorder

- Off-licence promethazine hydrochloride can be used on its own for the rapid tranquillisation of adults
- Dose: 25–50 mg oral promethazine hydrochloride OR 50 mg IM
- Oral is useful if the patient already takes a regular antipsychotic
- IM is useful in a benzodiazepine-tolerant patient
- Dilution of promethazine is not required before IM injection, dose may be repeated to a max of 100 mg/day
- Wait 1–2 hours post injection to assess response
- Off-licence promethazine hydrochloride can be used to increase the efficacy and tolerance of rapid tranquillisation with haloperidol in adults
- Dose: 25–50 mg promethazine hydrochloride together with 5–10 mg haloperidol IM/oral
- Sites of promethazine injection are the thigh, upper arm and gluteal region. There must be sufficient muscle mass at the site of injection
- Promethazine hydrochloride can be used to treat insomnia in drug and alcohol withdrawal where benzodiazepines are contraindicated due to the risk of dependence
- In other population of patients, promethazine has a role in the management of insomnia, however other interventions should be explored first

Overdose

- Promethazine in overdose has anticholinergic effects including: drowsiness, sedation, blurred vision, dizziness, urinary retention, delirium, hallucinations, agitation, tachycardia, dry mouth, constipation, reduced sweating and hyperthermia
- The most common effects of overdose are delirium and mild to moderate CNS depression. Coma requiring ventilation occurs rarely and supportive treatment is often required
- Promethazine has also been associated with dystonic reactions, psychosis and neuroleptic malignant syndrome
- The reported amount taken in overdose has been found to be associated with the probability of delirium; charcoal ingested within 2 hours can reduce the risk of delirium developing

Promethazine hydrochloride (Continued)

Long-Term Use
- Promethazine hydrochloride should be used in the short term
- In the long term its anticholinergic side effects outweigh the benefits of the drug
- It is also associated with neuroleptic malignant syndrome and dystonic reactions

Habit Forming
- No

How to Stop
- Taper generally not necessary

Pharmacokinetics

Absorption
- Bioavailability is 25% as there is a significant first-pass effect (75%)
- Tmax occurs after 2–3 hours
- Clinical effects are seen within 20 minutes and its effects last 4–6 hours

Distribution
- Widely distributed in the body, it crosses the blood–brain barrier and crosses the placenta
- Promethazine is highly bound to plasma proteins (80–90%)

Biotransformation
- CYP450 2D6 is the principal enzyme involved in the liver metabolism of promethazine hydrochloride
- The main metabolites of promethazine hydrochloride are promethazine sulphoxide and to a lesser extent desmethylpromethazine. These metabolites are inactive

Elimination
- Half-life about 5–14 hours
- Elimination of the inactive metabolites occurs via renal excretion and via bile
- About 2% is excreted as promethazine hydrochloride unchanged

 Drug Interactions
- CYP450 2D6 of the cytochrome P450 system is the principal enzyme involved in promethazine hydrochloride metabolism in the liver
- Drugs that inhibit CYP450 2D6 are likely to increase plasma concentrations of promethazine hydrochloride

- Some examples of CYP450 2D6 inhibitors include fluoxetine, paroxetine and quinidine
- CYP450 2D6 is not susceptible to enzyme induction thus other drugs are unlikely to increase the rate at which promethazine hydrochloride is metabolised
- CNS depressants: promethazine hydrochloride may intensify the effects of other CNS depressants such as alcohol, sedatives, anaesthetics, tricyclic antidepressants and tranquillisers. Avoid combining these therapies in patients
- Adrenaline: promethazine hydrochloride may decrease the vasopressor effects of adrenaline. Do not give in combination
- Anticholinergics: promethazine hydrochloride has anticholinergic side effects; care should be taken when prescribing promethazine hydrochloride in the presence of other anticholinergic agents
- Haloperidol: promethazine may inhibit the metabolism of haloperidol; haloperidol has the potential for QT prolongation. Single combined doses are unlikely to confer risk however caution should be taken with multiple combined dosing
- Monoamine oxidase inhibitors: when prescribed with promethazine hydrochloride, there is an increased incidence of extrapyramidal side effects

 Other Warnings/Precautions
- Promethazine hydrochloride should be used with care in patients with susceptibility to angle-closure glaucoma, prostatic hypertrophy, stenosing peptic ulcer, pyloroduodenal obstruction, bladder-neck obstruction, and urinary retention
- Use cautiously in patients with severe coronary artery disease
- Use with caution in patients with epilepsy
- Promethazine has been rarely reported to cause neuroleptic malignant syndrome as it is a weak dopamine antagonist

Do Not Use
- In neonates and children <2 years, except under specialist advice as the safety of promethazine hydrochloride has not been investigated in infants
- If there is a proven allergy to promethazine

Renal Impairment

- Dose reduction usually not necessary, however promethazine has a long half-life so monitor for excess sedative effects
- Interstitial nephritis has been reported in a patient who was a poor metaboliser of promethazine – use with caution

Hepatic Impairment

- Use with caution

Elderly

- Promethazine hydrochloride can impair cognitive and psychomotor performance which is potentially dangerous in the elderly as it can increase the risk of falls
- Promethazine can also trigger seizures, dyskinesia, dystonia and hallucinations. It should therefore only be used in the short term as a sedative to manage the behavioural and psychological symptoms of dementia

Children and Adolescents

- Children under 6 years should not be given over-the-counter cough and cold medicines containing promethazine
- Off-licence promethazine hydrochloride IM can be used for the rapid tranquillisation of children and adolescents if the oral route is refused
- Dose: <12 years: 5–25 mg (max 50 mg/day), >12 years: 25–50 mg (max 100 mg/day)
- Onset of action: up to 60 minutes
- It is an effective sedative and is useful if the cause of the behavioural disturbance is unknown and there is a concern about the use of antipsychotic medication
- Not licensed for use for sedation in children under 2 years

Before you prescribe – developmental considerations:

For insomnia:

- Sleep patterns change significantly during development. Careful assessment of history, expectations from child and parent, and exploration of possible causes are always required
- Sleep disturbance is often secondary to other issues such as psychiatric disorders, physical disorders, distress, lack of structure in family environment, other psychosocial problems, alcohol or substance use, other prescribed medication
- Treat underlying problems first or concurrently
- Sleep hygiene and behavioural measures should be attempted first (see above) and continued when prescribing
- If using promethazine for insomnia: only recommended for short-term use
- Consider causes such as other prescribed medications that may interfere with sleep, drug and alcohol use, physical causes such as pain, restless leg syndrome, sleep apnoea, underlying psychiatric disorders
- Refer to specialist services and offer CBT and sleep hygiene advice such as:
  ○ The environment should be conducive to sleep; sleep in cool, dark and comfortable environment
  ○ Establish bedtime routine; relax before bedtime and sleep and wake at the same time each day
  ○ Regular exercise (not before bedtime), exposure to sunlight
  ○ Only stay in bed when sleeping
  ○ Avoid caffeine late in the day
  ○ Reduce screen-time in evening or switch on night-mode
  ○ Avoid smoking and excessive alcohol
  ○ Avoid napping during the day

For sedation:

- Deal with causal problem: psychosocial distress and safeguarding concerns, trauma, psychiatric disorders. Initial short-term use might be appropriate where exploration of underlying cause would otherwise not be possible

Practical notes:

- Carefully weigh the risks and benefits of pharmacological treatment against the risks and benefits of non-treatment and make sure to document this in the patient's chart
- If it does not work: review child/young person's profile, consider new or changing individual or systemic contributing factors, such as peer or family conflict
- Consider dose adjustment before switching or augmentation. Be vigilant of polypharmacy especially in complex and highly vulnerable children/adolescents
- Consider non-concordance by parent or child/adolescent, address underlying reasons for non-concordance

- Children and adolescents who cannot swallow tablets can be given oral solution
- Re-evaluate the need for continued treatment regularly

Pregnancy

- Evidence suggests maternal promethazine use during pregnancy is not associated with an increased risk of congenital malformations
- Limited evidence does not show an association between maternal promethazine use and pre-term delivery, low birth weight or neurodevelopmental problems
- Manufacturer advises avoiding in the 2 weeks prior to delivery due to the risk of irritability and excitement in the newborn
- Neonates whose mothers have taken promethazine close to delivery should be monitored for these effects
- Maternal use of more than one CNS-acting medication is likely to lead to more severe symptoms in the neonate
- Use in pregnancy may be justified if the benefit of continued treatment exceeds any associated risk

Breastfeeding

- Evidence suggests insignificant amounts in mother's breast milk
- No published evidence of safety but extensive experience of safe use in breastfeeding
- Infants of women who choose to breastfeed should be monitored for possible adverse effects
- Mothers taking hypnotics should be warned about the risks of co-sleeping

THE ART OF PSYCHOPHARMACOLOGY

Potential Advantages

- It is an effective and safe sedative to use in adults and children >2 years
- Can be used in combination with haloperidol to increase the tolerance and efficacy of rapid tranquillisation in adults
- Can be used to treat insomnia in patients undergoing withdrawal from drugs or alcohol where dependence risk if offered benzodiazepine treatment is high

Potential Disadvantages

- Limited evidence of its efficacy as an agent to treat insomnia in the general population
- Long onset of action when used for rapid tranquillisation
- Antimuscarinic side effects are more pronounced in the elderly and can lead to increased risk of falls and worsen dementia/delirium

Primary Target Symptoms

- Agitation
- Angioedema; conjunctivitis, rash, urticaria
- Insomnia
- Motion sickness
- Nausea and vomiting
- Vertigo

Pearls

- NICE Guidelines recommend medication for insomnia only as a second-line treatment after non-pharmacological treatment options have been tried (e.g. cognitive behavioural therapy for insomnia)
- Promethazine is commonly prescribed in inpatient psychiatric setting and can help with reductions of levels of anxiety and agitation in patients as well as acting as a hypnotic
- It can be added to more activating antipsychotics such as aripiprazole to help reduce any agitation or insomnia
- Oral promethazine can be given as required or as regular tablets in the short term for agitation in preference to benzodiazepines
- Promethazine can be given as a short-acting IM injection for rapid tranquillisation as required for the control of agitation and aggression
- IM promethazine can be combined with IM haloperidol for rapid tranquillisation. The anticholinergic effects of promethazine can help to counteract any extrapyramidal side effects caused by haloperidol via potent D2 blockade

Promethazine hydrochloride (Continued)

Suggested Reading

Bak M, Weltens I, Bervoets C, et al. The pharmacological management of agitated and aggressive behaviour: a systematic review and meta-analysis. Eur Psychiatry 2019;57:78–100.

Huf G, Alexander J, Gandhi P, et al. Haloperidol plus promethazine for psychosis-induced aggression. Cochrane Database Syst Rev 2016;11(11):CD005146.

Muir-Cochrane E, Oster C, Gerace A, et al. The effectiveness of chemical restraint in managing acute agitation and aggression: a systematic review of randomized controlled trials. Int J Ment Health Nurs 2020;29(2):110–26.

Ostinelli EG, Brooke-Powney MJ, Li X, et al. Haloperidol for psychosis-induced aggression or agitation (rapid tranquillisation). Cochrane Database Syst Rev 2017;7(7):CD009377.

Patel MX, Sethi FN, Barnes TR, et al. Joint BAP NAPICU evidence-based consensus guidelines for the clinical management of acute disturbance: de-escalation and rapid tranquillisation. J Psychopharmacol 2018;32(6):601–40.

Zareifopoulos N, Panayiotakopoulos G. Treatment options for acute agitation in psychiatric patients: theoretical and empirical evidence. Cureus 2019;11(11):e6152.

Propranolol hydrochloride

Brands

- Bedranol
- Bedranol SR
- Beta-Prograne
- Half Beta-Prograne

Generic?

Yes

Class

- Beta blocker, antihypertensive

Commonly Prescribed for

(bold for BNF indication)
- **Thyrotoxicosis (adjunct)**
- **Thyrotoxic crisis**
- **Hypertension (not licensed in children under 12 years old)**
- **Prophylaxis of variceal bleeding in portal hypertension**
- **Phaeochromocytoma (only with an alpha-blocker) in preparation for surgery, or if unsuitable for surgery**
- **Angina**
- **Hypertrophic cardiomyopathy**
- **Anxiety tachycardia**
- **Anxiety with symptoms such as palpitation, sweating, and tremor**
- **Prophylaxis after myocardial infarction**
- **Essential tremor**
- **Migraine prophylaxis**
- **Arrhythmias**
- **Tetralogy of Fallot**
- **Hyperthyroidism with autonomic symptoms (in children)**
- **Infantile haemangioma [proliferating, with ulceration, risk of disfigurement, or functional impairment] (initiated under specialist supervision)**
- PTSD, prophylactic
- Akathisia (antipsychotic-induced)
- Generalised anxiety disorder
- Violence, aggression

 How the Drug Works

- For migraine, proposed mechanisms include inhibition of the adrenergic pathway, interaction with the serotonin system and receptors, inhibition of nitric oxide synthesis, and normalisation of contingent negative variation
- For tremor, antagonism of peripheral beta 2 receptors is the proposed mechanism
- For PTSD, blockade of beta 1 adrenergic receptors may theoretically prevent fear conditioning and reconsolidation of fear
- For violence/aggression, the mechanism is poorly established; presumed to be related to central actions at beta adrenergic and serotonin receptors

How Long Until It Works

- For migraine, can begin to work within 2 weeks, but may take up to 6–8 weeks on a stable dose to see full effect
- For tremor, can begin to work within days

If It Works

- For migraine, the goal is to treat those with 4 or more migraines per month and reduce the severity and frequency of attacks; consider gradual withdrawal after 6–12 months of effective prophylaxis
- For tremor, can cause reduction in the severity of tremor, allowing greater functioning with daily activities and clearer speech
- For PTSD, may theoretically block the effects of stress from prior traumatic experiences
- For aggression, may reduce aggression, agitation or uncooperativeness

If It Doesn't Work

- Increase to highest tolerated dose
- For migraine, address other issues such as medication overuse or other co-existing medical disorders; consider changing to another drug or adding a second drug
- For tremor, co-administration with primidone (up to 250 mg 3 times per day) or gabapentin (up to 600 mg twice per day) can augment response; otherwise move to second-line medications including benzodiazepines, topiramate, nadolol, and botulinum toxin; alternative treatments include wrist weights
- For truly refractory tremor, thalamotomy or deep brain stimulation of brain regions such as the thalamus, the globus pallidus and the subthalamic nucleus is an option
- For PTSD, consider initiating first-line pharmacotherapy (SSRI, SNRI) and psychotherapy
- For violence/aggression, switch to another agent, e.g. valproate or an antipsychotic

Propranolol hydrochloride (Continued)

Best Augmenting Combos for Partial Response or Treatment Resistance

- For migraine, low-dose polytherapy with 2 or more drugs might be better tolerated and more effective than high-dose monotherapy
- For tremor, can combine with primidone or second-line medications
- For aggression and violence, can combine with valproate and/or antipsychotics

Tests

- None for healthy individuals

SIDE EFFECTS

How Drug Causes Side Effects

- By blocking beta adrenergic receptors, it can cause dizziness, bradycardia, and hypotension

Notable Side Effects

- Bradycardia, hypotension, hyperglycaemia, hypoglycaemia, weight gain
- Bronchospasm, cold/flu symptoms, sinusitis, pneumonias
- Dizziness, vertigo, fatigue, depression, sleep disturbances
- Sexual dysfunction, decreased libido, dysuria, urinary retention, joint pain
- Exacerbation of symptoms in peripheral vascular disease and Raynaud's syndrome

Common or very common

- CNS/PNS: confusion, depression, headache, paraesthesia, sleep disorders, visual impairment
- CVS: bradycardia, heart failure, peripheral vascular disease, syncope
- GIT: abdominal discomfort, constipation, diarrhoea, nausea, vomiting
- Resp: bronchospasm, dyspnoea
- Other: dry eye, erectile dysfunction, fatigue, peripheral coldness, rash

Rare or very rare

- Blood disorders: thrombocytopenia
- CNS: altered mood, memory loss, neuromuscular dysfunction, psychosis
- CVS: postural hypotension
- Other: alopecia, skin reactions

Frequency not known

- Hypoglycaemia

Life-Threatening or Dangerous Side Effects

- In acute congestive heart failure may further depress myocardial contractility
- Can blunt premonitory symptoms of hypoglycaemia in diabetes and mask clinical symptoms of hyperthyroidism
- Risk of excessive myocardial depression in general anaesthesia

Weight Gain

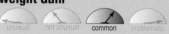

- Many experience and/or can be significant in amount

Sedation

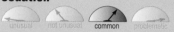

- Many experience and/or can be significant in amount

What To Do About Side Effects

- Lower dose, change to a modified-release formulation, or switch to another agent
- Disturbances are more common with lipophilic blockers like propranolol than with hydrophobic beta blockers (e.g. atenolol, sotalol)

Best Augmenting Agents for Side Effects

- Polytherapy and use of alternative therapies
- Excessive bradycardia may be countered with intravenous injection of atropine sulfate

DOSING AND USE

Usual Dosage Range

- For drug-induced akathisia 30–80 mg/day (start at 10 mg 3 times per day)
- For generalised anxiety disorder 40–120 mg/day in divided doses (start at 40 mg and titrate up)
- For PTSD 40–80 mg/day (start at 40 mg)

Dosage Forms

- Tablet 10 mg, 40 mg, 80 mg, 160 mg
- Modified-release capsule 80 mg, 160 mg
- Oral solution 5 mg/5 mL, 10 mg/5 mL, 40 mg/5 mL, 50 mg/5 mL
- Injection 1 mg/mL

How to Dose

- Dose depends on indication and age
- Hyperthyroidism:
  - Neonate: initial dose 250–500 mcg/kg every 6–8 hours, adjusted according to response
  - Child: initial dose 250–500 mcg/kg every 8 hours, adjusted according to response; increased as needed up to 1 mg/kg every 8 hours (max per dose 40 mg every 8 hours)
- Thyrotoxicosis (adjunct):
  - Neonate: initial dose 250–500 mcg/kg every 6–8 hours, adjusted according to response
  - Child: initial dose 250–500 mcg/kg every 8 hours, adjusted according to response; increased as needed up to 1 mg/kg every 8 hours (max per dose 40 mg every 8 hours)
  - Adult: oral 10–40 mg 3–4 times per day
- Thyrotoxic crisis:
  - Neonate: initial dose 250–500 mcg/kg every 6–8 hours, adjusted according to response
  - Child: initial dose 250–500 mcg/kg every 8 hours, adjusted according to response; increased as needed up to 1 mg/kg every 8 hours (max per dose 40 mg every 8 hours)
  - Adult: (intravenous injections) 1 mg over 1 minute, dose may be repeated as needed at intervals of 2 minutes, maximum total dose is 5 mg in anaesthesia; max 10 mg per course
- Hypertension:
  - Neonate: initial dose 250 mcg/kg 3 times a day, then increased as needed up to 2 mg/kg 3 times per day
  - Child 1 month–11 years: initial dose 0.25–1 mg/kg 3 times per day, then increased to 5 mg/kg/day in divided doses, dose should be increased at weekly intervals
  - Child 12–17 years: initial dose 80 mg twice per day, then increased as needed up to 160–320 mg/day; dose should be increased at weekly intervals, slow-release preparations may be used for once-daily administration
  - Adult: initial dose 80 mg twice per day, dose increased each week as needed; maintenance 160–320 mg/day

- Prophylaxis of variceal bleeding in portal hypertension: oral initial dose 40 mg twice per day, increased to 80 mg twice per day (max per dose 160 mg twice per day), dose to be adjusted according to heart rate
- Phaeochromocytoma (only with an alpha blocker) in preparation for surgery: oral 60 mg for 3 days before surgery; or if not suitable for surgery: 30 mg/day
- Angina: initial dose oral 40 mg 2–3 times per day; maintenance 120–240 mg/ day
- Hypertrophic cardiomyopathy; anxiety tachycardia: oral 10–40 mg 3–4 times per day
- Anxiety with symptoms such as palpitation, sweating and tremor: oral 40 mg/day, increased if needed to 40 mg 3 times per day
- Prophylaxis after myocardial infarction: initial dose oral 40 mg 4 times per day for 2–4 days, then 80 mg twice per day, treatment to be started 5–21 days after infarction
- Essential tremor: initial dose oral 40 mg 2–3 times per day; maintenance 80–160 mg/day
- Migraine prophylaxis:
  - Child 2–11 years: initial dose 200–500 mcg/kg twice per day; usual dose 10–20 mg twice per day (max per dose 2 mg/kg twice per day)
  - Child 12–17 years: initial dose 20–40 mg twice per day; usual dose 40–80 mg twice per day (max per dose 120 mg); max 4 mg/kg per day
  - Adult: 80–240 mg daily in divided doses
- Arrhythmias:
  - Neonate: (oral) 250–500 mcg/kg 3 times per day, adjusted according to response; (slow intravenous injections) 20–50 mcg/kg, then 20–50 mcg/kg every 6–8 hours as needed, ECG monitoring required
  - Child: (oral) 250–500 mcg/kg 3–4 times per day (max per dose 1 mg/kg 4 times per day), adjusted according to response; max 160 mg/day; (slow intravenous injections) 25–50 mcg/kg, then 25–50 mcg/kg every 6–8 hours if required, ECG monitoring required
  - Adult: (oral) 10–40 mg 3–4 times per day; (intravenous injection) 1 mg over 1 minute, dose repeat at 2 minute intervals, max 10 mg per course (5 mg in anaesthesia)

- Tetralogy of Fallot:
  - Neonate: (oral) 0.25–1 mg/kg 2–3 times per day (max per dose 2 mg/kg 3 times a day); (slow intravenous injections) initial dose 15–20 mcg/kg (max per dose 100 mcg/kg), then 15–20 mcg/kg every 12 hours if required, ECG monitoring is required
  - Child 1 month–11 years: (oral) 0.25–1 mg/kg 3–4 times per day (max dose to be given in divided doses; max 5 mg/kg per day); (slow intravenous injections) initial dose 15–20 mcg/kg (max per dose 100 mcg/kg), then 15–20 mcg/kg every 6–8 hours as needed, ECG monitoring is required

 Dosing Tips

- With administration by intravenous injection, excessive bradycardia can occur and may be countered with intravenous injection of atropine sulfate

Overdose

- Light-headedness, dizziness, possibly syncope as a result of bradycardia and hypotension; heart failure may be precipitated or exacerbated
- With intravenous administration, excessive bradycardia can occur; may be countered with intravenous injection of atropine sulfate

Long-Term Use

- Safe

Habit Forming

- No

How to Stop

- Should not be discontinued abruptly; instead gradually reduce dosage over 1–2 weeks
- May exacerbate angina, and there are reports of tachyarrhythmias or myocardial infarction with rapid discontinuation in patients with cardiac disease

Pharmacokinetics

- Apparent elimination half-life of immediate-release preparation is 3–6 hours
- Following oral dosing with the modified-release preparation of propranolol, the blood profile is flatter than after conventional propranolol, but the half-life is increased to 10–20 hours. The liver removes up to 90% of an oral dose and the elimination half-life is 3–6 hours

 Drug Interactions

- Cimetidine, oral contraceptives, ciprofloxacin, hydralazine, hydroxychloroquine, loop diuretics, certain SSRIs (with CYP 2D6 metabolism), and phenothiazines can increase levels and/or effects of propranolol
- Use with calcium channel blockers can be synergistic or additive, use with caution
- Barbiturates, penicillin, rifampin, calcium, aluminium salts, thyroid hormones, and cholestyramine can decrease effects of beta blockers
- NSAIDs, sulfinpyrazone, and salicylates inhibit prostaglandin synthesis and may inhibit the antihypertensive activity of beta blockers
- Propranolol can increase adverse effects of gabapentin and benzodiazepines
- Propranolol can increase levels of lidocaine, resulting in toxicity, and increase the anticoagulant effect of warfarin
- Increased postural hypotension with prazosin and peripheral ischaemia with ergot alkaloids
- Sudden discontinuation of clonidine while on beta blockers or when stopping together can cause life-threatening increases in blood pressure

 Other Warnings/Precautions

- Caution is advised in patients with a history of hypersensitivity – may increase sensitivity to allergens and result in more serious hypersensitivity response; may also reduce response to adrenaline
- Use with caution in patients with myasthenia gravis, diabetes, psoriasis or a history of obstructive airways disease (introduce cautiously)
- Symptoms of hypoglycaemia and thyrotoxicosis may be masked
- Caution in patients with first-degree AV block
- Caution in patients with portal hypertension (risk of deterioration in liver function)

Do Not Use

- In patients with asthma, bronchospasm, or history of obstructive airways disease
- In patients with cardiogenic shock; hypotension; marked bradycardia; metabolic acidosis; phaeochromocytoma (apart from specific use with alpha blockers)
- In patients with Prinzmetal's angina (in adults); second-degree AV block; severe peripheral arterial disease; sick sinus syndrome; third-degree AV block; uncontrolled heart failure
- If there is proven allergy to propranolol

SPECIAL POPULATIONS

Renal Impairment

- Caution; dose reduction may be required

Hepatic Impairment

- Reduce oral dose

Cardiac Impairment

- Do not use in cardiogenic shock, marked bradycardia, Prinzmetal's angina (in adults), second-degree AV block, sick sinus syndrome, third-degree AV block, uncontrolled heart failure

Elderly

- Use with caution
- Prescription potentially inappropriate in certain circumstances:
  - In combination with verapamil or diltiazem (risk of heart block)
  - In patients with bradycardia (heart rate less than 50 beats per minute), type II heart block or complete heart block (risk of complete heart block, asystole)
  - In diabetes mellitus patients with frequent hypoglycaemic episodes (risk of suppressing hypoglycaemic symptoms)
  - In a history of asthma requiring treatment (risk of increased bronchospasm)

 Children and Adolescents

- Adjust dose: see How to Dose section
- For slow intravenous injection, give over at least 3–5 minutes; rate of administration should not exceed 1 mg/min. May be diluted with sodium chloride 0.9% or glucose 5%; incompatible with bicarbonate
- Avoid abrupt withdrawal

 Pregnancy

- Controlled studies have not been conducted in pregnant women
- Very limited human data does not rule out foetal toxicity
- A meta-analysis suggests may increase cleft lip and/or palate and neural tube defects in the infant
- May cause adverse effects on foetal growth, risk of congenital heart defects
- May reduce perfusion of the placenta
- Use only if potential benefits outweigh the potential risks to the foetus
- Use near term may result in neonatal beta-adrenoceptor blockade leading to neonatal bradycardia, hypotension, and hypoglycaemia

Breastfeeding

- Small amounts found in mother's breast milk
- Considered compatible with breastfeeding
- Considered the beta blocker of choice in breastfeeding

THE ART OF PSYCHOPHARMACOLOGY

Potential Advantages

- Patients who do not respond to or tolerate other options
- Patients with autonomic hyperactivity

Potential Disadvantages

- Multiple potential undesirable adverse effects, including bradycardia, hypotension, and fatigue

Primary Target Symptoms

- Migraine frequency and severity
- Tremor
- Effects of stress from prior traumatic experience
- Aggression, agitation

Pearls

- Often used in combination with other drugs in migraine, which may allow patients to better tolerate medications that cause tremor, such as valproate

Propranolol hydrochloride (Continued)

- May worsen depression, but helpful for anxiety
- 50–70% of patients with essential tremor receive some relief, usually with about 50% improvement or greater

- May be used for lithium-induced tremor
- Propranolol may theoretically block the effects of stress from prior traumatic experiences, but this is unproven and data thus far are mixed

 Suggested Reading

Brunet A, Poundja J, Tremblay J, et al. Trauma reactivation under the influence of propranolol decreases posttraumatic stress symptoms and disorders: 3 open-label trials. J Clin Psychopharmacol 2011;31(4):547–50.

Cohen H, Kaplan Z, Koresh O, et al. Early post-stressor intervention with propranolol is ineffective in preventing posttraumatic stress responses in an animal model for PTSD. Eur Neuropsychopharmacol 2011;21(3):230–40.

Fleminger S, Greenwood RJ, Oliver DL. Pharmacological management for agitation and aggression in people with acquired brain injury. Cochrane Database Syst Rev 2003;(1):CD003299.

Lyons KE, Pahwa R. Pharmacotherapy of essential tremor: an overview of existing and upcoming agents. CNS Drugs 2008;22(12):1037–45.

Silberstein SD. Preventive migraine treatment. Neurol Clin 2009;27(2):429–43.

Quetiapine

Brands

- Atrolak XL
- Biquelle XL
- Brancico XL
- Mintreleq XL
- Sondate XL
- Seroquel; Seroquel XL
- Zaluron XL

Generic?

Yes

Class

- Neuroscience-based nomenclature: low-dose quetiapine: pharmacology domain – histamine; mode of action – receptor antagonist; middle-dose quetiapine: pharmacology domain – norepinephrine; mode of action: reuptake inhibitor and presynaptic receptor antagonist; upper-dose quetiapine: pharmacology domain – dopamine, serotonin, norepinephrine; mode of action – multimodal
- Atypical antipsychotic (serotonin-dopamine antagonist; second-generation antipsychotic; also a mood stabiliser)

Commonly Prescribed for

(bold for BNF indication)

- **Schizophrenia**
- **Treatment of mania in bipolar disorder**
- **Treatment of depression in bipolar disorder**
- **Prevention of mania and depression in bipolar disorder**
- **Adjunctive treatment of major depression**
- Mixed mania
- Behavioural disturbances in dementias
- Behavioural disturbances in Lewy body disease
- Psychosis associated with levodopa treatment in Parkinson's disease
- Behavioural disturbances in children and adolescents
- Disorders associated with problems with impulse control
- Severe treatment-resistant anxiety

How the Drug Works

- Blocks dopamine 2 receptors, reducing positive symptoms of psychosis and stabilising affective symptoms

- Blocks serotonin 2A receptors, causing enhancement of dopamine release in certain brain regions and thus reducing motor side effects and possibly improving cognitive and affective symptoms
- *Interactions at a myriad of other neurotransmitter receptors may contribute to quetiapine's efficacy in treatment-resistant depression or bipolar depression, especially 5HT1A partial agonist action, norepinephrine reuptake blockade and 5HT2C antagonist and 5HT7 antagonist properties
- *Specifically, actions at 5HT1A receptors may contribute to efficacy for cognitive and affective symptoms in some patients, especially at moderate to high doses
- Quetiapine is a dopamine D1, dopamine D2, 5HT2, alpha 1 adrenoceptor, and histamine 1 receptor antagonist

How Long Until It Works

- Psychotic and manic symptoms can improve within 1 week, but it may take several weeks for full effect on behaviour as well as on cognition and affective stabilisation
- Classically recommended to wait at least 4–6 weeks to determine efficacy of drug, but in practice some patients require up to 16–20 weeks to show a good response, especially on cognitive symptoms

If It Works

- Most often reduces positive symptoms in schizophrenia but does not eliminate them
- Can improve negative symptoms, as well as aggressive, cognitive, and affective symptoms in schizophrenia
- Most patients with schizophrenia do not have a total remission of symptoms but rather a reduction of symptoms by about a third
- Perhaps 5–15% of schizophrenic patients can experience an overall improvement of >50–60%, especially when receiving stable treatment for >1 year
- Such patients are considered super-responders or "awakeners" since they may be well enough to be employed, live independently, and sustain long-term relationships
- Many bipolar patients may experience a reduction of symptoms by half or more

- Continue treatment until reaching a plateau of improvement
- After reaching a satisfactory plateau, continue treatment for at least 1 year after first episode of psychosis, but it may be preferable to continue treatment indefinitely to avoid subsequent episodes
- After any subsequent episodes of psychosis, treatment may need to be indefinite
- Treatment may not only reduce mania but also prevent recurrences of mania in bipolar disorder

If It Doesn't Work

- Try one of the other atypical antipsychotics (risperidone or olanzapine should be considered first before considering other agents such as aripiprazole, amisulpride or lurasidone)
- If 2 or more antipsychotic monotherapies do not work, consider clozapine
- Some patients may require treatment with a conventional antipsychotic
- If no first-line atypical antipsychotic is effective, consider higher doses or augmentation with valproate or lamotrigine
- Consider non-concordance and switch to another antipsychotic with fewer side effects or to an antipsychotic that can be given by depot injection
- Consider initiating rehabilitation and psychotherapy such as cognitive remediation
- Consider presence of concomitant drug abuse

⚖ Best Augmenting Combos for Partial Response or Treatment Resistance

- Valproic acid (Depakote, Epilim)
- Other mood-stabilising anticonvulsants (carbamazepine, oxcarbazepine, lamotrigine)
- Lithium
- Benzodiazepines

Tests

Before starting an atypical antipsychotic

* Measure weight, BMI, and waist circumference
- Get baseline personal and family history of diabetes, obesity, dyslipidaemia, hypertension, and cardiovascular disease

* Check pulse and blood pressure, fasting plasma glucose or glycosylated haemoglobin (HbA1c), fasting lipid profile, and prolactin level
- Full blood count (FBC), urea and electrolytes (including creatinine and eGFR), liver function tests (LFTs)
- Assessment of nutritional status, diet, and level of physical activity
- Determine if the patient:
  - is overweight (BMI 25.0–29.9)
  - is obese (BMI ≥30)
  - has pre-diabetes – fasting plasma glucose: 5.5 mmol/L to 6.9 mmol/L or HbA1c: 42 to 47 mmol/mol (6.0 to 6.4%)
  - has diabetes – fasting plasma glucose: >7.0 mmol/L or HbA1c: ≥48 mmol/L (≥6.5%)
  - has hypertension (BP >140/90 mm Hg)
  - has dyslipidaemia (increased total cholesterol, LDL cholesterol, and triglycerides; decreased HDL cholesterol)
- Treat or refer such patients for treatment, including nutrition and weight management, physical activity counselling, smoking cessation, and medical management
- Baseline ECG for: inpatients; those with a personal history or risk factor for cardiac disease (quetiapine can cause QT-interval prolongation)

Children and adolescents:
- As for adults
- Also check history of congenital heart problems, history of dizziness when stressed or on exertion, history of long-QT syndrome, family history of long-QT syndrome, bradycardia, myocarditis, family history of cardiac myopathies, low K/low Mg/low Ca
- Measure weight, BMI, and waist circumference plotted on a growth chart
- Pulse, BP plotted on a percentile chart
- ECG: note for QTc interval: machine-generated may be incorrect in children as different formula needed if HR <60 or >100
- Baseline prolactin levels

Monitoring after starting an atypical antipsychotic

- FBC annually to detect chronic bone marrow suppression, stop treatment if neutrophils fall below 1.5x10⁹/L and refer to specialist care if neutrophils fall below 0.5x10⁹/L
- Urea and electrolytes (including creatinine and eGFR) annually
- LFTs annually

Quetiapine (Continued)

- Prolactin levels at 6 months and then annually (quetiapine is less likely to increase prolactin levels)
* Weight/BMI/waist circumference, weekly for the first 6 weeks, then at 12 weeks, at 1 year, and then annually
* Pulse and blood pressure at 12 weeks, 1 year, and then annually
* Fasting blood glucose, HbA1c, and blood lipids at 12 weeks, at 1 year, and then annually
* For patients with type 2 diabetes, measure HbA1c at 3–6 month intervals until stable, then every 6 months
* Even in patients without known diabetes, be vigilant for the rare but life-threatening onset of diabetic ketoacidosis, which always requires immediate treatment, by monitoring for the rapid onset of polyuria, polydipsia, weight loss, nausea, vomiting, dehydration, rapid respiration, weakness and clouding of sensorium, even coma
* If HbA1c remains ≥48 mmol/mol (6.5%) then drug therapy should be offered, e.g. metformin
- Treat or refer for treatment or consider switching to another atypical antipsychotic for patients who become overweight, obese, pre-diabetic, diabetic, hypertensive, or dyslipidaemic while receiving an atypical antipsychotic

Children and adolescents:
- As for adults
- Weight/BMI/waist circumference, weekly for the first 6 weeks, then at 12 weeks, then every 6 months, plotted on a growth/percentile chart
- Height every 6 months, plotted on a growth chart
- Pulse and blood pressure at 12 weeks, then every 6 months plotted on a percentile chart
- ECG prior to starting and 2 weeks after dose increase for monitoring of QTc interval. Machine-generated may be incorrect in children as different formula needed if HR <60 or >100
- Prolactin levels: prior to starting and after 12 weeks, 24 weeks, and 6-monthly thereafter. Consider additional monitoring in young adults (under 25) who have not yet reached peak bone mass. Quetiapine is only associated with marginal increase of prolactin
- In prepubertal children monitor sexual maturation
- Post-pubertal children and young persons monitor sexual side effects (both sexes: loss of libido, sexual dysfunction, galactorrhoea, infertility; male: diminished ejaculate gynaecomastia; female: oligorrhoea/amenorrhoea, reduced vaginal lubrication, dyspareunia, acne, hirsutism)

SIDE EFFECTS

How Drug Causes Side Effects
- By blocking histamine 1 receptors in the brain, it can cause sedation and possibly weight gain
- By blocking alpha 1 adrenergic receptors, it can cause dizziness, sedation, and hypotension
- By blocking muscarinic 1 receptors, it can cause dry mouth, constipation, and sedation
- By blocking dopamine 2 receptors in the striatum, it can cause motor side effects (rare)
- Mechanism of weight gain and increased incidence of diabetes and dyslipidaemia with atypical antipsychotics is unknown

Notable Side Effects
- Dose-dependent weight gain
* May increase risk for diabetes and dyslipidaemia
* Dizziness, sedation
- Dry mouth, constipation
- Dyspepsia, abdominal pain
- Tachycardia
- Orthostatic hypotension, usually during initial dose titration
- Theoretical risk of tardive dyskinesia

Common or very common
- CNS/PNS: blurred vision, dysarthria, headache, irritability, sleep disorders, suicidal behaviour (particularly on initiation), suicidal ideation (particularly on initiation)
- CVS: palpitations, syncope
- GIT: dyspepsia, increased appetite
- Resp: dyspnoea, rhinitis
- Other: asthenia, fever, hyperglycaemia, peripheral oedema, syncope, withdrawal syndrome

Uncommon
- Blood disorders: anaemia, thrombocytopenia
- Other: diabetes mellitus, dysphagia, hyponatraemia, hypothyroidism, sexual dysfunction, skin reactions

Rare or very rare
- GIT: gastrointestinal disorders, hepatic disorders, pancreatitis
- Other: angioedema, breast swelling, hypothermia, menstrual disorder, metabolic syndrome, rhabdomyolysis, severe cutaneous adverse reactions (SCARs), SIADH

Life-Threatening or Dangerous Side Effects
- Hyperglycaemia, in some cases extreme and associated with ketoacidosis or hyperosmolar coma or death
- Rare neuroleptic malignant syndrome
- Rare seizures
- Increased risk of death and cerebrovascular events in elderly patients with dementia-related psychosis
- Sudden death
- Neonatal withdrawal syndrome
- Agranulocytosis
- Embolism and thrombosis

Weight Gain

- Many patients experience and/or can be significant in amount at effective antipsychotic doses
- Can become a health problem in some
- May be less than for some antipsychotics, more than for others

Sedation

- Frequent and can be significant in amount
- Some patients may not tolerate it
- More than for some other antipsychotics, but never say always as not a problem in everyone
- Can wear off over time
- Can re-emerge as dose increases and then wear off again over time
- Not necessarily increased as dose is raised
- Drowsiness may affect performance of skilled tasks (e.g. driving or operating machinery), especially at start of treatment; effects of alcohol are enhanced

What To Do About Side Effects
- Wait
- Wait
- Wait
- Reduce the dose
- Low-dose benzodiazepine or beta blocker may reduce akathisia
- Take more of the dose at bedtime to help reduce daytime sedation
- Weight loss, exercise programmes, and medical management for high BMIs, diabetes, and dyslipidaemia
- Switch to another antipsychotic (atypical) – quetiapine or clozapine are best in cases of tardive dyskinesia

Best Augmenting Agents for Side Effects
- Dystonia: antimuscarinic drugs (e.g. procyclidine) as oral or IM depending on the severity; botulinum toxin if antimuscarinics not effective
- Parkinsonism: antimuscarinic drugs (e.g. procyclidine)
- Akathisia: beta blocker propranolol (30–80 mg/day) or low-dose benzodiazepine (e.g. 0.5–3.0 mg/day of clonazepam) may help; other agents that may be tried include the 5HT2 antagonists such as cyproheptadine (16 mg/day) or mirtazapine (15 mg at night – caution in bipolar disorder); clonidine (0.2–0.8 mg/day) may be tried if the above ineffective
- Tardive dyskinesia: stop any antimuscarinic, consider tetrabenazine
- Addition of low doses (2.5–5 mg) of aripiprazole can reverse the hyperprolactinaemia/galactorrhoea caused by other antipsychotics
- Addition of aripiprazole (5–15 mg/day) or metformin (500–2000 mg/day) to weight-inducing atypical antipsychotics such as olanzapine and clozapine can help mitigate against weight gain

DOSING AND USE

Usual Dosage Range
- Schizophrenia: 300–750 mg/day in 2 divided doses (quetiapine IR); 300–800 mg once daily (quetiapine MR)

- Treatment of mania in bipolar disorder: 400–800 mg/day in 2 divided doses (quetiapine IR); 400–800 mg once daily (quetiapine MR)
- Treatment of depression in bipolar disorder: 300–600 mg/day
- Prevention of mania and depression in bipolar disorder: 300–800 mg/day in divided doses (quetiapine IR); 300–800 mg once daily (quetiapine MR)
- Adjunctive treatment of major depression: 150–300 mg once daily (quetiapine MR)

Dosage Forms

- Immediate-release (IR) tablet 25 mg, 100 mg, 150 mg, 200 mg, 300 mg, 400 mg
- Modified-release (MR) tablet 50 mg, 150 mg, 200 mg, 300 mg, 400 mg, 600 mg
- Oral suspension 20 mg/mL

How to Dose

Adults:

* Schizophrenia:
- Quetiapine IR: initial dose 25 mg twice per day; increase by 25–50 mg twice per day each day until desired efficacy is reached; max 750 mg/day; in elderly the rate of dose titration may need to be slower and the daily dose lower
- Quetiapine MR: 300 mg once daily for day 1, then 600 mg once daily for day 2, then, adjusted according to response, usual dose 600 mg once daily, max dose under specialist supervision; max 800 mg/day; in elderly initially 50 mg/day adjusted according to response by increments of 50 mg/day
- In practice, can start adults with schizophrenia under age 65 with same doses as recommended for acute bipolar mania

* Bipolar mania:
- Quetiapine IR: initiate in twice-daily doses, totalling 100 mg/day on day 1, increasing to 400 mg/day on day 4 in increments of up to 100 mg/day; further dosage adjustments up to 800 mg/day by day 6 should be in increments of no greater than 200 mg/day; in elderly the rate of dose titration may need to be slower and the daily dose lower (starting dose in 12.5–25 mg daily; usual maintenance dose is 75–125 mg/day; max dose 200–300 mg/day)

- Quetiapine MR: 300 mg once daily for day 1, then 600 mg once daily for day 2, then, adjusted according to response, usual dose 400–800 mg once daily; in elderly initially 50 mg/day adjusted according to response by increments of 50 mg/day

* Bipolar depression:
- Quetiapine IR or quetiapine MR: 50 mg at bedtime; titrate as needed to reach 300 mg/day by day 4; adjust dose according to response up to a max dose of 600 mg/day; in elderly the rate of dose titration may need to be slower and daily dose lower

* Prevention of mania and depression in bipolar disorder:
- Quetiapine IR: continue at the dose effective for treatment of bipolar disorder and adjust to lowest effective dose; usual dose 300–800 mg/day in 2 divided doses
- Quetiapine IR or quetiapine MR: continue at the dose effective for treatment of bipolar disorder and adjust to lowest effective dose; usual dose 300–800 mg once daily

* Adjunctive treatment of major depression:
- Quetiapine MR: 50 mg (evening dose) for 2 days, then 150 mg/day for 2 days, then, adjusted according to response, usual dose 150–300 mg/day; in elderly initial dose 50 mg/day for 3 days, then increased as needed to 100 mg/day for 4 days, then adjusted by increments of 50 mg, adjusted according to response, usual dose 50–300 mg/day, dose of 300 mg should not be reached before 22nd day of treatment

Children and adolescents:

* Schizophrenia:
- Quetiapine IR: initial dose 25 mg twice per day, adjusted according to response by 25–50 mg; max 750 mg/day; quetiapine MR: initial dose 50 mg once daily, adjusted according to response by 50 mg/day, usual dose 400–800 mg/day; max 800 mg/day

* Mania:
- Quetiapine IR: 25 mg twice per day for day 1, 50 mg twice per day for day 2, 100 mg twice per day for day 3, 150 mg twice per day for day 4, 200 mg twice per day for day 5, then adjusted according to response by up to 100 mg/day, usual dose 400–600 mg/day in 2 divided doses
- See also The Art of Switching section, after Pearls

Quetiapine (Continued)

Dosing Tips

- First episode, minimum effective dose in schizophrenia: 150 mg/day (estimate, as too few data available); for subsequent episodes 300 mg/day
- Max dose for schizophrenia 750 mg/day
- Max dose for bipolar affective disorder 800 mg/day
- To treat drug-induced akathisia: switch antipsychotic to quetiapine (lowest dose possible)
- *More may be much more: clinical practice suggests quetiapine often underdosed, then switched prior to adequate trials
- Clinical practice suggests that at low doses it may be a sedative hypnotic, possibly due to potent H1 antihistamine actions, but this can risk numerous antipsychotic-related side effects and there are many other options
- *Initial target dose of 400–800 mg/day should be reached in most cases to optimise the chances of success in treating acute psychosis and acute mania, but many patients are not adequately dosed in clinical practice
- Many patients do well with immediate-release as a single daily oral dose, usually at bedtime
- Recommended titration to 400 mg/day by the fourth day can often be achieved when necessary to control acute symptoms
- Rapid dose escalation in manic or psychotic patients may lessen sedative side effects
- *Higher doses generally achieve greater response for manic or psychotic symptoms
- In contrast, some patients with bipolar depression may respond well to doses less than 300 mg/day and as little as 25 mg/day
- Dosing in major depression may be even lower than in bipolar depression, and dosing may be even lower still in anxiety disorders
- *Occasional patients may require more than 800–1200 mg/day for psychosis or mania
- Rather than raise the dose above these levels in acutely agitated patients requiring acute antipsychotic actions, consider augmentation with a benzodiazepine or conventional antipsychotic, either orally or intramuscularly
- Rather than raise the dose above these levels in partial responders, consider augmentation with a mood-stabilising anticonvulsant such as valproate or lamotrigine
- Children and elderly should generally be dosed at the lower end of the dosage spectrum
- MR preparations should not be chewed or crushed but rather should be swallowed whole
- MR preparations may theoretically generate increased concentrations of active metabolite norquetiapine, with theoretically improved profile for affective and anxiety disorders
- Treatment should be suspended if absolute neutrophil count falls below 1.5×10^9/L
- Patients can be switched from immediate-release to modified-release tablets at the equivalent daily dose; to maintain clinical response, dose titration may be required

Overdose

- Can be fatal; signs and symptoms may include lethargy, delirium, sedation, slurred speech, hypotension, hypothermia, sinus tachycardia, arrhythmias and QT prolongation, respiratory depression, rhabdomyolysis, NMS
- Arrhythmias may respond to correction of hypoxia, acidosis, and other biochemical abnormalities, but specialist advice should be sought if arrhythmias result from a prolonged QT interval; the use of some anti-arrhythmic drugs can worsen such arrhythmias
- Dystonic reactions are rapidly abolished by injection of drugs such as procyclidine hydrochloride or diazepam (emulsion preferred)

Long-Term Use

- Approved for long-term maintenance in schizophrenia and bipolar disorder

Habit Forming

- No

How to Stop

- See also the Switching section of individual agents for how to stop quetiapine
- Rapid discontinuation may lead to rebound psychosis and worsening of symptoms and insomnia

- There is a high risk of relapse if medication is stopped after 1–2 years. Withdrawal of antipsychotic drugs after long-term therapy should always be gradual and closely monitored to avoid the risk of acute withdrawal syndromes or rapid relapse. Patients should be monitored for 2 years after withdrawal of antipsychotic medication for signs and symptoms of relapse

Pharmacokinetics

- Half-life of quetiapine about 7 hours, and norquetiapine about 12 hours
- Quetiapine is a substrate for CYP450 3A4
- Food may slightly increase absorption

 Drug Interactions

- CYP450 3A4 inhibitors and CYP450 2D6 inhibitors may reduce clearance of quetiapine and thus raise quetiapine plasma levels
- Concomitant use of quetiapine with CYP450 3A4 inhibitors such as ketaconazole is contraindicated; it is also not recommended to consume grapefruit juice while on quetiapine therapy
- CYP450 3A4 inducers such as carbamazepine can significantly reduce the plasma levels of quetiapine rendering it less effective
- May increase effect of anti-hypertensive agents
- Caution should be exercised when quetiapine is used concomitantly with medicinal products known to cause electrolyte imbalance or that increase the QT interval

 Other Warnings/Precautions

- All antipsychotics should be used with caution in patients with angle-closure glaucoma, blood disorders, cardiovascular disease, depression, diabetes, epilepsy and susceptibility to seizures, history of jaundice, myasthenia gravis, Parkinson's disease, photosensitivity, prostatic hypertrophy, severe respiratory disorders
- Quetiapine should be used cautiously in patients at risk for aspiration pneumonia, as dysphagia has been reported
- Priapism has been reported

- Use with caution in patients with known cardiovascular disease or cerebrovascular disease
- Use with caution in patients with conditions that predispose to hypotension (dehydration, overheating)
- Monitor patients for activation of suicidal ideation, especially children and adolescents
- Avoid use with drugs that increase the QT interval and in patients with risk factors for prolonged QT interval
- Increased risk of stroke in patients with dementia
- Has been linked to cases of new onset diabetes and ketoacidosis. Risks may be dose-related with daily doses of 400 mg or more clearly being linked to changes in HbA1c
- May increase seizure threshold up to two-fold and linked to higher rates of drug-related seizure
- Use with caution in patients with a history of sleep apnoea or with risk factors for sleep apnoea

Do Not Use

- With concomitant administration of CYP450 3A4 inhibitors, such as HIV-protease inhibitors, azole-antifungal agents, erythromycin; clarithromycin is contraindicated
- If there is a proven allergy to quetiapine

Renal Impairment

- No dose adjustment required

Hepatic Impairment

- Downward dose adjustment may be necessary
- Extensively metabolised by the liver but short half-life. Clearance reduced on average by 30% in hepatic impairment so small adjustments in dose may be necessary. Caution recommended in hepatic impairment
- Caution – risk of increased plasma concentrations. Quetiapine IR: initial dose 25 mg/day, increased daily by increments of 25–50 mg/day; quetiapine MR: initial dose 50 mg/day, increased daily by increments of 50 mg/day

Quetiapine (Continued)

Cardiac Impairment

- Drug should be used with caution because of risk of orthostatic hypotension
- Quetiapine can cause QT-interval prolongation
- An ECG required, particularly if physical examination identifies cardiovascular risk factors, personal history of cardiovascular disease, or if the patient is being admitted as an inpatient

Elderly

- Lower doses are generally used (e.g. 25–100 mg twice per day), although higher doses may be used if tolerated
- Delirium: oral 12.5–50 mg twice per day. This may be increased every 12 hours to 200 mg daily if it is tolerated
- Agitation/ psychosis in dementia: starting dose is 12.5–25 mg/day. Usual maintenance dose is 50–100 mg/day and max dose is 100–300 mg/day
- Although atypical antipsychotics are commonly used for behavioural disturbances in dementia, no agent has been approved for treatment of elderly patients with dementia-related psychosis
- Elderly patients with dementia-related psychosis treated with atypical antipsychotics are at an increased risk of death compared to placebo, and also have an increased risk of cerebrovascular events

Children and Adolescents

- Not licensed for use in children in UK, nevertheless approved for use under expert supervision for children with schizophrenia or mania aged 12–17 years
- Licensed in other countries for children with schizophrenia ages 13–17 years and for children with acute mania ages 10 to 17 years
- Clinical experience and early data suggest quetiapine may be safe and effective for behavioural disturbances in children and adolescents

Before you prescribe:

- Do not offer antipsychotic medication when transient or attenuated psychotic symptoms or other mental state changes associated with distress, impairment, or help-seeking behaviour are not sufficient for a diagnosis of psychosis or schizophrenia. Consider individual CBT with or without family therapy and other treatments recommended for anxiety, depression, substance use, or emerging personality disorder
- For first-episode psychosis (FEP) antipsychotic medication should only be started by a specialist following a comprehensive multidisciplinary assessment and in conjunction with recommended psychological interventions (CBT, family therapy)
- As first-line treatment: allow patient to choose from aripiprazole, olanzapine or risperidone. As second-line treatment switch to alternative from list. Consider quetiapine depending on desired profile
- For bipolar disorder: if bipolar disorder is suspected in primary care in children or adolescents refer them to a specialist service
- Choice of antipsychotic medication should be an informed choice depending on individual factors and side-effect profile (metabolic, cardiovascular, extrapyramidal, hormonal, other)
- All children and young people with FEP/ bipolar should be supported with sleep management, anxiety management, exercise and activation schedules, and healthy diet
- Where a child or young person presents with self-harm and suicidal thoughts the immediate risk management may take first priority
- Short-term treatment of behavioural disturbances in children and adolescents (under expert supervision). There are many reasons for challenging behaviours and consideration should be given to possible physical, psychosocial and environmental causes. These should be addressed first. Consider behavioural interventions and family support. Consider trauma-informed practice. Pharmacological treatment can be offered alongside the above
- A risk management plan is important prior to start of medication because of the possible increase in suicidal ideation and behaviours in adolescents and young adults

Practical notes:

- Carefully weigh the risks and benefits of pharmacological treatment against the risks and benefits of non-treatment and make sure to document this in the patient's chart
- Monitor weight, weekly for the first 6 weeks, then at 12 weeks, and then every 6 months (plotted on a growth chart)
- Monitor height every 6 months (plotted on a growth chart)

- Monitor waist circumference every 6 months (plotted on a percentile chart)
- Monitor pulse and blood pressure (plotted on a percentile chart) at 12 weeks and then every 6 months
- Monitor fasting blood glucose, HbA1c, blood lipid and prolactin levels at 12 weeks and then every 6 months
- Monitor for activation of suicidal ideation at the beginning of treatment. Inform parents or guardians of this risk so they can help observe child or adolescent patients
- If it does not work: review child's/young person's profile, consider new/changing contributing individual or systemic factors such as peer or family conflict. Consider drug/substance misuse. Consider dose adjustment before switching or augmentation. Be vigilant of polypharmacy especially in complex and highly vulnerable children/adolescents
- Consider non-concordance by parent or child, consider non-concordance in adolescents, address underlying reasons for non-concordance
- Children are more sensitive to most side effects
  ○ There is an inverse relationship between age and incidence of EPS
  ○ Exposure to antipsychotics during childhood and young age is associated with a three-fold increase of diabetes mellitus
  ○ Treatment with all second-generation antipsychotics (SGAs) has been associated with changes in most lipid parameters
  ○ Weight gain correlates with time on treatment. Any childhood obesity is associated with obesity in adults
- May tolerate lower doses better
- Dose adjustments may be necessary in the presence of interacting drugs
- Re-evaluate the need for continued treatment regularly
- Provide Medicines for Children leaflet for quetiapine for schizophrenia-bipolar-disorder-and-agitation
- Monitoring of endocrine function (weight, height, sexual maturation and menses) is required when a child is taking an antipsychotic drug that is known to cause hyperprolactinaemia

Pregnancy

- Human data does not suggest increased risk of malformations but is not conclusive
- Some animal studies have shown reproductive toxicity
- There is a risk of abnormal muscle movements and withdrawal symptoms in newborns whose mothers took an antipsychotic during the third trimester; symptoms may include agitation, abnormally increased or decreased muscle tone, tremor, sleepiness, severe difficulty breathing, and difficulty feeding
- Psychotic symptoms may worsen during pregnancy and some form of treatment may be necessary
- Olanzapine and clozapine have been associated with maternal hyperglycaemia which may lead to developmental toxicity, risk may also apply for other atypical antipsychotics
- Psychotic symptoms may worsen during pregnancy and some form of treatment may be necessary
- Use in pregnancy may be justified if the benefit of continued treatment exceeds any associated risk
- Switching antipsychotics may increase the risk of relapse
- Quetiapine may be preferable to anticonvulsant mood stabilisers if treatment or prophylaxis are required during pregnancy

Breastfeeding

- Very small amounts expected in mother's breast milk
- Haloperidol is considered to be the preferred first-generation antipsychotic, and quetiapine the preferred second-generation antipsychotic
- Infants of women who choose to breastfeed should be monitored for possible adverse effects

THE ART OF PSYCHOPHARMACOLOGY
Potential Advantages

- Bipolar depression
- Some cases of psychosis and bipolar disorder refractory to treatment with other antipsychotics

∗ Patients with Parkinson's disease who need an antipsychotic or mood stabiliser

∗ Patients with Lewy body dementias who need an antipsychotic or mood stabiliser

• Children and adolescents: can provide more sedation than some other atypical antipsychotics if that is desired

• No extrapyramidal symptoms, little effect on prolactin

Potential Disadvantages

• Patients requiring rapid onset of action

• Patients who have difficulty tolerating sedation

• Children and adolescents: can result in more sedation than some other atypical antipsychotics if that is NOT desired

Primary Target Symptoms

• Positive symptoms of psychosis

• Negative symptoms of psychosis

• Cognitive symptoms

• Unstable mood (both depression and mania)

• Aggressive symptoms

• Insomnia and anxiety

 Pearls

∗ May be the preferred antipsychotic for psychosis in Lewy body disease

• Anecdotal reports of efficacy in treatment-refractory cases and positive symptoms of psychoses other than schizophrenia

∗ Efficacy may be underestimated for psychosis and mania since quetiapine is often under-dosed in clinical practice

∗ Approved in bipolar depression

• The active metabolite of quetiapine, norquetiapine, has the additional properties of norepinephrine reuptake inhibition and antagonism of 5HT2C receptors, which may contribute to therapeutic effects for mood and cognition

• Dosing differs depending on the indication, with high-dose mechanisms including robust blockade of D2 receptors above 60% occupancy and equal or greater 5HT2A blockade; medium-dose mechanisms including moderate amounts of NET inhibition combined with 5HT2C antagonism and 5HT1A partial agonism; and low-dose mechanisms including H1 antagonism and 5HT1A partial agonism and, to a lesser extent, NET inhibition and 5HT2C antagonism

• More sedation than some other antipsychotics, which may be of benefit in acutely manic or psychotic patients but not for stabilised patients in long-term maintenance

∗ Essentially limited motor side effects or prolactin elevation

• May have less weight gain than some antipsychotics, more than others

∗ Controversial as to whether quetiapine has more or less risk of diabetes and dyslipidaemia than some other antipsychotics

• Commonly used at low doses to augment other atypical antipsychotics, but such antipsychotic polypharmacy has not been systematically studied

• Commonly used at low doses to help reduce distress and agitation in anxiety disorders and emotionally unstable personality disorder

• Anecdotal reports of efficacy in PTSD, including symptoms of sleep disturbance and anxiety

• Patients with inadequate responses to atypical antipsychotics may benefit from determination of plasma drug levels and, if low, a dosage increase even beyond the usual prescribing limits

• For treatment-resistant patients, especially those with impulsivity, aggression, violence, and self-harm, long-term polypharmacy with 2 atypical antipsychotics or with 1 atypical antipsychotic and 1 conventional antipsychotic may be useful or even necessary while closely monitoring

• In such cases, it may be beneficial to combine 1 depot antipsychotic with 1 oral antipsychotic

• Quetiapine has robust efficacy in all aspects of bipolar disorder including prevention of bipolar depression

• Quetiapine has the best supporting data and may be considered treatment of choice in rapid cycling bipolar disorder

• RCTs have demonstrated clear efficacy for doses of 300–600 mg/day as monotherapy for bipolar depression; may be superior to both lithium and paroxetine

• Quetiapine also prevents relapse into depression and mania

• Quetiapine is not associated with switching to mania

• Quetiapine may be effective in choreiform movements in Huntington's disease

THE ART OF SWITCHING

 **Switching from Oral Antipsychotics to Quetiapine**

- With aripiprazole, amisulpride, and paliperidone, immediate stop is possible; begin quetiapine at middle dose
- With risperidone and lurasidone, it is generally advisable to begin quetiapine gradually, titrating over at least 2 weeks to allow patients to become tolerant to the sedating effect
- For more convenient dosing, patients who are currently being treated with divided doses of immediate-release tablets may be switched to extended-release quetiapine at the equivalent total daily dose taken once daily

*May need to taper clozapine slowly over 4 weeks or longer

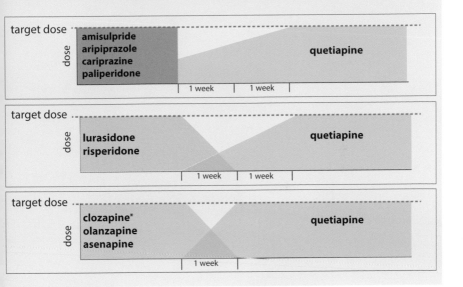

Suggested Reading

Citrome L. Adjunctive aripiprazole, olanzapine, or quetiapine for major depressive disorder: an analysis of number needed to treat, number needed to harm, and likelihood to be helped or harmed. Postgrad Med 2010;122(4):39–48.

Huhn M, Nikolakopoulou A, Schneider-Thoma J, et al. Comparative efficacy and tolerability of 32 oral antipsychotics for the acute treatment of adults with multi-episode schizophrenia: a systematic review and network meta-analysis. Lancet 2019;394(10202):939–51.

Keating GM, Robinson DM. Quetiapine: a review of its use in the treatment of bipolar depression. Drugs 2007;67(7):1077–95.

Komossa K, Rummel-Kluge C, Schmid F, et al. Quetiapine versus other atypical antipsychotics for schizophrenia. Cochrane Database Syst Rev 2010;20(1):CD006625.

Lieberman JA, Stroup TS, McEvoy JP. Effectiveness of antipsychotic drugs in patients with chronic schizophrenia. N Engl J Med 2005;353(12):1209–23.

Nasrallah HA. Atypical antipsychotic-induced metabolic side effects: insights from receptor-binding profiles. Mol Psychiatry 2008;13(1):27–35.

Quetiapine (Continued)

Pillinger T, McCutcheon RA, Vano L, et al. Comparative effects of 18 antipsychotics on metabolic function in patients with schizophrenia, predictors of metabolic dysregulation, and association with psychopathology: a systematic review and network meta-analysis. Lancet Psychiatry 2020;7(1):64–77.

Smith LA, Cornelius V, Warnock A, et al. Pharmacological interventions for acute bipolar mania: a systematic review of randomized placebo-controlled trials. Bipolar Disord 2007;9(6):551–60.

Suttajit S, Srisurapanont M, Maneeton N, et al. Quetiapine for acute bipolar depression: a systematic review and meta-analysis. Drug Des Devel Ther 2014;8:827–38.

Suttajit S, Srisurapanont M, Xia J, et al. Quetiapine versus typical antipsychotic medications for schizophrenia. Cochrane Database Syst Rev 2013;(5):CD007815.

Reboxetine

THERAPEUTICS

Brands
- Edronax

Generic?
No, not in UK

Class
- Neuroscience-based nomenclature: pharmacology domain – norepinephrine; mode of action – reuptake inhibitor
- Selective norepinephrine reuptake inhibitor (SNRI); antidepressant

Commonly Prescribed for
(bold for BNF indication)
- **Major depression**
- Dysthymia
- Panic disorder
- Attention deficit hyperactivity disorder (ADHD)

 How the Drug Works
- Boosts neurotransmitter noradrenaline and may also increase dopamine in prefrontal cortex
- Blocks noradrenaline reuptake pump (noradrenaline transporter)
- Presumably this increases noradrenergic neurotransmission
- Since dopamine is inactivated by noradrenaline reuptake in frontal cortex which largely lacks dopamine transporters, reboxetine can increase dopamine neurotransmission in this part of the brain

How Long Until It Works
- Onset of therapeutic actions with some antidepressants can be seen within 1–2 weeks, but often delayed 2–4 weeks
- If it is not working within 3–4 weeks for depression, it may require a dosage increase or it may not work at all
- May continue to work for many years to prevent relapse of symptoms

If It Works
- The goal of treatment is complete remission of current symptoms as well as prevention of future relapses
- Treatment most often reduces or even eliminates symptoms, but is not a cure since symptoms can recur after medicine is stopped

- Continue treatment until all symptoms are gone (remission), especially in depression and whenever possible in anxiety disorders
- Once symptoms are gone, continue treating for at least 6–9 months for the first episode of depression or >12 months if relapse indicators present
- If >5 episodes and/or 2 episodes in the last few years then need to continue for at least 2 years or indefinitely

If It Doesn't Work
- Important to recognise non-response to treatment early on (3–4 weeks)
- Many patients have only a partial response where some symptoms are improved but others persist (especially insomnia, fatigue, and problems concentrating)
- Other patients may be non-responders, sometimes called treatment-resistant or treatment-refractory
- Some patients who have an initial response may relapse even though they continue treatment
- Consider increasing dose, switching to another agent, or adding an appropriate augmenting agent
- Lithium may be added for suicidal patients or those at high risk of relapse
- Consider psychotherapy
- Consider ECT
- Consider evaluation for another diagnosis or for a co-morbid condition (e.g. medical illness, substance abuse, etc.)
- Some patients may experience a switch into mania and so would require antidepressant discontinuation and initiation of a mood stabiliser

 Best Augmenting Combos for Partial Response or Treatment Resistance
- Mood stabilisers or atypical antipsychotics for bipolar depression
- Atypical antipsychotics for psychotic depression
- Atypical antipsychotics as first-line augmenting agents (quetiapine MR 300 mg/day or aripiprazole at 2.5–10 mg/day) for treatment-resistant depression
- Atypical antipsychotics as second-line augmenting agents (risperidone 0.5–2 mg/day or olanzapine 2.5–10 mg/day) for treatment-resistant depression

- Mirtazapine at 30–45 mg/day as another second-line augmenting agent (a dual serotonin and noradrenaline combination, but observe for switch into mania, increase in suicidal ideation)
- Although T3 (20–50 mcg/day) is another second-line augmenting agent the evidence suggests that it works best with tricyclic antidepressants
- Other augmenting agents but with less evidence include bupropion (up to 400 mg/day), buspirone (up to 60 mg/day) and lamotrigine (up to 400 mg/day)
- Benzodiazepines if agitation present
- Hypnotics or trazodone for insomnia
- Augmenting agents reserved for specialist use include: modafinil for sleepiness, fatigue and lack of concentration; stimulants, oestrogens, testosterone
- Lithium is particularly useful for suicidal patients and those at high risk of relapse including with factors such as severe depression, psychomotor retardation, repeated episodes (>3), significant weight loss, or a family history of major depression (aim for lithium plasma levels 0.6–1.0 mmol/L)
- For elderly patients lithium is a very effective augmenting agent
- For severely ill patients other combinations may be tried especially in specialist centres
- Augmenting agents that may be tried include omega-3, SAM-e, L-methylfolate
- Additional non-pharmacological treatments such as exercise, mindfulness, CBT, and IPT can also be helpful
- If present after treatment response (4–8 weeks) or remission (6–12 weeks), the most common residual symptoms of depression include cognitive impairments, reduced energy and problems with sleep

Tests

- None for healthy individuals

SIDE EFFECTS

How Drug Causes Side Effects

- Noradrenaline increases in parts of the brain and body and at receptors other than those that cause therapeutic actions (e.g. unwanted actions of noradrenaline on acetylcholine release causing constipation and dry mouth, etc.)

- Most side effects are immediate but often go away with time

Notable Side Effects

- Insomnia, dizziness, anxiety, agitation
- Dry mouth, constipation
- Urinary hesitancy, urinary retention
- Sexual dysfunction (impotence)
- Dose-dependent hypotension

Common or very common
- CNS/PNS: akathisia, anxiety, dizziness, headache, insomnia, paraesthesia
- CVS: hypertension, hypotension, palpitations, tachycardia, vasodilation
- GIT: altered taste, constipation, decreased appetite, dry mouth, nausea, vomiting
- Other: accommodation disorder, chills, hyperhidrosis, sexual dysfunction, skin reactions, urinary disorders, urinary tract infection

Uncommon
- Mydriasis, vertigo

Rare or very rare
- Glaucoma

Frequency not known
- CNS: aggression, hallucination, irritability, suicidal tendencies
- Other: hyponatraemia, peripheral coldness, potassium depletion (long-term use), Raynaud's phenomenon, testicular pain

 Life-Threatening or Dangerous Side Effects
- Rare seizures
- Rare induction of mania
- Rare increase in suicidal ideation and behaviours in adolescents and young adults (up to age 25), hence patients should be warned of this potential adverse event

Weight Gain

 unusual not unusual common problematic

- Reported but not expected

Sedation

 unusual not unusual common problematic

- Reported but not expected

What to Do About Side Effects

- Wait

- Wait
- Wait
- Lower the dose
- In a few weeks, switch or add other drugs

Best Augmenting Agents for Side Effects

- Many side effects are dose-dependent (i.e. they increase as dose increases, or they re-emerge until tolerance redevelops)
- Many side effects are time-dependent (i.e. they start immediately upon dosing and upon each dose increase, but go away with time)
- Often best to try another antidepressant monotherapy prior to resorting to augmentation strategies to treat side effects
- Trazodone or a hypnotic for insomnia
- For sexual dysfunction: can augment with bupropion for women, sildenafil for men; or otherwise switch to another antidepressant
- Urinary retention can be treated with an alpha 1 blocker, e.g. tamsulosin
- Mirtazapine for insomnia, agitation, and gastrointestinal side effects
- Benzodiazepines for jitteriness and anxiety, especially at initiation of treatment and especially for anxious patients
- Increased activation or agitation may represent the induction of a bipolar state, especially a mixed dysphoric bipolar condition sometimes associated with suicidal ideation, and requires the addition of lithium, a mood stabiliser or an atypical antipsychotic, and/or discontinuation of reboxetine

DOSING AND USE

Usual Dosage Range
- 8 mg/day in 2 doses (12 mg max daily dose)

Dosage Forms
- Tablet 4 mg

How to Dose
- Initial dose 4 mg twice per day for 3–4 weeks, then increased as needed to 10 mg/day in divided doses

 Dosing Tips
- Minimum effective dose 8 mg/day

- When switching from another antidepressant or adding to another antidepressant, dosing may need to be lower and titration slower to prevent activating side effects (e.g. 2 mg in the daytime for 2–3 days, then 2 mg twice per day for 1–2 weeks)
- Give second daily dose in late afternoon rather than at bedtime to avoid undesired activation or insomnia in the evening
- May not need full dose of 8 mg/day when given in conjunction with another antidepressant
- Some patients may need 10 mg/day or more if well tolerated without orthostatic hypotension and if additional efficacy is seen at high doses in difficult cases
- Early dosing in patients with panic and anxiety may need to be lower and titration slower, perhaps with the use of concomitant short-term benzodiazepines to increase tolerability

Overdose
- Postural hypotension, anxiety, hypertension

Long-Term Use
- Safe

Habit Forming
- No

How to Stop
- Avoid abrupt withdrawal

Pharmacokinetics
- Metabolised by CYP450 3A4
- Inhibits CYP450 2D6 and 3A4 at high doses
- Elimination half-life about 13 hours

 Drug Interactions
- Tramadol increases the risk of seizures in patients taking an antidepressant
- May need to reduce reboxetine dose or avoid concomitant use with inhibitors of CYP450 3A4, such as azole and antifungals, macrolide antibiotics, fluvoxamine, fluoxetine, sertraline, etc.
- Use with ergotamine may increase blood pressure
- Reboxetine may increase the risk of hypokalaemia when given with thiazide diuretics
- Use with caution with MAO inhibitors, including 14 days after MAOIs are stopped

• Risk of hypertensive crisis when used with linezolid antibiotic

Other Warnings/Precautions

• Use with caution in patients with bipolar disorder unless treated with concomitant mood-stabiliser
• Use with caution in patients with urinary retention, benign prostatic hypertrophy, susceptibility to angle-closure glaucoma, history of epilepsy
• Use with caution with drugs that lower blood pressure
• Use with caution in patients with a history of cardiovascular disease
• Monitor patients for activation of suicidal ideation, especially those up to age 25

Do Not Use

• If patient is taking an MAOI (except as noted under drug interactions)
• If patient is taking pimozide
• If there is a proven allergy to reboxetine

• Must weigh the risk of treatment (first trimester foetal development, third trimester newborn delivery) to the child against the risk of no treatment (recurrence of depression, maternal health, infant bonding) to the mother and child
• For many patients this may mean continuing treatment during pregnancy

Breastfeeding

• Small amounts found in mother's breast milk
• Immediate postpartum period is a high-risk time for depression, especially in women who have had prior depressive episodes, so drug may need to be reinstituted late in the third trimester or shortly after childbirth to prevent a recurrence during the postpartum period
• Must weigh benefits of breastfeeding with risks and benefits of antidepressant treatment versus nontreatment to both the infant and the mother
• For many patients, this may mean continuing treatment during breastfeeding
• Other antidepressants may be preferable, e.g. paroxetine, sertraline, imipramine, or nortriptyline

SPECIAL POPULATIONS

Renal Impairment

• Plasma concentrations are increased (10% renal excretion)
• May need to lower dose (50%)

Hepatic Impairment

• Plasma concentrations are increased
• May need to lower dose (50%)

Cardiac Impairment

• Use with caution

Elderly

• Not recommended

Children and Adolescents

• No guidelines for children; safety and efficacy have not been established

Pregnancy

• Controlled studies have not been conducted in pregnant women
• Not generally recommended for use during pregnancy, especially during first trimester

THE ART OF PSYCHOPHARMACOLOGY

Potential Advantages

• Tired, unmotivated patients who have not responded to SSRIs
• Patients with cognitive disturbances
• Patients with psychomotor retardation
• May be helpful to attenuate weight gain in patients taking olanzapine

Potential Disadvantages

• Patients unable to comply with twice-daily dosing
• Patients unable to tolerate activation

Primary Target Symptoms

• Depressed mood
• Energy, motivation, and interest
• Suicidal ideation
• Cognitive disturbance
• Psychomotor retardation

Pearls

• May be effective if SSRIs have failed
*May be more likely than SSRIs to improve social and work functioning

- Reboxetine is a mixture of an active and an inactive enantiomer, and the active enantiomer may be developed in future clinical testing
*Side effects may appear "anticholinergic," but reboxetine does not directly block muscarinic receptors
- Constipation, dry mouth, and urinary retention are noradrenergic, due in part to peripheral alpha 1 receptor stimulation causing decreased acetylcholine release
*Thus, antidotes for these side effects can be alpha 1 antagonists such as tamsulosin, especially for urinary retention in men over 50 with borderline urine flow
- Novel use of reboxetine may be for attention deficit disorder, analogous to the actions of another norepinephrine selective reuptake inhibitor, atomoxetine, but few controlled studies
- Another novel use may be for neuropathic pain, alone or in combination with other antidepressants, but few controlled studies
- Some studies suggest efficacy in panic disorder

 ## Suggested Reading

Cipriani A, Furukawa TA, Salanti G, et al. Comparative efficacy and acceptability of 21 antidepressant drugs for the acute treatment of adults with major depressive disorder: a systematic review and network meta-analysis. Lancet 2018;391(10128):1357–66.

Eyding D, Lelgemann M, Grouven U, et al. Reboxetine for acute treatment of major depression: systematic review and meta-analysis of published and unpublished placebo and selective serotonin reuptake inhibitor controlled trials. BMJ 2010;341:c4737.

Fleishaker JC. Clinical pharmacokinetics of reboxetine, a selective norepinephrine reuptake inhibitor for the treatment of patients with depression. Clin Pharmacokinet 2000;39(6):413–27.

Kasper S, el Giamal N, Hilger E. Reboxetine: the first selective noradrenaline re-uptake inhibitor. Expert Opin Pharmacother 2000;1(4):771–82.

Keller M. Role of serotonin and noradrenaline in social dysfunction: a review of data on reboxetine and the Social Adaptation Self-evaluation Scale (SASS). Gen Hosp Psychiatry 2001;23(1):15–19.

Tanum L. Reboxetine: tolerability and safety profile in patients with major depression. Acta Psychiatr Scand Suppl 2000;402:37–40.

Risperidone

THERAPEUTICS

Brands
- Okedi
- Risperdal Consta

Generic?
Yes

Class
- Neuroscience-based nomenclature: low-dose risperidone: pharmacology domain – dopamine, serotonin; mode of action – antagonist; upper-dose risperidone: pharmacology domain – dopamine, serotonin, norepinephrine; mode of action – antagonist
- Atypical antipsychotic (serotonin dopamine antagonist; second-generation antipsychotics; also a mood stabiliser)

Commonly Prescribed for
(bold for BNF indication)
- **Schizophrenia and other psychoses**
- **Acute and chronic psychosis**
- **Mania**
- **Short-term treatment (up to 6 weeks) of persistent aggression in patients with moderate-severe Alzheimer's dementia unresponsive to non-pharmacological interventions and when there is a risk of harm to self or others**
- **Short-term treatment (up to 6 weeks) of persistent aggression in conduct disorder (under expert supervision)**
- **Short-term treatment of severe aggression in autism (under expert supervision)**

 ### How the Drug Works
- Blocks dopamine 2 receptors, reducing positive symptoms of psychosis and stabilising affective symptoms
- Blocks serotonin 2A receptors, causing enhancement of dopamine release in certain brain regions and thus reducing motor side effects and possibly improving cognitive and affective symptoms
- *Serotonin 7 antagonist properties may contribute to antidepressant actions

How Long Until It Works
- Within 1 week psychotic symptoms can improve but may take several weeks to see improvements in behaviour, cognition and affect
- The drug should be trialled for at least 4–6 weeks to determine its efficacy, unless there is an adverse reaction, but it has been reported that patients require up to 20 weeks to show a good response especially on cognitive symptoms
- It will take about 3 weeks before risperidone is absorbed at an adequate level to begin treating symptoms if using long-acting injection

If It Works
- Reduces positive symptoms but does not eliminate them
- Improves negative, affective, aggressive behaviour and cognitive symptoms
- A super-responder, representing 5–15% of patients with schizophrenia, can experience an overall improvement of 50–60% when receiving stable treatment for more than a year
- A substantial number of patients with bipolar disorder may experience a reduction of symptoms by more than a half and indeed treatment may prevent recurrences of mania in bipolar disorder
- Continue treatment until reaching a plateau of improvement
- After reaching a satisfactory plateau, continue treatment for at least 1 year after first episode of psychosis, but it may be preferable to continue treatment indefinitely to avoid subsequent episodes
- After any subsequent episodes of psychosis, treatment may need to be indefinite

If It Doesn't Work
- Try one of the other atypical antipsychotics (olanzapine should be considered first before considering other agents such as quetiapine, aripiprazole, amisulpride or lurasidone)
- If 2 or more antipsychotic monotherapies do not work, consider clozapine
- Some patients may require treatment with a conventional antipsychotic
- If no first-line atypical antipsychotic is effective, consider higher doses or augmentation with valproate or lamotrigine
- Consider non-concordance and switch to another antipsychotic with fewer side effects or to an antipsychotic that can be given by depot injection

Risperidone (Continued)

- Consider initiating rehabilitation and psychotherapy such as cognitive remediation
- Consider presence of concomitant drug abuse

⚖ Best Augmenting Combos for Partial Response or Treatment Resistance

- Valproic acid (Depakote, Epilim); risperidone plus valproic acid can help to reduce hostility in patients with schizophrenia
- Other mood-stabilising anticonvulsants (carbamazepine, oxcarbazepine, lamotrigine)
- Lithium
- Benzodiazepines

Tests

Before starting an atypical antipsychotic

* Measure weight, BMI, and waist circumference
- Get baseline personal and family history of diabetes, obesity, dyslipidaemia, hypertension, and cardiovascular disease
* Check pulse and blood pressure, fasting plasma glucose or glycosylated haemoglobin (HbA1c), fasting lipid profile, and prolactin level
- Full blood count (FBC), urea and electrolytes (including creatinine and eGFR), liver function tests (LFTs)
- Assessment of nutritional status, diet, and level of physical activity
- Determine if the patient is:
  - overweight (BMI 25.0–29.9)
  - obese (BMI ≥30)
  - has pre-diabetes – fasting plasma glucose: 5.5 mmol/L to 6.9 mmol/L or HbA1c: 42 to 47 mmol/mol (6.0 to 6.4%)
  - has diabetes – fasting plasma glucose: >7.0 mmol/L or HbA1c: ≥48 mmol/L (≥6.5%)
  - has hypertension (BP >140/90 mm Hg)
  - has dyslipidaemia (increased total cholesterol, LDL cholesterol, and triglycerides; decreased HDL cholesterol)
- Treat or refer such patients for treatment, including nutrition and weight management, physical activity counselling, smoking cessation, and medical management

- Baseline ECG for: inpatients; those with a personal history or risk factor for cardiac disease

Children and adolescents:
- As for adults
- Also check history of congenital heart problems, history of dizziness when stressed or on exertion, history of long-QT syndrome, family history of long-QT syndrome, bradycardia, myocarditis, family history of cardiac myopathies, low K/low Mg/low Ca++
- Measure weight, BMI, and waist circumference plotted on a growth chart
- Pulse, BP plotted on a percentile chart
- ECG: note for QTc interval: machine-generated may be incorrect in children as different formula needed if HR <60 or >100
- Baseline prolactin levels

Monitoring after starting an atypical antipsychotic

- FBC annually to detect chronic bone marrow suppression, stop treatment if neutrophils fall below 1.5x10⁹/L and refer to specialist care if neutrophils fall below 0.5x10⁹/L
- Urea and electrolytes (including creatinine and eGFR) annually
- LFTs annually
- Prolactin levels at 6 months and then annually (risperidone is likely to increase prolactin levels)
* Weight/BMI/waist circumference, weekly for the first 6 weeks, then at 12 weeks, at 1 year and then annually
* Pulse and blood pressure at 12 weeks, 1 year, and then annually
* Fasting blood glucose, HbA1c, and blood lipids at 12 weeks, at 1 year, and then annually
* For patients with type 2 diabetes, measure HbA1c at 3–6 month intervals until stable, then every 6 months
* Even in patients without known diabetes, be vigilant for the rare but life-threatening onset of diabetic ketoacidosis, which always requires immediate treatment, by monitoring for the rapid onset of polyuria, polydipsia, weight loss, nausea, vomiting, dehydration, rapid respiration, weakness and clouding of sensorium, even coma
- If HbA1c remains ≥48 mmol/mol (6.5%) then drug therapy should be offered, e.g. metformin

- Treat or refer for treatment or consider switching to another atypical antipsychotic for patients who become overweight, obese, pre-diabetic, diabetic, hypertensive, or dyslipidaemic while receiving an atypical antipsychotic

Children and adolescents:
- As for adults
- Weight/BMI /waist circumference, weekly for the first 6 weeks, then at 12 weeks, then every 6 months, plotted on a growth/percentile chart
- Height every 6 months, plotted on a growth chart
- Pulse and blood pressure at 12 weeks, then every 6 months plotted on a percentile chart
- ECG prior to starting and 2 weeks after dose increase for monitoring of QTc interval. Machine-generated may be incorrect in children as different formula needed if HR <60 or >100
- Prolactin levels: prior to starting and after 12 weeks, 24 weeks, and 6-monthly thereafter. Consider additional monitoring in young adults (under 25) who have not yet reached peak bone mass
- In prepubertal children monitor sexual maturation
- In post-pubertal children and young persons monitor sexual side effects (both sexes: loss of libido, sexual dysfunction, galactorrhoea, infertility; male: diminished ejaculate, gynaecomastia; female: oligorrhoea/amenorrhoea, reduced vaginal lubrication, dyspareunia, acne, hirsutism)

SIDE EFFECTS

How Drug Causes Side Effects
- By blocking alpha 1 adrenergic receptors, it can cause dizziness, sedation, and hypotension
- By blocking dopamine 2 receptors in the striatum, it can cause motor side effects, especially at high doses
- By blocking dopamine 2 receptors in the pituitary, it can cause elevations in prolactin
- Mechanism of weight gain and increased incidence of diabetes and dyslipidaemia with atypical antipsychotics is unknown

Notable Side Effects
* May increase risk for diabetes and dyslipidaemia
* Dose-dependent extrapyramidal symptoms
* Dose-related hyperprolactinaemia
* Dose-dependent dizziness, insomnia, anxiety, sedation

Common or very common
- CNS/PNS: anxiety, depression, headache, sleep disorders, vision disorders
- CVS: chest discomfort, hypertension
- Endocrine: hyperglycaemia
- GIT: abnormal appetite, decreased weight, diarrhoea, gastrointestinal discomfort, nausea, oral disorders
- Resp: cough, dyspnoea, nasal congestion
- Other: anaemia, asthenia, conjunctivitis, epistaxis, fall, fever, increased risk of infection, joint disorders, laryngeal pain, muscle spasms, oedema, pain, sexual dysfunction, skin reactions, urinary disorders

Uncommon
- CNS/PNS: abnormal gait, abnormal posture, abnormal sensation, altered mood, cerebrovascular insufficiency, coma, confusion, impaired concentration, impaired consciousness, dysarthria, dysphonia, tinnitus, vertigo
- CVS: cardiac conduction disorders, palpitations, syncope
- Endocrine: diabetes mellitus
- GIT: altered taste, dysphagia, gastrointestinal disorders, polydipsia and thirst
- Resp: respiratory disorders
- Other: alopecia, breast abnormalities, chills, cystitis, dry eye, ear pain, eye disorders, flushing, malaise, menstrual cycle irregularities, muscle weakness, procedural pain, thrombocytopenia, vaginal discharge

Rare or very rare
- CNS: sleep apnoea
- GIT: jaundice, pancreatitis
- Endocrine: diabetic ketoacidosis, hypoglycaemia
- Other: angioedema, dandruff, eyelid crusting, glaucoma, hypothermia, peripheral coldness, rhabdomyolysis, SIADH, water intoxication, withdrawal syndrome

Frequency not known
- Cardiac arrest

Risperidone (Continued)

 Life-Threatening or Dangerous Side Effects

- Hyperglycaemia, in some cases extreme and associated with ketoacidosis or hyperosmolar coma or death, has been reported in patients taking atypical antipsychotics
- Increased risk of death and cerebrovascular events in elderly patients with dementia-related psychosis
- Rare neuroleptic malignant syndrome (much reduced risk compared to conventional antipsychotics)
- Rare seizures

Weight Gain

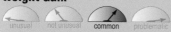

- Many patients experience and/or can be significant in amount

Sedation

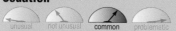

- Many patients experience and/or can be significant in amount
- Usually transient

What To Do About Side Effects

- Wait
- Wait
- Wait
- Reduce the dose
- Low-dose benzodiazepine or beta blocker may reduce akathisia
- Take more of the dose at bedtime to help reduce daytime sedation
- Weight loss, exercise programmes, and medical management for high BMIs, diabetes, and dyslipidaemia
- Switch to another antipsychotic (atypical) – quetiapine or clozapine are best in cases of tardive dyskinesia

Best Augmenting Agents for Side Effects

- Dystonia: antimuscarinic drugs (e.g. procyclidine) as oral or IM depending on the severity; botulinum toxin if antimuscarinics not effective
- Parkinsonism: antimuscarinic drugs (e.g. procyclidine)

- Akathisia: beta blocker propranolol (30–80 mg/day) or low-dose benzodiazepine (e.g. 0.5–3.0 mg/day of clonazepam) may help; other agents that may be tried include the 5HT2 antagonists such as cyproheptadine (16 mg/day) or mirtazapine (15 mg at night – caution in bipolar disorder); clonidine (0.2–0.8 mg/day) may be tried if the above ineffective
- Tardive dyskinesia: stop any antimuscarinic, consider tetrabenazine
- Addition of low doses (2.5–5 mg) of aripiprazole can reverse the hyperprolactinaemia/galactorrhoea caused by other antipsychotics
- Addition of aripiprazole (5–15 mg/day) or metformin (500–2000 mg/day) to weight-inducing atypical antipsychotics such as olanzapine and clozapine can help mitigate against weight gain

DOSING AND USE

Usual Dosage Range

- Schizophrenia and other psychoses in patients tolerant to risperidone by mouth: IM injection 25–50 mg every 2 weeks
- Acute and chronic psychosis: 2–16 mg/day
- Mania: 1–6 mg/day
- Short-term treatment (up to 6 weeks) of persistent aggression in patients with moderate-severe Alzheimer's dementia unresponsive to non-pharmacological interventions and when there is a risk of harm to self or others: 0.5–2 mg/day in divided doses

Dosage Forms

- Tablet 0.25 mg, 0.5 mg, 1 mg, 2 mg, 3 mg, 4 mg, 6 mg
- Orodispersible tablet 0.5 mg, 1 mg, 2 mg, 3 mg, 4 mg
- Oral solution 1 mg/mL
- Powder and solvent for suspension for injection 25 mg, 37.5 mg, 50 mg

How to Dose
Adults:

*Schizophrenia and other psychoses in patients tolerant to oral risperidone (up to 4 mg/day):
- IM injection (deltoid or gluteal) – initial dose 25 mg every 2 weeks, adjusted by

increments of 12.5 mg at least every 4 weeks (max 50 mg every 2 weeks)
- Oral risperidone may need to continue on initiation (for 4–6 weeks) and when depot dose is being adjusted

∗Schizophrenia and other psychoses in patients tolerant to oral risperidone (over 4 mg/day):
- IM injection – initial dose 37.5 mg every 2 weeks, adjusted by increments of 12.5 mg at least every 4 weeks (max 50 mg every 2 weeks)
- Oral risperidone may need to continue on initiation (for 4–6 weeks) and when depot dose is being adjusted

∗Acute and chronic psychosis:
- 2 mg/day in 1–2 divided doses for day 1, then 4 mg/day in 1–2 divided doses for day 2; some patients may require a slower titration
- Usual dose 4–6 mg/day, doses >10 mg/day only if benefit outweighs risk; max 16 mg/day

∗Mania:
- Initial dose 2 mg/day, increased by increments of 1 mg/day as needed; usual dose 1–6 mg/day

∗Short-term treatment of persistent aggression in patients in moderate-severe Alzheimer's dementia:
- Up to 6 weeks only
- Only to be used when non-pharmacological means have not helped and there is associated risk of harm to self and others
- Initial dose 0.25 mg twice per day, increased by increments of 0.25 mg twice per day every other day and adjusted according to response; usual dose 0.5 mg twice per day (max 1 mg twice per day)

Children and Adolescents:
- Under expert supervision

∗Acute and chronic psychosis:
- Child 12–17 years: 2 mg/day in 1–2 divided doses for day 1, then 4 mg/day in 1–2 divided doses for day 2; some patients may require a slower titration
- Usual dose 4–6 mg/day, doses >10 mg/day only if benefit outweighs risk; max 16 mg/day

∗Short-term monotherapy of mania in bipolar disorder:
- Child 12–17 years: initial dose 500 mcg/day, adjusted by increments of 0.5–1 mg/day according to response; usual dose 2.5 mg/day in 1–2 divided doses; max 6 mg/day

∗Short-term treatment of persistent aggression in conduct disorder:
- Up to 6 weeks only
- Child 5–17 years (body weight <50 kg): initial dose 0.25 mg/day, increased by increments of 0.25 mg/day every other day adjusted according to response; usual dose 0.5 mg/day; max 0.75 mg/day
- Child 5–17 years (body weight ≥50 kg): initial dose 0.5 mg/day, increased by increments of 0.5 mg/day every other day adjusted according to response; usual dose 1 mg/day; max 1.5 mg/day

∗Short-term treatment of severe aggression in autism:
- Child 5–17 years (body weight 15–20 kg): initial dose 0.25 mg/day for at least 4 days, increased as needed to 0.5 mg/day, then increased by increments of 0.25 mg/day every 2 weeks with a review of benefits versus side-effects after 3–4 weeks; discontinue at 6 weeks if no response; max 1 mg/day
- Child 5–17 years (body weight 20–45 kg): initial dose 0.5 mg/day for at least 4 days, increased as needed to 1 mg/day, then increased by increments of 0.5 mg/day every 2 weeks with a review of benefits versus side effects after 3–4 weeks; discontinue at 6 weeks if no response; max 2.5 mg/day
- Child 5–17 years (body weight ≥45 kg): initial dose 0.5 mg/day for at least 4 days, increased as needed to 1 mg/day, then increased by increments of 0.5 mg/day every 2 weeks with a review of benefits versus side-effects after 3–4 weeks; discontinue at 6 weeks if no response; max 3 mg/day

 Dosing Tips
- Use oral risperidone before giving injection to assure good tolerability. Those stabilised on 2 mg/day start on 25 mg/2 weeks. Those on higher doses start on 37.5 mg/2 weeks and be prepared to use 50 mg/2 weeks
- The therapeutic threshold for risperidone plasma levels is 20 ng/mL
- When transferring from oral to depot therapy, the dose by mouth should be reduced gradually

Risperidone (Continued)

Overdose
- Signs and symptoms include lethargy, tachycardia, QT-prolongation, changes in BP
- Toxicity in overdose is low with the lowest dose to cause overdose unclear, but overall fatality is rare in those taking risperidone on its own
- Causes less depression of consciousness and respiration than other sedatives
- Hypotension, hyperthermia, sinus tachycardia and arrhythmias may complicate poisoning

Long-Term Use
- No long-term adverse effects are noted
- Often used for long-term maintenance treatment in schizophrenia or bipolar disorder

Habit Forming
- No

How to Stop
- High risk of relapse if medication is stopped after 1–2 years withdrawal of antipsychotic drugs after long-term therapy; should always be gradual and closely monitored to avoid the risk of acute withdrawal syndromes or relapse
- Patients should be monitored for 2 years after withdrawal for signs and symptoms of relapse

Pharmacokinetics
- Metabolites are active including 9-OH risperidone (paliperidone)
- Metabolised mostly by CYP450 2D6 and to lesser extent by 3A4
- Long-acting risperidone has elimination phase of about 7–8 weeks after last injection
- Food does not affect absorption
- Half-life for parent drug of oral formulation is about 20–24 hours
- Half-life for long-acting risperidone is about 3–6 days

 Drug Interactions
- Risperidone plasma levels may increase in the presence of CYP450 2D6 inhibitors (e.g. paroxetine, fluoxetine, duloxetine, bupropion) – especially at higher doses of the inhibitor)
- Risperidone plasma levels may reduce when used with CYP450 3A4 inducers (e.g. rifampicin, carbamazepine, phenytoin)

- Risperidone plasma levels may increase when used with CYP450 3A4 inhibitors (e.g. ketaconazole, paroxetine, fluoxetine, fluvoxamine, ciprofloxacin, cimetidine)
- Plasma levels of risperidone may also increase in the presence of phenothiazines, beta blockers, calcium channel blockers such as verapamil, and some TCAs
- Increased mortality has been observed in elderly patients with dementia concomitantly receiving furosemide

 Other Warnings/Precautions
- All antipsychotics should be used with caution in patients with angle-closure glaucoma, blood disorders, cardiovascular disease, depression, diabetes, epilepsy and susceptibility to seizures, history of jaundice, myasthenia gravis, Parkinson's disease, photosensitivity, prostatic hypertrophy, severe respiratory disorders
- May increase effects of antihypertensive agents
- May antagonise levodopa, dopamine agonists
- May enhance QTc prolongation of other drugs capable of prolonging QTc interval
- Increased risk of sedation when used with CNS depressants such as alcohol
- The combined use with psychostimulants such as methylphenidate can lead to extrapyramidal symptoms
- Concomitant use with paliperidone is not recommended
- Risperidone has been confused with ropinirole; care must be taken to ensure the correct drug is prescribed and dispensed
- Use with caution in a dehydrated patient
- Use is problematic in dementia with Lewy bodies, in cataract surgery due to the risk of floppy iris syndrome and in patients with a prolactin-dependent tumour

Do Not Use
- Intramuscular formulation in children
- In a patient with acute porphyrias
- In elderly patients with dementia concomitantly receiving furosemide
- If there is a proven allergy to risperidone or paliperidone

Renal Impairment
- With oral use: initial and subsequent doses should be halved

Hepatic Impairment

- With oral use: initial and subsequent doses should be halved and titrate more slowly
- With IM use: if an oral dose of at least 2 mg/day is tolerated, 25 mg as a depot injection can be given every 2 weeks

Cardiac Impairment

- In cardiac impairment, use with caution due to risk of orthostatic hypotension
- An ECG may be required, particularly if physical examination identifies cardiovascular risk factors, personal history of cardiovascular disease, or if the patient is being admitted as an inpatient

Elderly

- Chronic and acute psychosis: initial dose 500 mcg twice per day, then increased by increments of 500 mcg twice per day, increased to 1–2 mg twice per day
- Mania: initial dose 500 mcg twice per day, then increased by increments of 500 mcg twice per day, increased to 1–2 mg twice per day
- Increased risk of stroke in the elderly with atrial fibrillation

Children and Adolescents

- Not licensed for use in children for psychosis, mania or autism
- Risperidone is licensed for short-term (up to 6 weeks) use in persistent aggression in conduct disorder under expert supervision in children above 5 years
- Unlicensed use includes: acute and chronic psychosis under expert supervision, manic episodes, short-term (up to 6 weeks) severe aggression associated with autism, severe tics, and Tourette syndrome

Before you prescribe:

- Do not offer antipsychotic medication when transient or attenuated psychotic symptoms or other mental state changes associated with distress, impairment, or help-seeking behaviour are not sufficient for a diagnosis of psychosis or schizophrenia. Consider individual CBT with or without family therapy and other treatments recommended for anxiety, depression, substance use, or emerging personality disorder
- For first-episode psychosis (FEP) antipsychotic medication should only be started by a specialist following a comprehensive multidisciplinary assessment and in conjunction with recommended psychological interventions (CBT, family therapy)
- As first-line treatment: allow patient to choose from aripiprazole, olanzapine or risperidone. As second-line treatment switch to alternative from list. Consider quetiapine depending on desired profile
- For bipolar disorder: if bipolar disorder is suspected in primary care in children or adolescents refer them to a specialist service
- Choice of antipsychotic medication should be an informed choice depending on individual factors and side-effect profile (metabolic, cardiovascular, extrapyramidal, hormonal, other)
- All children and young people with FEP/ bipolar should be supported with sleep management, anxiety management, exercise and activation schedules, and healthy diet
- Where a child or young person presents with self-harm and suicidal thoughts the immediate risk management may take first priority
- Short-term treatment of behavioural disturbances in children and adolescents with conduct disorder (under expert supervision). There are many reasons for challenging behaviours and consideration should be given to possible physical, psychosocial and, environmental causes. These should be addressed first. Consider behavioural interventions and family support. Consider trauma-informed practice. Pharmacological treatment can be offered alongside the above
- Short-term use (up to 6 weeks) in autism-related severe aggression in children aged 6 to 17 years (under expert supervision): there are many reasons for challenging behaviours in ASD and consideration should be given to possible physical, psychosocial, environmental or ASD-specific causes (e.g. sensory processing difficulties, communication). These should be addressed first. Consider behavioural interventions and family support. Pharmacological treatment can be offered alongside the above. It may be prudent to periodically discontinue the prescriptions if symptoms are well controlled, as irritability

can change as the patient goes through neurodevelopmental changes

- Severe tics and Tourette syndrome in children aged 6 to 18: transient tics occur in up to 20% of children. Tourette syndrome occurs in 1% of children. Tics wax and wane over time and may be exacerbated by factors such as fatigue, inactivity, stress. Tics are a lifelong disorder, but often get better over time. As many as 65% of young people with Tourette syndrome have only mild tics in adult life. Psychoeducation and evidence-based psychological interventions (habit reversal therapy (HRT) or exposure and response prevention (ERP)) should be offered first. Pharmacological treatment may be considered in conjunction with psychological interventions where tics result in significant impairment or psychosocial consequences, and/or where psychological interventions have been ineffective. If co-morbid with ADHD other choices (clonidine/guanfacine) may be better options to avoid polypharmacy
- A risk management plan is important prior to start of medication because of the possible increase in suicidal ideation and behaviours in adolescents and young adults

Practical notes:

- Carefully weigh the risks and benefits of pharmacological treatment against the risks and benefits of non-treatment and make sure to document this in the patient's chart
- Monitor weight, weekly for the first 6 weeks, then at 12 weeks, and then every 6 months (plotted on a growth chart)
- Height every 6 months (plotted on a growth chart)
- Waist circumference every 6 months (plotted on a percentile chart)
- Pulse and blood pressure (plotted on a percentile chart) at 12 weeks and then every 6 months
- Fasting blood glucose, HbA1c, blood lipid and prolactin levels at 12 weeks and then every 6 months
- Monitor for activation of suicidal ideation at the beginning of treatment. Inform parents or guardians of this risk so they can help observe child or adolescent patients
- If it does not work: review child's/young person's profile, consider new/changing contributing individual or systemic factors such as peer or family conflict. Consider drug/substance misuse. Consider

dose adjustment before switching or augmentation. Be vigilant of polypharmacy especially in complex and highly vulnerable children/adolescents

- Consider non-concordance by parent or child, consider non-concordance in adolescents, address underlying reasons for non-concordance
- Children are more sensitive to most side effects
  - There is an inverse relationship between age and incidence of extrapyramidal symptoms
  - Exposure to antipsychotics during childhood and young age is associated with a three-fold increase of diabetes mellitus
  - Treatment with all second-generation antipsychotics has been associated with changes in most lipid parameters
  - Weight gain correlates with time on treatment. Any childhood obesity is associated with obesity in adults
- Dose adjustments may be necessary in the presence of interacting drugs
- Re-evaluate the need for continued treatment regularly
- Provide Medicines for Children leaflet for risperidone for schizophrenia-bipolar-disorder-and-agitation
- Monitoring of endocrine function (weight, height, sexual maturation and menses) is required when a child is taking an antipsychotic drug that is known to cause hyperprolactinaemia

 Pregnancy

- One large cohort study has found an increased risk of major malformations, although absolute risk remains low
- There is a risk of abnormal muscle movements and withdrawal symptoms in newborns whose mothers took an antipsychotic during the third trimester; symptoms may include agitation, abnormally increased or decreased muscle tone, tremor, sleepiness, severe difficulty breathing, and difficulty feeding
- Psychotic symptoms may worsen during pregnancy and some form of treatment may be necessary
- Use in pregnancy may be justified if the benefit of continued treatment exceeds any associated risk

- Switching antipsychotics may increase the risk of relapse
- Risperidone may be preferable to anticonvulsant mood stabilisers if treatment or prophylaxis are required during pregnancy
- Effects of hyperprolactinaemia on the foetus are unknown
- Olanzapine and clozapine have been associated with maternal hyperglycaemia which may lead to developmental toxicity; risk may also apply for other atypical antipsychotics
- Depot antipsychotics should only be used when there is a good response to the depot and a history of non-concordance with oral medication

Breastfeeding

- Small amounts expected in mother's breast milk
- Risk of accumulation in infant due to long half-life
- Haloperidol is considered to be the preferred first-generation antipsychotic, and quetiapine the preferred second-generation antipsychotic
- Infants of women who choose to breastfeed should be monitored for possible adverse effects

THE ART OF PSYCHOPHARMACOLOGY

Potential Advantages

- Some cases of psychosis and mania refractory to treatment with other antipsychotics
- Often a preferred treatment for dementia with aggressive features
- Often a preferred atypical antipsychotic for children with behavioural disturbances of multiple causes
- Non-concordant patients (long-acting injection risperidone)
- Long-term outcomes may be improved when concordance enhanced (long-acting injection risperidone)

Potential Disadvantages

- Patients for whom elevated prolactin may not be desired (e.g. pregnant patients, pubescent girls with amenorrhoea, post-menopausal women with low oestrogen who do not take oestrogen replacement therapy)

Primary Target Symptoms

- Positive and negative symptoms of psychosis
- Cognitive functioning
- Unstable mood
- Aggressive symptoms

 Pearls

* Well accepted for treatment of behavioural symptoms in children and adolescents, but may cause more sedation and weight gain in this population
* Well accepted for the short-term treatment of persistent aggression in Alzheimer's disease
- Some patients respond to or tolerate risperidone better than paliperidone and vice versa
- Hyperprolactinaemia in women with low oestrogen may accelerate osteoporosis
- Less sedation and weight gain in comparison to some atypicals such as olanzapine
- May cause motor side effects especially in Lewy body disease
- Long-acting injection requires simultaneous oral medication and in some cases for several weeks
- Long-acting injection may be well tolerated
- Therapeutic drug monitoring may be helpful

RISPERIDONE LONG-ACTION INJECTION

Risperdal Consta Properties

Vehicle	Water
Tmax	21 days
T1/2 with multiple dosing	3–6 days
Time to steady state	About 6–8 weeks
Able to be loaded	No
Dosing schedule (maintenance)	2 weeks
Injection site	IM
Needle gauge	20 or 21
Dosage forms (25 mg, 37.5 mg, 50 mg)	Powder and solvent for suspension for injection
Injection volume	1 vial; range 0.5–1 vial

Risperidone (Continued)

Usual Dosage Range
- 25–50 mg every 2 weeks

How to Dose
- Not recommended for patients who have not first demonstrated tolerability to oral risperidone
- Conversion from oral: oral coverage is required for 3–4 weeks; 2 mg oral risperidone is about 25 mg long-acting injection every 2 weeks

 Dosing Tips

- With long-acting injections, the absorption rate constant is slower than the elimination rate constant, thus resulting in "flip-flop" kinetics – i.e. time to steady state is a function of absorption rate, while concentration at steady state is a function of elimination rate
- The rate-limiting step for plasma drug levels for long-acting injections is not drug metabolism, but rather slow absorption from the injection site
- In general, 5 half-lives of any medication are needed to achieve 97% of steady-state levels
- The long half-life of depot/long-acting injection antipsychotics means that one must either adequately load the dose (if possible) or provide oral supplementation
- The failure to adequately load the dose leads either to prolonged cross-titration from oral antipsychotic or to sub-therapeutic antipsychotic plasma levels for weeks or months in patients who are not receiving (or adhering to) oral supplementation
- Because plasma antipsychotic levels increase gradually over time, dose requirements may ultimately decrease; if possible obtaining periodic plasma levels can be beneficial to prevent unnecessary plasma level creep
- The time to get a blood level for patients receiving long-acting injection is the morning of the day they will receive their next injection
- Advantages: also used for affective psychoses; kinetics are linear and stable over time
- Disadvantages: Tmax is long (21 days) and loading is not possible thus necessitating oral coverage for 3–4 weeks; split doses are not possible since drug is not in a solution (i.e. half a syringe is not necessarily half the drug dose); vials require refrigeration storage
- Response threshold is generally 20 ng/mL; the tolerability threshold is poorly defined
- The therapeutic range to aim for is 28–112 ng/mL; aim for the upper part of the therapeutic range in treatment-resistant cases
- Changes in blood levels due to dosage changes (missed dose) are not apparent for 3–4 weeks, so titration should occur at intervals of no less than 4 weeks
- Two different dosage strengths of long-acting injection risperidone should not be combined in a single administration
- Missed dose: if dose is 2 or more weeks late, oral coverage for 3 weeks while restarting injections may be necessary
- Steady-state plasma concentrations are maintained for 4–6 weeks after the last injection

THE ART OF SWITCHING

Switching from Oral Antipsychotics to Risperidone Long-Acting Injection

- Discontinuation of oral antipsychotic can begin immediately if adequate loading is pursued
- How to discontinue oral formulations:
  - Down-titration is not required for: amisulpride, aripiprazole, cariprazine, paliperidone
  - 1 week down-titration is required for: lurasidone, risperidone
  - 3–4 week down-titration is required for: asenapine, olanzapine, quetiapine
  - 4+-week down-titration is required for: clozapine
- For patients taking benzodiazepine or anticholinergic medication, this can be continued during cross-titration to help alleviate side effects such as insomnia, agitation, and/or psychosis. Once the patient is stable on long-acting injections, these can be tapered one at a time as appropriate

Switching from Oral Antipsychotics to Risperidone

- With some antipsychotics, namely aripiprazole, amisulpride, and paliperidone, immediate stop is possible. Following this one can begin risperidone at an intermediate dose
- Paliperidone is the active metabolite of risperidone and therefore concomitant use is not advised
- Quetiapine, olanzapine, and asenapine should be titrated down over 3–4 weeks to allow patients to cope with the withdrawal symptoms
- Clozapine should be tapered off slowly over 4+ weeks – you might want to change to risperidone in case of hypertriglyceridaemia; has been shown to reverse this
*Benzodiazepines or anticholinergics can be administered during cross-titration to help alleviate side effects such as insomnia, agitation, and/or psychosis

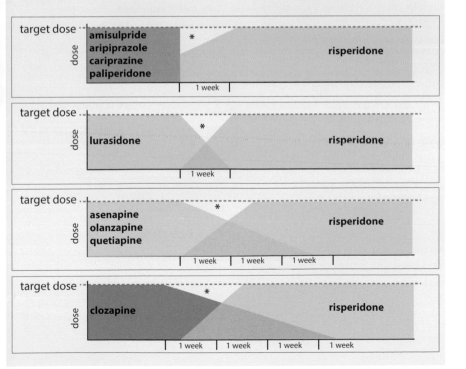

Risperidone (Continued)

 Suggested Reading

Byerly MJ, Marcus RN, Tran Q-V, et al. Effects of aripiprazole on prolactin levels in subjects with schizophrenia during cross-titration with risperidone or olanzapine: analysis of a randomized, open-label study. Schizophr Res 2009;107:218–22.

Citrome L. Sustained-release risperidone via subcutaneous injection: a systematic review of RBP-7000 (PERSERIS ™) for the treatment of schizophrenia. Clin Schizophr Relat Psychoses 2018;12(3):130–41.

Huhn M, Nikolakopoulou A, Schneider-Thoma J, et al. Comparative efficacy and tolerability of 32 oral antipsychotics for the acute treatment of adults with multi-episode schizophrenia: a systematic review and network meta-analysis. Lancet 2019;394(10202):939–51.

Knegtering R, Castelein S, Bous H, et al. A randomized open-label study of the impact of quetiapine versus risperidone on sexual functioning. J Clin Psychopharmacol 2004;24:56–61.

Mall GD, Hake L, Benjamin AB, et al. Catatonia and mild neuroleptic malignant syndrome after initiation of long-acting injectable risperidone: case report. J Clin Psychopharmacol 2008;28:572–3.

Moller H-J. Long-acting injectable risperidone for the treatment of schizophrenia: clinical perspectives. Drugs 2007;67(11):1541–66.

Nasrallah HA. Atypical antipsychotic-induced metabolic side effects: insights from receptor-binding profiles. Mol Psychiatry 2008;13(1):27–35.

Nelson MW, Reynolds RR, Kelly DL, et al. Adjunctive quetiapine decreases symptoms of tardive dyskinesia in a patient taking risperidone. Clin Neuropharmacol 2003;26:297–8.

Pillinger T, McCutcheon RA, Vano L, et al. Comparative effects of 18 antipsychotics on metabolic function in patients with schizophrenia, predictors of metabolic dysregulation, and association with psychopathology: a systematic review and network meta-analysis. Lancet Psychiatry 2020;7(1):64–77.

Smith LA, Cornelius V, Warnock A, et al. Pharmacological interventions for acute bipolar mania: a systematic review of randomized placebo-controlled trials. Bipolar Disord 2007;9(6):551–60.

Wilson WH. A visual guide to expected blood levels of long-acting injectable risperidone in clinical practice. J Psychiatr Pract 2004;10(6):393–401.

Rivastigmine

Brands
- Nimvastid
- Almuriva
- Alzest
- Exelon
- Erastig
- Prometax

Generic?
Yes

Class
- Neuroscience-based nomenclature: pharmacology domain – acetylcholine; mode of action – enzyme inhibitor
- Cholinesterase inhibitor (acetylcholinesterase inhibitor and butyrylcholinesterase inhibitor); cognitive enhancer

Commonly Prescribed for
(bold for BNF indication)
- **Alzheimer's disease (mild-moderate)**
- **Parkinson's disease dementia (mild-moderate)**
- Dementia with Lewy bodies
- Alzheimer's disease of atypical or mixed type

How the Drug Works
∗ Pseudo-irreversibly inhibits centrally active acetylcholinesterase (AChE), making more acetylcholine available
- Increased availability of acetylcholine compensates in part for degenerating cholinergic neurons in neocortex that regulate memory
∗ Inhibits butyrylcholinesterase (BuChE)
- May release growth factors or interfere with amyloid deposition

How Long Until It Works
- Takes up to 6 weeks before any improvement in baseline memory or behaviour is evident
- Can take up to 6 months before any stabilisation in degenerative course is evident
- Patients on rivastigmine (6–12 mg/day by mouth or 9.5 mg/day by skin patch) versus placebo were better on three outcomes after 6 months of treatment

If It Works
- May improve symptoms of disease, or slow progression, but does not reverse the degenerative process

If It Doesn't Work
- Consider adjusting dose, switching to a different cholinesterase inhibitor or consider adding memantine in moderate or severe Alzheimer's disease
- Reconsider diagnosis and rule out other conditions such as depression or a dementia other than Alzheimer's disease

 Best Augmenting Combos for Partial Response or Treatment Resistance
- Augmenting agents may help with managing non-cognitive symptoms
∗ Memantine for moderate to severe Alzheimer's disease
∗ Atypical antipsychotics should only be used for severe aggression or psychosis when this is causing significant distress
- Careful consideration needs to be undertaken for co-morbid conditions and to the benefits and risks of treatment in view of the increased risk of stroke and death with antipsychotic drugs in dementia
∗ Antidepressants if concomitant depression, apathy, or lack of interest, however efficacy may be limited
- Not rational to combine with another cholinesterase inhibitor

Tests
- Baseline ECG may be useful
- Monitor body weight

How Drug Causes Side Effects
- Peripheral inhibition of acetylcholinesterase can cause gastrointestinal side effects
- Central inhibition of acetylcholinesterase may contribute to nausea, vomiting, weight loss, and sleep disturbances

Notable Side Effects
∗ Nausea, diarrhoea, vomiting, appetite loss, weight loss, dyspepsia, increased gastric acid secretion

- Headache, dizziness
- Fatigue, asthenia, sweating

Common or very common
- CNS/PNS: anxiety, depression, dizziness, drowsiness, fall, headache, movement disorders, tremor
- CVS: arrhythmias, hypertension, syncope
- GIT: decreased appetite, diarrhoea, gastrointestinal discomfort, hypersalivation, nausea, vomiting, weight decreased
- Other: asthenia, dehydration, hyperhidrosis, skin reactions, urinary incontinence, urinary tract infection
- Specific to oral use: abnormal gait, confusion, hallucinations, malaise, parkinsonism, sleep disorders

Uncommon
- Aggression, atrioventricular block
- Specific to oral use: hypotension
- Specific to transdermal use: gastric ulcer

Rare or very rare
- Pancreatitis, seizure
- Specific to oral use: angina pectoris, gastrointestinal disorders, gastrointestinal haemorrhage

Frequency not known
- Hepatitis
- Specific to transdermal use: hallucination, nightmare
- Transdermal administration is less likely to cause side effects

 Life-Threatening or Dangerous Side Effects
- Syncope
- Pancreatitis
- Seizures
- Gastrointestinal haemorrhage

Weight Gain

unusual   not unusual   common   problematic
- Weight loss is common

Sedation

unusual   not unusual   common   problematic
- Reported but not expected

What To Do About Side Effects
- Wait

- Side effects such as nausea improve with time
- Take in daytime to reduce insomnia or take with food to reduce nausea
- Use slower dose titration
- Consider lowering dose, switching to a different agent, or adding an appropriate augmenting agent

Best Augmenting Agents for Side Effects
- Many side effects cannot be improved with an augmenting agent

DOSING AND USE

Usual Dosage Range
* Mild-moderate dementia in Alzheimer's and Parkinson's disease:
- Oral: 3–6mg twice per day (max per dose 6 mg twice per day)

* Mild dementia for Alzheimer's:
- Transdermal patch: 9.5 mg/24 hours, but can go up to 13.3 mg/24 hours daily if well tolerated and cognitive deterioration or functional decline demonstrated

Dosage Forms
- Capsule 1.5 mg, 3 mg, 4.5 mg, 6 mg
- Liquid 2 mg/mL (120 mL bottle)
- Transdermal patch 4.6 mg/24 hours, 9.5 mg/24 hours, 13.3 mg/24 hours (each box has 30 units)

How to Dose
* Mild-moderate dementia in Alzheimer's disease or Parkinson's disease:
- Oral: initial dose 1.5 mg twice per day, increased by increments of 1.5 mg twice per day, at least every 2 weeks depending on response and tolerance; usual dose 3–6 mg twice per day (max per dose 6 mg twice per day), if treatment interrupted for longer than several days, re-titrate from 1.5 mg twice per day

* Mild-moderate dementia in Alzheimer's disease:
- Transdermal patch: 4.6 mg/24 hours daily for a minimum of 4 weeks, increased if tolerated to 9.5 mg/24 hours daily for a further 6 months, then increased if required to 13.3 mg/24 hours daily if tolerated well and cognitive deterioration or functional

decline present; caution in patients with body weight < 50 kg, if treatment interrupted for more than 3 days, re-titrate from 4.6 mg/24 hours patch

Dosing Tips

Switching from oral to transdermal therapy:

- When switching from oral to transdermal therapy, patients taking 3–6 mg by mouth daily should initially switch to 4.6 mg/24 hours patch, then titrate. Patients taking 9 mg by mouth daily should switch to 9.5 mg/24 hours patch if oral dose stable and well tolerated. If oral dose not stable or well tolerated patients should switch to 4.6 mg/24 hours patch, then titrate. Patients taking 12 mg by mouth daily should switch to 9.5 mg/24 hours patch. The first patch should be applied on the day following the last oral dose

With transdermal use:

- Apply patches to clean, dry, non-hairy, non-irritated skin on back, upper arm or chest, removing after 24 hours and siting a replacement patch on a different area
- New application site should be selected for each day; patch should be applied at about the same time every day; only one patch should be applied at a time; patches should not be cut; new patch should not be applied to the same spot for at least 14 days
- Plasma exposure with transdermal rivastigmine is 20–30% lower when applied to the abdomen or thigh as compared to the upper back, chest, or upper arm
- Advise patients and carers of patch administration instructions, particularly to remove the previous day's patch before applying the new patch
- For transdermal formulation, dose increases should occur after a minimum of 4 weeks at the previous dose and only if the previous dose was well tolerated
- Avoid touching the exposed (sticky) side of the patch, and after application, wash hands with soap and water; do not touch eyes until after hands have been washed
- A rivastigmine transdermal patch (9.5 mg/24 hours) has been shown to be as effective as the highest dose of capsules but with a superior tolerability profile in a 6-month double-blind, placebo-controlled RCT

- Incidence of nausea is generally higher during the titration phase than during maintenance treatment
- If restarting treatment after a lapse of several days or more, dose titration should occur as when starting drug for the first time
- Oral doses between 6–12 mg/day have been shown to be more effective than doses between 1–4 mg/day
- Recommended to take oral rivastigmine with food
- Rapid dose titration increases the incidence of gastrointestinal side effects
- Probably best to utilise highest tolerated dose within the usual dosage range
- If a person is intolerant to rivastigmine switching to another agent should be done after complete resolution of side effects; if there is a lack of efficacy, switching can be done more quickly

Overdose

- Can be lethal; nausea, vomiting, excess salivation, sweating, hypotension, bradycardia, collapse, convulsions, muscle weakness (weakness of respiratory muscles can lead to death)

Long-Term Use

- Drug may lose effectiveness in slowing degenerative course of Alzheimer's disease after 6 months
- Can be effective in some patients for several years and stopping medication is not recommended if the disease becomes severe and the medication is well tolerated

Habit Forming

- No

How to Stop

- Will need tapering due to its short half-life (reduce dose by 1.5–3.0 mg every 2–4 weeks)
- Discontinuation may lead to notable deterioration in memory and behaviour, which may not be restored when drug is restarted or another cholinesterase inhibitor is initiated

Pharmacokinetics

- Half-life for oral formulation about 1 hour

- Half-life for transdermal patch about 3.4 hours
- Not hepatically metabolised; no CYP450-mediated pharmacokinetic drug interactions

 Drug Interactions

- Rivastigmine may increase the effects of anaesthetics and should be discontinued prior to surgery
- Rivastigmine may interact with anticholinergic agents and the combination may decrease the efficacy of both
- Antagonistic effects with competitive neuromuscular blockers (e.g. tubocurarine)
- Clearance of rivastigmine may be increased by nicotine
- Potential for synergistic activity with cholinomimetics such as depolarising neuromuscular blocking agents (e.g. succinylcholine), cholinergic agonists (e.g. bethanechol) or peripherally acting cholinesterase inhibitors (e.g. neostigmine)
- Synergistic effects on cardiac conduction with beta blockers, amiodarone, calcium channel blockers
- Bradycardia may occur if combined with beta blockers
- Theoretically, could reduce the efficacy of levodopa in Parkinson's disease
- Not recommended in combination with metoclopramide due to risk of additive extrapyramidal effects
- Not rational to combine with another cholinesterase inhibitor
- Rivastigmine may inhibit the butyrylcholinesterase-mediated metabolism of other substances, e.g. cocaine
- Smoking tobacco increases the clearance of rivastigmine
- Caution with concomitant use of drugs known to induce QT prolongation and/or torsades de pointes
- Movement disorders and neuroleptic malignant syndrome have occurred with concomitant use of antipsychotics and cholinesterase inhibitors
- Concurrent use with metoclopramide may result in increased risk of extrapyramidal symptoms

 Other Warnings/Precautions

- May exacerbate asthma or other chronic obstructive pulmonary disease
- Increased gastric acid secretion may increase the risk of ulcers, therefore use with caution in patients with duodenal or gastric ulcers or with a susceptibility to ulcers
- Bradycardia or heart block may occur in patients with or without cardiac impairments
- Use with caution in patients with conduction abnormalities or sick sinus syndrome
- Use with caution in patients with bladder outflow obstruction
- Use with caution in patients with a history of seizures
- Severe vomiting with oesophageal rupture may occur if rivastigmine therapy is resumed without re-titrating the drug to full dosing
- Individuals with low body weight may be at greater risk for adverse effects
- Risk of fatal overdose with patch administration errors

Do Not Use

- If there is a proven allergy to rivastigmine or other carbamates

SPECIAL POPULATIONS

Renal Impairment

- Adjust dose according to individual tolerability

Hepatic Impairment

- Titrate according to individual tolerability in mild to moderate hepatic impairment
- Use with caution in severe impairment

Cardiac Impairment

- Use with caution with cardiac impairment as acetylcholinesterase inhibitors can have vagotonic effects on heart rate (i.e. bradycardia): may be of importance in patients with "sick sinus syndrome" or other supraventricular cardiac disturbances, such as sinoatrial or atrioventricular block
- Acetylcholinesterase inhibitors should be used with caution in patients taking medication that reduce heart rate (e.g. digoxin or beta blockers)

Elderly

- Some patients may tolerate lower doses better
- Use of cholinesterase inhibitors may be associated with increased rates of syncope, bradycardia, pacemaker insertion, and hip fracture in older adults with dementia
- Not recommended for elderly patients with a history of bradycardia, heart block, recurrent unexplained syncope
- Not for use with concurrent drugs that reduce heart rate (risk of cardiac conduction failure, syncope and injury)

Children and Adolescents

- Safety and efficacy have not been established

Pregnancy

- Controlled studies have not been conducted in pregnant women
- Animal studies do not show adverse effects
- *Not recommended for use in pregnant women or women of childbearing potential

Breastfeeding

- Unknown if rivastigmine is secreted in human breast milk, but all psychotropics assumed to be secreted in breast milk
- *Recommended either to discontinue drug or bottle feed
- Rivastigmine is not recommended for use in nursing women

THE ART OF PSYCHOPHARMACOLOGY

Potential Advantages

- Theoretically, butyrylcholinesterase inhibition centrally could enhance therapeutic efficacy
- May be useful in some patients who do not respond to or do not tolerate other cholinesterase inhibitors

Potential Disadvantages

- Theoretically, butyrylcholinesterase inhibition peripherally could enhance side effects

Primary Target Symptoms

- Memory loss in Alzheimer's disease
- Behavioural symptoms in Alzheimer's disease
- Memory loss in dementia in Parkinson's disease

Pearls

- Dramatic reversal of symptoms of Alzheimer's disease is not generally seen with cholinesterase inhibitors
- Can lead to therapeutic nihilism among prescribers and lack of an appropriate trial of a cholinesterase inhibitor
- Perhaps only 50% of Alzheimer's patients are diagnosed, and only 50% of those diagnosed are treated, and only 50% of those treated are given a cholinesterase inhibitor, and then only for 200 days in a disease that lasts 7–10 years
- Must evaluate lack of efficacy and loss of efficacy over months, not weeks
- Cholinesterase inhibitors have at best a modest impact on non-cognitive features of dementia such as apathy, disinhibition, delusions, anxiety, lack of cooperation, pacing; however, in the absence of safe and effective alternatives a trial of a cholinesterase inhibitor is appropriate
- Treat the patient but ask the caregiver about efficacy
- What to expect from a cholinesterase inhibitor:
  - Patients do not generally improve dramatically although this can be observed in a significant minority of patients
  - Onset of behavioural problems and nursing home placement can be delayed
  - Functional outcomes, including activities of daily living, can be preserved
  - Caregiver burden and stress can be reduced
- Delay in progression in Alzheimer's disease is not evidence of disease-modifying actions of cholinesterase inhibition
- Cholinesterase inhibitors like rivastigmine depend upon the presence of intact targets for acetylcholine for maximum effectiveness and thus may be most effective in the early stages of Alzheimer's disease
- The most prominent side effects of rivastigmine are gastrointestinal effects, which are usually mild and transient

Rivastigmine (Continued)

- May cause more gastrointestinal side effects than some other cholinesterase inhibitors, especially if not slowly titrated
- At recommended doses, transdermal formulation may have lower incidence of gastrointestinal side effects than oral formulation
- Use with caution in underweight or frail patients
- Weight loss can be a problem in Alzheimer's patients with debilitation and muscle wasting
- Women over 85, particularly with low body weights, may experience more adverse effects
- For patients with intolerable side effects, generally allow a washout period with resolution of side effects prior to switching to another cholinesterase inhibitor
- Cognitive improvement may be linked to substantial (> 65%) inhibition of acetylcholinesterase
- Rivastigmine's effects on butyrylcholinesterase may be more relevant in later stages of Alzheimer's disease, when gliosis is occurring
- Butyrylcholinesterase actively could interfere with amyloid plaque formation, which contains this enzyme
- Some Alzheimer's patients who fail to respond to another cholinesterase inhibitor may respond when switched to rivastigmine
- Some Alzheimer's patients who fail to respond to rivastigmine may respond to another cholinesterase inhibitor
- To prevent potential clinical deterioration, generally switch from long-term treatment with one cholinesterase inhibitor to another without a washout period
- May slow the progression of mild cognitive impairment to Alzheimer's disease
- May be useful for dementia with Lewy bodies (DLB, constituted by early loss of attentiveness and visual perception with possible hallucinations, Parkinson-like movement problems, fluctuating cognition such as daytime drowsiness and lethargy, staring into space for long periods, episodes of disorganised speech)
- May decrease delusion, apathy, agitation, and hallucinations in dementia with Lewy bodies
- Only consider AChE inhibitors or memantine for people with vascular dementia if they have suspected co-morbid Alzheimer's disease, Parkinson's disease dementia or dementia with Lewy bodies
- Do not offer AChE inhibitors or memantine to people with frontotemporal dementia
- Do not offer AChE inhibitors or memantine to people with cognitive impairment caused by multiple sclerosis
- May be helpful for dementia in Down's syndrome

 Suggested Reading

Bentue-Ferrer D, Tribut O, Polard E, et al. Clinically significant drug interactions with cholinesterase inhibitors: a guide for neurologists. CNS Drugs 2003;17:947–63.

Birks JS, Chong LY, Grimley Evans J. Rivastigmine for Alzheimer's disease. Cochrane Database Syst Rev 2015;9(9):CD001191.

Dhillon S. Rivastigmine transdermal patch: a review of its use in the management of dementia of the Alzheimer's type. Drugs 2011;71(9):1209–31.

Jones RW. Have cholinergic therapies reached their clinical boundary in Alzheimer's disease? Int J Geriatr Psychiatry 2003;18(Suppl 1):S7–13.

Sertraline

THERAPEUTICS

Brands
• Lustral

Generic?
Yes

Class
• Neuroscience-based nomenclature: pharmacology domain – serotonin; mode of action – reuptake inhibitor
• SSRI (selective serotonin reuptake inhibitor); often classified as an antidepressant, but it is not just an antidepressant

Commonly Prescribed for
(Bold for BNF indication)
• **Depressive illness**
• **Obsessive-compulsive disorder**
• **Panic disorder**
• **Post-traumatic stress disorder**
• **Social anxiety disorder**
• Premenstrual dysphoric disorder (PMDD)
• Generalised anxiety disorder (GAD)
• Agoraphobia

 ### How the Drug Works
• Boosts neurotransmitter serotonin
• Blocks serotonin reuptake pump (serotonin transporter)
• Desensitises serotonin receptors, especially serotonin 1A receptors
• Presumably increases serotonergic neurotransmission
∗Sertraline also has some ability to block dopamine reuptake pump (dopamine transporter), which could increase dopamine neurotransmission and contribute to its therapeutic actions
• Sertraline also binds at sigma 1 receptors

How Long Until It Works
∗Some patients may experience increased energy or activation early after initiation of treatment
• Onset of therapeutic actions with some antidepressants can be seen within 1–2 weeks, but often delayed 2–4 weeks
• If it is not working within 3–4 weeks for depression, it may require a dosage increase or it may not work at all

• By contrast, for generalised anxiety, onset of response and increases in remission rates may still occur after 8 weeks, and for up to 6 months after initiating dosing
• For OCD if no improvement within about 10–12 weeks, then treatment may need to be reconsidered
• May continue to work for many years to prevent relapse of symptoms

If It Works
• The goal of treatment is complete remission of current symptoms as well as prevention of future relapses
• Treatment most often reduces or even eliminates symptoms, but is not a cure since symptoms can recur after medicine is stopped
• Continue treatment until all symptoms are gone (remission), especially in depression and whenever possible in anxiety disorders (e.g. OCD, PTSD)
• Once symptoms are gone, continue treating for at least 6–9 months for the first episode of depression or >12 months if relapse indicators present
• If >5 episodes and/or 2 episodes in the last few years then need to continue for at least 2 years or indefinitely
• Use in anxiety disorders may also need to be indefinite

If It Doesn't Work
• Important to recognise non-response to treatment early on (3–4 weeks)
• Many patients have only a partial response where some symptoms are improved but others persist (especially insomnia, fatigue, and problems concentrating in depression)
• Other patients may be non-responders, sometimes called treatment-resistant or treatment-refractory
• Some patients who have an initial response may relapse even though they continue treatment
• Consider increasing dose, switching to another agent or adding an appropriate augmenting agent
• Lithium may be added for suicidal patients or those at high risk of relapse
• Consider psychotherapy
• Consider ECT
• Consider evaluation for another diagnosis or for a co-morbid condition (e.g. medical illness, substance abuse, etc.)

Sertraline (Continued)

- Some patients may experience a switch into mania and so would require antidepressant discontinuation and initiation of a mood stabiliser

 Best Augmenting Combos for Partial Response or Treatment Resistance

In OCD:
- Consider cautious addition of an antipsychotic (risperidone, quetiapine, olanzapine, aripiprazole or haloperidol) as augmenting agent
- Alternative augmenting agents may include ondansetron, granisetron, topiramate, lamotrigine
- A switch to clomipramine may be a better option in treatment-resistant cases
- Combine an SSRI or clomipramine with an evidence-based psychological treatment

In depression:
- Mood stabilisers or atypical antipsychotics for bipolar depression
- Atypical antipsychotics for psychotic depression
- Atypical antipsychotics as first-line augmenting agents (quetiapine MR 300 mg/day or aripiprazole at 2.5–10 mg/day) for treatment-resistant depression
- Atypical antipsychotics as second-line augmenting agents (risperidone 0.5–2 mg/day or olanzapine 2.5–10 mg/day) for treatment-resistant depression
- Mirtazapine at 30–45 mg/day as another second-line augmenting agent (a dual serotonin and noradrenaline combination, but observe for switch into mania, increase in suicidal ideation or rare risk of non-fatal serotonin syndrome)
- Although T3 (20–50 mcg/day) is another second-line augmenting agent the evidence suggests that it works best with tricyclic antidepressants
- Other augmenting agents but with less evidence include bupropion (up to 400 mg/day), buspirone (up to 60 mg/day) and lamotrigine (up to 400 mg/day)
- Benzodiazepines if agitation present
- Hypnotics or trazodone for insomnia (but there is a rare risk of non-fatal serotonin syndrome with trazodone)
- Augmenting agents reserved for specialist use include: modafinil for sleepiness, fatigue and lack of concentration; stimulants, oestrogens, testosterone
- Lithium is particularly useful for suicidal patients and those at high risk of relapse including with factors such as severe depression, psychomotor retardation, repeated episodes (>3), significant weight loss, or a family history of major depression (aim for lithium plasma levels 0.6–1.0 mmol/L)
- For elderly patients lithium is a very effective augmenting agent
- For severely ill patients other combinations may be tried especially in specialist centres
- Augmenting agents that may be tried include omega-3, SAM-e, L-methylfolate
- Additional non-pharmacological treatments such as exercise, mindfulness, CBT, and IPT can also be helpful
- If present after treatment response (4–8 weeks) or remission (6–12 weeks), the most common residual symptoms of depression include cognitive impairments, reduced energy and problems with sleep

Tests
- None for healthy individuals

SIDE EFFECTS

How Drug Causes Side Effects
- Theoretically, due to increases in serotonin concentrations at serotonin receptors in parts of the brain and body other than those that cause therapeutic actions (e.g. unwanted actions of serotonin in sleep centres causing insomnia, unwanted actions of serotonin in the gut causing diarrhoea, etc.)
- *Increasing serotonin can cause diminished dopamine release and might contribute to emotional flattening, cognitive slowing, and apathy in some patients, although this could theoretically be diminished by sertraline's dopamine reuptake blocking properties
- Most side effects are immediate but often go away with time, in contrast to most therapeutic effects which are delayed and are enhanced over time
- Sertraline's possible dopamine reuptake blocking properties could contribute to agitation, anxiety, and undesirable activation, especially early in dosing

Notable Side Effects

- CNS: insomnia but also sedation, agitation, tremors, headache, dizziness
- GIT: decreased appetite, nausea, diarrhoea, constipation, dry mouth
- Sexual dysfunction (men: delayed ejaculation, erectile dysfunction; men and women: decreased sexual desire, anorgasmia)
- SIADH (syndrome of inappropriate antidiuretic hormone secretion)
- Mood elevation in diagnosed or undiagnosed bipolar disorder
- Sweating (dose-dependent)
- Bruising and rare bleeding

Common or very common

- CNS: depression, neuromuscular dysfunction
- Other: chest pain, gastrointestinal disorders, increased risk of infection, vasodilation

Uncommon

- CNS/PNS: abnormal sensation, abnormal thinking, euphoric mood, migraine, speech disorder
- CVS: hypertension
- GIT: burping, dysphagia, thirst
- Resp: dyspnoea, respiratory disorders
- Other: back pain, chills, cold sweat, ear pain, hypothyroidism, muscle complaints, muscle weakness, periorbital oedema

Rare or very rare

- CNS/PNS: abnormal gait, coma, conversion disorder, drug dependence, dysphonia, eye disorders, glaucoma, psychotic disorder, vision disorders
- CVS: cardiac disorder, myocardial infarction, peripheral ischaemia
- Endocrine/metabolic: diabetes mellitus, hypercholesterolaemia, hypoglycaemia
- GIT: hepatic disorders, hiccups
- Other: abnormal hair texture, balanoposthitis, bone disorder, genital discharge, lymphadenopathy, neoplasms, oliguria, vulvovaginal atrophy

Frequency not known

- Cerebrovascular insufficiency, gynaecomastia, hyperglycaemia, leucopenia, neuroleptic malignant syndrome, pancreatitis

 Life-Threatening or Dangerous Side Effects

- Rare seizures

- Rare induction of mania
- Rare increase in suicidal ideation and behaviours in adolescents and young adults (up to age 25), hence patients should be warned of this potential adverse event

Weight Gain

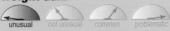

- Weight changes may be seen
- Some patients may experience weight loss

Sedation

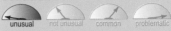

- Reported but not expected
- Possibly activating in some patients

What To Do About Side Effects

- Wait
- Wait
- Wait
- If sertraline is activating, take in the morning to help reduce insomnia
- Reduce dose to 25 mg or even 12.5 mg until side effects abate, then increase dose as tolerated, usually to at least 50 mg/day
- In a few weeks, switch or add other drugs

Best Augmenting Agents for Side Effects

- Many side effects are dose-dependent (i.e. they increase as dose increases, or they re-emerge until tolerance redevelops)
- Many side effects are time-dependent (i.e. they start immediately upon dosing and upon each dose increase, but go away with time)
- Often best to try another antidepressant monotherapy prior to resorting to augmentation strategies to treat side effects
- Trazodone, mirtazapine or hypnotic for insomnia
- Mirtazapine for agitation, and gastrointestinal side effects
- Bupropion for emotional flattening, cognitive slowing, or apathy
- For sexual dysfunction: can augment with bupropion for women, sildenafil for men; or otherwise switch to another antidepressant
- Benzodiazepines for jitteriness and anxiety, especially at initiation of treatment and especially for anxious patients
- Increased activation or agitation may represent the induction of a bipolar state,

especially a mixed dysphoric bipolar condition sometimes associated with suicidal ideation, and requires the addition of lithium, a mood stabiliser or an atypical antipsychotic, and/or discontinuation of the SSRI

DOSING AND USE

Usual Dosage Range
• 50–200 mg/day

Dosage Forms
• Tablet 25 mg, 50 mg, 100 mg

How to Dose
∗Depression and OCD:
• Initial dose 50 mg/day; can be increased by increments of 50 mg once per week; max dose generally 200 mg/day; single dose
∗Panic, PTSD, and agoraphobia:
• Initial dose 25 mg/day; increase to 50 mg/day after 1 week thereafter, usually wait a few weeks to assess drug effects before increasing dose; max dose generally 200 mg/day; single dose
∗Social anxiety:
• 50 mg–200 mg/day
∗PMDD:
• Initial dose 50 mg/day; can dose daily through the menstrual cycle or limit to the luteal phase
∗OCD (under specialist supervision in children 6–12 years):
• Starting dose 25 mg/day (children 6–12 years), 50 mg/day (adolescents/adults). Can be increased by increments of 50 mg per week, max dose 200 mg/day
∗PTSD (children):
• Starting dose 12.5–25 mg/day, and 50–200 mg/day, can be increased by increments of 50 mg per week
∗GAD:
• Prescribed at half the normal starting dose for depression; titrate up into the normal antidepressant dose range as tolerated; initial worsening of anxiety may be seen; response usually seen within 6 weeks and continues to increase over time; optimal duration of treatment should be at least 1 year
• In children and adolescents: starting dose is 25–50 mg and the effective dose is 50–100 mg, sometimes higher

Dosing Tips
• Give once daily, often in the mornings to reduce chances of insomnia
• Many patients ultimately require more than 50 mg dose per day
• Some patients are dosed above 200 mg
• Evidence that some treatment-resistant OCD patients may respond safely to doses up to 400 mg/day, but this is for experts and use with caution
• The more anxious and agitated the patient, the lower the starting dose, the slower the titration, and the more likely the need for a concomitant agent such as trazodone or a benzodiazepine
• If intolerable anxiety, insomnia, agitation, akathisia, or activation occur either upon dosing initiation or discontinuation, consider the possibility of activated bipolar disorder and switch to a mood stabiliser or atypical antipsychotic
• Utilise half a 25-mg tablet (12.5 mg) when initiating treatment in patients with a history of intolerance to previous antidepressants

Overdose
• Rarely lethal in monotherapy overdose; vomiting, sedation, heart rhythm disturbances, dilated pupils, agitation; fatalities have been reported in sertraline overdose combined with other drugs or alcohol
• Rarely, severe poisoning may result in serotonin syndrome, with marked neuropsychiatric effects, neuromuscular hyperactivity, and autonomic instability; hyperthermia, rhabdomyolysis, renal failure, and coagulopathies may develop
• Management is supportive; activated charcoal given within 1 hour of the overdose reduces absorption of the drug
• Convulsions can be treated with lorazepam, diazepam, or midazolam oromucosal solution
• Seek specialist input for the management of hyperthermia or serotonin syndrome

Long-Term Use
• Safe

Habit Forming
• No

How to Stop

- If taking SSRIs for more than 6–8 weeks, it is not recommended to stop them suddenly due to the risk of withdrawal effects (dizziness, nausea, stomach cramps, sweating, tingling, dysaesthesias)
- Taper dose gradually over 4 weeks, or longer if withdrawal symptoms emerge
- Inform all patients of the risk of withdrawal symptoms
- If withdrawal symptoms emerge, raise dose to stop symptoms and then restart withdrawal much more slowly

Pharmacokinetics

- Half-life of parent drug 22–36 hours
- Half-life of metabolite N-desmethylsertraline 62–104 hours
- Inhibits CYP450 2D6 (weakly at low doses)
- Inhibits CYP450 3A4 (weakly at low doses)

 Drug Interactions

- Tramadol increases the risk of seizures in patients taking an antidepressant
- Can increase TCA levels; use with caution with TCAs or when switching from a TCA to sertraline
- Can cause a fatal "serotonin syndrome" when combined with MAOIs, so do not use with MAOIs or for at least 14 days after MAOIs are stopped
- Do not start an MAOI for at least 5 half-lives (5 to 7 days for most drugs) after discontinuing sertraline
- Can rarely cause weakness, hyperreflexia, and incoordination when combined with sumatriptan or possibly with other triptans, requiring careful monitoring of patient
- Increased risk of bleeding when used in combination with NSAIDs, aspirin, alteplase, anti-platelets, and anticoagulants
- NSAIDs may impair effectiveness of SSRIs
- Increased risk of hyponatraemia when sertraline is used in combination with other agents that cause hyponatraemia, e.g. thiazides
- Via CYP450 3A4 inhibition, sertraline could theoretically increase the concentrations of pimozide and cause QTc prolongation and dangerous cardiac arrhythmias
- False-positive urine immunoassay screening tests for benzodiazepine have been reported in patients taking sertraline

due to a lack of specificity of the screening tests; false-positive results may be expected for several days following discontinuation of sertraline

 Other Warnings/Precautions

- Add or initiate other antidepressants with caution for up to 2 weeks after discontinuing sertraline
- Use with caution in patients with diabetes
- Use with caution in patients with susceptibility to angle-closure glaucoma
- Use with caution in patients receiving ECT or with a history of seizures
- Use with caution in patients with a history of bleeding disorders
- Use with caution in patients with bipolar disorder unless treated with concomitant mood-stabilising agent
- When treating children, carefully weigh the risks and benefits of pharmacological treatment against the risks and benefits of nontreatment with antidepressants and make sure to document this in the patient's chart
- Warn patients and their caregivers about the possibility of activating side effects and advise them to report such symptoms immediately
- Monitor patients for activation of suicidal ideation, especially children and adolescents

Do Not Use

- If patient has poorly controlled epilepsy
- If patient enters a manic phase
- If patient is already taking an MAOI (risk of serotonin syndrome)
- If patient is taking pimozide
- If there is a proven allergy to sertraline

Renal Impairment

- No dose adjustment
- Not removed by haemodialysis
- Use with caution
- Sertraline has been used to treat dialysis-associated hypotension and uraemia pruritus, however should be used with caution as acute renal failure has been reported

- Has been associated with serotonin syndrome when used in patients on haemodialysis

Hepatic Impairment

- Lower dose or give less frequently, perhaps by half in mild to moderate impairment
- Avoid in severe impairment (prolonged half-life)

Cardiac Impairment

- Proven cardiovascular safety in depressed patients with recent myocardial infarction or angina
- Treating depression with SSRIs in patients with acute angina or following myocardial infarction may reduce cardiac events and improve survival as well as mood

Elderly

- Some patients may tolerate lower doses and/or slower titration better
- Risk of SIADH with SSRIs is higher in the elderly
- Reduction in the risk of suicidality with antidepressants compared to placebo in adults age 65 and older
- Max dose in elderly is 100 mg/day

Children and Adolescents

- Sertraline is licensed for the treatment of obsessive-compulsive disorder in children
- It has also been shown to be effective in anxiety disorders; only small effect size for depression

Before you prescribe:

- Carefully weigh the risks and benefits of pharmacological treatment against the risks and benefits of nontreatment with antidepressants and make sure to document this in the patient's chart
- For OCD, children and young people should be offered CBT (including ERP) that involves the family or carers and is adapted to suit the developmental age of the child as the treatment of choice
- For anxiety disorders evidence-based psychological treatments should be offered as first-line treatment including psychoeducation and skills training for parents, particularly of young children, to promote and reinforce the child's exposure to feared or avoided social situations and development of skills

- Monotherapy with sertraline (55% response) is as effective as CBT for anxiety (60% response) compared with placebo (24% response), and combined therapy with CBT and sertraline is most likely to be successful (81% response)
- For mild to moderate depression, psychotherapy (individual or systemic) should be the first-line treatment. For moderate to severe depression, pharmacological treatment may be offered when the young person is unresponsive after 4–6 sessions of psychological therapy. Combined initial therapy (SSRI and psychological therapy) may be considered
- Sertraline may be considered as second-line option, or first-line in co-morbid anxiety disorder
- For both severe depression and anxiety disorders, pharmacological interventions may have to commence prior to psychological treatments to enable the child/young person to engage in psychological therapy
- Where a child or young person presents with self-harm and suicidal thoughts the immediate risk management may take first priority
- All children and young people presenting with depression/anxiety should be supported with sleep management, anxiety management, exercise and activation schedules, and healthy diet

Practical notes:

- Inform parents and child/young person that improvements may take several weeks to emerge
- The earliest effects may only be apparent to outsiders
- A risk management plan should be discussed prior to start of medication because of the possible increase in suicidal ideation and behaviours in adolescents and young adults
- Monitor patients face-to-face regularly, and weekly during the first 2–3 weeks of treatment or after increase
- Monitor for activation of suicidal ideation at the beginning of treatment
- Use with caution, observing for activation of known or unknown bipolar disorder and/or suicidal ideation, and inform parents or guardians of this risk so they can help observe child or adolescent patients

If it does not work:
- Review child's/young person's profile, consider new/changing contributing individual or systemic factors such as peer or family conflict. Consider physical health problems
- Consider non-concordance, especially in adolescents. In all children consider non-concordance by parent or child, address underlying reasons for non-concordance
- Consider dose adjustment before switching or augmentation. Be vigilant of polypharmacy especially in complex and highly vulnerable children/adolescents
- Sertraline is metabolised quickly by children and twice-daily dosing should be considered. It should be used cautiously and only by specialists
- For all SSRIs children can have a two-to three-fold higher incidence of behavioural activation and vomiting than adolescents, who also have a somewhat higher incidence than adults
- Recommended max dose is 200 mg/day
- Adolescents often receive adult dose, but doses slightly lower for children
- Effect of sertraline on growth has not been investigated; long-term effects are unknown
- Re-evaluate the need for continued treatment regularly

Pregnancy

- Not generally recommended for use during pregnancy, especially during first trimester
- Nonetheless, continuous treatment during pregnancy may be necessary and has not been proven to be harmful to the foetus
- Must weigh the risk of treatment (first trimester foetal development, third trimester newborn delivery) to the child against the risk of no treatment (recurrence of depression, maternal health, infant bonding) to the mother and child
- For many patients, this may mean continuing treatment during pregnancy
- Exposure to SSRIs in pregnancy has been associated with cardiac malformations, however recent studies have suggested that these findings may be due to other patient factors

- Exposure to SSRIs in pregnancy has been associated with an increased risk of spontaneous abortion, low birth weight and preterm delivery. Data is conflicting and the effects of depression cannot be ruled out from some studies
- SSRI use beyond the 20th week of pregnancy may be associated with increased risk of persistent pulmonary hypertension (PPHN) in newborns. Whilst the risk of PPHN remains low it presents potentially serious complications
- SSRI/SNRI antidepressant use in the month before delivery may result in a small increased risk of postpartum haemorrhage
- Neonates exposed to SSRIs or SNRIs late in the third trimester have developed complications requiring prolonged hospitalisation, respiratory support, and tube feeding; reported symptoms are consistent with either a direct toxic effect of SSRIs and SNRIs or, possibly, a drug discontinuation syndrome, and include respiratory distress, cyanosis, apnoea, seizures, temperature instability, feeding difficulty, vomiting, hypoglycaemia, hypotonia, hypertonia, hyperreflexia, tremor, jitteriness, irritability, and constant crying

Breastfeeding

- Small amounts found in mother's breast milk
- Trace amounts may be present in nursing children whose mothers are taking sertraline
- If child becomes irritable or sedated, breastfeeding or drug may need to be discontinued
- Immediate postpartum period is a high-risk time for depression, especially in women who have had prior depressive episodes, so drug may need to be reinstituted late in the third trimester or shortly after childbirth to prevent a recurrence during the postpartum period
- Must weigh benefits of breastfeeding with risks and benefits of antidepressant treatment versus nontreatment to both the infant and the mother
- For many patients, this may mean continuing treatment during breastfeeding
- Sertraline or paroxetine are the preferred SSRIs for breastfeeding mothers

THE ART OF PSYCHOPHARMACOLOGY

Potential Advantages

- Patients with atypical depression (hypersomnia, increased appetite)
- Patients with fatigue and low energy
- Patients who wish to avoid hyperprolactinaemia (e.g. pubescent children, girls and women with galactorrhoea, girls and women with unexplained amenorrhoea, postmenopausal women who are not taking oestrogen replacement therapy)
- Patients who are sensitive to the prolactin-elevating properties of other SSRIs
- Licensed for treatment of obsessive-compulsive disorder in children and adolescents

Potential Disadvantages

- Initiating treatment in anxious patients with some insomnia
- Patients with co-morbid irritable bowel syndrome
- Can require dosage titration
- Data from placebo-controlled trials in paediatric populations with MDD were not sufficient to support an indication for sertraline in this age group, though clinical experience suggests some effectiveness
- In children: those who already show psychomotor agitation, anger, irritability, or who do not have a psychiatric diagnosis

Primary Target Symptoms

- Depressed mood
- Anxiety
- Sleep disturbance, both insomnia and hypersomnia (eventually, but may actually cause insomnia, especially short-term)
- Panic attacks, avoidant behaviour, re-experiencing, hyperarousal

 Pearls

- * May be a type of "dual action" agent with both potent serotonin reuptake inhibition and less potent dopamine reuptake inhibition, but the clinical significance of this is unknown
- Cognitive and affective "flattening" may theoretically be diminished in some patients

by sertraline's dopamine reuptake blocking properties

- * May be a first-line choice for atypical depression (e.g. hypersomnia, hyperphagia, low energy, mood reactivity)
- Best-documented cardiovascular safety of any antidepressant, proven safe for depressed patients with recent myocardial infarction or angina
- May bind to sigma 1 receptors, enhancing sertraline's anxiolytic actions
- Can have more gastrointestinal effects, particularly diarrhoea, than some other antidepressants
- May be more effective treatment for women with PTSD or depression than for men with PTSD or depression, but the clinical significance of this is unknown
- SSRIs may be useful for hot flushes in perimenopausal women
- For sexual dysfunction, can augment with bupropion or switch to a non-SSRI such as bupropion or mirtazapine
- Some postmenopausal women's depression will respond better to sertraline plus oestrogen augmentation than to sertraline alone
- Non-response to sertraline in elderly may require consideration of mild cognitive impairment or Alzheimer's disease
- Not as well tolerated as some SSRIs for panic, especially when dosing is initiated, unless given with benzodiazepines or trazodone
- Relative lack of effect on prolactin may make it a preferred agent for some children, adolescents, and women
- Some evidence suggests that sertraline treatment during only the luteal phase may be more effective than continuous treatment for patients with PMDD
- Sertraline 200 mg/day and naltrexone 100 mg/day had improved drinking outcomes and better mood than placebo/drug alone as relapse prevention medication
- Sertraline is safe post MI and in heart failure
- Sertraline has been reported to prolong the QTc interval in overdose but the clinical consequences of this are uncertain
- Sertraline is the best-tolerated SSRI for GAD

Suggested Reading

Cipriani A, Furukawa TA, Salanti G, et al. Comparative efficacy and acceptability of 21 antidepressant drugs for the acute treatment of adults with major depressive disorder: a systematic review and network meta-analysis. Lancet 2018;391(10128):1357–66.

Cipriani A, La Ferla T, Furukawa TA, et al. Sertraline versus other antidepressive agents for depression. Cochrane Database Syst Rev 2010;14(4):CD006117.

DeVane CL, Liston HL, Markowitz JS. Clinical pharmacokinetics of sertraline. Clin Pharmacokinet 2002;41:1247–66.

Flament MF, Lane RM, Zhu R, et al. Predictors of an acute antidepressant response to fluoxetine and sertraline. Int Clin Psychopharmacol 1999;14:259–75.

Khouzam HR, Emes R, Gill T, et al. The antidepressant sertraline: a review of its uses in a range of psychiatric and medical conditions. Compr Ther 2003;29:47–53.

McRae AL, Brady KT. Review of sertraline and its clinical applications in psychiatric disorders. Expert Opin Pharmacother 2001;2:883–92.

Sodium oxybate

Brands
- Xyrem

Generic?
Yes

Class
- Neuroscience-based nomenclature: pharmacology domain – GABA; mode of action – agonist
- CNS depressant; GABA-B receptor partial agonist

Commonly Prescribed for
(bold for BNF indication)
- **Narcolepsy with cataplexy (under expert supervision)**
- Fibromyalgia
- Chronic pain/neuropathic pain
- Reducing excessive sleepiness in patients with narcolepsy

How the Drug Works
- Gamma hydroxybutyrate (GHB) is an endogenous putative neurotransmitter synthesised from its parent compound, GABA; sodium oxybate is the sodium salt of GHB and is administered exogenously
- Has agonist actions at GHB receptors and partial agonist actions at GABA-B receptors
- Improves slow-wave sleep at night, presumably leaving patients better rested and more alert during the day

How Long Until It Works
- Can immediately reduce daytime sleepiness
- Can take several days to optimise dosing and clinical improvement

If It Works
- Improves daytime sleepiness and may improve fatigue in patients with narcolepsy
- Reduces frequency of cataplexy attacks
- May improve sleep physiology and subjective experience of pain and fatigue in patients with fibromyalgia and other chronic pain conditions

If It Doesn't Work
- Increase dose
- Consider an alternative treatment

Best Augmenting Combos for Partial Response or Treatment Resistance
- Sodium oxybate may itself act as an augmenting agent to stimulants or modafinil for excessive sleepiness in narcolepsy
- *The majority of patients taking sodium oxybate in clinical trials for narcolepsy and cataplexy were taking a concomitant stimulant
- Can be used as an augmenting agent for fibromyalgia with SNRIs (e.g. duloxetine) and alpha 2 delta ligands (e.g. gabapentin, pregabalin), but has not been well studied in combination with these agents

Tests
- None for healthy individuals

How Drug Causes Side Effects
- Unknown
- CNS side effects presumably due to excessive CNS actions on various neurotransmitter systems

Notable Side Effects
- Headache, dizziness, sedation
- Nausea, vomiting
- Enuresis

Common or very common
- CNS/PNS: abnormal sensation, anxiety, blurred vision, confusion, depression, dizziness, fall, feeling drunk, headache, impaired concentration, movement disorders, sedation, sleep disorders, sleep paralysis, tremor, vertigo
- CVS: hypertension, palpitations
- GIT: abnormal appetite, altered taste, decreased weight, diarrhoea, nausea, upper abdominal pain, vomiting
- Other: arthralgia, asthenia, back pain, dyspnoea, hyperhidrosis, increased risk of infection, muscle spasms, nasal congestion, peripheral oedema, skin reactions, snoring, urinary disorders

Uncommon
- CNS: abnormal behaviour, abnormal thinking, hallucination, memory loss, psychosis, suicidal behaviours

- Other: faecal incontinence

Frequency not known
- CNS: altered mood, delusions, homicidal ideation, loss of consciousness, seizure, sleep apnoea
- Other: angioedema, dehydration, dry mouth, respiratory depression

 Life-Threatening or Dangerous Side Effects
- Respiratory depression, especially when taken in overdose
- Neuropsychiatric events (psychosis, depression, paranoia, agitation)
- Confusion and wandering at night (unclear if this is true somnambulism)
- Homicidal ideation
- Seizures

Weight Gain

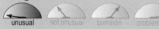

- Weight loss is a very common side effect

Sedation

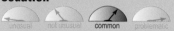

- Sedation is a very common side effect

What To Do About Side Effects
- Wait
- Lower the dose
- If unacceptable side effects persist, discontinue use
- Discontinue concomitant medications that might be contributing to sedation

Best Augmenting Agents for Side Effects
- Many side effects cannot be improved with an augmenting agent

---

DOSING AND USE

Usual Dosage Range
- 2.25 g/day–9 g/day

Dosage Forms
- Oral solution 500 mg/mL

How to Dose
- Adult: initial dose 2.25 g on retiring at bedtime followed by 2.25 g after 2.5–4

hours, then increased by increments of 1.5 g/day in 2 divided doses, dose further adjusted according to response at intervals of 1–2 weeks; re-titrate dose if restarting after an interval of more than 2 weeks, max 9 g/day in 2 divided doses

 Dosing Tips
- *Both nightly doses of sodium oxybate should be prepared prior to bedtime, and the prepared second dose should be placed in close proximity to the patient's bed before the first dose is ingested
- Each dose must be diluted with 60 mL of water in a child-resistant cup that is supplied by the pharmacist
- The patient will probably need to set an alarm clock in order to wake up for the second dose
- Once prepared, the solution containing sodium oxybate should be consumed within 24 hours in order to minimise bacterial growth and contamination
- Food significantly reduces the bioavailability of sodium oxybate, so the patient should wait at least 2 hours after eating before taking the first dose of sodium oxybate
- It is best to minimise variability in the timing of dosing in relation to meals
- Once-nightly dosing has been studied and found effective in fibromyalgia
- Reduce dose by 20% with concurrent use of sodium valproate or valproic acid

Overdose
- Depressed consciousness with rapid fluctuations: confusion, agitation, ataxia, coma (especially at higher doses)
- Blurred vision, emesis, diaphoresis, headache, impaired psychomotor, myoclonus and tonic-clonic seizures
- Severe respiratory depression, Cheyne-Stokes respiration, apnoea
- Bradycardia, hypothermia, unconsciousness, muscular hypotonia but with tendon reflexes
- Gastric lavage and airway protection may be considered

Long-Term Use
- The need for continued treatment needs to be periodically evaluated
- For some patients this will be a life-long treatment

Habit Forming

- Sodium oxybate is a Schedule 2 controlled drug which means the patient may be required to prove their identity when collecting their prescription and must store the drug securely
- Risk of developing dependence and/or tolerance; risk may be greater with higher doses
- History of drug addiction may increase risk of dependence

How to Stop

- There is a risk of discontinuation effects including rebound cataplexy and withdrawal symptoms in some patients so a slower taper may be recommended

Pharmacokinetics

- Metabolised by the liver
- Elimination half-life about 30–60 minutes
- Absorption is delayed and decreased by high-fat meals
- Excretion is almost entirely via biotransformation to carbon dioxide, which is then eliminated by expiration

 Drug Interactions

- Should not be used in combination with CNS depressants or sedative hypnotics
- The dose of sodium oxybate needs to be reduced by 20% when used with sodium valproate or valproic acid

 Other Warnings/Precautions

- *Because of the rapid onset of CNS-depressant effects, sodium oxybate should only be ingested at bedtime and while in bed
- Sodium oxybate should not be used with alcohol or other CNS depressants, including opiates
- Use only with extreme caution in patients with impaired respiratory function or obstructive sleep apnoea
- Use with caution in morbidly obese patients (body mass index 40 kg/m²)
- Use with caution in patients with a history of depression
- Use with caution in the elderly
- Use with caution in patients with epilepsy

- Use with caution in patients with heart failure or hypertension due to the high sodium content
- Patients with history of drug abuse should be monitored closely
- Sodium oxybate may cause CNS effects similar to those caused by other CNS agents (e.g. confusion, psychosis, paranoia, agitation, depression, and suicidality)

Do Not Use

- In patients with major depression
- In patients with succinic semi-aldehyde dehydrogenase deficiency
- In patients taking sedative hypnotics
- If there is a proven allergy to sodium oxybate (gamma hydroxybutyrate)

Renal Impairment

- Caution – contains 3.96 mmol Na+ per mL
- Dose adjustment is not necessary
- Not excreted renally

Hepatic Impairment

- Halve initial dose

Cardiac Impairment

- Because sodium oxybate has sodium content, this may need to be considered in patients with hypertension or heart failure

Elderly

- Higher risk of side effects in elderly

 Children and Adolescents

- Not licensed for use in children and adolescents
- Has been widely used off-label to treat narcolepsy symptoms in children and adolescents (aged 7–19 years) with paediatric Type 1 narcolepsy (NT1) in non-controlled studies, showing a similar safety profile and therapeutic response to adult patients
- Ongoing paediatric therapy is based only on observational data shared among sleep disorder clinicians
- Study has shown clinical efficacy of sodium oxybate for the treatment of both excessive daytime sleepiness and cataplexy in narcolepsy in children

Sodium oxybate (Continued)

Pregnancy

- Human data extremely limited, animal studies do not show adverse effects
- Data from a limited number of pregnant women exposed in the first trimester indicate a possible increased risk of spontaneous abortions
- Use in women of childbearing potential requires weighing potential benefits to the mother against potential risks to the foetus
- *Generally, sodium oxybate should be discontinued prior to anticipated pregnancies

Breastfeeding

- Unknown if sodium oxybate is secreted in human breast milk, but all psychotropics assumed to be secreted in breast milk
- Short half-life should limit the amount excreted into breast milk
- Waiting for 5 hours after taking before breastfeeding likely to prevent any significant exposure
- If drug is continued while breastfeeding, infant should be monitored for possible adverse effects
- If infant becomes irritable or sedated, breastfeeding or drug may need to be discontinued

THE ART OF PSYCHOPHARMACOLOGY

Potential Advantages

- Less activating than stimulants
- For narcolepsy, may help patients insufficiently responsive to stimulants
- Has the biggest effect size on pain, fatigue, and sleep in fibromyalgia

Potential Disadvantages

- Has abuse potential
- Requires a second dose in the middle of the night
- Potentially more dangerous than other treatments, especially for fibromyalgia or chronic pain, and especially if taken with sedative hypnotics and/or opiates
- Risk of tolerance, dependence and misuse

Primary Target Symptoms

- Sleepiness, fatigue
- Cataplexy
- Painful physical symptoms
- Lack of nonrestorative sleep in fibromyalgia and chronic pain

Pearls

- Sodium oxybate increases slow-wave sleep, thereby improving sleep quality at night and allowing individuals to feel more rested during the day
- Sodium oxybate also increases growth hormone, which is one of the reasons that it has been abused by athletes
- *There are positive trials for efficacy in fibromyalgia, with improvement in sleep, pain, and fatigue, but not licensed for this due to safety concerns
- *Sodium oxybate is the sodium salt of gamma-hydroxybutyric acid (GHB). GHB is illegally used recreationally as a club drug and has also been implicated in several cases as a "date rape drug"

 Suggested Reading

Carter LP, Pardi D, Gorsline J, et al. Illicit gamma-hydroxybutyrate (GHB) and pharmaceutical sodium oxybate (Xyrem): differences in characteristics and misuse. Drug Alcohol Depend 2009;104(1–2):1–10.

Moldofsky H, Inhaber NH, Guinta DR, et al. Effects of sodium oxybate on sleep physiology and sleep/wake-related symptoms in patients with fibromyalgia syndrome: a double-blind, randomized, placebo-controlled study. J Rheumatol 2010;37(10):2156–66.

Owen RT. Sodium oxybate: efficacy, safety and tolerability in the treatment of narcolepsy with or without cataplexy. Drugs Today (Barc) 2008;44(3):197–204.

Russell IJ, Perkins AT, Michalek JE, et al. Sodium oxybate relieves pain and improves function in fibromyalgia syndrome: a randomized, double-blind, placebo-controlled, multicenter clinical trial. Arthritis Rheum 2009;60(1):299–309.

Wang YG, Swich TJ, Carter LP, et al. Safety overview of post marketing and clinical experience of sodium oxybate (Xyrem): abuse, misuse, dependence, and diversion. J Clin Sleep Med 2009;15(4):365–71.

Sulpiride

Brands
• Non-proprietary

Generic?
Yes

Class
• Neuroscience-based nomenclature: pharmacology domain – dopamine; mode of action – antagonist
• Conventional antipsychotic (neuroleptic, benzamide, dopamine 2 antagonist)

Commonly Prescribed for
(bold for BNF indication)
• **Schizophrenia with predominantly negative symptoms**
• **Schizophrenia with mainly positive symptoms**
• **Tourette syndrome (children – under expert supervision)**
• Depression

 How the Drug Works
• Blocks dopamine 2 receptors, reducing positive symptoms of psychosis
• Blocks dopamine 3 and 4 receptors, which may contribute to sulpiride's actions
• Possibly blocks presynaptic dopamine 2 autoreceptors more potently at low doses, which could theoretically contribute to improving negative symptoms of schizophrenia as well as depression

How Long Until It Works
• Psychotic symptoms can improve within 1 week, but it may take several weeks for full effect on behaviour

If It Works
• Most often reduces positive symptoms in schizophrenia but does not eliminate them
• Most patients with schizophrenia do not have a total remission of symptoms but rather a reduction of symptoms by about a third
• Continue treatment in schizophrenia until reaching a plateau of improvement
• After reaching a satisfactory plateau, continue treatment for at least a year after first episode of psychosis in schizophrenia
• For second and subsequent episodes of psychosis in schizophrenia, treatment may need to be indefinite

If It Doesn't Work
• Consider trying one of the first-line atypical antipsychotics (risperidone, olanzapine, quetiapine, aripiprazole, paliperidone, amisulpride)
• Consider trying another conventional antipsychotic
• If two or more antipsychotic monotherapies do not work, consider clozapine

 Best Augmenting Combos for Partial Response or Treatment Resistance
• Augmentation of conventional antipsychotics has not been systematically studied
• Addition of an anticonvulsant such as valproate, carbamazepine, or lamotrigine may be helpful
• Addition of a benzodiazepine, especially short-term for agitation
• Sulpiride itself can act as an augmenting agent when added to clozapine in partial or non-responders

Tests
Baseline
∗Measure weight, BMI, and waist circumference
• Get baseline personal and family history of diabetes, obesity, dyslipidaemia, hypertension, and cardiovascular disease
• Check for personal history of drug-induced leucopenia/neutropenia
∗Check pulse and blood pressure, fasting plasma glucose or glycosylated haemoglobin (HbA1c), fasting lipid profile, and prolactin levels
• Full blood count (FBC)
• Assessment of nutritional status, diet, and level of physical activity
• Determine if the patient:
  • is overweight (BMI 25.0–29.9)
  • is obese (BMI ≥30)
  • has pre-diabetes – fasting plasma glucose: 5.5 mmol/L to 6.9 mmol/L or HbA1c: 42 to 47 mmol/mol (6.0 to 6.4%)
  • has diabetes – fasting plasma glucose: >7.0 mmol/L or HbA1c: ≥48 mmol/L (≥6.5%)

- has hypertension (BP >140/90 mm Hg)
- has dyslipidaemia (increased total cholesterol, LDL cholesterol, and triglycerides; decreased HDL cholesterol)
- Treat or refer such patients for treatment, including nutrition and weight management, physical activity counselling, smoking cessation, and medical management
- Baseline ECG for: inpatients; those with a personal history or risk factor for cardiac disease

Monitoring

- Monitor weight and BMI during treatment
- Consider monitoring fasting triglycerides monthly for several months in patients at high risk for metabolic complications and when initiating or switching antipsychotics
- While giving a drug to a patient who has gained >5% of initial weight, consider evaluating for the presence of pre-diabetes, diabetes, or dyslipidaemia, or consider switching to a different antipsychotic
- Patients with low white blood cell count (WBC) or history of drug-induced leucopenia/neutropenia should have full blood count (FBC) monitored frequently during the first few months and sulpiride should be discontinued at the first sign of decline of WBC in the absence of other causative factors
- Monitor prolactin levels and for signs and symptoms of hyperprolactinaemia

---

SIDE EFFECTS

How Drug Causes Side Effects

- By blocking dopamine 2 receptors in the striatum, it can cause motor side effects
- By blocking dopamine 2 receptors in the pituitary, it can cause elevations in prolactin
- By blocking dopamine 2 receptors excessively in the mesocortical and mesolimbic dopamine pathways, especially at high doses, it can cause worsening of negative and cognitive symptoms (neuroleptic-induced deficit syndrome)
- Anticholinergic actions may cause sedation, blurred vision, constipation, dry mouth
- Antihistaminergic actions may cause sedation, weight gain
- By blocking alpha 1 adrenergic receptors, it can cause dizziness, sedation, and hypotension

- Mechanism of weight gain and any possible increased incidence of diabetes or dyslipidaemia with conventional antipsychotics is unknown

Notable Side Effects

*Extrapyramidal symptoms, akathisia
*Prolactin elevation, galactorrhoea, amenorrhoea
- Sedation, dizziness, sleep disturbance, headache, impaired concentration
- Dry mouth, nausea, vomiting, constipation, anorexia
- Impotence
- Rare tardive dyskinesia
- Rare hypomania
- Palpitations
- Weight gain

Common or very common

- Breast abnormalities

Uncommon

- Abnormal orgasm, increased muscle tone, increased salivation

Rare or very rare

- Oculogyric crisis

Frequency not known

- Cardiac arrest, confusion, dyspnoea, hyponatraemia, SIADH, trismus, urticaria

 Life-Threatening or Dangerous Side Effects

- Neuroleptic malignant syndrome
- Oculogyric crisis
- Cardiac arrest
- Hyponatraemia

Weight Gain

- Many experience and/or can be significant in amount

Sedation

- Many experience and/or can be significant in amount, especially at high doses

What To Do About Side Effects

- Wait
- Wait
- Wait

- Reduce the dose
- Low-dose benzodiazepine or beta blocker may reduce akathisia
- Take more of the dose at bedtime to help reduce daytime sedation
- Weight loss, exercise programmes, and medical management for high BMIs, diabetes, and dyslipidaemia
- Switch to another antipsychotic (atypical) – quetiapine or clozapine are best in cases of tardive dyskinesia

Best Augmenting Agents for Side Effects

- Dystonia: antimuscarinic drugs (e.g. procyclidine) as oral or IM depending on the severity; botulinum toxin if antimuscarinics not effective
- Parkinsonism: antimuscarinic drugs (e.g. procyclidine)
- Akathisia: beta blocker propranolol (30–80 mg/day) or low-dose benzodiazepine (e.g. 0.5–3.0 mg/day of clonazepam) may help; other agents that may be tried include the 5HT2 antagonists such as cyproheptadine (16 mg/day) or mirtazapine (15 mg at night – caution in bipolar disorder); clonidine (0.2–0.8 mg/day) may be tried if the above ineffective
- Tardive dyskinesia: stop any antimuscarinic, consider tetrabenazine

DOSING AND USE

Usual Dosage Range

- Schizophrenia with predominantly negative symptoms: 200–800 mg/day in divided doses
- Schizophrenia with predominantly positive symptoms: 200–2400 mg/day in divided doses

Dosage Forms

- Tablet 200 mg, 400 mg
- Oral solution 200 mg/5 mL

How to Dose

Adults:
* Schizophrenia with negative symptoms:
- 200–400 mg twice per day; max 800 mg/day
* Schizophrenia with positive symptoms:
- 200–400 mg twice per day; max 2.4 g/day

Children and adolescents:
- Under expert supervision only
* Schizophrenia with negative symptoms:
- Child 14–17 years 200–400 mg twice per day; max 800 mg/day
* Schizophrenia with positive symptoms:
- Child 14–17 years 200–400 mg twice per day; max 2400 mg/day
* Tourette syndrome (unlicensed):
- Child 2–11 years 50–400 mg twice per day
- Child 12–17 years 100–400 mg twice per day

 Dosing Tips

* Low doses of sulpiride may be more effective at reducing negative symptoms than positive symptoms in schizophrenia; high doses may be equally effective at reducing both symptom dimensions
* Lower doses are more likely to be activating: higher doses are more likely to be sedating
- Some patients receive more than 2400 mg/day
- Stop treatment if neutrophils fall below 1.5×10^9/L and refer to specialist care if neutrophils fall below 0.5×10^9/L

Overdose

- Agitation, restlessness, clouding of consciousness or confusion, extrapyramidal symptoms, arrhythmias
- Hypotension and coma at higher doses; can be fatal

Long-Term Use

- Can in rare cases lead to tardive dyskinesia with long-term use

Habit Forming

- No

How to Stop

- Recommended to reduce dose over a week
- Slow down-titration (over 6–8 weeks), especially when simultaneously beginning a new antipsychotic while switching (i.e. cross-titration)
- Rapid discontinuation may lead to rebound psychosis and worsening of symptoms
- If anti-Parkinson agents are being used, they should be continued for a few weeks after sulpiride is discontinued

Pharmacokinetics
- Elimination half-life about 6–8 hours
- Excreted largely unchanged

Drug Interactions
- Sulpiride may decrease the effects of levodopa and dopamine agonists
- Sulpiride may increase the effects of anti-hypertensives
- CNS effects may be increased if sulpiride is used with other CNS depressants
- Antacids or sucralfate may reduce the absorption of sulpiride
- QT prolongation may occur when combined with bradycardia-inducing medications (beta blockers, diltiazem and verapamil, clonidine, digitalis) or medications which induce electrolyte imbalance, in particular those causing hypokalaemia (hypokalaemic diuretics, stimulant laxatives, IV amphotericin B, glucocorticoids, tetracosactides), or antiarrhythmics (quinidine, disopyramide, amiodarone, sotalol), or other agents (pimozide, haloperidol, methadone, imipramine antidepressants, lithium, cisapride, thioridazine, IV erythromycin, halofantrine, pentamidine)
- Some patients taking a neuroleptic and lithium have developed encephalopathic syndrome similar to neuroleptic malignant syndrome

Other Warnings/Precautions
- All antipsychotics should be used with caution in patients with blood dyscrasias, cardiovascular disease, conditions predisposing to seizures, depression, diabetes, epilepsy, history of jaundice, myasthenia gravis, Parkinson's disease, photosensitisation, prostatic hypertrophy, severe respiratory disease, susceptibility to angle-closure glaucoma
- Use with caution in aggressive, agitated or excited patients as even small doses may worsen condition
- May exacerbate symptoms of mania or hypomania

- If signs of neuroleptic malignant syndrome develop, treatment should be immediately discontinued
- Use cautiously in patients with alcohol withdrawal or convulsive disorders because of possible lowering of seizure threshold
- Use with caution in patients with hypertension, cardiovascular disease, pulmonary disease, hyperthyroidism
- Antiemetic effect of sulpiride may mask signs of other disorders or overdose; suppression of cough reflex may cause asphyxia
- Use only with caution, if at all, in Lewy body disease

Do Not Use
- If there is CNS depression
- If the patient is in a comatose state
- If the patient has phaeochromocytoma
- If the patient has concomitant prolactin-dependent tumours, e.g. pituitary gland prolactinomas and breast cancer
- If there is a proven allergy to sulpiride

SPECIAL POPULATIONS

Renal Impairment
- Start with small doses in severe renal impairment because of increased cerebral sensitivity

Hepatic Impairment
- Use with caution

Cardiac Impairment
- Use with caution

Elderly
- Start on a lower initial dose and titrate upwards according to response
- Although conventional antipsychotics are commonly used for behavioural disturbances in dementia, no agent has been approved for treatment of elderly patients with dementia-related psychosis
- Elderly patients with dementia-related psychosis treated with antipsychotics are at an increased risk of death compared to placebo, and have an increased risk of cerebrovascular events

Children and Adolescents

- Licensed for use in children above the age of 14 for schizophrenia under expert supervision
- Used to treat Tourette syndrome in children above 2 years of age (not licensed and under expert supervision)

Pregnancy

- Very limited data for the use of sulpiride in pregnancy
- There is a risk of abnormal muscle movements and withdrawal symptoms in newborns whose mothers took an antipsychotic during the third trimester; symptoms may include agitation, abnormally increased or decreased muscle tone, tremor, sleepiness, severe difficulty breathing, and difficulty feeding
- Potential risks should be weighed against the potential benefits, and sulpiride should be used only if deemed necessary
- Psychotic symptoms may worsen during pregnancy and some form of treatment may be necessary
- Use in pregnancy may be justified if the benefit of continued treatment exceeds any associated risk
- Switching antipsychotics may increase the risk of relapse
- Antipsychotics may be preferable to anticonvulsant mood stabilisers if treatment is required for mania during pregnancy
- Effects of hyperprolactinaemia on the foetus are unknown

Breastfeeding

- Significant amounts expected in mother's breast milk
- Haloperidol is considered to be the preferred first-generation antipsychotic, and quetiapine the preferred second-generation antipsychotic
- Infants of women who choose to breastfeed should be monitored for possible adverse effects

THE ART OF PSYCHOPHARMACOLOGY

Potential Advantages

- For negative symptoms of psychosis in some patients

Potential Disadvantages

- Aggravated or aggressive patients
- Patients with severe renal impairment
- Patients who cannot tolerate sedation at high doses

Primary Target Symptoms

- Positive symptoms of psychosis
- Negative symptoms of psychosis
- Cognitive functioning
- Depressive symptoms

Pearls

- Sulpiride has been added to clozapine as an augmenting agent for treatment-resistant schizophrenia
- Variable gastrointestinal absorption may lead to highly variable clinical responses especially at low doses
- When mild to moderate tics are associated with obsessive-compulsive symptoms, depression, or anxiety, sulpiride monotherapy can be helpful
- Patients have very similar antipsychotic responses when treated with any of the conventional antipsychotics, which is different from atypical antipsychotics where antipsychotic responses of individual patients can occasionally vary greatly from one atypical to another
- Patients with inadequate responses to atypical antipsychotics may benefit from a trial of augmentation with a conventional antipsychotic such as sulpiride or from switching to a conventional antipsychotic such as sulpiride
- However, long-term polypharmacy with a combination of a conventional antipsychotic such as sulpiride with an atypical antipsychotic may combine their side effects without clearly augmenting the efficacy of either

Sulpiride (Continued)

- For treatment-resistant patients, especially those with impulsivity, aggression, violence, and self-harm, long-term polypharmacy with 2 atypical antipsychotics and 1
- conventional antipsychotic may be useful or even necessary while closely monitoring
- In such cases, it may be beneficial to combine 1 depot antipsychotic with 1 oral antipsychotic

 Suggested Reading

Barber S, Olotu U, Corsi M, et al. Clozapine combined with different antipsychotic drugs for treatment-resistant schizophrenia. Cochrane Database Syst Rev 2017;3(3):CD006324.

Huhn M, Nikolakopoulou A, Schneider-Thoma J, et al. Comparative efficacy and tolerability of 32 oral antipsychotics for the acute treatment of adults with multi-episode schizophrenia: a systematic review and network meta-analysis. Lancet 2019;394(10202):939–51.

Roessner V, Schoenefeld K, Buse J, et al. Pharmacological treatment of tic disorders and Tourette syndrome. Neuropharmacology 2013;68:143–9.

Shiloh R, Zemishlany Z, Aizenberg D, et al. Sulpiride augmentation in people with schizophrenia partially responsive to clozapine. A double-blind, placebo-controlled study. Br J Psychiatry 1997;171:569–73.

Wang J, Sampson S. Sulpiride versus placebo for schizophrenia. Cochrane Database Syst Rev 2014;(4):CD007811.

Temazepam

Brands
• Non-proprietary

Generic?
Yes

Class
• Neuroscience-based nomenclature: pharmacology domain – GABA; mode of action – positive allosteric modulator (PAM)
• Benzodiazepine (hypnotic)

Commonly Prescribed for
(bold for BNF indication)
• **Insomnia (short-term use)**
• **Conscious sedation for dental procedures**
• **Premedication before surgery or investigatory procedures**
• Catatonia

How the Drug Works
• Binds to benzodiazepine receptors at the GABA-A ligand-gated chloride channel complex
• Enhances the inhibitory effects of GABA
• Boosts chloride conductance through GABA-regulated channels
• Inhibitory actions in sleep centres may provide sedative hypnotic effects

How Long Until It Works
• Generally takes effect in less than an hour, but can take longer in some patients

If It Works
• Improves quality of sleep
• Effects on total wake-time and number of night time awakenings may be decreased over time

If It Doesn't Work
• If insomnia does not improve after 7–10 days, it may be a manifestation of a primary psychiatric or physical illness such as obstructive sleep apnoea or restless leg syndrome, which requires independent evaluation
• Increase the dose
• Improve sleep hygiene
• Switch to another agent

Best Augmenting Combos for Partial Response or Treatment Resistance
• Generally best to switch to another agent
• RCTs support the effectiveness of Z-hypnotics over a period of at least 6 months
• Trazodone
• Agents with antihistamine actions (e.g. promethazine, TCAs)
• Use melatonin and melatonin-related drugs (adults over the age of 55)

Tests
• In patients with seizure disorders, concomitant medical illness, and/or those with multiple concomitant long-term medications, periodic liver tests and blood counts may be prudent

How Drug Causes Side Effects
• Same mechanism for side effects as for therapeutic effects – namely due to excessive actions at benzodiazepine receptors
• Actions at benzodiazepine receptors that carry over to the next day can cause daytime sedation, amnesia, and ataxia
• Long-term adaptations in benzodiazepine receptors may explain the development of dependence, tolerance, and withdrawal

Notable Side Effects
∗ Sedation, fatigue, depression
∗ Dizziness, ataxia, slurred speech, weakness
∗ Forgetfulness, confusion
∗ Hyperexcitability, nervousness
• Rare hallucinations, mania
• Rare hypotension
• Hypersalivation, dry mouth
• Rebound insomnia when withdrawing from long-term treatment

Frequency not known
• Drug abuse, dry mouth, increased salivation, slurred speech

Life-Threatening or Dangerous Side Effects

- Respiratory depression (particularly with high dose)
- Suicidal ideation
- Withdrawal syndrome
- Rare hepatic dysfunction, renal dysfunction, blood dyscrasias

Weight Gain

- Reported but not expected

Sedation

- Many experience and/or can be significant in amount

What To Do About Side Effects

- Wait
- To avoid problems with memory, only take temazepam if planning to have a full night's sleep
- Lower the dose
- Switch to a shorter-acting sedative hypnotic
- Switch to a non-benzodiazepine hypnotic
- Administer flumazenil if side effects are severe or life-threatening

Best Augmenting Agents for Side Effects

- Many side effects cannot be improved with an augmenting agent

---

DOSING AND USE

Usual Dosage Range

- 10–20 mg/day for treatment of insomnia

Dosage Forms

- Oral solution 10 mg/5 mL
- Tablet 10 mg, 20 mg

How to Dose

∗ Insomnia (short-term use)
- Adult: 10–20 mg at bedtime, alternatively 30–40 mg at bedtime, higher dose range only to be administered in exceptional circumstances; for debilitated patients use elderly dose
- Elderly: 10 mg at bedtime, alternatively 20 mg at bedtime, higher dose only to be administered in exceptional circumstances
∗ Conscious sedation for dental procedures
- Adult: 15–30 mg, to be administered 30–60 minutes before procedure
∗ Premedication before surgery or investigatory procedures
- Adult: 10–20 mg, to be taken 1–2 hours before procedure, alternatively 30 mg, to be taken 1–2 hours before procedure, higher alternate dose only administered in exceptional circumstances
- Elderly: 10 mg, to be taken 1–2 hours before procedure, alternatively 20 mg, to be taken 1–2 hours before procedure, higher alternate dose only administered in exceptional circumstances

 Dosing Tips

- Use lowest possible effective dose and assess need for continued treatment regularly
- Temazepam should generally not be prescribed in quantities greater than 2–4 weeks' supply
- Patients with lower body weights may require lower doses
∗ Because temazepam is slowly absorbed, administering the dose 1–2 hours before bedtime may improve onset of action and shorter sleep latency
- Risk of dependence may increase with dose and duration of treatment
- Use intermittent dosing (alternate nights or less) where possible
- Discontinue slowly after medium- to long-term use
- At a dose of 15 mg temazepam reduces sleep latency by 37 minutes, increases total sleep time by 99 minutes, and helps to improve sleep quality to a small extent

Overdose

- Can be fatal in monotherapy; slurred speech, poor coordination, respiratory depression, sedation, confusion, coma
- Temazepam had the highest rate of drug intoxication, including overdose, among the most common benzodiazepines in cases with and without combination with alcohol in many studies in the 1980s and 1990s

Long-Term Use
- Not generally intended for long-term use

Habit Forming
- Temazepam is a Class C/Schedule 3 drug
- Some patients may develop dependence and/or tolerance; risk may be greater with higher doses
- History of drug addiction may increase risk of dependence

How to Stop
- If taken for more than a few weeks, taper to reduce chances of withdrawal effects
- Patients with history of seizure may seize upon sudden withdrawal
- Rebound insomnia may occur the first 1–2 nights after stopping
- For patients with severe problems discontinuing a benzodiazepine, dosing may need to be tapered over many months (i.e. reduce dose by 1% every 3 days by crushing tablet and suspending or dissolving in 100 mL of fruit juice and then disposing of 1 mL while drinking the rest; 3–7 days later, dispose of 2 mL, and so on). This is both a form of very slow biological tapering and a form of behavioural desensitisation

Pharmacokinetics
- Rapid absorption with significant blood levels achieved in less than 30 minutes
- Peak levels at 2–3 hours
- Metabolism mainly in the liver. No active metabolites
- Half-life about 8–20 hours
- Excretion mainly via kidneys

 Drug Interactions
- Increased depressive effects when taken with other CNS depressants
- If temazepam is used with kava, clearance of either drug may be affected
- Advise patients of interactions with alcohol

 Other Warnings/Precautions
- Warning regarding the increased risk of CNS-depressant effects when benzodiazepines and opioid medications are used together, including specifically the risk of slowed or difficulty breathing and death

- If alternatives to the combined use of benzodiazepines and opioids are not available, clinicians should limit the dosage and duration of each drug to the minimum possible while still achieving therapeutic efficacy
- Patients and their caregivers should be warned to seek medical attention if unusual dizziness, lightheadedness, sedation, slowed or difficulty breathing, or unresponsiveness occur
- Dosage changes should be made in collaboration with prescriber
- History of drug or alcohol abuse often creates greater risk for dependency
- Some depressed patients may experience a worsening of suicidal ideation
- Some patients may exhibit abnormal thinking or behavioural changes similar to those caused by other CNS depressants (i.e. either depressant actions or disinhibiting actions)
- Avoid prolonged use and abrupt cessation
- Use lower doses in debilitated patients and the elderly
- Use with caution in patients with myasthenia gravis; respiratory disease
- Use with caution in patients with hypoalbuminaemia
- Use with caution in patients with personality disorder (dependent/avoidant or anankastic types) as may increase risk of dependence
- Use with caution in patients with a history of alcohol or drug dependence/abuse
- Benzodiazepines may cause a range of paradoxical effects including aggression, antisocial behaviours, anxiety, overexcitement, perceptual abnormalities and talkativeness. Adjustment of dose may reduce impulses
- Use with caution as temazepam can cause muscle weakness and organic brain changes
- Insomnia may be a symptom of a primary disorder, rather than a primary disorder itself
- Temazepam should only be administered at bedtime
- Temazepam is a popular drug of misuse – avoid in addiction-prone individuals

Do Not Use
- If patient has acute pulmonary insufficiency, respiratory depression, significant neuromuscular respiratory weakness, sleep

Temazepam (Continued)

apnoea syndrome or unstable myasthenia gravis
- If patient has CNS depression
- If patient has compromised airway
- Alone in chronic psychosis in adults
- On its own to try to treat depression, anxiety associated with depression, obsessional states or phobic states
- In addiction-prone individuals
- If patient is acutely intoxicated with alcohol, narcotics, or other psychoactive substances
- In patient with acute narrow-angle glaucoma
- If there is a proven allergy to temazepam or any benzodiazepine

Renal Impairment
- Increased cerebral sensitivity to benzodiazepines
- Start with small doses in severe impairment

Hepatic Impairment
- Temazepam may be preferred to some other benzodiazepines to use as a sedative as it has a short half-life and no active metabolites
- Nevertheless, dose reduction recommended in mild to moderate impairment, adjust dose according to response
- When used for insomnia: initiate at 5 mg at bedtime, increase to 10 mg or 20 mg at bedtime in extreme cases
- Note that even low doses may precipitate hepatic encephalopathy
- Severe hepatic deficiencies (hepatitis and liver cirrhosis) can decrease the elimination of temazepam by a factor of two

Cardiac Impairment
- Dosage adjustment may not be necessary
- Benzodiazepines have been used to treat insomnia associated with acute myocardial infarction

Elderly
- Quarter to half the adult dose recommended

Children and Adolescents
- Can be used as premedication before surgery or investigatory procedures:

10–20 mg, to be taken 1 hour before procedure
- Tablets not licensed for use in children

Pregnancy
- Possible increased risk of birth defects when benzodiazepines taken during pregnancy
- Because of the potential risks, temazepam is not generally recommended as treatment for insomnia during pregnancy, especially during the first trimester
- Drug should be tapered if discontinued
- Infants whose mothers received a benzodiazepine late in pregnancy may experience withdrawal effects
- Neonatal flaccidity has been reported in infants whose mothers took a benzodiazepine during pregnancy
- Seizures, even mild seizures, may cause harm to the embryo/foetus

Breastfeeding
- Small amounts found in mother's breast milk
- Effects of benzodiazepines on infant have been observed and include feeding difficulties, sedation, and weight loss
- Caution should be taken with the use of benzodiazepines in breastfeeding mothers; seek to use low doses for short periods to reduce infant exposure
- Use of shorter-acting 'Z' drugs zopiclone or zolpidem preferred
- Considered not to pose a risk to the infant when given as a single dose (e.g. for premedication)
- Mothers taking hypnotics should be warned about the risks of co-sleeping

Potential Advantages
- Patients with middle insomnia (nocturnal awakening)
- Significantly decreases the number of nightly awakenings

Potential Disadvantages
- Patients with early insomnia (problems falling asleep)
- May distort the normal sleep pattern

Primary Target Symptoms

- Time to sleep onset
- Total sleep time
- Night time awakenings

Pearls

- NICE Guidelines recommend medication for insomnia only as a second-line treatment after non-pharmacological treatment options have been tried (e.g. cognitive behavioural therapy for insomnia)
- Temazepam is not only sleep-promoting, but also has anxiolytic, muscle relaxant and anticonvulsant properties
- If tolerance develops, it may result in increased anxiety during the day and/or increased wakefulness during the latter part of the night

*Slow gastrointestinal absorption compared to other sedative benzodiazepines, so may be more effective for nocturnal awakening than for initial insomnia unless dosed 1–2 hours prior to bedtime
*Notable for delayed onset of action compared to some other sedative hypnotics
- Though not systematically studied, benzodiazepines have been used effectively to treat catatonia and are the initial recommended treatment
- Temazepam significantly decreases the number of nightly awakenings, but has the drawback of distorting the normal sleep pattern
- Temazepam had the highest rate of drug intoxication, including overdose, among the most common benzodiazepines in cases with and without combination with alcohol in many studies in the 1980s and 1990s

 Suggested Reading

Ashton H. Guidelines for the rational use of benzodiazepines. When and what to use. Drugs 1994;48:25–40.

Fraschini F, Stankov B. Temazepam: pharmacological profile of a benzodiazepine and new trends in its clinical application. Pharmacol Res 1993;27:97–113.

Heel RC, Brogden RN, Speight TM, et al. Temazepam: a review of its pharmacological properties and therapeutic efficacy as an hypnotic. Drugs 1981;21:321–40.

McElnay JC, Jones ME, Alexander B. Temazepam (Restoril, Sandoz Pharmaceuticals). Drug Intell Clin Pharm 1982;16:650–6.

Tetrabenazine

Brands
• Xenazine

Generic?
Yes

Class
• Vesicular monoamine transporter 2 (VMAT2) inhibitor

Commonly Prescribed for
(bold for BNF indication)
• **Moderate-severe tardive dyskinesia**
• **Movement disorders due to Huntington's chorea, hemiballismus, senile chorea, and related neurological conditions**

 How the Drug Works
• Tetrabenazine is a selective and reversible inhibitor of VMAT2 which packages monoamines, including dopamine, into synaptic vesicles of presynaptic neurons in the CNS

How Long Until It Works
• As early as 2–4 weeks

If It Works
• Patients should experience a significant reduction in the total Abnormal Involuntary Movement Scale (AIMS) score

If It Doesn't Work
• If tardive dyskinesia does not reverse with tetrabenazine, then other management options include reserpine (rarely used), benzodiazepines (clonazepam 1–4 mg/day or diazepam 6–25 mg/day), vitamin E (400–1600 IU/day), ginkgo biloba, propranolol (40–120 mg/day if no contraindications)
• Other potential treatments that are less commonly prescribed include: amantadine (100–300 mg/day), botulinum toxin (useful for focal symptoms), melatonin (10 mg/day)

 Best Augmenting Combos for Partial Response or Treatment Resistance
• Tetrabenazine itself is an augmenting agent to treat side effects of antipsychotic drugs

Tests
• None for healthy individuals
• For patients at risk of QTc prolongation: assess QTc interval at baseline and at doses at the higher end of the therapeutic range

How Drug Causes Side Effects
• Theoretically due to increases in monoamine concentrations at receptors in parts of the brain and body other than those that cause therapeutic actions
• Depletion of dopamine due to long-term inhibition of VMAT2 may also be responsible for some side effects

Notable Side Effects
• Drowsiness
• Parkinsonism
• Akathisia
• Depression

Common or very common
• CNS/PNS: anxiety, confusion, depression, drowsiness, insomnia, parkinsonism
• CVS: hypotension
• GIT: constipation, diarrhoea, nausea, vomiting

Uncommon
• Hyperthermia, impaired consciousness

Rare or very rare
• Neuroleptic malignant syndrome, skeletal muscle damage

Frequency not known
• CNS: dizziness, suicidal ideation
• Other: bradycardia, dry mouth, epigastric pain

Life-Threatening or Dangerous Side Effects

- QTc prolongation
- Neuroleptic malignant syndrome
- Depression and suicidal ideas

Weight Gain

- Reported but not expected

Sedation

- Many experience and/or can be significant in amount

What To Do About Side Effects

- Wait
- Wait
- Wait
- Reduce dose or discontinue if agitation, akathisia, restlessness, or parkinsonism occurs

Best Augmenting Agents for Side Effects

- Tetrabenazine is itself an augmenting agent to treat a side effect of antipsychotic drugs

DOSING AND USE

Usual Dosage Range

- Moderate-severe tardive dyskinesia: 25–200 mg/day
- Movement disorders due to Huntington's chorea, hemiballismus, senile chorea, and related neurological conditions: 75–200 mg/day

Dosage Forms

- Tablet 25 mg

How to Dose

*Moderate-severe tardive dyskinesia:
- Initial dose 12.5 mg/day, increased gradually according to response

*Movement disorders due to Huntington's chorea, hemiballismus, senile chorea, and related neurological conditions:
- Initial dose 25 mg 3 times per day, increased if tolerated by increments of 25 mg every 3–4 days; max 200 mg/day

- Elderly: may need a lower initial dose

Dosing Tips

- Treatment requires dose titration
- Once a stable dose has been reached, treatment should be reassessed periodically in the context of the underlying condition and concomitant medications
- If switching from reserpine: at least 20 days need to elapse after stopping reserpine before starting tetrabenazine

Overdose

- Limited experience
- Overdose with tetrabenazine: acute dystonia, confusion, diarrhoea, hypotension, hallucinations, hypothermia, nausea, oculogyric crisis, rubor, sedation, sweating, tremor, vomiting

Long-Term Use

- Long-term improvement in chorea

Habit Forming

- No

How to Stop

- Avoid abrupt withdrawal

Pharmacokinetics

- Tetrabenazine has a low and erratic bioavailability
- It is extensively metabolised by first-pass mechanisms
- Almost all of tetrabenazine is metabolised to metabolites; these include the active metabolites dihydrotetrabenazine and hydroxytetrabenazine
- The major metabolite, hydroxytetrabenazine, is reported to be as active as tetrabenazine in depleting brain amines – it is likely that this is the major therapeutic agent
- Half-life of about 1.9 hours

Drug Interactions

- Tetrabenazine and reserpine should not be taken concomitantly as tetrabenazine can block the action of reserpine
- Caution when combining with medications that can prolong QTc interval (e.g. amisulpride, chlorpromazine, zuclopenthixol)

- Tetrabenazine potentially increases the risk of CNS excitation and hypertension when given with MAOIs. Should avoid for 14 days after stopping the MAOI
- Levodopa should be administered with caution in presence of tetrabenazine
- Concomitant use with TCAs, alcohol, opioids, beta blockers, antihypertensives, hypnotics, and neuroleptics is not recommended
- Tetrabenazine can act as a CYP2D6 inhibitor and therefore may cause increased plasma concentrations of agents metabolised by CYP2D6
- Inhibitors of CYP2D6 (e.g. fluoxetine, paroxetine, terbinafine, moclobemide, and quinidine) may result in increased plasma concentrations of the active metabolite dihydrotetrabenazine; a reduction in tetrabenazine dose may be necessary
- Concomitant use with alcohol and other sedating drugs can cause additive sedative effects

 Other Warnings/Precautions

- May cause QTc interval prolongation
- Caution in patients with susceptibility to QTc interval prolongation
- Due to increased risk of depression and suicidality in patients with Huntingdon's disease who take tetrabenazine, one should monitor for emergence or worsening of depression, suicidality, or unusual changes in behaviour; patients and caregivers should be informed of the risk of depression and suicidality and told to report behaviours of concern promptly

Do Not Use

- If patient has untreated depression or is actively suicidal
- If patient has parkinsonism
- If patient has phaeochromocytoma
- If patient has a prolactin-dependent tumour
- If there is a proven allergy to tetrabenazine

SPECIAL POPULATIONS

Renal Impairment
- Use with caution

Hepatic Impairment
- Mild-moderate impairment: initial dose reduction of 50% and slower dose titration

- Severe impairment: caution due to increased risk of exposure

Cardiac Impairment
- May cause QTc interval prolongation – monitor QTc
- Caution in patients with susceptibility to QTc interval prolongation

Elderly
- Some patients may tolerate lower doses better

 Children and Adolescents
- Safety and efficacy have not been established

 Pregnancy
- Avoid unless essential
- Extremely limited evidence of safety in humans
- Toxicity in animal studies

Breastfeeding
- Some drug or metabolite expected in mother's breast milk
- No evidence of safety
- Avoid
- If drug is continued while breastfeeding, infant should be monitored for side effects seen in adults

THE ART OF PSYCHOPHARMACOLOGY

Potential Advantages
- Flexible dosing
- No CYP450 3A4 drug interactions

Potential Disadvantages
- Requires multiple daily dosing
- Risk of depression and suicidality

Primary Target Symptoms
- Repetitive involuntary movements of tardive dyskinesia (usually associated with lower facial and distal extremity musculature, e.g. tongue protrusion, writhing of tongue, lip smacking, chewing, blinking, and grimacing)

Tetrabenazine (Continued)

Pearls

- Depression and suicidal ideas have been reported from clinical trials of tetrabenazine
- Tetrabenazine is almost 100% metabolised
- Active metabolites include dihydrotetrabenazine and hydroxytetrabenazine

- Hydroxytetrabenazine acts to deplete brain amines and is likely to be the major therapeutic agent
- Deutetrabenazine (deuterated form of tetrabenazine) is a more expensive alternative available in USA and is less likely to cause depression and suicidal ideation

Suggested Reading

Meyer JM. Forgotten but not gone: new developments in the understanding and treatment of tardive dyskinesia. CNS Spectr 2016;21(S1):13–24.

Ricciardi L, Pringsheim T, Barnes TRE, et al. Treatment recommendations for tardive dyskinesia. Can J Psychiatry 2019;64(6):388–99.

Schneider F, Stamler D, Bradbury M, et al. Pharmacokinetics of deutetrabenazine and tetrabenazine: dose proportionality and food effect. Clin Pharmacol Drug Dev 2021;10(6):647–59.

Solmi M, Pigato G, Kane JM, et al. Treatment of tardive dyskinesia with VMAT-2 inhibitors: a systematic review and meta-analysis of randomized controlled trials. Drug Des Devel Ther 2018;12:1215–38.

Tranylcypromine

Brands
• Non-proprietary

Generic?
Yes

Class
• Neuroscience-based nomenclature: pharmacology domain – serotonin, norepinephrine, dopamine; mode of action – multimodal
• Monoamine oxidase inhibitor (MAOI)

Commonly Prescribed for
(bold for BNF indication)
• **Depressive illness**
• Treatment-resistant depression
• Treatment-resistant panic disorder
• Treatment-resistant social anxiety disorder

 How the Drug Works
• Irreversibly blocks monoamine oxidase (MAO) from breaking down noradrenaline, serotonin, and dopamine
• This presumably boosts noradrenergic, serotonergic, and dopaminergic neurotransmission
∗As the drug is structurally related to amfetamine, it may have some stimulant-like actions due to monoamine release and reuptake inhibition

How Long Until It Works
• Some patients may experience stimulant-like actions early in dosing
• Onset of therapeutic actions usually not immediate, but often delayed 2–4 weeks
• If it is not working within 3–4 weeks, it may require a dosage increase or it may not work at all
• May continue to work for many years to prevent relapse of symptoms

If It Works
• The goal of treatment is complete remission of current symptoms as well as prevention of future relapses
• Treatment most often reduces or even eliminates symptoms, but is not a cure since symptoms can recur after medicine is stopped

• Continue treatment until all symptoms are gone (remission), especially in depression and whenever possible in anxiety disorders
• Once symptoms are gone, continue treating for at least 6–9 months for the first episode of depression or >12 months if relapse indicators present
• If >5 episodes and/or 2 episodes in the last few years then need to continue for at least 2 years or indefinitely
• Use in anxiety disorders may also need to be indefinite

If It Doesn't Work
• Important to recognise non-response to treatment early on (3–4 weeks)
• Many patients have only a partial response where some symptoms are improved but others persist (especially insomnia, fatigue, and problems concentrating)
• Other patients may be non-responders, sometimes called treatment-resistant or treatment-refractory
• Some patients who have an initial response may relapse even though they continue treatment
• Consider increasing dose, switching to another agent, or adding an appropriate augmenting agent
• Lithium may be added for suicidal patients or those at high risk of relapse
• Consider psychotherapy
• Consider ECT
• Consider evaluation for another diagnosis or for a co-morbid condition (e.g. medical illness, substance abuse, etc.)
• Some patients may experience a switch into mania and so would require antidepressant discontinuation and initiation of a mood stabiliser

 Best Augmenting Combos for Partial Response or Treatment Resistance
∗Augmentation of MAOIs has not been systematically studied, and this is something for the expert, to be done with caution and with careful monitoring
• Lithium is particularly useful for suicidal patients and those at high risk of relapse including with factors such as severe

Tranylcypromine (Continued)

depression, psychomotor retardation, repeated episodes (>3), significant weight loss, or a family history of major depression (aim for lithium plasma levels 0.6–1.0 mmol/L)
- Atypical antipsychotics (with special caution for those agents with monoamine reuptake blocking properties)
- Mood-stabilising anticonvulsants
- *A stimulant such as dexamfetamine or methylphenidate (with caution; may activate bipolar disorder and suicidal ideation; may elevate blood pressure)

Tests
- Patients should be monitored for changes in blood pressure
- Patients receiving high doses or long-term treatment should have hepatic function evaluated periodically

SIDE EFFECTS

How Drug Causes Side Effects
- Theoretically due to increases in monoamines in parts of the brain and body and at receptors other than those that cause therapeutic actions (e.g. unwanted actions of serotonin in sleep causing insomnia, unwanted actions of norepinephrine on vascular smooth muscle causing hypertension, etc.)
- Side effects are generally immediate, but immediate side effects often disappear in time

Notable Side Effects
- Agitation, anxiety, insomnia, weakness, sedation, dizziness
- Constipation, dry mouth, nausea, change in appetite, weight gain
- Sexual dysfunction
- Orthostatic hypotension (dose-related), syncope may develop at higher doses

Rare or very rare
- Hepatocellular injury

Frequency not known
- CNS/PNS: drug dependence, headache (throbbing), hypomania, mydriasis, photophobia, sleep disorder
- CVS: chest pain, extrasystole, hypertension
- Other: diarrhoea, flushing, pain, pallor

Life-Threatening or Dangerous Side Effects
- Hypertensive crisis (especially when MAOIs are used with certain tyramine-containing foods or prohibited drugs)
- Blood dyscrasias
- Induction of mania
- Rare increase in suicidal ideation and behaviours in adolescents and young adults (up to age 25), hence patients should be warned of this potential adverse event
- Seizures
- Hepatotoxicity

Weight Gain
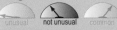
- Occurs in significant minority

Sedation
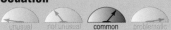
- Many experience and/or can be significant in amount
- Can also cause activation

What to Do About Side Effects
- Wait
- Wait
- Wait
- Lower the dose
- Take at night if daytime sedation; take in daytime if overstimulated at night
- Switch after appropriate washout to an SSRI or newer antidepressant

Best Augmenting Agents for Side Effects
- Trazodone (with caution) for insomnia
- Benzodiazepines for insomnia
- Many side effects cannot be improved with an augmenting agent

DOSING AND USE

Usual Dosage Range
- 10–30 mg/day (in divided doses)

Dosage Forms
- Tablet 10 mg

How to Dose
- Initial dose 10 mg twice per day, last dose at no later than 3 pm, dose may be increased as needed after 7 days to 30 mg/day (10 mg morning, 20 mg afternoon), doses above 30 mg/day only under close supervision; maintenance dose 10 mg/day

 Dosing Tips
- Orthostatic hypotension, especially at high doses, may require splitting into 3–4 daily doses
- Patients receiving high doses may need to be evaluated periodically for effects on the liver

Overdose
- Tremor, dizziness, sedation, sweating, ataxia, headache, insomnia, restlessness, weakness, anxiety, irritability; cardiovascular effects, confusion, respiratory depression, or coma may also occur

Long-Term Use
- May require periodic evaluation of hepatic function
- MAOIs may lose efficacy long-term

Habit Forming
- Some patients have developed dependence on MAOIs, may relate to amfetamine-like action

How to Stop
- The dose should preferably be reduced gradually over about 4 weeks, or longer if withdrawal symptoms emerge (6 months in patients who have been on long-term maintenance treatment)

Pharmacokinetics
- Clinical duration of action may be up to 14 days due to irreversible enzyme inhibition
- Half-life of about 2 hours

 Drug Interactions
- Tramadol may increase the risk of seizures in patients taking an MAOI
- Can cause a fatal "serotonin syndrome" when combined with drugs that block serotonin reuptake, so do not use with a serotonin reuptake inhibitor or for half-lives of the SSRI after stopping the serotonin reuptake inhibitor (see Table 1 after Pearls)
- Hypertensive crisis with headache, intracranial bleeding, and death may result from combining MAOIs with sympathomimetic drugs (e.g. amfetamines, methylphenidate, cocaine, dopamine, epinephrine, norepinephrine, and related compounds methyldopa, levodopa, L-tryptophan, L-tyrosine, and phenylalanine)
- Do not combine with another MAOI, alcohol, or guanethidine
- Adverse drug reactions can result from combining MAOIs with tricyclic/tetracyclic antidepressants and related compounds, including carbamazepine and mirtazapine, and should be avoided except by experts to treat difficult cases
- MAOIs in combination with spinal anaesthesia may cause combined hypotensive effects
- Combination of MAOIs and CNS depressants may enhance sedation and hypotension

 Other Warnings/Precautions
- Use requires low-tyramine diet (see Table 2 after Pearls)
- Patient and prescriber must be vigilant to potential interactions with any drug, including antihypertensives and over-the-counter cough/cold preparations
- Over-the-counter medications to avoid include cough and cold preparations, including those containing dextromethorphan, nasal decongestants (tablets, drops, or spray), hay-fever medications, sinus medications, asthma inhalant medications, anti-appetite medications, weight-reducing preparations, "pep" pills (see Table 3 after Pearls)
- Hypoglycaemia may occur in diabetic patients receiving insulin or oral antidiabetic agents
- Use cautiously in patients receiving reserpine, anaesthetics, disulfiram, anticholinergic agents

Tranylcypromine (Continued)

- Tranylcypromine is not recommended for use in patients who cannot be monitored closely
- Use with caution in patients with acute porphyrias, blood disorders, cardiovascular disease, diabetes, epilepsy
- Use with caution in patients undergoing ECT
- Use with great caution in the elderly
- Use with caution in patients undergoing surgery
- When treating children, carefully weigh the risks and benefits of pharmacological treatment against the risks and benefits of nontreatment with antidepressants and make sure to document this in the patient's chart
- Ensure low-tyramine diet sheet is given and understood
- Warn patients and their caregivers about the possibility of activating side effects and advise them to report such symptoms immediately
- Monitor patients for activation of suicidal ideation, especially those up to the age of 25

Do Not Use

- In agitated patients or in the manic phase
- If patient is taking pethidine
- If patient is taking a sympathomimetic agent or taking guanethidine
- If patient is taking another MAOI
- If patient is taking any agent that can inhibit serotonin reuptake (e.g. SSRIs, sibutramine, tramadol, duloxetine, venlafaxine, clomipramine, etc.)
- If patient is taking diuretic
- If patient has phaeochromocytoma
- If patient has cardiovascular or cerebrovascular disease
- If patient has frequent or severe headaches
- If patient is undergoing elective surgery and requires general anaesthesia
- If patient has a history of liver disease or abnormal liver function tests
- If patient is taking a prohibited drug
- If patient is not adherent to a low-tyramine diet
- If patient has hyperthyroidism
- If there is a proven allergy to tranylcypromine

Renal Impairment

- Use with caution – drug may accumulate in plasma
- May require lower than usual adult dose

Hepatic Impairment

- Tranylcypromine should not be used in patients with history of hepatic impairment or in patients with abnormal liver function tests

Cardiac Impairment

- Contraindicated in patients with any cardiac impairment

Elderly

- Initial dose lower than usual adult dose
- Elderly patients may have greater sensitivity to adverse effects
- Reduction in the risk of suicidality with antidepressants compared to placebo in adults age 65 and older

 ## Children and Adolescents

- Not generally recommended for use in children and adolescents under age 18

 ## Pregnancy

- Controlled studies have not been conducted in pregnant women
- Not generally recommended for use during pregnancy, especially during first and third trimesters
- Should evaluate patient for treatment with an antidepressant with a better risk/benefit ratio

Breastfeeding

- Some drug is found in mother's breast milk
- Effects on infant unknown
- Immediate postpartum period is a high-risk time for depression, especially in women who have had prior depressive episodes, so drug may need to be reinstituted shortly after childbirth to prevent a recurrence during the postpartum period
- Should evaluate patient for treatment with an antidepressant with a better risk/benefit ratio

THE ART OF PSYCHOPHARMACOLOGY

Potential Advantages
- Atypical depression
- Severe depression
- Treatment-resistant depression or anxiety disorders

Potential Disadvantages
- Requires compliance to dietary restrictions, concomitant drug restrictions
- Patients with cardiac problems or hypertension
- Multiple daily doses

Primary Target Symptoms
- Depressed mood
- Somatic symptoms
- Sleep and eating disturbances
- Psychomotor retardation
- Morbid preoccupation

 Pearls

- MAOIs are generally reserved for use after SSRIs, SNRIs, TCAs or combinations of newer antidepressants have failed
- Patient should be advised not to take any prescription or over-the-counter drugs without consulting their doctor because of possible drug interactions with the MAOI
- Headache is often the first symptom of hypertensive crisis
- The rigid dietary restrictions may reduce compliance (see Table 2 after Pearls)
- Mood disorders can be associated with eating disorders (especially in adolescent females), and tranylcypromine can be used to treat both depression and bulimia
- MAOIs are viable treatment options in depression when other classes of antidepressants have not worked, but they are not frequently used
- *Myths about the danger of dietary tyramine can be exaggerated, but prohibitions against concomitant drugs often not followed closely enough
- Orthostatic hypotension, insomnia, and sexual dysfunction are often the most troublesome side effects
- *MAOIs should be for the expert, especially if combining with agents of potential risk (e.g. stimulants, trazodone, TCAs)
- *MAOIs should not be neglected as therapeutic agents for the treatment-resistant
- Although generally prohibited, a heroic but potentially dangerous treatment for severely treatment-resistant patients is for an expert to give a tricyclic/tetracyclic antidepressant other than clomipramine simultaneously with an MAOI for patients who fail to respond to numerous other antidepressants
- Use of MAOIs with clomipramine is always prohibited because of the risk of serotonin syndrome and death
- Start the MAOI with the tricyclic/tetracyclic antidepressant simultaneously at low doses after appropriate drug washout, then alternately increase doses of these agents every few days to a week as tolerated
- Although very strict dietary and concomitant drug restrictions must be observed to prevent hypertensive crises and serotonin syndrome, the most common side effects of MAOI and tricyclic/tetracyclic combinations may be weight gain and orthostatic hypotension

Table 1. Drugs contraindicated due to risk of serotonin syndrome/toxicity

Do Not Use:			
Antidepressants	Drugs of Abuse	Opioids	Other
SSRIs	MDMA (ecstasy)	Pethidine	Non-subcutaneous sumatriptan
SNRIs	Cocaine	Tramadol	Chlorphenamine
Clomipramine	Metamfetamine	Methadone	Procarbazine?
St. John's wort	High-dose or injected amfetamine	Fentanyl	Morphinan-containing compounds

Table 2. Dietary guidelines for patients taking MAOIs

Foods to avoid*	Foods allowed
Dried, aged, smoked, fermented, spoiled, or improperly stored meat, poultry, and fish including game	Fresh or processed meat, poultry, and fish; properly stored pickled or smoked fish
Broad bean pods	All other vegetables
Aged cheeses	Processed cheese slices, cottage cheese, ricotta cheese, yoghurt, cream cheese
Tap and unpasteurised beer	Canned or bottled beer and alcohol
Marmite	Brewer's and baker's yeast
Sauerkraut, kimchi	
Soy products/tofu	Peanuts
Banana peel	Bananas, avocados, raspberries
Tyramine-containing nutritional supplement	

*Not necessary for 6-mg transdermal or low-dose oral selegiline

Table 3. Drugs that boost norepinephrine: should only be used with caution with MAOIs

Use With Caution:			
Decongestants	Stimulants	Antidepressants with norepinephrine reuptake inhibition	Other
Phenylephrine	Amfetamines	Most tricyclics	Local anaesthetics containing vasoconstrictors
Pseudoephedrine	Methylphenidate	NRIs	Tapentadol
	Cocaine	NDRIs	
	Metamfetamine		
	Modafinil		

Suggested Reading

Amsterdam JD, Kim TT. Relative effectiveness of monoamine oxidase inhibitor and tricyclic antidepressant combination therapy for treatment-resistant depression. J Clin Psychopharmacol 2019;39(6):649–52.

Baker GB, Coutts RT, McKenna KF, et al. Insights into the mechanisms of action of the MAO inhibitors phenelzine and tranylcypromine: a review. J Psychiatry Neurosci 1992;17:206–14.

Gillman PK. A reassessment of the safety profile of monoamine oxidase inhibitors: elucidating tired old tyramine myths. J Neural Transm (Vienna) 2018;125(11):1707–17.

Kennedy SH. Continuation and maintenance treatments in major depression: the neglected role of monoamine oxidase inhibitors. J Psychiatry Neurosci 1997;22:127–31.

Kim T, Xu C, Amsterdam JD. Relative effectiveness of tricyclic antidepressant versus monoamine oxidase inhibitor monotherapy for treatment-resistant depression. J Affect Disord 2019;250:199–203.

Lippman SB, Nash K. Monoamine oxidase inhibitor update. Potential adverse food and drug interactions. Drug Saf 1990;5:195–204.

Ricken R, Ulrich S, Schlattmann P, Adli M. Tranylcypromine in mind (part II): Review of clinical pharmacology and meta-analysis of controlled studies in depression. Eur Neuropsychopharmacol 2017;27(8):714–31.

Thase ME, Triyedi MH, Rush AJ. MAOIs in the contemporary treatment of depression. Neuropsychopharmacology 1995;12:185–219.

Ulrich S, Ricken R, Adli M. Tranylcypromine in mind (part I): review of pharmacology. Eur Neuropsychopharmacol 2017;27(8):697–713.

Ulrich S, Ricken R, Buspavanich P, et al. Efficacy and adverse effects of tranylcypromine and tricyclic antidepressants in the treatment of depression: a systematic review and comprehensive meta-analysis. J Clin Psychopharmacol 2020;40(1):63–74.

Trazodone hydrochloride

Brands

• Molipaxin

Generic?

Yes

Class

• Neuroscience-based nomenclature: pharmacology domain – serotonin; mode of action – multimodal
• SARI (serotonin 2 antagonist/reuptake inhibitor); antidepressant; hypnotic

Commonly Prescribed for

(bold for BNF indication)
• **Depressive illness (particularly where sedation is required)**
• **Anxiety**

 ## How the Drug Works

• Potent receptor antagonist (serotonin 2A)
• Relatively weaker serotonin reuptake pump (serotonin transporter) blockade
• Receptor agonist (serotonin 1A)

How Long Until It Works

∗Onset of therapeutic actions in insomnia is immediate if dosing is correct
• Onset of therapeutic actions in depression usually not immediate, but often delayed 2–4 weeks whether given as an adjunct to another antidepressant or as a monotherapy
• If it is not working within 3–4 weeks for depression, it may require a dosage increase or it may not work at all
• By contrast, for generalised anxiety, onset of response and increases in remission rates may still occur after 8 weeks, and for up to 6 months after initiating dosing
• May continue to work for many years to prevent relapse of symptoms in depression and to reduce symptoms of chronic insomnia

If It Works

∗For insomnia, use possibly can be indefinite as there is no reliable evidence of tolerance, dependence, or withdrawal, but few long-term studies
• For secondary insomnia, if underlying condition (e.g. depression, anxiety disorder) is in remission, trazodone treatment may be discontinued if insomnia does not re-emerge
• The goal of treatment for depression is complete remission of current symptoms of depression as well as prevention of future relapses
• Treatment most often reduces or even eliminates symptoms of depression, but is not a cure since symptoms can recur after medicine stopped
• Continue treatment until all symptoms are gone (remission), especially in depression and whenever possible in anxiety disorders
• Once symptoms of depression are gone, continue treating for at least 6–9 months for the first episode of depression or >12 months if relapse indicators present
• If >5 episodes and/or 2 episodes in the last few years then need to continue for at least 2 years or indefinitely
• Use in anxiety disorders may also need to be indefinite, but long-term treatment is not well studied in these conditions

If It Doesn't Work

• For insomnia, try escalating doses or switch to another agent
• It is important to recognise non-response to treatment for depression early on (3–4 weeks)
• Many patients have only a partial response where some symptoms are improved but others persist (especially insomnia, fatigue, and problems concentrating)
• Other patients may be non-responders, sometimes called treatment-resistant or treatment-refractory
• Some patients who have an initial response may relapse even though they continue treatment
• Consider increasing dose, switching to another agent, or adding an appropriate augmenting agent for treatment of depression
• Lithium may be added for suicidal patients or those at high risk of relapse
• Consider psychotherapy
• Consider ECT
• Consider evaluation for another diagnosis or for a co-morbid condition (e.g. medical illness, substance abuse, etc.)
• Some patients may experience a switch into mania and so would require antidepressant discontinuation and initiation of a mood stabiliser

Trazodone hydrochloride (Continued)

⚖️ Best Augmenting Combos for Partial Response or Treatment Resistance

- Trazodone is not frequently used as a monotherapy for insomnia, but can be combined with sedative hypnotic benzodiazepines in difficult cases
- Trazodone can also improve insomnia in numerous other psychiatric conditions (e.g. bipolar disorder, schizophrenia, alcohol withdrawal) and be added to numerous other psychotropic drugs (e.g. lithium, mood stabilisers, antipsychotics)
- Trazodone is most frequently used in depression as an augmenting agent to numerous psychotropic drugs
- Trazodone can not only improve insomnia in depressed patients treated with antidepressants, but can also be an effective booster of antidepressant actions of other antidepressants (use combinations of antidepressants with caution as this may activate bipolar disorder and suicidal ideation)
- Mood stabilisers or atypical antipsychotics for bipolar depression
- Atypical antipsychotics for psychotic depression
- Atypical antipsychotics as first-line augmenting agents (quetiapine MR 300 mg/day or aripiprazole at 2.5–10 mg/day) for treatment-resistant depression
- Atypical antipsychotics as second-line augmenting agents (risperidone 0.5–2 mg/day or olanzapine 2.5–10 mg/day) for treatment-resistant depression
- Although T3 (20–50 mcg/day) is another second-line augmenting agent the evidence suggests that it works best with tricyclic antidepressants
- Other augmenting agents but with less evidence include bupropion (up to 400 mg/day), buspirone (up to 60 mg/day) and lamotrigine (up to 400 mg/day)
- Benzodiazepines if agitation present
- Hypnotics for insomnia
- Augmenting agents reserved for specialist use include: modafinil for sleepiness, fatigue and lack of concentration; stimulants, oestrogens, testosterone
- Lithium is particularly useful for suicidal patients and those at high risk of relapse including with factors such as severe depression, psychomotor retardation, repeated episodes (>3), significant weight loss, or a family history of major depression (aim for lithium plasma levels 0.6–1.0 mmol/L)
- For elderly patients lithium is a very effective augmenting agent
- For severely ill patients other combinations may be tried especially in specialist centres
- Augmenting agents that may be tried include omega-3, SAM-e, L-methylfolate
- Additional non-pharmacological treatments such as exercise, mindfulness, CBT, and IPT can also be helpful
- If present after treatment response (4–8 weeks) or remission (6–12 weeks), the most common residual symptoms of depression include cognitive impairments, reduced energy and problems with sleep

Tests

- None for healthy individuals

SIDE EFFECTS

How Drug Causes Side Effects

- Sedative effects may be due to antihistamine properties
- Blockade of alpha adrenergic 1 receptors may explain dizziness, sedation, and hypotension
- Most side effects are immediate but often go away with time

Notable Side Effects

- Sedation, dizziness, fatigue, headache, incoordination, tremor
- Nausea, vomiting, oedema, blurred vision, constipation, dry mouth
- Hypotension, syncope
- Occasional sinus bradycardia (long-term)

Frequency not known

- Blood disorders: agranulocytosis, anaemia, eosinophilia, leucopenia, thrombocytopenia
- CNS/PNS: aggression, anxiety, aphasia, blurred vision, confusion, decreased alertness, delirium, delusions, dizziness, drowsiness, hallucination, headache, mania, memory loss, movement disorders, paraesthesia, seizure, sleep disorders, suicidal behaviours, tremor, vertigo
- CVS: arrhythmias, hypertension, palpitations, QT interval prolongation, syncope
- GIT: abnormal appetite, altered taste, constipation, decreased weight, diarrhoea, dry mouth, gastroenteritis,

gastrointestinal discomfort, hepatic disorder, hypersalivation, jaundice (discontinue), nausea, paralytic ileus, vomiting
• Other: arthralgia, asthenia, chest pain, decreased libido, dyspnoea, fever, hyperhidrosis, hyponatraemia, influenza-like illness, myalgia, nasal congestion, neuroleptic malignant syndrome, oedema, pain, postural hypotension, priapism (discontinue), serotonin syndrome, SIADH, skin reactions, urinary disorder, withdrawal syndrome

 Life-Threatening or Dangerous Side Effects
• Priapism
• Seizures
• Rare rash
• Rare induction of mania
• Rare increase in suicidal ideation and behaviours in adolescents and young adults (up to age 25), hence patients should be warned of this potential adverse event

Weight Gain

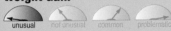
unusual   not unusual   common   problematic

• Reported but not expected

Sedation

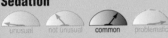
unusual   not unusual   common   problematic

• Many experience and/or can be significant in amount

What to Do About Side Effects
• Wait
• Wait
• Wait
• The risk of side effects is reduced by titrating slowly to the minimum effective dose (every 2–3 days)
• Consider using a lower starting dose in elderly patients
• Manage side effects that are likely to be transient (e.g. drowsiness) by explanation, reassurance and, if necessary, dose reduction and re-titration
• Giving patients simple strategies for managing mild side effects (e.g. dry mouth) may be useful
• For persistent, severe or distressing side effects the options are:
  • Dose reduction and re-titration if possible
  • Switching to an antidepressant with a lower propensity to cause that side effect

• Non-drug management of the side effect (e.g. diet and exercise for weight gain)
• Take larger dose at night to prevent daytime sedation

Best Augmenting Agents for Side Effects
• Many side effects cannot be improved with an augmenting agent

DOSING AND USE

Usual Dosage Range
• 150–600 mg/day

Dosage Forms
• Tablet 50 mg, 100 mg, 150 mg
• Capsule 50 mg, 100 mg
• Oral solution 50 mg/5 mL, 100 mg/5 mL

How to Dose
✴ Depressive illness:
• Monotherapy in adults: initial dose 150 mg/day in divided doses, dose to be taken after food or at bedtime; can increase every 3–4 days by 50 mg/day as needed; max 400 mg/day (outpatient) or 600 mg/day (inpatient), split into 2 daily doses
• Monotherapy in elderly: initial dose 100 mg/day in divided doses, dose to be taken after food or at bedtime; can increase to 300 mg/day in divided doses (outpatient) or 600 mg/day in divided doses
✴ Anxiety:
• 75 mg/day; can increase to 300 mg/day as needed

 Dosing Tips
• Start low and go slow
✴ Patients can have carryover sedation, ataxia, and intoxicated-like feeling if dosed too aggressively, particularly when initiating dosing
✴ Do not discontinue trials if ineffective at low doses (<50 mg) as many patients with difficult cases may respond to higher doses (150–300 mg, even up to 600 mg in some cases)
• For relief of daytime anxiety, can give part of the dose in the daytime if not too sedating
• Although use as a monotherapy for depression is usually in divided doses due to its short half-life, use as an adjunct is

often effective and best tolerated once daily at bedtime

Overdose
• Rarely lethal; sedation, vomiting, priapism, respiratory arrest, seizure, ECG changes

Long-Term Use
• Safe

Habit Forming
• No

How to Stop
• Taper is prudent to avoid withdrawal effects, but tolerance, dependence, and withdrawal effects have not been reliably demonstrated

Pharmacokinetics
• Metabolised by CYP450 3A4
• The elimination of trazodone is biphasic, with a terminal elimination half-life of 5 to 13 hours

 Drug Interactions
• Tramadol increases the risk of seizures in patients taking an antidepressant
• Fluoxetine and other SSRIs may raise trazodone plasma levels
• Trazodone may block the hypotensive effects of some antihypertensive drugs
• Trazodone may increase digoxin or phenytoin concentrations
• Trazodone may interfere with the antihypertensive effects of clonidine
• Generally, do not use with MAOIs, including 14 days after MAOIs are stopped
• Reports of increased and decreased prothrombin time in patients taking warfarin and trazodone
• Activation and agitation may represent the induction of a bipolar state, especially a mixed dysphoric bipolar condition sometimes associated with suicidal ideation, and require the addition of lithium, a mood stabiliser or an atypical antipsychotic, and/or discontinuation of trazodone

 Other Warnings/Precautions
• Possibility of additive effects if trazodone is used with other CNS depressants

• Treatment should be discontinued if prolonged penile erection occurs because of the risk of permanent erectile dysfunction
• Advise patients to seek medical attention immediately if painful erections occur lasting more than 1 hour
• Generally, priapism reverses spontaneously while penile blood flow and other signs are being monitored, but in urgent cases, local phenylephrine injections or even surgery may be indicated
• Use with caution in patients with history of seizures
• Use with caution in patients with chronic constipation, increased intra-ocular pressure, prostatic hypertrophy, susceptibility to angle-closure glaucoma, urinary retention
• Use with caution in patients with arrhythmias, cardiovascular disease, hyperthyroidism (risk of arrhythmias)
• Use with caution in patients with a significant risk of suicide
• Use with caution in patients with bipolar disorder unless treated with concomitant mood-stabilising agent
• Treatment with trazodone should be stopped if the patient enters a manic phase
• Use with caution in patients with a history of psychosis
• When treating children, carefully weigh the risks and benefits of pharmacological treatment against the risks and benefits of nontreatment with antidepressants and make sure to document this in the patient's record
• Warn patients and their caregivers about the possibility of activating side effects and advise them to report such symptoms immediately
• Monitor patients for activation of suicidal ideation, especially children and adolescents

Do Not Use
• In patients during a manic phase
• In the recovery period after an acute myocardial infarction
• If patient is taking an MAOI, but also see Pearls
• If there is a proven allergy to trazodone

SPECIAL POPULATIONS

Renal Impairment
- Use with caution; start with low dose and increase gradually in severe impairment

Hepatic Impairment
- Use with caution, particularly in severe impairment (increased risk of side effects)

Cardiac Impairment
- Trazodone may be arrhythmogenic
- Should only be used with caution in patients with cardiovascular disease
- Monitor patients closely
- Not recommended for use during recovery from myocardial infarction

Elderly
- Elderly patients may be more sensitive to adverse effects and may require lower doses
- Reduction in the risk of suicidality with antidepressants compared to placebo in adults age 65 and older

 ### Children and Adolescents
- Trazodone is not licensed for use in children and adolescents
- Safety and efficacy have not been established, but trazodone has been used for behavioural disturbances, depression, and night terrors
- Children require lower initial dose and slow titration
- Boys may be even more sensitive to having prolonged erections than adult men
- Carefully weigh the risks and benefits of pharmacological treatment against the risks and benefits of nontreatment with antidepressants and make sure to document this in the patient's record
- Monitor patients face-to-face regularly, particularly during the first several weeks of treatment
- Use with caution, observing for activation of known or unknown bipolar disorder and/or suicidal ideation, and inform parents or guardians of this risk so they can help observe child or adolescent patients

 ### Pregnancy
- Controlled studies have not been conducted in pregnant women
- Very limited evidence does not suggest increased risk of congenital malformations, intrauterine death, preterm delivery or low birth weight
- Poor neonatal adaptation syndrome and/ or withdrawal has been reported in infants whose mothers took other antidepressants during pregnancy or near delivery
- Maternal use of more than one CNS-acting medication is likely to lead to more severe symptoms in the neonate
- Must weigh the risk of treatment (first trimester foetal development, third trimester newborn delivery) to the child against the risk of no treatment (recurrence of depression, maternal health, infant bonding) to the mother and child
- For many patients this may mean continuing treatment during pregnancy

Breastfeeding
- Small amounts found in mother's breast milk
- If child becomes irritable or sedated, breastfeeding or drug may need to be discontinued
- Immediate postpartum period is a high-risk time for depression, especially in women who have had prior depressive episodes, so drug may need to be reinstituted late in the third trimester or shortly after childbirth to prevent a recurrence during the postpartum period
- Must weigh benefits of breastfeeding with risks and benefits of antidepressant treatment versus nontreatment to both the infant and the mother
- For many patients, this may mean continuing treatment during breastfeeding
- Other antidepressants may be preferable, e.g. imipramine or nortriptyline

Trazodone hydrochloride (Continued)

THE ART OF PSYCHOPHARMACOLOGY

Potential Advantages
- For insomnia when it is preferred to avoid the use of dependence-forming agents
- As an adjunct to the treatment of residual anxiety and insomnia with other antidepressants
- Depressed patients with anxiety
- Patients concerned about sexual side effects or weight gain

Potential Disadvantages
- For patients with fatigue, hypersomnia
- For patients intolerant to sedating effects

Primary Target Symptoms
- Depression
- Anxiety
- Sleep disturbances

 Pearls
- May be less likely than some antidepressants to precipitate hypomania or mania
- Preliminary data suggest that trazodone may be effective treatment for drug-induced dyskinesias, perhaps in part because it reduces accompanying anxiety
- Trazodone may have some efficacy in treating agitation and aggression associated with dementia

* May cause sexual dysfunction only infrequently
- Can cause carryover sedation, sometimes severe, if dosed too high
- Often not tolerated as a monotherapy for moderate to severe cases of depression, as many patients cannot tolerate high doses (>150 mg)
- Do not forget to try at high doses, up to 600 mg/day, if lower doses well tolerated but ineffective
* For the expert psychopharmacologist, trazodone can be used cautiously for insomnia associated with MAOIs, despite the warning – must be attempted only if patients closely monitored and by experts experienced in the use of MAOIs
- Priapism may occur in 1 in 8000 men
- Early indications of impending priapism may be slow penile detumescence when awakening from REM sleep
- When using to treat insomnia, remember that insomnia may be a symptom of some other primary disorder, and not a primary disorder itself, and thus warrant consideration for co-morbid psychiatric and/or medical conditions
- Rarely, patients may complain of visual "trails" or after-images on trazodone

 Suggested Reading

Cipriani A, Furukawa TA, Salanti G, et al. Comparative efficacy and acceptability of 21 antidepressant drugs for the acute treatment of adults with major depressive disorder: a systematic review and network meta-analysis. Lancet 2018;391(10128):1357–66.

DeVane CL. Differential pharmacology of newer antidepressants. J Clin Psychiatry 1998;59 (Suppl 20):S85–93.

Haria M, Fitton A, McTavish D. Trazodone. A review of its pharmacology, therapeutic use in depression and therapeutic potential in other disorders. Drugs Aging 1994;4:331–55.

Rotzinger S, Bourin M, Akimoto Y, et al. Metabolism of some "second"- and "fourth"-generation antidepressants: iprindole, viloxazine, bupropion, mianserin, maprotiline, trazodone, nefazodone, and venlafaxine. Cell Mol Neurobiol 1999;19:427–42.

Stahl SM. Mechanism of action of trazodone: a multifunctional drug. CNS Spectr 2009;14(10):536–46.

Trifluoperazine

THERAPEUTICS

Brands
- Non-proprietary

Generic?
Yes

Class
- Neuroscience-based nomenclature: pharmacology domain – dopamine, serotonin; mode of action – antagonist
- Conventional antipsychotic (neuroleptic, phenothiazine, dopamine 2 antagonist)

Commonly Prescribed for
(bold for BNF indication)
- **Schizophrenia and other psychoses**
- **Short-term adjunctive management of psychomotor agitation, excitement, and violent or dangerously impulsive behaviour**
- **Short-term adjunctive management of severe anxiety**
- **Severe nausea and vomiting**
- Bipolar disorder

 ### How the Drug Works
- Blocks dopamine D2 receptors, reducing positive symptoms of psychosis
- Dopamine D2 in the vomiting centre may reduce nausea and vomiting

How Long Until It Works
- Psychotic symptoms can improve within 1 week, but it may take several weeks for full effect on behaviour
- Actions on nausea and vomiting are immediate

If It Works
- Most often reduces positive symptoms in schizophrenia but does not eliminate them
- Most patients with schizophrenia do not have a total remission of symptoms but rather a reduction of symptoms by about a third
- Continue treatment in schizophrenia until reaching a plateau of improvement
- After reaching a satisfactory plateau, continue treatment for at least a year after first episode of psychosis in schizophrenia

- For second and subsequent episodes of psychosis in schizophrenia, treatment may need to be indefinite
- Reduces symptoms of acute psychotic mania but not proven as a mood stabiliser or as an effective maintenance treatment in bipolar disorder
- After reducing acute psychotic symptoms in mania, switch to a mood stabiliser and/or an atypical antipsychotic for mood stabilisation and maintenance

If It Doesn't Work
- Consider trying one of the first-line atypical antipsychotics (risperidone, olanzapine, quetiapine, aripiprazole, paliperidone, amisulpride)
- Consider trying another conventional antipsychotic
- If two or more antipsychotic monotherapies do not work, consider clozapine

 ### Best Augmenting Combos for Partial Response or Treatment Resistance
- Augmentation of conventional antipsychotics has not been systematically studied
- Addition of a mood-stabilising anticonvulsant such as valproate, carbamazepine, or lamotrigine may be helpful in both schizophrenia and bipolar mania
- Augmentation with lithium in bipolar mania may be helpful
- Addition of a benzodiazepine, especially short term for agitation

Tests
Baseline
- *Measure weight, BMI, and waist circumference
- Get baseline personal and family history of diabetes, obesity, dyslipidaemia, hypertension, and cardiovascular disease
- Check for personal history of drug-induced leucopenia/neutropenia
- *Check pulse and blood pressure, fasting plasma glucose or glycosylated haemoglobin (HbA1c), fasting lipid profile, and prolactin levels
- Full blood count (FBC)
- Assessment of nutritional status, diet, and level of physical activity

- Determine if the patient:
  - is overweight (BMI 25.0–29.9)
  - is obese (BMI ≥30)
  - has pre-diabetes – fasting plasma glucose: 5.5 mmol/L to 6.9 mmol/L or HbA1c: 42 to 47 mmol/mol (6.0 to 6.4%)
  - has diabetes – fasting plasma glucose: >7.0 mmol/L or HbA1c: ≥48 mmol/L (≥6.5%)
  - has hypertension (BP >140/90 mm Hg)
  - has dyslipidaemia (increased total cholesterol, LDL cholesterol, and triglycerides; decreased HDL cholesterol)
- Treat or refer such patients for treatment, including nutrition and weight management, physical activity counselling, smoking cessation, and medical management
- Baseline ECG for: inpatients; those with a personal history or risk factor for cardiac disease

Monitoring

- Monitor weight and BMI during treatment
- Consider monitoring fasting triglycerides monthly for several months in patients at high risk for metabolic complications and when initiating or switching antipsychotics
- While giving a drug to a patient who has gained >5% of initial weight, consider evaluating for the presence of pre-diabetes, diabetes, or dyslipidaemia, or consider switching to a different antipsychotic
- Patients with low white blood cell count (WBC) or history of drug-induced leucopenia/neutropenia should have full blood count (FBC) monitored frequently during the first few months and trifluoperazine should be discontinued at the first sign of decline of WBC in the absence of other causative factors
- Monitor prolactin levels and for signs and symptoms of hyperprolactinaemia

SIDE EFFECTS

How Drug Causes Side Effects

- By blocking dopamine 2 receptors in the striatum, it can cause motor side effects
- By blocking dopamine 2 receptors in the pituitary, it can cause elevations in prolactin
- By blocking dopamine 2 receptors excessively in the mesocortical and mesolimbic dopamine pathways, especially at high doses, it can cause worsening of negative and cognitive symptoms (neuroleptic-induced deficit syndrome)
- Anticholinergic actions may cause sedation, blurred vision, constipation, dry mouth
- Antihistaminergic actions may cause sedation, weight gain
- By blocking alpha 1 adrenergic receptors, it can cause dizziness, sedation, and hypotension
- Mechanism of weight gain and any possible increased incidence of diabetes or dyslipidaemia with conventional antipsychotics is unknown

Notable Side Effects

* Neuroleptic-induced deficit syndrome
* Akathisia
* Rash
* Extrapyramidal side effects (more frequent at doses greater than 6 mg)
* Acute dystonias (the risk is increased in men, young adults, children, antipsychotic-naive patients, rapid dose escalation, and abrupt treatment discontinuation)
* Parkinsonism, tardive dyskinesia, tardive dystonia
* Galactorrhoea, amenorrhoea
- Dizziness, sedation
- Dry mouth, constipation, urinary retention, blurred vision
- Decreased sweating
- Sexual dysfunction
- Hypotension

Frequency not known

- Blood disorders: pancytopenia, thrombocytopenia
- CNS/PNS: anxiety, blurred vision, confusion, decreased alertness
- CVS: cardiac arrest, postural hypotension (dose-related)
- GIT: cholestatic jaundice, decreased appetite
- Other: fatigue, hyperpyrexia, lens opacity, muscle weakness, oedema, photosensitivity, skin reactions, urinary hesitation, withdrawal syndrome

 ### Life-Threatening or Dangerous Side Effects

- Rare neuroleptic malignant syndrome
- Rare agranulocytosis
- Rare embolism and thrombosis
- Very rare sudden death

Weight Gain

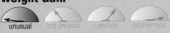
unusual   not unusual   common   problematic

- Though not expected has been reported more frequently in recent studies

Sedation

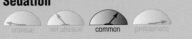
unusual   not unusual   common   problematic

- Many experience and/or can be significant in amount
- Sedation is usually transient

What to Do About Side Effects

- Wait
- Wait
- Wait
- Reduce the dose
- Low-dose benzodiazepine or beta blocker may reduce akathisia
- Take more of the dose at bedtime to help reduce daytime sedation
- Weight loss, exercise programmes, and medical management for high BMIs, diabetes, and dyslipidaemia
- Switch to another antipsychotic (atypical) – quetiapine or clozapine are best in cases of tardive dyskinesia

Best Augmenting Agents for Side Effects

- Dystonia: antimuscarinic drugs (e.g. procyclidine) as oral or IM depending on the severity; botulinum toxin if antimuscarinics not effective
- Parkinsonism: antimuscarinic drugs (e.g. procyclidine)
- Akathisia: beta blocker propranolol (30–80 mg/day) or low-dose benzodiazepine (e.g. 0.5–3.0 mg/day of clonazepam) may help; other agents that may be tried include the 5HT2 antagonists such as cyproheptadine (16 mg/day) or mirtazapine (15 mg at night – caution in bipolar disorder); clonidine (0.2–0.8 mg/day) may be tried if the above ineffective
- Tardive dyskinesia: stop any antimuscarinic, consider tetrabenazine

DOSING AND USE

Usual Dosage Range

- Schizophrenia and other psychoses: 10–20 mg/day
- Short-term adjunctive management of severe anxiety: 2–6 mg/day
- Severe nausea and vomiting: 2–6 mg/day

Dosage Forms

- Tablet 1 mg, 5 mg
- Oral solution: 1 mg/5 mL, 5 mg/5 mL

How to Dose

Adults:

*Schizophrenia and other psychoses:
- Initial dose 5 mg twice per day, may be increased by 5 mg/day after 7 days, with further increments of 5 mg after every 3 days. When acute symptoms under control, dose may be lowered to allow for maintenance treatment

*Short-term adjunctive management of severe anxiety:
- 2–4 mg/day in divided doses, increased as needed to 6 mg/day

*Severe nausea and vomiting:
- 2–4 mg/day in divided doses; max 6 mg/day

Children and adolescents:

*Schizophrenia and other psychoses:
- Under expert supervision
- Child 12–17 years: initial dose 5 mg twice per day, daily dose may be increased by 5 mg after 7 days with further increments of 5 mg every 3 days.
- When acute symptoms under control, dose may be lowered to allow for maintenance treatment

*Short-term adjunctive management of severe anxiety:
- Under expert supervision
- Child 3–5 years: up to 500 mcg twice per day
- Child 6–11 years: up to 2 mg twice per day
- Child 12–17 years: 1–2 mg twice per day, increased as needed to 3 mg twice per day

*Severe nausea and vomiting unresponsive to other antiemetics:
- Child 3–5 years: up to 500 mcg twice per day

- Child 6–11 years: up to 2 mg twice per day
- Child 12–17 years: 1–2 mg twice per day (max 3 mg twice per day)

 Dosing Tips

* Use only low doses and short term for anxiety because trifluoperazine is not a first-line agent for anxiety and has the risk of tardive dyskinesia
- Many patients can be dosed once a day
- Stop treatment if neutrophils fall below 1.5×10^9/L and refer to specialist care if neutrophils fall below 0.5×10^9/L

Overdose

- Extrapyramidal symptoms, sedation, seizures, coma, hypotension, respiratory depression
- Treat hypotension with fluid replacement, plus noradrenaline or dobutamine; adrenaline is contraindicated

Long-Term Use

- Some side effects may be irreversible (e.g. tardive dyskinesia)
- Not intended to treat anxiety long-term (i.e. longer than 12 weeks)

Habit Forming

- No

How to Stop

- There is a high risk of relapse if medication is stopped after 1–2 years. Withdrawal of antipsychotic drugs after long-term therapy should always be gradual and closely monitored to avoid the risk of acute withdrawal syndromes or rapid relapse. Patients should be monitored for 2 years after withdrawal of antipsychotic medication for signs and symptoms of relapse
- Slow down-titration of oral formulation (over 6–8 weeks), especially when simultaneously beginning a new antipsychotic while switching (i.e. cross-titration)
- Rapid oral discontinuation may lead to rebound psychosis and worsening of symptoms
- If anti-Parkinson agents are being used, they should be continued for a few weeks after trifluoperazine is discontinued

Pharmacokinetics

- Mean elimination half-life about 12.5 hours

 Drug Interactions

- May decrease the effects of levodopa, dopamine agonists
- May increase the effects of antihypertensive drugs except for guanethidine, whose antihypertensive actions trifluoperazine may antagonise
- Additive effects may occur if used with CNS depressants
- Alcohol and diuretics may increase the risk of hypotension; adrenaline may lower blood pressure
- Phenothiazines may reduce effects of anticoagulants
- Some patients taking a neuroleptic and lithium have developed an encephalopathic syndrome similar to neuroleptic malignant syndrome
- If used with propranolol, plasma levels of both drugs may rise

 Other Warnings/Precautions

- All antipsychotics should be used with caution in patients with angle-closure glaucoma, blood disorders, cardiovascular disease, depression, diabetes, epilepsy and susceptibility to seizures, history of jaundice, myasthenia gravis, Parkinson's disease, photosensitivity, prostatic hypertrophy, severe respiratory disorders
- Skin photosensitivity may occur at higher doses. Advise to avoid undue exposure to sunlight and use sun screen if necessary
- If signs of neuroleptic malignant syndrome develop, treatment should be immediately discontinued
- Use cautiously in patients with alcohol withdrawal or convulsive disorders because of possible lowering of seizure threshold
- Avoid extreme heat exposure
- Antiemetic effect of trifluoperazine may mask signs of other disorders or overdose; suppression of cough reflex may cause asphyxia
- Use with caution, if at all in Lewy body disease

Do Not Use

- If there is CNS depression
- If the patient is in a comatose state
- If the patient has phaeochromocytoma
- Do not use adrenaline in event of overdose as interaction with some pressor agents may lower blood pressure
- If there is a proven allergy to trifluoperazine
- If there is a known sensitivity to any phenothiazine

SPECIAL POPULATIONS

Renal Impairment

- Start with small doses in severe renal impairment because of increased cerebral sensitivity

Hepatic Impairment

- Can precipitate coma; phenothiazines are hepatotoxic

Cardiac Impairment

- Cardiovascular toxicity can occur, especially postural hypotension

Elderly

- Schizophrenia and other psychoses: initial dose up to 2.5 mg twice per day, may be increased by 5 mg/day in divided doses after 7 days. May be further increased by increments of 5 mg every 3 days as needed. Once stabilised, gradually reduce to achieve an effective maintenance dose
- Short-term adjunct for severe anxiety: up to 2 mg/day in divided doses, increased as needed to 6 mg/day
- Should check blood pressure in the elderly before starting and for the first few weeks of treatment

Children and Adolescents

- Licensed for use in schizophrenia and other psychoses for children and adolescents aged 12–17 years (under expert supervision)
- Licensed for use for the short-term adjunctive management of severe anxiety in children and adolescents aged 3–17 years (under expert supervision)
- Licensed for use for severe nausea and vomiting unresponsive to other antiemetics for children and adolescents aged 3–17 years

Pregnancy

- Controlled studies have not been conducted in pregnant women
- There is a risk of abnormal muscle movements and withdrawal symptoms in newborns whose mothers took an antipsychotic during the third trimester; symptoms may include agitation, abnormally increased or decreased muscle tone, tremor, sleepiness, severe difficulty breathing, and difficulty feeding
- Reports of extrapyramidal symptoms, jaundice, hyperreflexia, hyporeflexia in infants whose mothers took a phenothiazine during pregnancy
- Psychotic symptoms may worsen during pregnancy and some form of treatment may be necessary
- Use in pregnancy may be justified if the benefit of continued treatment exceeds any associated risk
- Switching antipsychotics may increase the risk of relapse
- Effects of hyperprolactinaemia on the foetus are unknown

Breastfeeding

- Small amounts in mother's breast milk
- Risk of accumulation in infant due to long half-life
- Haloperidol is considered to be the preferred first-generation antipsychotic, and quetiapine is the preferred second generation antipsychotic
- Infants of women who choose to breastfeed should be monitored for possible adverse effects

THE ART OF PSYCHOPHARMACOLOGY

Potential Advantages

- Less risk of sedation
- Less risk of orthostatic hypotension

Potential Disadvantages

- Patients with tardive dyskinesia
- Children
- Elderly

Trifluoperazine (Continued)

Primary Target Symptoms
- Positive symptoms of psychosis
- Motor and autonomic hyperactivity
- Violent or aggressive behaviour

Pearls
- Trifluoperazine is a higher potency phenothiazine and can cause more movement disorders versus chlorpromazine
- Less risk of sedation, orthostatic hypotension and seizure induction versus chlorpromazine
- Patients have very similar antipsychotic responses to any conventional antipsychotic, which is different from atypical antipsychotics where antipsychotic responses of individual patients can occasionally vary greatly from one atypical antipsychotic to another
- Patients with inadequate responses to atypical antipsychotics may benefit from a trial of augmentation with a conventional antipsychotic such as trifluoperazine or from switching to a conventional antipsychotic such as trifluoperazine
- However, long-term polypharmacy with a combination of a conventional antipsychotic such as trifluoperazine with an atypical antipsychotic may combine their side effects without clearly augmenting the efficacy of either
- For treatment-resistant patients, especially those with impulsivity, aggression, violence, and self-harm, long-term polypharmacy with 2 atypical antipsychotics or with 1 atypical antipsychotic and 1 conventional antipsychotic may be useful or even necessary while closely monitoring
- In such cases, it may be beneficial to combine 1 depot antipsychotic with 1 oral antipsychotic
- Although a frequent practice by some prescribers, adding 2 conventional antipsychotics together has little rationale and may reduce tolerability without clearly enhancing efficacy

 Suggested Reading

Alonso-Pedero L, Bes-Rastrollo, Marti A. Effects of antidepressant and antipsychotic use on weight gain: a systematic review. Obes Rev 2019;20(12):1680–90.

Doongaji DR, Satoskar RS, Sheth AS, et al. Centbutindole vs trifluoperazine: a double-blind controlled clinical study in acute schizophrenia. J Postgrad Med 1989;35:3–8.

Frankenburg FR. Choices in antipsychotic therapy in schizophrenia. Harv Rev Psychiatry 1999;6:241–9.

Huhn M, Nikolakopoulou A, Schneider-Thoma J, et al. Comparative efficacy and tolerability of 32 oral antipsychotics for the acute treatment of adults with multi-episode schizophrenia: a systematic review and network meta-analysis. Lancet 2019;394(10202):939–51.

Kiloh LG, Williams SE, Grant DA, Whetton PS. A double-blind comparative trial of loxapine and trifluoperazine in acute and chronic schizophrenic patients. J Int Med Res 1976;4:441–8.

Marques LO, Lima MS, Soares BG. Trifluoperazine for schizophrenia. Cochrane Database Syst Rev 2004;(1):CD003545.

Trihexyphenidyl hydrochloride

THERAPEUTICS

Brands
• Non-proprietary

Generic?
Yes

Class
• Antiparkinson agent; anticholinergic

Commonly Prescribed for
(bold for BNF indication)
• **Parkinson's disease (if used in combination with co-careldopa or co-beneldopa)**
• **Parkinsonism**
• **Drug-induced extrapyramidal symptoms (but not tardive dyskinesia)**
• **Dystonia (unlicensed use in children)**

 How the Drug Works
• Muscarinic acetylcholine receptor antagonist (generally non-selective but binds with higher affinity to the M1 subtype)
• Has a higher affinity for central muscarinic receptors located in the cerebral cortex and lower affinity for those located peripherally
• May modify nicotinic acetylcholine receptor neurotransmission, leading indirectly to enhanced dopamine release in the striatum

How Long Until It Works
• For extrapyramidal disorders and parkinsonism, onset of action can be within minutes or hours

If It Works
• Reduces motor side effects
• Does not lessen the ability of antipsychotics to cause tardive dyskinesia

If It Doesn't Work
• For extrapyramidal disorders, increase to highest tolerated dose
• Consider switching to procyclidine, or a benzodiazepine
• Disorders that develop after prolonged antipsychotic use may not respond to treatment

• Consider discontinuing the agent that precipitated the extrapyramidal side effects (EPS)

 Best Augmenting Combos for Partial Response or Treatment Resistance
• If ineffective, switch to another agent rather than augment
• Trihexyphenidyl itself has been used as an augmenting agent to antipsychotics

Tests
• None for healthy individuals

SIDE EFFECTS

How Drug Causes Side Effects
• Prevents the action of acetylcholine on muscarinic receptors

Notable Side Effects
• Dry mouth, blurred vision
• Confusion, hallucinations
• Constipation, nausea, vomiting
• Urinary retention

Frequency not known
• CNS/PNS: aggravated myasthenia gravis, anxiety, confusion, delusions, dizziness, euphoric mood, hallucination, insomnia, memory loss, vision disorders
• GIT: constipation, dry mouth, dysphagia, nausea, thirst, vomiting
• Other: decreased bronchial secretion, fever, flushing, mydriasis, skin reactions, tachycardia, urinary disorders

 Life-Threatening or Dangerous Side Effects
• Angle-closure glaucoma
• Heat stroke, especially in the elderly
• Tachycardia, cardiac arrhythmias, hypotension
• Urinary retention
• Anticholinergic agents such as trihexyphenidyl can exacerbate or unmask tardive dyskinesia
• Myasthenia gravis aggravated

Weight Gain

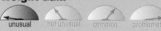

unusual   not unusual   common   problematic

• Reported but not expected

Sedation

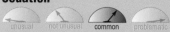

unusual   not unusual   common   problematic

• Many experience and/or can be significant in amount

What To Do About Side Effects

• For confusion or hallucination, discontinue use
• For sedation, lower the dose and/or take the entire dose at night
• For dry mouth, chew gum or drink water
• For urinary retention, obtain a urological evaluation; may need to discontinue use

Best Augmenting Agents for Side Effects

• Many side effects cannot be improved with an augmenting agent

DOSING AND USE

Usual Dosage Range

• Parkinson's disease: 2–6 mg/day in divided doses
• Parkinsonism, drug-induced extrapyramidal symptoms (but not tardive dyskinesia): 5–20 mg/day

Dosage Forms

• Oral solution 5 mg/5 mL (200 mL bottle)
• Tablet 2 mg, 5 mg

How to Dose

∗ Parkinson's disease (if used in combination with co-careldopa or co-beneldopa):
• Adult: maintenance 2–6 mg/day in divided doses
• Elderly: not recommended – increased toxicity and can aggravate dementia
∗ Parkinsonism, drug induced extrapyramidal symptoms (but not tardive dyskinesia):
• Adult: 1 mg/day, then increased by increments of 2 mg every 3–5 days, adjusted according to response; maintenance 5–15 mg/day in 3–4 divided doses; max dose 20 mg/day

• Elderly: lower doses preferred
Children and adolescents:
∗ Dystonia (unlicensed):
• Child 3 months–17 years: initial dose 1–2 mg/day in 1–2 divided doses, then increased by increments of 1 mg every 3–7 days, dose adjusted according to response and side effects; max 2 mg/kg/day

 Dosing Tips

• If drug-induced EPS occur soon after initiation of a neuroleptic drug, they are likely to be transient; thus, attempt to withdraw trihexyphenidyl after 1–2 weeks to determine if still needed
• To achieve more rapid relief, temporarily lower the dose of the offending agent (phenothiazine, thioxanthene, or butyrophenone) when starting trihexyphenidyl
• Taking trihexyphenidyl with meals can reduce side effects

Overdose

• Dilated pupils, dry mouth, dry skin, flushing, nausea, hyperpyrexia, hypertension, rapid respiration, rash, tachycardia, vomiting
• CNS stimulation: confusion, convulsions, delirium, hallucinations, incoordination, psychosis, restlessness
• In severe overdose: CNS depression with coma, circulatory collapse, respiratory failure and death

Long-Term Use

• Safe
• Effectiveness may decrease over time (years) and side effects such as sedation and cognitive impairment may worsen

Habit Forming

• No, but may be liable to abuse

How to Stop

• Taper not necessary but avoid abrupt withdrawal in patients taking long-term treatment

Pharmacokinetics

• Elimination half-life is about 3–4 hours

Drug Interactions

- Use with amantadine may increase anticholinergic side effects
- Anticholinergic agents may increase serum levels and effects of digoxin
- Additive anticholinergic side effects may be seen in combination with some antipsychotics and promethazine
- Anticholinergics can decrease gastric motility, resulting in increased gastric deactivation of levodopa and reduction in efficacy

Other Warnings/Precautions

- Caution in patients with cardiovascular disease, hypertension
- Caution in patients with prostatic hypertrophy or susceptible to angle-closure glaucoma
- Use with caution in patients with psychotic disorders
- Use with caution in patients with pyrexia
- Use with caution in the elderly
- Drug is also liable to abuse
- Anticholinergic agents can have additive effects when used with drugs of abuse such as cannabinoids, barbiturates, opioids and alcohol
- Use with caution in hot weather, as trihexyphenidyl may increase susceptibility to heat stroke

Do Not Use

- In elderly patient with Parkinson's disease due to risk of toxicity and of aggravating dementia
- In patient with myasthenia gravis
- In patient with gastrointestinal obstruction
- If there is proven allergy to trihexyphenidyl

Renal Impairment
- Use with caution

Hepatic Impairment
- Use with caution

Cardiac Impairment
- Use with caution in patients with hypertension or cardiovascular disease including known arrhythmias, especially tachycardia

Elderly

- Not recommended for use in Parkinson's disease in the elderly because of toxicity and risk of aggravating dementia
- For other indications use lower end of the dose range

Children and Adolescents

- Not licensed for use in children and adolescents
- Used to treat dystonia in children aged 3 months–17 years

Pregnancy

- Controlled studies have not been conducted in pregnant women
- Use of centrally acting drugs throughout pregnancy or around time of delivery is associated with an increased risk of poor neonatal adaptation syndrome
- Maternal exposure prior to delivery may cause anticholinergic side effects in the newborn

Breastfeeding

- Unknown if trihexyphenidyl is secreted in human breast milk, but all psychotropics assumed to be secreted in breast milk
- *Recommended either to discontinue drug or bottle feed unless the potential benefit to the mother justifies the potential risk to the child
- Infants of women who choose to breastfeed while on trihexyphenidyl should be monitored for possible adverse effects

THE ART OF PSYCHOPHARMACOLOGY

Potential Advantages
- Extrapyramidal disorders related to antipsychotic use
- Generalised dystonias (well tolerated in younger age groups)

Potential Disadvantages
- Patients with long-standing extrapyramidal disorders may not respond to treatment
- Multiple dose-dependent side effects may limit use

Primary Target Symptoms
- Tremor, akinesia, rigidity, drooling, dystonia

Trihexyphenidyl hydrochloride (Continued)

Pearls

- May be abused for its euphoric and sedative/hypnotic action, especially at high doses
- Has dopamine-enhancing actions
- Useful adjunct in younger Parkinson's patients with tremor
- Useful in the treatment of post-encephalitic Parkinson's disease and for extrapyramidal reactions, other than tardive dyskinesias
- Post-encephalitic Parkinson's patients usually tolerate higher doses better than idiopathic Parkinson's patients
- Generalised dystonias are more likely to benefit from anticholinergic therapy than focal dystonias; trihexyphenidyl is used more commonly than benztropine
- Sedation limits use, especially in older patients

- Patients with mental impairment do poorly
- Dystonias related to cerebral palsy, head injuries, and stroke may improve with trihexyphenidyl, especially in younger, cognitively normal patients
- Schizophrenia patients may abuse trihexyphenidyl and other anticholinergic medications to relieve negative symptoms, for a stimulant effect or to improve symptoms of drug-induced parkinsonism
- Can cause cognitive side effects with chronic use, so periodic trials of discontinuation may be useful to justify continuous use, especially in institutional settings as adjunct to antipsychotics
- Can be used for clozapine-induced hypersalivation at a dose range of 2–15 mg/day, but with the higher doses there is an increased risk of cognitive impairment

 Suggested Reading

Brocks DR. Anticholinergic drugs used in Parkinson' s disease: an overlooked class of drugs from a pharmacokinetic perspective. J Pharm Pharm Sci 1999;2(2):39–46.

Colosimo C, Gori MC, Inghilleri M. Postencephalitic tremor and delayed-onset parkinsonism. Parkinsonism Relat Disord 1999;5(3):123–4.

Costa J, Espírito-Santo C, Borges A, et al. Botulinum toxin type A versus anticholinergics for cervical dystonia. Cochrane Database Syst Rev 2005;(1):CD004312.

Sanger TD, Bastian A, Brunstrom J, et al. Prospective open-label clinical trial of trihexyphenidyl in children with secondary dystonia due to cerebral palsy. J Child Neurol 2007;22(5):530–7.

Zemishlany Z, Aizenberg D, Weiner Z, et al. Trihexyphenidyl (Artane) abuse in schizophrenic patients. Int Clin Psychopharmacol 1996;11(3):199–202.

Trimipramine

Brands
• Non-proprietary

Generic?
Yes

Class
• Neuroscience-based nomenclature: pharmacology domain – serotonin, dopamine; mode of action – antagonist
• Tricyclic antidepressant (TCA)
• Serotonin and noradrenaline reuptake inhibitor

Commonly Prescribed for
(bold for BNF indication)
• **Depressive illness (particularly where sedation is required)**
• Anxiety
• Insomnia
• Neuropathic pain/chronic pain

 ## How the Drug Works
• Boosts neurotransmitters serotonin and noradrenaline
• Blocks serotonin reuptake pump (serotonin transporter), presumably increasing serotonergic neurotransmission
• Blocks noradrenaline reuptake pump (noradrenaline transporter), presumably increasing noradrenergic neurotransmission
• Presumably desensitises both serotonin 1A receptors and beta adrenergic receptors
• Since dopamine is inactivated by noradrenaline reuptake in frontal cortex, which largely lacks dopamine transporters, trimipramine can increase dopamine neurotransmission in this part of the brain

How Long Until It Works
• May have immediate effects in treating insomnia or anxiety
• Onset of therapeutic actions with some antidepressants can be seen within 1–2 weeks, but often delayed up to 2–4 weeks
• If it is not working within 3–4 weeks for depression, it may require a dosage increase or it may not work at all
• By contrast, for generalised anxiety, onset of response and increases in remission rates may still occur after 8 weeks, and for up to 6 months after initiating dosing

• May continue to work for many years to prevent relapse of symptoms

If It Works
• The goal of treatment is complete remission of current symptoms as well as prevention of future relapses
• Treatment most often reduces or even eliminates symptoms, but is not a cure since symptoms can recur after medicine is stopped
• Continue treatment until all symptoms are gone (remission), especially in depression and whenever possible in anxiety disorders
• Once symptoms are gone, continue treating for at least 6–9 months for the first episode of depression or >12 months if relapse indicators present
• If >5 episodes and/or 2 episodes in the last few years then need to continue for at least 2 years or indefinitely
• The goal of treatment in chronic neuropathic pain is to reduce symptoms as much as possible, especially in combination with other treatments
• Treatment of chronic neuropathic pain may reduce symptoms, but rarely eliminates them completely, and is not a cure since symptoms can recur after medicine has been stopped
• Use in anxiety disorders and chronic pain may also need to be indefinite, but long-term treatment is not well studied in these conditions

If It Doesn't Work
• Important to recognise non-response to treatment early on (3–4 weeks)
• Many patients have only a partial response where some symptoms are improved but others persist (especially insomnia, fatigue, and problems concentrating)
• Other patients may be non-responders, sometimes called treatment-resistant or treatment-refractory
• Some patients who have an initial response may relapse even though they continue treatment
• Consider increasing dose, switching to another agent, or adding an appropriate augmenting agent
• Lithium may be added for suicidal patients or those at high risk of relapse
• Consider psychotherapy
• Consider ECT

- Consider evaluation for another diagnosis or for a co-morbid condition (e.g. medical illness, substance abuse, etc.)
- Some patients may experience a switch into mania and so would require antidepressant discontinuation and initiation of a mood stabiliser

⚖ Best Augmenting Combos for Partial Response or Treatment Resistance

- Mood stabilisers or atypical antipsychotics for bipolar depression
- Atypical antipsychotics for psychotic depression
- Atypical antipsychotics as first-line augmenting agents (quetiapine MR 300 mg/day or aripiprazole at 2.5–10 mg/day) for treatment-resistant depression
- Atypical antipsychotics as second-line augmenting agents (risperidone 0.5–2 mg/day or olanzapine 2.5–10 mg/day) for treatment-resistant depression
- Mirtazapine at 30–45 mg/day as another second-line augmenting agent (a dual serotonin and noradrenaline combination, but observe for switch into mania, increase in suicidal ideation or serotonin syndrome)
- T3 (20–50 mcg/day) is another second-line augmenting agent that works best with tricyclic antidepressants
- Other augmenting agents but with less evidence include bupropion (up to 400 mg/day), buspirone (up to 60 mg/day) and lamotrigine (up to 400 mg/day)
- Benzodiazepines if agitation present
- Hypnotics or trazodone for insomnia (but beware of serotonin syndrome with trazodone)
- Augmenting agents reserved for specialist use include: modafinil for sleepiness, fatigue and lack of concentration; stimulants, oestrogens, testosterone
- Lithium is particularly useful for suicidal patients and those at high risk of relapse including with factors such as severe depression, psychomotor retardation, repeated episodes (>3), significant weight loss, or a family history of major depression (aim for lithium plasma levels 0.6–1.0 mmol/L)
- For elderly patients lithium is a very effective augmenting agent

- For severely ill patients other combinations may be tried especially in specialist centres
- Augmenting agents that may be tried include omega-3, SAM-e, L-methylfolate
- Additional non-pharmacological treatments such as exercise, mindfulness, CBT, and IPT can also be helpful
- If present after treatment response (4–8 weeks) or remission (6–12 weeks), the most common residual symptoms of depression include cognitive impairments, reduced energy and problems with sleep
- For chronic pain: gabapentin, other anticonvulsants, or opiates if done by experts while monitoring carefully in difficult cases

Tests

- Baseline ECG is useful for patients over age 50
- ECGs may be useful for selected patients (e.g. those with personal or family history of QTc prolongation; cardiac arrhythmia; recent myocardial infarction; decompensated heart failure; or taking agents that prolong QTc interval such as pimozide, thioridazine, selected antiarrhythmics, moxifloxacin etc.)
- *Since tricyclic and tetracyclic antidepressants are frequently associated with weight gain, before starting treatment, weigh all patients and determine if the patient is already overweight (BMI 25.0–29.9) or obese (BMI ≥30)
- Before giving a drug that can cause weight gain to an overweight or obese patient, consider determining whether the patient already has:
  - Pre-diabetes – fasting plasma glucose: 5.5 mmol/L to 6.9 mmol/L or HbA1c: 42 to 47 mmol/mol (6.0 to 6.4%)
  - Diabetes – fasting plasma glucose: >7.0 mmol/L or HbA1c: ≥48 mmol/L (≥6.5%)
  - Hypertension (BP >140/90 mm Hg)
  - Dyslipidaemia (increased total cholesterol, LDL cholesterol, and triglycerides; decreased HDL cholesterol)
- Treat or refer such patients for treatment, including nutrition and weight management, physical activity counselling, smoking cessation, and medical management
- *Monitor weight and BMI during treatment
- *While giving a drug to a patient who has gained >5% of initial weight, consider evaluating for the presence of pre-diabetes,

diabetes, dyslipidaemia, or consider switching to a different antidepressant
- Patients at risk for electrolyte disturbances (e.g. patients aged >60, patients on diuretic therapy) should have baseline and periodic serum potassium and magnesium measurements

SIDE EFFECTS

How Drug Causes Side Effects
- Anticholinergic activity may explain sedative effects, dry mouth, constipation, and blurred vision
- Sedative effects and weight gain may be due to antihistaminergic properties
- Blockade of alpha adrenergic 1 receptors may explain dizziness, sedation, and hypotension
- Cardiac arrhythmias and seizures, especially in overdose, may be caused by blockade of ion channels

Notable Side Effects
- Blurred vision, constipation, urinary retention, dry mouth, increased appetite, weight gain
- Fatigue, weakness, dizziness, hypotension, sedation, headache, anxiety, restlessness, agitation
- Sexual dysfunction (impotence, change in libido)
- Sweating, rash, itching

Frequency not known
- CNS/PNS: agitation, altered mood, drowsiness, paranoid delusions, peripheral neuropathy, seizure, suicidal tendencies, tremor
- CVS: arrhythmias, hypotension
- GIT: cholestatic jaundice, constipation, dry mouth, jaundice
- Other: accommodation disorder, agranulocytosis, anticholinergic syndrome, bone fracture, bone marrow depression, hyperglycaemia, hyperhidrosis, rash, respiratory depression, sexual dysfunction, urinary hesitation, withdrawal syndrome

☠ Life-Threatening or Dangerous Side Effects
- Paralytic ileus, hyperthermia (TCAs + anticholinergic agents)

- Lowered seizure threshold and rare seizures
- Orthostatic hypotension, sudden death, arrhythmias, tachycardia
- QTc prolongation
- Hepatic failure, extrapyramidal symptoms
- Increased intraocular pressure
- Rare induction of mania and paranoid delusions
- Rare increase in suicidal ideation and behaviours in adolescents and young adults (up to age 25), hence patients should be warned of this potential adverse event

Weight Gain

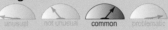

- Many experience and/or can be significant in amount
- Can increase appetite and carbohydrate craving

Sedation

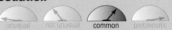

- Many experience and/or can be significant in amount
- Tolerance to sedative effects may develop with long-term use

What to Do About Side Effects
- Wait
- Wait
- Wait
- The risk of side effects is reduced by titrating slowly to the minimum effective dose (every 2–3 days)
- Consider using a lower starting dose in elderly patients
- Manage side effects that are likely to be transient (e.g. drowsiness) by explanation, reassurance and, if necessary, dose reduction and re-titration
- Giving patients simple strategies for managing mild side effects (e.g. dry mouth) may be useful
- For persistent, severe or distressing side effects the options are:
  - Dose reduction and re-titration if possible
  - Switching to an antidepressant with a lower propensity to cause that side effect
  - Non-drug management of the side effect (e.g. diet and exercise for weight gain)

Best Augmenting Agents for Side Effects

- Many side effects cannot be improved with an augmenting agent

DOSING AND USE

Usual Dosage Range
- 50–300 mg/day

Dosage Forms
- Tablet 10 mg, 25 mg
- Capsule 50 mg

How to Dose
- Adult: initial dose either 50–75 mg/day in divided doses or once daily at bedtime, increased as needed to 150–300 mg/day
- Elderly: initial dose 10–25 mg 3 times per day, maintenance 75–150 mg/day

Dosing Tips
- If given in a single dose, should generally be administered at bedtime because of its sedative properties
- If given in split doses, largest dose should generally be given at bedtime because of its sedative properties
- If patients experience nightmares, split dose and do not give large dose at bedtime
- Patients treated for chronic pain may only require lower doses
- If intolerable anxiety, insomnia, agitation, akathisia, or activation occur either upon dosing initiation or discontinuation, consider the possibility of activated bipolar disorder, and switch to a mood stabiliser or an atypical antipsychotic

Overdose
- Can be fatal; coma, CNS depression, convulsions, hyperreflexia, extensor plantar responses, dilated pupils, cardiac arrhythmias, severe hypotension, ECG changes, hypothermia, respiratory failure, urinary retention

Long-Term Use
- Safe

Habit Forming
- No

How to Stop
- Taper gradually to avoid withdrawal effects
- Even with gradual dose reduction some withdrawal symptoms may appear within the first 2 weeks
- It is best to reduce the dose gradually over 4 weeks or longer if withdrawal symptoms emerge
- If severe withdrawal symptoms emerge during discontinuation, raise dose to stop symptoms and then restart withdrawal much more slowly (over at least 6 months in patients on long-term maintenance treatment)

Pharmacokinetics
- Substrate for CYP450 2D6, 2C19, and 2C9
- Half-life is about 23 hours

Drug Interactions
- Tramadol increases the risk of seizures in patients taking TCAs
- Use of TCAs with anticholinergic drugs may result in paralytic ileus or hyperthermia
- Fluoxetine, paroxetine, bupropion, duloxetine, terbinafine and other CYP450 2D6 inhibitors may increase TCA concentrations
- Cimetidine may increase plasma concentrations of TCAs and cause anticholinergic symptoms
- Phenothiazines or haloperidol may raise TCA blood concentrations
- May alter effects of antihypertensive drugs; may inhibit hypotensive effects of clonidine
- Use with sympathomimetic agents may increase sympathetic activity
- Methylphenidate may inhibit metabolism of TCAs
- Trimipramine can increase the effects of adrenaline/epinephrine
- Carbamazepine decreases the exposure to trimipramine
- Both trimipramine and carbamazepine can increase the risk of hyponatraemia
- Trimipramine is predicted to increase the risk of severe toxic reaction when given with MAOIs; avoid and for 14 days after stopping the MAOI
- Both trimipramine and MAOIs can increase the risk of hypotension
- Do not start an MAOI for at least 5 half-lives (5 to 7 days for most drugs) after discontinuing trimipramine
- Activation and agitation, especially following switching or adding antidepressants,

may represent the induction of a bipolar state, especially a mixed dysphoric bipolar condition sometimes associated with suicidal ideation, and require the addition of lithium, a mood stabiliser or an atypical antipsychotic, and/or discontinuation of trimipramine

 Other Warnings/Precautions

- Can possibly increase QTc interval at higher doses
- Arrhythmias may occur at higher doses, but are rare
- Increased risk of arryhthmias in patients with hyperthyroidism or phaeochromocytoma
- Caution if patient is taking agents capable of significantly prolonging QTc interval or if there is a history of QTc prolongation
- Caution if the patient is taking drugs that inhibit TCA metabolism, including CYP450 2D6 inhibitors
- Because TCAs can prolong QTc interval, use with caution in patients who have bradycardia or who are taking drugs that can induce bradycardia (e.g. beta blockers, calcium channel blockers, clonidine, digitalis)
- Because TCAs can prolong QTc interval, use with caution in patients who have hypokalaemia and/or hypomagnesaemia or who are taking drugs that can induce hypokalaemia and/or hypo-magnesaemia (e.g. diuretics, stimulant laxatives, intravenous amphotericin B, glucocorticoids, tetracosactide)
- Caution if there is reduced CYP450 2D6 function, such as patients who are poor 2D6 metabolisers
- Can exacerbate chronic constipation
- Use caution when treating patients with epilepsy
- Use caution in patients with diabetes
- Use with caution in patients with a history of bipolar disorder, psychosis or significant risk of suicide
- Use with caution in patients with increased intra-ocular pressure or susceptibility to angle-closure glaucoma
- Use with caution in patients with prostatic hypertrophy or urinary retention

Do Not Use

- In patients during a manic phase

- If there is a history of cardiac arrhythmia, recent acute myocardial infarction, heart block
- In patients with acute porphyrias
- If there is a proven allergy to trimipramine

Renal Impairment

- Use with caution; may need to lower dose

Hepatic Impairment

- Use with caution; may need to lower dose
- Avoid in severe impairment

Cardiac Impairment

- Baseline ECG is recommended
- TCAs have been reported to cause arrhythmias, prolongation of conduction time, postural hypotension, sinus tachycardia, and heart failure, especially in the diseased heart
- Myocardial infarction and stroke have been reported with TCAs
- TCAs produce QTc prolongation, which may be enhanced by the existence of bradycardia, hypokalaemia, congenital or acquired long QTc interval, which should be evaluated prior to administering trimipramine
- Use with caution if treating concomitantly with a medication likely to produce prolonged bradycardia, hypokalaemia, heart block, or prolongation of the QTc interval
- Avoid TCAs in patients with a known history of QTc prolongation, recent acute myocardial infarction, and decompensated heart failure
- TCAs may cause a sustained increase in heart rate in patients with ischaemic heart disease and may worsen (decrease) heart rate variability, an independent risk of mortality in cardiac populations
- Since SSRIs may improve (increase) heart rate variability in patients following a myocardial infarct and may improve survival as well as mood in patients with acute angina or following a myocardial infarction, these are more appropriate agents for cardiac population than tricyclic/tetracyclic antidepressants
- *Risk/benefit ratio may not justify use of TCAs in cardiac impairment

Trimipramine (Continued)

Elderly
- Baseline ECG is recommended for patients over age 50
- May be more sensitive to anticholinergic, cardiovascular, hypotensive, and sedative effects
- Initial dose 10–25 mg 3 times per day
- Initial dose should be increased with caution and under close supervision
- Reduction in the risk of suicidality with antidepressants compared to placebo in adults age 65 and older

Children and Adolescents
- Not licensed for use in children and adolescents

Pregnancy
- No strong evidence of TCA maternal use during pregnancy being associated with an increased risk of congenital malformations
- Risk of malformations cannot be ruled out due to limited information on specific TCAs
- Poor neonatal adaptation syndrome and/or withdrawal has been reported in infants whose mothers took a TCA during pregnancy or near delivery
- Maternal use of more than one CNS-acting medication is likely to lead to more severe symptoms in the neonate
- Must weigh the risk of treatment (first trimester foetal development, third trimester newborn delivery) to the child against the risk of no treatment (recurrence of depression, maternal health, infant bonding) to the mother and child
- For many patients this may mean continuing treatment during pregnancy

Breastfeeding
- Small amounts expected in mother's breast milk
- Infant should be monitored for sedation and poor feeding
- Immediate postpartum period is a high-risk time for depression, especially in women who have had prior depressive episodes; antidepressants may need to be reinstituted late in the third trimester or shortly after childbirth to prevent a recurrence during the postpartum period
- Must weigh benefits of breastfeeding with risks and benefits of antidepressant treatment versus nontreatment to both the infant and the mother
- For many patients this may mean continuing treatment during breastfeeding
- Other antidepressants may be preferable, e.g. imipramine or nortriptyline

THE ART OF PSYCHOPHARMACOLOGY

Potential Advantages
- Patients with insomnia, anxiety
- Severe or treatment-resistant depression

Potential Disadvantages
- Paediatric and geriatric patients
- Patients concerned with weight gain and sedation

Primary Target Symptoms
- Depressed mood
- Symptoms of anxiety
- Somatic symptoms

Pearls
* May be more useful than some other TCAs for patients with anxiety, sleep disturbance, and depression with physical illness
* May be more sedating than some other TCAs
- TCAs are often a first-line treatment option for chronic pain
- TCAs are no longer generally considered a first-line option for depression because of their side-effect profile
- TCAs continue to be useful for severe or treatment-resistant depression
- TCAs may aggravate psychotic symptoms
- Use with alcohol can cause additive CNS-depressant effects
- Underweight patients may be more susceptible to adverse cardiovascular effects
- Patients with inadequate hydration and patients with cardiac disease may be more susceptible to TCA-induced cardiotoxicity than healthy adults
- Patients on tricyclics should be aware that they may experience symptoms such as photosensitivity or blue-green urine
- SSRIs may be more effective than TCAs in women, and TCAs may be more effective than SSRIs in men

- Since tricyclic/tetracyclic antidepressants are substrates for CYP450 2D6, and 7% of the population (especially Whites) may have a genetic variant leading to reduced activity of 2D6, such patients may not safely tolerate normal doses of tricyclic/tetracyclic antidepressants and may require dose reduction
- Patients who seem to have extraordinarily severe side effects at normal or low doses may have this phenotypic CYP450 2D6 variant and require low doses or switching to another antidepressant not metabolised by 2D6

THE ART OF SWITCHING

 **Switching**

- Consider switching to another agent or adding an appropriate augmenting agent if it doesn't work
- Consider switching to a different antidepressant if the patient has gained >5% of initial weight
- With patients with significant side effects at normal or low doses, they may have the phenotypic CYP450 2D6 variant; consider low doses or switching to another antidepressant not metabolised by 2D6

Suggested Reading

Anderson IM. Selective serotonin reuptake inhibitors versus tricyclic antidepressants: a meta-analysis of efficacy and tolerability. J Affect Disord 2000;58(1):19–36.

Anderson IM. Meta-analytical studies on new antidepressants. Br Med Bull 2001;57:161–78.

Berger M, Gastpar M. Trimipramine: a challenge to current concepts on antidepressives. Eur Arch Psychiatry Clin Neurosci 1996;246(5):235–9.

Lapierre YD. A review of trimipramine. 30 years of clinical use. Drugs 1989;38(Suppl 1):S17–24; discussion 49–50.

Tryptophan

Brands
• Optimax

Generic?
No, not in UK

Class
• Neuroscience-based nomenclature: Serotonin/melatonin (indolamine) precursor
• Essential amino acid

Commonly Prescribed for
(bold for BNF indication)
• **Treatment-resistant depression**
• Insomnia
• Seasonal affective disorder
• Premenstrual syndrome
• Fibromyalgia

 How the Drug Works
• The sole precursor to serotonin and melatonin
• Availability of tryptophan is the rate-limiting factor in serotonin synthesis
• Oral tryptophan is absorbed into the systemic circulation and transported across the blood–brain barrier
• Increasing levels of tryptophan, and therefore serotonin, presumably influence serotonin signalling in the brain
• The effect of tryptophan on sleep is thought to follow an increase in (peripheral) melatonin synthesis

How Long Until It Works
• Many patients may experience an acute improvement in mood
• May have immediate effect in treating insomnia
• Onset of therapeutic action not always immediate, and often delayed 2–4 weeks
• If it is not working within 3–4 weeks for depression, it may require a dosage increase or it may not work at all

If It Works
• The goal of treatment is complete remission of current symptoms as well as prevention of future relapses
• Treatment most often reduces or even eliminates symptoms, but is not a cure since symptoms can recur after medicine is stopped

• Once symptoms are gone, continue treating for at least 6–9 months for the first episode of depression or >12 months if relapse indicators present
• If >5 episodes and/or 2 episodes in the last few years then need to continue for at least 2 years or indefinitely
• In patients with acute sleep disturbance (e.g. jet lag), treatment may only be required for a short period until normal circadian rhythms and sleep-wake cycle are re-established

If It Doesn't Work
• Important to recognise non-response to treatment early on (3–4 weeks)
• Many depressed patients have only a partial response where some symptoms are improved but others persist (especially fatigue and problems concentrating)
• Consider supplementing pyridoxine (vitamin B6), especially in those with risk factors for deficiency (e.g. anticonvulsants, isoniazid, alcohol); pyridoxine is a cofactor required for the synthesis of serotonin from tryptophan
• Consider alternative augmenting agents such as atypical antipsychotics, lithium (for suicidal patients or those at high risk of relapse), mirtazapine or T3 (added to TCAs)
• Consider psychotherapy
• Consider ECT
• Consider evaluation for another diagnosis or for a co-morbid condition (e.g. medical illness, substance abuse, etc.)
• Some patients may experience a switch into mania and so would require antidepressant discontinuation and initiation of a mood stabiliser
• If insomnia does not improve after 7–10 days, it may be a manifestation of a primary psychiatric or physical illness such as obstructive sleep apnoea or restless leg syndrome, which requires independent evaluation
• Improve sleep hygiene
• Switch to another agent

 Best Augmenting Combos for Partial Response or Treatment Resistance
• If tryptophan monotherapy is ineffective, switch to another agent rather than augment
• Tryptophan is itself a second-line augmenting agent to antidepressants and lithium

- Tryptophan is itself an augmenting agent for treatment-resistant depression

Tests

- None for healthy individuals
- FBC should be conducted if any features of eosinophilia-myalgia syndrome arise (incapacitating myalgia, muscle cramps, dyspnoea, peripheral oedema)
- As of 2005, patients do not need to be registered with the eosinophilia-myalgia syndrome monitoring scheme (OPTICS)

SIDE EFFECTS

How Drug Causes Side Effects

- Adverse reactions are usually mild and occur within the first few days of treatment
- Peripheral conversion of tryptophan to serotonin likely accounts for the gastrointestinal side effects
- Increase in daytime melatonin synthesis may contribute to drowsiness

Notable Side Effects

- Sedation
- Nausea

Frequency not known

- CNS: dizziness, drowsiness, headache, suicidal tendencies
- Other: asthenia, eosinophilia-myalgia syndrome (EMS), myalgia, myopathy, nausea, oedema

 Life-Threatening or Dangerous Side Effects

- EMS, a rare complication linked to contaminated supply of tryptophan in the late 1980s; the current risk is seen as low
- The potential for (uncontaminated) tryptophan to cause EMS has not been established and is not clear

Weight Gain

unusual   not unusual   common   problematic

- Reported but not expected

Sedation

unusual   not unusual   common   problematic

- Many experience and/or can be significant in amount

- These effects may be offset by the overall benefit to sleep

What To Do About Side Effects

- Wait
- Observe
- Adjust dose
- If side effects persist, discontinue use
- Owing to its short half-life, side effects typically subside rapidly with the withdrawal of treatment

Best Augmenting Agents for Side Effects

- Most side effects typically subside within a few days of initiating treatment
- Many side effects cannot be improved with an augmenting agent

DOSING AND USE

Usual Dosage Range

- Depression: 3–6 g/day in divided doses
- Insomnia: 1–6 g/day at bedtime

Dosage Forms

- Capsule 500 mg (special order)

How to Dose

*Depression:
- Tryptophan should be started at 3 g/day divided into 3 doses
- Gradually increase dose to achieve desired therapeutic effect; max dose 6 g/day
*Insomnia:
- A single 1g dose taken 1 hr before bedtime

 Dosing Tips

- Requires dosing 3 times per day for full antidepressant effect
- If side effects are poorly tolerated, consider a regime of 1.5 g/day divided into 3 doses
- Efficacy is affected by food, so administration with or without food should be consistent

Overdose

- Limited data
- Nausea and vomiting

Long-Term Use

- Limited data suggest that it is safe

Habit Forming

- No

How to Stop

- No known withdrawal symptoms
- Theoretically, discontinuation could lead to a rapid decline in mood as observed in studies of tryptophan depletion

Pharmacokinetics

- Half-life is about 2 hours
- Undergoes significant metabolism in the gut (via the serotonin pathway), and in the liver (via the kynurenine pathway)
- Under inflammatory conditions the extra-hepatic metabolism of tryptophan to kynurenine is increased; reducing the availability of tryptophan for serotonin synthesis
- In the plasma, tryptophan competes with other large-neutral amino acids for transport across the blood–brain barrier
- Metabolised in serotonergic neurons to 5-hydroxy-tryptophan which is rapidly converted into serotonin
- Serotonin may be subsequently metabolised to the sleep-promoting hormone melatonin

 Drug Interactions

- No interactions with drugs metabolised by CYP450 enzymes
- Can cause "serotonin syndrome" when combined with other agents: antidepressants such as MAOIs (may be fatal), SSRIs or TCAs, lithium, methadone
- Tryptophan greatly decreases the effective concentration of levodopa through competition at the blood–brain barrier; caution is advised

 Other Warnings/Precautions

- If symptoms of eosinophilia-myalgia syndrome (incapacitating myalgia, muscle cramps, dyspnoea, peripheral oedema) are present, stop tryptophan immediately
- Use with caution in patients with bipolar disorder unless treated with a concomitant mood-stabilising agent
- Monitor patients for activation of suicidal ideation, especially children and adolescents
- Tryptophan should be used cautiously in patients being treated with phenothiazines or benzodiazepines as isolated cases of sexual disinhibition have been reported

Do Not Use

- In patients with a history of eosinophilia-myalgia syndrome
- If there is a proven allergy to tryptophan

SPECIAL POPULATIONS

Renal Impairment

- Little data available but dose adjustment may be necessary

Hepatic Impairment

- Use with caution in patients with moderate-severe hepatic impairment
- Serum tryptophan levels may be elevated in patients with liver cirrhosis

Cardiac Impairment

- Limited data available

Elderly

- May require lower initial dose and slower titration

 Children and Adolescents

- Safety and efficacy have not been established

 Pregnancy

- Controlled studies have not been conducted in pregnant women
- Safety in pregnancy has not been established
- Must weigh the risk of treatment (first trimester foetal development, third trimester newborn delivery) to the child against the risk of no treatment (recurrence of depression, maternal health, infant bonding) to the mother and child

Breastfeeding

- Tryptophan natural component of breast milk
- Immediate postpartum period is a high-risk time for depression, especially in women who have had prior depressive episodes; antidepressants may need to be reinstituted late in the third trimester or shortly after childbirth to prevent a recurrence during the postpartum period
- Must weigh benefits of breastfeeding with risks and benefits of antidepressant

treatment versus nontreatment to both the infant and the mother
- For many patients this may mean continuing treatment during breastfeeding
- Theoretical risk that tryptophan therapy may increase serotonin levels in the infant
- Other antidepressants may be preferable, e.g. paroxetine, sertraline, imipramine, or nortriptyline

THE ART OF PSYCHOPHARMACOLOGY

Potential Advantages
- Patients who would rather take a "natural supplement"
- No known abuse potential; not a controlled substance
- Side effects are uncommon even at higher doses

Potential Disadvantages
- Uncertainties around the link between tryptophan and eosinophilia-myalgia syndrome
- Three-times-daily dosing may limit compliance
- Limited data available regarding long-term use

Primary Target Symptoms
- Depressed mood
- Insomnia

 Pearls
- Tryptophan has been found to be effective in the treatment of depression on its own, with lithium or with other antidepressants

- Typical dietary intake of tryptophan is 800–1000 mg/day; but may be lower in the elderly or those with a co-morbid eating disorder
- Tryptophan competes with other large neutral amino acids at blood–brain barrier; the effective dose is reduced when taken alongside a protein-rich meal
- The insulin release associated with a carbohydrate-rich meal promotes the peripheral uptake of amino acids other than tryptophan; increasing transport of tryptophan into the brain
- Tryptophan may act through the entrainment-maintenance of circadian rhythms underlying a normal sleep-wake cycle
- Thus, tryptophan may also prove effective for treatment of circadian rhythm disturbances such as shift work sleep disorder and jet lag
- Tryptophan depletion, through the use of tryptophan-free dietary substitutes, has been successfully employed in the treatment of acute mania; but there is limited data to support its use

THE ART OF SWITCHING

 **Switching**
- Little available evidence to inform switching, but no data to suggest that there is a significant risk of interaction with other psychiatric medications
- Given the short half-life of tryptophan (about 2 hours), the risk of interaction when switching from tryptophan to other medications is likely to be small
- When switching from a serotonin reuptake inhibitor consider allowing for appropriate washout before starting tryptophan given the small risk of serotonin syndrome

Suggested Reading

pplebaum J, Bersudsky Y, Klein E. Rapid tryptophan depletion as a treatment for acute mania: double-blind, pilot-controlled study. Bipolar Disord 2007;9(8):884–7.

artzema AG, Porta MS, Tilson HH, et al. Tryptophan toxicity: a pharmacoepidemiologic review f eosinophilia-myalgia syndrome. Dicp 1991;25(11):1259–62.

nott PJ, Curzon G. Free tryptophan in plasma and brain tryptophan metabolism. Nature 972;239(5373):452–3.

1aes M, Leonard BE, Myint AM, et al. The new '5-HT' hypothesis of depression: cell-mediated ımune activation induces indoleamine 2, 3-dioxygenase, which leads to lower plasma ryptophan and an increased synthesis of detrimental tryptophan catabolites (TRYCATs), both f which contribute to the onset of depression. Prog Neuropsychopharmacol Biol Psychiatry 011;35(3):702–21.

chneider-Helmert D, Spinweber CL. Evaluation of L-tryptophan for treatment of insomnia: a eview. Psychopharmacology (Berl) 1986;89(1):1–7.

haw KA, Turner J, Del Mar C. Tryptophan and 5-hydroxytryptophan for depression. Cochrane atabase Syst Rev 2002;(1):CD003198.

oung SN. Use of tryptophan in combination with other antidepressant treatments: a review. J sychiatry Neurosci 1991;16(5):241–6.

'oung SN, Smith SE, Pihl RO, et al. Tryptophan depletion causes a rapid lowering of mood in ormal males. Psychopharmacology (Berl) 1985;87(2):173–7.

Valproate

Brands

- Depakote (valproic acid)
- Epilim (sodium valproate); Epilim Chrono; Epilim Chronosphere MR
- Convulex (valproic acid)
- Dyzantil (sodium valproate)
- Episenta (sodium valproate)
- Epival CR (sodium valproate)
- Belvo (valproic acid)
- Syonell (valproic acid)
- Depakin (sodium valproate – imported from Italy)

Generic?

Yes

Class

- Neuroscience-based nomenclature: pharmacology domain – glutamate; mode of action – unclear
- Anticonvulsant, mood stabiliser, migraine prophylaxis, voltage-sensitive sodium channel modulator

Commonly Prescribed for

(bold for BNF indication)

- **Treatment of manic episodes associated with bipolar disorder**
- **Migraine prophylaxis**
- **Epilepsy**
- Maintenance treatment of bipolar disorder
- Mixed episodes
- Bipolar depression
- Psychosis, schizophrenia (adjunctive)
- Aggressive behaviour
- Generalised anxiety disorder

 How the Drug Works

- * Blocks voltage-sensitive sodium channels by an unknown mechanism
- Increases brain concentrations of gamma-aminobutyric acid (GABA) by an unknown mechanism

How Long Until It Works

- For acute mania, effects should occur within a few days depending on the formulation of the drug

- May take several weeks to months to optimise an effect on mood stabilisation
- Should also reduce seizures and improve migraine within a few weeks

If It Works

- The goal of treatment is complete remission of symptoms (e.g. mania, seizures, migraine)
- Continue treatment until all symptoms are gone or until improvement is stable and then continue treating indefinitely as long as improvement persists
- Continue treatment indefinitely to avoid recurrence of mania, depression, seizures, and headaches

If It Doesn't Work

- * Many patients have only a partial response where some symptoms are improved but others persist or continue to wax and wane without stabilisation of mood
- Other patients may be non-responders, sometimes called treatment-resistant or treatment-refractory
- Consider checking plasma drug levels, increasing dose, switching to another agent, or adding an appropriate augmenting agent
- Consider adding psychotherapy
- Consider the presence of non-concordance and counsel patient
- Switch to another mood stabiliser with fewer side effects
- Consider evaluation for another diagnosis or for a co-morbid condition (e.g. medical illness, substance abuse, etc.)

 Best Augmenting Combos for Partial Response or Treatment Resistance

- Lithium
- Atypical antipsychotics (especially risperidone, olanzapine, quetiapine and aripiprazole)
- * Lamotrigine (with caution and at half the dose in the presence of valproate because valproate can double lamotrigine levels)
- * Antidepressants (with caution because antidepressants can destabilise mood in

some patients, including induction of rapid cycling or suicidal ideation; in particular consider bupropion; also SSRIs, SNRIs, others; generally avoid TCAs, MAOIs)

Tests

* Full blood count and liver function tests, repeated after 6 months and then annually
* BMI
* Consider coagulation tests prior to planned surgery or if there is a history of bleeding
* Plasma drug levels may assist in monitoring of efficacy, concordance or toxicity
* Since valproate is frequently associated with weight gain, before starting treatment, weigh all patients and determine if the patient is already overweight (BMI 25.0–29.9) or obese (BMI ≥30)
* Before giving a drug that can cause weight gain to an overweight or obese patient, consider determining whether the patient already has pre-diabetes – fasting plasma glucose: 5.5 mmol/L to 6.9 mmol/L or HbA1c: 42 to 47 mmol/mol (6.0 to 6.4%), diabetes – fasting plasma glucose: >7.0 mmol/L or HbA1c: ≥48 mmol/L (≥6.5%), or dyslipidaemia (increased total cholesterol, LDL cholesterol, and triglycerides; decreased HDL cholesterol), and treat or refer such patients for treatment, including nutrition and weight management, physical activity counselling, smoking cessation, and medical management
* Monitor weight and BMI during treatment
* While giving a drug to a patient who has gained >5% of initial weight, consider evaluating for the presence of pre-diabetes, diabetes, or dyslipidaemia, or consider switching to a different agent
* Effects on laboratory tests: false-positive urine test for ketones
* Women of childbearing age should be registered and under a Pregnancy Prevention Programme (pregnancy should be excluded before treatment initiation and highly effective contraception must be used during treatment) and reviewed on an annual basis with an Annual Risk Acknowledgement Form (see also under Other Warnings/Precautions section)

SIDE EFFECTS

How Drug Causes Side Effects

* CNS side effects theoretically due to excessive actions at voltage-sensitive sodium channels

Notable Side Effects

* Sedation, dose-dependent tremor, dizziness, ataxia, asthenia, headache
* Abdominal pain, nausea, vomiting, diarrhoea, reduced appetite, constipation, dyspepsia, weight gain
* Alopecia
* Polycystic ovaries (controversial)
* Hyperandrogenism, hyperinsulinaemia, lipid dysregulation (controversial)
* Decreased bone mineral density
* Hyperammonaemia
* Hyponatraemia
* Thrombocytopenia
* Aggression, behavioural disturbance
* Confusion, hallucinations, dementia (very rare)

Frequency not known

* Blood disorder: anaemia, haemorrhage, leucopenia, pancytopenia, thrombocytopenia
* CNS/PNS: abnormal behaviour, alertness, cerebral atrophy, coma, confusion, dementia, diplopia, drowsiness, encephalopathy, fine postural tremor, hallucination, hearing loss, impaired consciousness, movement disorders, parkinsonism, seizure, suicidal behaviours
* GIT: abdominal pain, diarrhoea, gastrointestinal disorder, hepatic disorders, nausea, vomiting, weight increased
* Other: alopecia (regrowth may be curly), bone disorders, bone fracture, gynaecomastia, hirsutism, hyperammonaemia, menstrual cycle irregularities, nail disorder, obesity, pancreatitis, peripheral oedema, severe cutaneous adverse reactions (SCARs), skin reactions, urine abnormalities, vasculitis

 Life-Threatening or Dangerous Side Effects

* Can cause tachycardia or bradycardia
* Rare hepatotoxicity with liver failure sometimes severe and fatal, particularly in children under 2 years old (withdraw

treatment immediately if persistent vomiting and abdominal pain, anorexia, jaundice, oedema, malaise, drowsiness, or loss of seizure control)
- Coma
- Encephalopathy
- Rare pancreatitis, sometimes fatal (discontinue treatment if symptoms of pancreatitis develop)
- Severe cutaneous adverse reactions (SCARs)
- Rare activation of suicidal ideation and behaviour (suicidality)

Weight Gain

- Many experience and/or can be significant in amount
- Can become a health problem in some

Sedation

- Frequent and can be significant in amount
- Some patients may not tolerate it
- Can wear off over time
- Can re-emerge as dose increases and then wear off again over time

What to Do About Side Effects

- Wait
- Wait
- Wait
- Take at night to reduce daytime sedation
- Lower the dose
- Switch to another agent

Best Augmenting Agents for Side Effects

* Propranolol 20–30 mg 2–3 times per day may reduce tremor
* Multivitamins fortified with zinc and selenium may help reduce alopecia
- Many side effects cannot be improved with an augmenting agent

DOSING AND USE

Usual Dosage Range

- Mania: 750–2000 mg/day in divided doses
- Migraine prophylaxis: 500–1000 mg/day in divided doses
- Epilepsy: 600–2500 mg/day in divided doses

Dosage Forms

- Valproate is available in UK in different forms: semi-sodium valproate (Depakote) is licensed for the treatment of acute mania (not licensed for use in children). Sodium valproate (Epilim) and valproic acid (Convulex) are both unlicensed for the treatment of bipolar disorder
- Semi-sodium valproate is a combined form of sodium valproate and valproic acid in 1:1 ratio
- Sodium valproate is metabolised to valproic acid, which is responsible for its pharmacological activity

Valproic acid/semi-sodium valproate:
- Tablet gastro-resistant (valproic acid as semi-sodium valproate) 250 mg, 500 mg
- Capsule gastro-resistant (valproic acid/ semi-sodium valproate) 125 mg, 150 mg, 300 mg, 500 mg

Sodium valproate:
- Tablet (sodium valproate) 100 mg
- Tablet modified-release (sodium valproate) 200 mg, 300 mg, 500 mg
- Tablet gastro-resistant (sodium valproate) 200 mg, 500 mg
- Capsule modified-release (sodium valproate) 150 mg, 300 mg
- Modified-release granules (sodium valproate) 50 mg, 100 mg, 250 mg, 500 mg, 750 mg, 1000 mg
- Oral solution (sodium valproate) 200 mg/5 mL, 200 mg/mL (Depakin imported from Italy)
- Solution for injection (sodium valproate) 300 mg/3 mL, 400 mg/4 mL
- Powder and solvent for solution for injection (sodium valproate) 400 mg

How to Dose

Adult:
* Treatment of manic episodes associated with bipolar disorder:
- Initial dose 750 mg/day in 2–3 divided doses, increased to 1–2 g/day, adjusted according to response, doses above 45 mg/ kg/day require careful monitoring
* Migraine prophylaxis:
- Initial dose 500 mg in 2 divided doses, increased as needed to 1 g/day in divided doses
* Epilepsy:
- Initial dose 600 mg/day in 2–4 divided doses, increased by increments of 150–300 mg every 3 days; maintenance 1–2 g/day in 2–4 divided doses, max 2.5 g/day in 2–4 divided doses (for Convulex)

Dosing Tips

∗Oral loading with 20–30 mg/kg per day may reduce onset of action to 5 days or less and may be especially useful for treatment of acute mania in inpatient settings
• Given the half-life of immediate-release valproate (e.g. Depakote), twice-daily dosing is necessary
• Modified-release sodium valproate tablets (e.g. Epilim Chrono) can be given once daily
• However, Epilim Chrono is only about 80% as bioavailable as Depakote, producing plasma drug levels 10–20% lower
∗Thus, Epilim Chrono is dosed about 8–20% higher when converting patients from Depakote
• Valproate levels are not routinely measured unless there is evidence of ineffectiveness, poor concordance, or toxicity is suspected
• Monitor closely if dose greater than 45 mg/kg/day

Overdose

• Fatalities have been reported; coma, restlessness, hallucinations, sedation, heart block

Long-Term Use

• Requires regular liver function tests and platelet counts

Habit Forming

• No

How to Stop

• Taper; may need to adjust dosage of concurrent medications as valproate is being discontinued
• Patients may seize upon withdrawal, especially if withdrawal is abrupt
∗Rapid discontinuation increases the risk of relapse in bipolar disorder
• Discontinuation symptoms uncommon

Pharmacokinetics

• Semi-sodium valproate (Depakote) mean terminal half-life about 14 hours
• Sodium valproate (Epilim) half-life about 8–20 hours (usually shorter in children)
• Metabolised primarily by the liver, about 25% dependent upon CYP450 system (CYP450 2C9 and 2C19)
• Inhibits CYP450 2C9
• Food slows rate but not extent of absorption

Drug Interactions

∗Lamotrigine dose should be reduced by about 50% if used with valproate, as valproate inhibits metabolism of lamotrigine and raises lamotrigine plasma levels, theoretically increasing the risk of rash
• Plasma levels of valproate may be lowered by carbamazepine, phenytoin, ethosuximide, phenobarbital, rifampicin
• Aspirin may inhibit metabolism of valproate and increase valproate plasma levels
• Plasma levels of valproate may also be increased by felbamate, chlorpromazine, quetiapine, fluoxetine, tricyclic antidepressants, fluvoxamine, topiramate, cimetidine, erythromycin, ibuprofen and warfarin
• Valproate inhibits metabolism of ethosuximide, phenobarbital, and phenytoin, and can thus increase their plasma levels
• No significant pharmacokinetic interactions of valproate with lithium or atypical antipsychotics
• Use of valproate with clonazepam may cause absence status
• Reports of hyperammonaemia with or without encephalopathy in patients taking topiramate combined with valproate, though this is not due to a pharmacokinetic interaction; in patients who develop unexplained lethargy, vomiting, or change in mental status, an ammonia level should be measured

Other Warnings/Precautions

∗Valproate is highly teratogenic and use in pregnancy leads to neurodevelopmental disorders (about 30–40% risk) and congenital malformations (about 10% risk)
∗Valproate must not be used in women and girls of childbearing potential unless the conditions of the Pregnancy Prevention Programme are met and only if other treatments are ineffective or not tolerated, as judged by an experienced specialist
∗Use of valproate in pregnancy is contra-indicated for migraine prophylaxis and bipolar disorder; it must only be considered for epilepsy if there is no suitable alternative treatment

∗ Women and girls (and their carers) must be fully informed of the risks and the need to avoid exposure to valproate medicines in pregnancy; supporting materials are available for use in the implementation of the Pregnancy Prevention Programme

∗ Specialists must book in review appointments at least annually with women and girls under the Pregnancy Prevention Programme, re-evaluate treatment as necessary, explain clearly the conditions as outlined in the supporting materials and complete and sign the Risk Acknowledgement Form – copies of the form must be given to the patient or carer and sent to their GP

∗ Specialists should comply with guidance given on the Annual Risk Acknowledgement form if they consider the patient is not at risk of pregnancy, including the need for review in case her risk status changes

∗ Be alert to the following symptoms of hepatotoxicity that require immediate attention: malaise, weakness, lethargy, facial oedema, anorexia, vomiting, yellowing of the skin and eyes

∗ Be alert to the following symptoms of pancreatitis that require immediate attention: abdominal pain, nausea, vomiting, anorexia

∗ Teratogenic effects in developing foetus such as neural tube defects may occur with valproate use

∗ Somnolence may be more common in the elderly and may be associated with dehydration, reduced nutritional intake, and weight loss, requiring slower dosage increases, lower doses, and monitoring of fluid and nutritional intake

• Use in patients with thrombocytopenia is not recommended; patients should report easy bruising or bleeding

• Evaluate for urea cycle disorders, as hyperammonaemic encephalopathy, sometimes fatal, has been associated with valproate administration in these uncommon disorders; urea cycle disorders, such as ornithine transcarbamylase deficiency, are associated with unexplained encephalopathy, intellectual disabilities, elevated plasma ammonia, cyclical vomiting, and lethargy

• Valproate is associated with severe cutaneous adverse reactions (SCARs) with potentially high mortality rates

• Warn patients and their caregivers about the possibility of activation of suicidal ideation and advise them to report such side effects immediately

• Use with caution in systemic lupus erythematosus

Do Not Use

• If patient has an acute porphyria, pancreatitis, suspected or known mitochondrial disorders

• If patient has a personal or family history of serious liver disease

• If patient has urea cycle disorder

• If there is a proven allergy to valproic acid or valproate

SPECIAL POPULATIONS

Renal Impairment

• May need to reduce dose

Hepatic Impairment

• Contraindicated

Cardiac Impairment

• No dose adjustment necessary

Elderly

• Reduce starting dose and titrate slowly; dosing is generally lower than in healthy adults

∗ Sedation in the elderly may be more common and associated with dehydration, reduced nutritional intake, and weight loss

• Monitor fluid and nutritional intake

• 1 in 3 elderly patients in long-term care who receive valproate may ultimately develop thrombocytopenia

Children and Adolescents

∗ Not generally recommended for use in children under age 10 for bipolar disorder except by experts and when other options have been considered

• Children under age 2 have significantly increased risk of hepatotoxicity, as they have a markedly decreased ability to eliminate valproate compared to older children and adults

• Use requires close medical supervision

• Indicated for the treatment of epilepsy in children and adolescents

Valproate (Continued)

Pregnancy

* Use of valproate in pregnancy is contra-indicated for migraine prophylaxis (unlicensed) and bipolar disorder; it must only be considered for epilepsy if there is no suitable alternative treatment

* Must only be used in women and girls of childbearing potential if other treatments are ineffective or not tolerated

* Use in girls and women of childbearing potential requires a Pregnancy Prevention Programme to be in place. This includes the completion of a signed risk acknowledgement form which should be completed before treatment is commenced and at an annual specialist review. See https://www.gov.uk/guidance/valproate-use-by-women-and-girls

* Birth defects seen in approximately 1 in 10 babies. Defects include spina bifida, facial and skull malformations and other congenital anomalies

* Rates of defects may be dose-dependent, reports of defect rates of 62.1% at doses of 3 g per day

* Cases of developmental delay associated with foetal exposure have been identified in 3–4 in 10 children. These may be in the absence of teratogenicity

* Women who present with unplanned pregnancies should have their treatment switched

* When stopping valproate it is usually necessary to taper the dose

* Women who have continued valproate during pregnancy should be referred for specialist monitoring and should be offered detailed anomaly scanning

* If prescribed for epilepsy the patient should be referred to a specialist to consider alternative treatment options

* If drug is continued, start on folate 5 mg/day early in pregnancy to reduce risk of neural tube defects

* For bipolar patients, given the risk of relapse in the postpartum period, mood stabiliser treatment should generally be restarted immediately after delivery if patient is unmedicated during pregnancy

* Antipsychotics may be preferable to lithium or anticonvulsants such as valproate if treatment of bipolar disorder is required during pregnancy

• Bipolar symptoms may recur or worsen during pregnancy and some form of treatment may be necessary

Breastfeeding

• Small amounts found in mother's breast milk

* Generally considered safe to breastfeed while taking valproate

• If drug is continued while breastfeeding, infant should be monitored for possible adverse effects including jaundice, bruising and bleeding

• If infant shows signs of irritability or sedation, drug may need to be discontinued

* Bipolar disorder may recur during the postpartum period, particularly if there is a history of prior postpartum episodes of either depression or psychosis

* Relapse rates may be lower in women who receive prophylactic treatment for postpartum episodes of bipolar disorder

• Due to the restrictions on the use of valproate in women and children of childbearing age, carbamazepine or antipsychotics are preferable to valproate during the postpartum period

Potential Advantages

• Manic phase of bipolar disorder
• Works well in combination with lithium and/or atypical antipsychotics

Potential Disadvantages

• Depressed phase of bipolar disorder
• Patients unable to tolerate sedation or weight gain
• Multiple drug interactions
• Multiple side-effect risks
• Pregnant patients
• Women and girls with childbearing potential

Primary Target Symptoms

• Unstable mood
• Incidence of migraine
• Incidence of partial complex seizures

Pearls

* Valproate must not be used in women and girls of childbearing potential unless the conditions of the Pregnancy Prevention

Programme are met and only if other treatments are ineffective or not tolerated, as judged by an experienced specialist

* Valproate is a treatment option that may be used for patients with mixed states of bipolar disorder or for patients with rapid-cycling bipolar disorder
* Seems to be more effective in treating manic episodes than depressive episodes in bipolar disorder (treats from above better than it treats from below)
* May also be more effective in preventing manic relapses than in preventing depressive episodes (stabilises from above better than it stabilises from below)
* Only a third of bipolar patients experience adequate relief with a monotherapy, so most patients need multiple medications for best control
* Useful in combination with atypical antipsychotics and/or lithium for acute mania
* May also be useful for bipolar disorder in combination with lamotrigine, but must reduce lamotrigine dose by half when combined with valproate
* Usefulness for bipolar disorder in combination with anticonvulsants other than lamotrigine is not well demonstrated

* May be useful as an adjunct to atypical antipsychotics for rapid onset of action in schizophrenia
* Can be used to treat aggression, agitation, and impulsivity not only in bipolar disorder and schizophrenia, but also in many other disorders, including dementia, personality disorders, and brain injury
* Patients with acute mania tend to tolerate side effects better than patients with hypomania or depression
* Multivitamins fortified with zinc and selenium may help reduce alopecia
* Association of valproate with polycystic ovaries is controversial and may be related to weight gain, obesity, or epilepsy
* Association of valproate with decreased bone mass is controversial and may be related to activity levels, exposure to sunlight, and epilepsy, and might be prevented by supplemental vitamin D 2000 IU/day and calcium 600–1000 mg/day
* The Commission on Human Medicines has advised The Medicines and Healthcare Products Regulatory Agency to recommend that no one under the age of 55 should be initiated on valproate unless two specialists independently consider and document that there is no other effective or tolerated treatment available

 ## Suggested Reading

Bowden CL. Valproate. Bipolar Disord 2003;5(3):189–202.

Gill D, Derry S, Wiffen PJ, et al. Valproic acid and sodium valproate for neuropathic pain and fibromyalgia in adults. Cochrane Database Syst Rev 2011;(10):CD009183.

Iacobucci G. MHRA bans valproate prescribing for women not in pregnancy prevention programme. BMJ 2018;361:k1823.

Landy SH, McGinnis J. Divalproex sodium–review of prophylactic migraine efficacy, safety and dosage, with recommendations. Tenn Med 1999;92(4):135–6.

Macritchie KA, Geddes JR, Scott J, et al. Valproic acid, valproate and divalproex in the maintenance treatment of bipolar disorder. Cochrane Database Syst Rev 2001;(3):CD003196.

Morgan S, Raine J, Hudson I. Valproate and the Pregnancy Prevention Programme. Br J Gen Pract 2019;69(682):229.

Smith LA, Cornelius V, Warnock A, et al. Pharmacological interventions for acute bipolar mania: a systematic review of randomized placebo-controlled trials. Bipolar Disord 2007;9(6):551–60.

Varenicline

THERAPEUTICS

Brands
- Champix

Generic?
No, not in UK

Class
- Neuroscience-based nomenclature: pharmacology domain – acetylcholine; mode of action – partial agonist
- Smoking cessation treatment; alpha 4 beta 2 partial agonist at nicotinic acetylcholine receptors

Commonly Prescribed for
(bold for BNF indication)
- **To aid smoking cessation**

 How the Drug Works
- Causes sustained but small amounts of dopamine release (less than with nicotine), reducing the reward and reinforcement of smoking
- Specifically, as a partial agonist at alpha 4 beta 2 nicotinic acetylcholine receptors, varenicline activates these receptors to a lesser extent than the full agonist nicotine and also prevents nicotine from binding to these receptors
- Its binding both alleviates symptoms of craving and withdrawal, and reduces the rewarding and reinforcing effects of smoking
- Most prominent actions are on mesolimbic dopaminergic neurons in the ventral tegmental area

How Long Until It Works
- Varenicline should normally be prescribed only as part of a programme of behavioural support
- Smokers should set a date to stop smoking and treatment with varenicline should start 1 to 2 weeks before this date
- Recommended initial treatment trial is 12 weeks; an additional 12-week trial in individuals who stop smoking after 12 weeks may increase likelihood of long-term abstinence

If It Works
- Reduces withdrawal symptoms and the urge to smoke; increases abstinence

If It Doesn't Work
- Evaluate for and address contributing factors, then reattempt treatment
- Consider switching to another agent

 Best Augmenting Combos for Partial Response or Treatment Resistance
- Best to attempt other monotherapies

Tests
- None for healthy individuals

SIDE EFFECTS

How Drug Causes Side Effects
- Theoretically due to increases in dopamine concentrations at receptors in parts of the brain and body other than those that cause therapeutic actions

Notable Side Effects
- Dose-dependent nausea, vomiting, constipation, flatulence
- Insomnia, headache, abnormal dreams

Common or very common
- CNS/PNS: dizziness, drowsiness, headache, sleep disorders
- GIT: abnormal appetite, constipation, diarrhoea, dry mouth, gastrointestinal discomfort, gastrointestinal disorders, nausea, oral disorders, vomiting, weight increased
- Other: asthenia, chest discomfort, joint disorders, muscle complaints, pain, skin reactions

Uncommon
- CNS/PNS: abnormal behaviour, abnormal thinking, anxiety, depression, hallucination, mood swings, numbness, seizure, suicidal ideation, tinnitus, tremor
- CVS: arrhythmias, palpitations
- GIT: burping
- Other: allergic rhinitis, conjunctivitis, eye pain, fever, fungal infection, haemorrhage,

Varenicline (Continued)

hot flush, hyperglycaemia, influenza-like illness, malaise, menorrhagia, sexual dysfunction, sweat changes, urinary disorders

Rare or very rare
- CNS/PNS: abnormal coordination, bradyphrenia, dysarthria, increased muscle tone, psychosis, snoring, vision disorders
- Other: angioedema, costochondritis, cyst, diabetes mellitus, eye disorders, feeling cold, glycosuria, polydipsia, scleral discolouration, severe cutaneous adverse reactions (SCARs), vaginal discharge

Frequency not known
- Loss of consciousness

 Life-Threatening or Dangerous Side Effects
- Activation of agitation, depressed mood, suicidal ideation, suicidal behaviour
- Seizures
- Rare reports of life-threatening angioedema causing respiratory compromise and severe cutaneous reactions such as Stevens-Johnson syndrome and erythema multiforme

Weight Gain

- Reported but not expected
- Some patients report weight loss

Sedation

- Reported but not expected
- Some patients report activation and insomnia

What to Do About Side Effects
- Wait
- Adjust dose to 0.5 mg twice daily temporarily or permanently
- If side effects persist, discontinue use

Best Augmenting Agents for Side Effects
- Dose reduction or switching to another agent may be more effective since most side effects cannot be improved with an augmenting agent

Usual Dosage Range
- 0.5–2.0 mg/day

Dosage Forms
- Tablet 0.5 mg, 1 mg

How to Dose
- The patient should set a date to stop smoking. Dosing should usually start at 1–2 weeks before this date
- Patients should be treated with varenicline for 12 weeks
- Initial dose 0.5 mg/day; after 3 days increase to 0.5 mg twice per day; after 4 days can increase to 1 mg twice per day for 11 weeks

 Dosing Tips
- Varenicline should be taken following a meal and with a full glass of water
- Behavioural support in combination with varenicline treatment should be routine as this can increase the chances of success
- Initial recommended treatment duration is 12 weeks; for individuals who have stopped smoking after 12 weeks continued treatment for an additional 12 weeks can increase the likelihood of long-term abstinence
- For patients who are unsuccessful in their attempt to quit following 12 weeks of treatment or those who relapse following treatment, it is best to attempt to address factors contributing to the failed attempt and then reintroduce treatment
- Incidence of nausea is dose-dependent

Overdose
- Limited available data

Long-Term Use
- Treatment for up to 24 weeks has been found effective

Habit Forming
- No

How to Stop
- Risk of relapse, irritability, depression, and insomnia on discontinuation
- Taper to avoid withdrawal effects, but no well-documented tolerance or dependence

Pharmacokinetics
- Elimination half-life 24 hours
- Excretion: kidneys 81–92%

Drug Interactions
- Does not inhibit hepatic enzymes or renal transport proteins, and thus is unlikely to affect plasma concentrations of other drugs
- Is not hepatically metabolised and thus is unlikely to be affected by other drugs
- Side effects may be increased if varenicline is taken with nicotine replacement therapy
- Varenicline may alter one's reaction to alcohol, with case reports showing decreased tolerance to alcohol, increased drunkenness, unusual or aggressive behaviour, or no memory of things that happened

Other Warnings/Precautions
- Monitor patients for changes in behaviour, agitation, depressed mood, worsening of pre-existing psychiatric illness, and suicidality
- Use cautiously in individuals with known psychiatric illness. May exacerbate underlying illness including depression
- Use cautiously in patients with a history of seizures or other factors that can lower the seizure threshold
- Use cautiously in patients with a history of cardiovascular disease
- Discontinuing smoking may lead to pharmacokinetic or pharmacodynamic changes in other drugs the patient is taking, which could potentially require dose adjustment
- Smoking induces CYP450 1A2, thus smoking cessation can increase the level of CYP450 1A2 substrates
- Due to increased risk of dizziness, somnolence and transient loss of consciousness, patients should be cautioned on the effects on driving and performance of skilled tasks

Do Not Use
- In combination with NRT or bupropion
- If there is a proven allergy to varenicline

Renal Impairment
- For severe impairment, maximum recommended dose is 0.5 mg twice per day
- For patients with end-stage renal disease undergoing haemodialysis, max recommended dose is 0.5 mg once per day
- Removed by haemodialysis

Hepatic Impairment
- Dose adjustment not generally necessary

Cardiac Impairment
- Effective in patients with cardiovascular disease; small increased risk of certain cardiovascular adverse effects in these patients

Elderly
- No special requirements but lower doses may be needed due to increased likelihood of decreased renal function

Children and Adolescents
- Safety and efficacy have not been established

Pregnancy
- Very limited data on evidence of safety in pregnancy
- Controlled studies do not currently indicate a risk of spontaneous abortion, major congenital malformation or intrauterine death
- Pregnant women wishing to stop smoking may consider behavioural therapy before pharmacotherapy
- Not generally recommended for use during pregnancy, especially during first trimester

Breastfeeding
- Varenicline is expected to be secreted in human breast milk
- Long half-life risks accumulation in the breastfed infant
- Recommended either to discontinue drug or bottle feed

Varenicline (Continued)

Potential Advantages

- More effective than other pharmacotherapies for smoking cessation

Potential Disadvantages

- Not well studied in patients with co-morbid psychiatric disorders

Primary Target Symptoms

- Cravings associated with nicotine withdrawal

Pearls

- More effective than nicotine or bupropion
- Usually well tolerated and accepted
- Nausea is a common side effect – the incidence is dose-dependent
- All smoking cessation medications are best used with a stop smoking programme that includes behavioural support
- Unlike nicotine or bupropion, the patient cannot "smoke over" varenicline since varenicline, but not the others, will block the effects of additional smoked nicotine if the patient decides to smoke during treatment

- Less than 20% of people treated with varenicline remain abstinent from smoking at 1 year
- Although tested in the general population excluding psychiatric patients, there is great unmet need for smoking cessation treatments in patients with psychiatric disorders, especially attention deficit hyperactivity disorder and schizophrenia
- Smoking cessation treatment in patients with co-morbid psychiatric disorders is not well studied
- Preliminary results suggest that varenicline is not associated with worsening of psychiatric symptoms in stable patients with schizophrenia, schizoaffective disorder, or depression
- Nevertheless, patients with co-morbid psychiatric disorders should be closely monitored in terms of their psychiatric symptoms, especially suicidality
- In a large multinational study there was no significant increase in moderate-to-severe neuropsychiatric adverse events with varenicline relative to nicotine patch or placebo in participants with or without history of psychiatric disorder

 Suggested Reading

Anthenelli RM, Benowitz N, West R, et al. Neuropsychiatric safety and efficacy of varenicline, bupropion, and nicotine patch in smokers with and without psychiatric disorders (EAGLES): a double-blind, randomised, placebo-controlled clinical trial. The Lancet 2016;387(10037):2507–20.

Cerimele JM, Durango A. Does varenicline worsen psychiatric symptoms in patients with schizophrenia or schizoaffective disorder? A review of published studies. J Clin Psychiatry 2012;73(8):e1039–47.

Jorenby DE, Hays JT, Rigotti NA. Efficacy of varenicline, an alpha4beta2 nicotinic acetylcholine receptor partial agonist, vs placebo or sustained-release bupropion for smoking cessation: a randomized controlled trial. JAMA 2006;296(1):56–63.

Meszaros ZS, Abdul-Malak Y, Dimmock JA, et al. Varenicline treatment of concurrent alcohol and nicotine dependence in schizophrenia: a randomized, placebo-controlled pilot trial. J Clin Psychopharmacol 2013;33(2):243–7.

Rollema H, Coe JW, Chambers LK, et al. Rationale, pharmacology and clinical efficacy of partial agonists of alpha4beta2 nACh receptors for smoking cessation. Trends Pharmacol Sci 2007;28(7):316–25.

Rosen LJ, Galili T, Kott J, et al. Diminishing benefit of smoking cessation medications during the first year: a meta-analysis of randomized controlled trials. Addiction 2018;113(5):805–16.

Wu P, Wilson K, Dimoulas P, et al. Effectiveness of smoking cessation therapies: a systematic review and meta-analysis. BMC Public Health 2006;6:300.

Venlafaxine

Brands
- Efexor XL
- Sunveniz XL

see index for additional brand names

Generic?
Yes

Class
- Neuroscience-based nomenclature: pharmacology domain – serotonin, norepinephrine; mode of action – reuptake inhibitor
- SNRI (dual serotonin and noradrenaline reuptake inhibitor); often classified as an antidepressant, but it is not just an antidepressant

Commonly Prescribed for
(bold for BNF indication)
- **Major depression**
- **Generalised anxiety disorder (GAD)**
- **Social anxiety disorder (social phobia)**
- **Panic disorder**
- **Menopausal symptoms, particularly hot flushes, in women with breast cancer (unlicensed)**
- Post-traumatic stress disorder (PTSD)
- Premenstrual dysphoric disorder (PMDD)

 How the Drug Works
- Boosts neurotransmitters serotonin, noradrenaline, and dopamine
- Blocks serotonin reuptake pump (serotonin transporter), presumably increasing serotonergic neurotransmission
- Blocks norepinephrine reuptake pump (noradrenaline transporter), presumably increasing noradrenergic neurotransmission
- Presumably desensitises both serotonin 1A receptors and beta adrenergic receptors
- Since dopamine is inactivated by noradrenergic reuptake in frontal cortex, which largely lacks dopamine transporters, venlafaxine can increase dopamine neurotransmission in this part of the brain
- Weakly blocks dopamine reuptake pump (dopamine transporter), and may increase dopamine neurotransmission

How Long Until It Works
- Onset of therapeutic actions with some antidepressants can be seen within 1–2 weeks, but often delayed 2–4 weeks
- If it is not working within 3–4 weeks for depression, it may require a dosage increase or it may not work at all
- By contrast, for generalised anxiety, onset of response and increases in remission rates may still occur after 8 weeks, and for up to 6 months after initiating dosing
- May continue to work for many years to prevent relapse of symptoms

If It Works
- The goal of treatment is complete remission of current symptoms as well as prevention of future relapses
- Treatment most often reduces or even eliminates symptoms, but is not a cure since symptoms can recur after medicine is stopped
- Continue treatment until all symptoms are gone (remission), especially in depression and whenever possible in anxiety disorders
- Once symptoms are gone, continue treating for at least 6–9 months for the first episode of depression or >12 months if relapse indicators present
- If >5 episodes and/or 2 episodes in the last few years then need to continue for at least 2 years or indefinitely
- Use in anxiety disorders may also need to be indefinite

If It Doesn't Work
- Important to recognise non-response to treatment early on (3–4 weeks)
- Many patients have only a partial response where some symptoms are improved but others persist (especially insomnia, fatigue, and problems concentrating)
- Other patients may be non-responders, sometimes called treatment-resistant or treatment-refractory
- Some patients who have an initial response may relapse even though they continue treatment
- Consider increasing dose, switching to another agent, or adding an appropriate augmenting agent
- Lithium may be added for suicidal patients or those at high risk of relapse
- Consider psychotherapy

Venlafaxine (Continued)

- Consider ECT
- Consider evaluation for another diagnosis or for a co-morbid condition (e.g. medical illness, substance abuse, etc.)
- Some patients may experience a switch into mania and so would require antidepressant discontinuation and initiation of a mood stabiliser

Best Augmenting Combos for Partial Response or Treatment Resistance

- Mood stabilisers or atypical antipsychotics for bipolar depression
- Atypical antipsychotics for psychotic depression
- Atypical antipsychotics as first-line augmenting agents (quetiapine MR 300 mg/day or aripiprazole at 2.5–10 mg/day) for treatment-resistant depression
- Atypical antipsychotics as second-line augmenting agents (risperidone 0.5–2 mg/day or olanzapine 2.5–10 mg/day) for treatment-resistant depression
- Mirtazapine at 30–45 mg/day as another second-line augmenting agent (a dual serotonin and noradrenaline combination, but observe for switch into mania, increase in suicidal ideation or rare risk of non-fatal serotonin syndrome)
- Although T3 (20–50 mcg/day) is another second-line augmenting agent the evidence suggests that it works best with tricyclic antidepressants
- Other augmenting agents but with less evidence include bupropion (up to 400 mg/day), buspirone (up to 60 mg/day) and lamotrigine (up to 400 mg/day)
- Benzodiazepines if agitation present
- Hypnotics or trazodone for insomnia (but there is a rare risk of non-fatal serotonin syndrome with trazodone)
- Augmenting agents reserved for specialist use include: modafinil for sleepiness, fatigue and lack of concentration; stimulants, oestrogens, testosterone
- Lithium is particularly useful for suicidal patients and those at high risk of relapse including with factors such as severe depression, psychomotor retardation, repeated episodes (>3), significant weight loss, or a family history of major depression (aim for lithium plasma levels 0.6–1.0 mmol/L)

- For elderly patients lithium is a very effective augmenting agent, but another option could be the combination of venlafaxine with selegiline
- For severely ill patients other combinations may be tried especially in specialist centres
- Augmenting agents that may be tried include omega-3, SAM-e, L-methylfolate
- Additional non-pharmacological treatments such as exercise, mindfulness, CBT, and IPT can also be helpful
- If present after treatment response (4–8 weeks) or remission (6–12 weeks), the most common residual symptoms of depression include cognitive impairments, reduced energy and problems with sleep

Tests

- Usually none required
- Baseline blood pressure could be useful in case of further dose titrations
- Baseline prolactin levels could be useful as venlafaxine may increase prolactin levels in some patients

SIDE EFFECTS
How Drug Causes Side Effects

- Theoretically due to increases in serotonin and norepinephrine concentrations at receptors in parts of the brain and body other than those that cause therapeutic actions (e.g. unwanted actions of serotonin in sleep centres causing insomnia, unwanted actions of norepinephrine on acetylcholine release causing constipation and dry mouth, etc.)
- Most side effects are immediate but often go away with time
- Most side effects increase with higher doses, at least transiently

Notable Side Effects

- Headache, nervousness, insomnia, sedation
- Nausea, diarrhoea, decreased appetite
- Sexual dysfunction (abnormal ejaculation/orgasm, impotence). Symptoms of sexual dysfunction may persist after treatment has stopped
- Asthenia, sweating
- SIADH (syndrome of inappropriate antidiuretic hormone secretion)

- Hyponatraemia
- Dose-dependent increase in blood pressure

Common or very common
- CNS/PNS: anxiety, confusion, depersonalisation, dizziness, headache, movement disorders, paraesthesia, sedation, sleep disorders, tinnitus, tremor, vision disorders
- CVS: arrhythmias, hypertension, palpitations
- GIT: altered taste, constipation, decreased appetite, diarrhoea, dry mouth, nausea, vomiting, weight changes
- Other: asthenia, chills, dyspnoea, hot flush, increased muscle tone, menstrual cycle irregularities, mydriasis, sexual dysfunction, skin reactions, sweat changes, urinary disorders, yawning

Uncommon
- Abnormal behaviours, alopecia, altered mood, angioedema, apathy, derealisation, haemorrhage, hallucination, hypotension, photosensitivity, syncope

Rare or very rare
- Blood disorders: agranulocytosis, neutropenia, thrombocytopenia
- Other: angle-closure glaucoma, bone marrow disorders, delirium, hepatitis, hyponatraemia, neuroleptic malignant syndrome, pancreatitis, QT interval prolongation, respiratory disorders, rhabdomyolysis, seizure, serotonin syndrome, severe cutaneous adverse reactions (SCARs), SIADH

Frequency not known
- Suicidal tendencies, vertigo, withdrawal syndrome

 Life-Threatening or Dangerous Side Effects
- Rare seizures
- Neuroleptic malignant syndrome
- Serotonin syndrome
- Pancreatitis
- Rare induction of mania
- Severe cutaneous adverse reactions (SCARs)
- Rare increase in suicidal ideation and behaviours in adolescents and young adults (up to age 25), hence patients

should be warned of this potential adverse event

Weight Gain

- Reported but not expected
- Possible weight loss, especially short term

Sedation

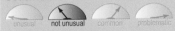

- Occurs in significant minority
- May be activating in some patients

What to Do About Side Effects
- Wait
- Wait
- Wait
- Lower the dose
- In a few weeks, switch or add other drugs

Best Augmenting Agents for Side Effects
- Many side effects are dose-dependent (i.e. they increase as dose increases, or they re-emerge until tolerance redevelops)
- Many side effects are time-dependent (i.e. they start immediately upon dosing and upon each dose increase, but go away with time)
- Often best to try another antidepressant monotherapy prior to resorting to augmentation strategies to treat side effects
- Trazodone or a hypnotic for insomnia
- For sexual dysfunction: can augment with bupropion for women, sildenafil for men; or otherwise switch to another antidepressant
- Urinary retention can be treated with an alpha 1 blocker, e.g. tamsulosin
- Mirtazapine for insomnia, agitation, and gastrointestinal side effects
- Benzodiazepines for jitteriness and anxiety, especially at initiation of treatment and especially for anxious patients
- Increased activation or agitation may represent the induction of a bipolar state, especially a mixed dysphoric bipolar condition sometimes associated with suicidal ideation, and requires the addition of lithium, a mood stabiliser or an atypical antipsychotic, and/or discontinuation of venlafaxine

DOSING AND USE

Usual Dosage Range

- Depression: 75–375 mg/day, once daily (modified-release) or divided into 2 doses (immediate-release)
- GAD and social anxiety disorder: 75–225 mg/day (modified-release)
- Panic disorder: 37.5–225 mg/day (modified-release)
- Menopause: 37.5–75 mg (modified-release)

Dosage Forms

- Tablet (immediate-release) 37.5 mg, 50 mg
- Tablet (modified-release) 37.5 mg, 75 mg, 150 mg, 225 mg, 300 mg
- Capsule (modified-release) 37.5 mg, 75 mg, 150 mg, 225 mg

How to Dose

* Depression:
- Initial dose 75 mg/day (modified-release) or 75 mg divided into 2 doses (immediate-release) for at least 2 weeks if side effects tolerated
- Increase daily dose no faster than 75 mg every 2 weeks until desired efficacy reached; max dose generally 375 mg/day; faster titration may be required in some patients

* GAD or social anxiety disorder:
- Initial dose 75 mg/day (modified-release), may be increased by 75 mg every 2 weeks up to a max of 225 mg/day; for social anxiety 75 mg/day may be adequate

* Panic disorder:
- Initial dose 37.5 mg/day (modified-release) for 1 week, increased to 75mg/day, may be increased every 2 weeks to 225 mg/day; max 225 mg/day

* Menopausal symptoms:
- 37.5 mg/day for 1 week, may be increased to 75 mg/day

Dosing Tips

- If symptoms are very severe, dose increases can be made at more frequent intervals, but not less than 4 days
- At all doses, potent serotonin reuptake blockade
- 75–225 mg/day may be predominantly serotonergic in some patients, and dual serotonin- and noradrenaline-acting in other patients

- 225–375 mg/day is dual serotonin- and noradrenaline-acting in most patients
* Thus, non-responders at lower doses should try higher doses to be assured of the benefits of dual SNRI action
- At very high doses (e.g. >375 mg/day), dopamine reuptake blocked as well in some patients
- Up to 600 mg/day has been given for heroic cases
- Venlafaxine has an active metabolite O-desmethylvenlafaxine (ODV), which is formed as the result of CYP450 2D6
- Thus, CYP450 2D6 inhibition reduces the formation of ODV, but this is of uncertain clinical significance
* If facilities available can consider checking plasma levels of ODV and venlafaxine in non-responders who tolerate high doses, and if plasma levels are low, experts can prudently prescribe doses above 375 mg/ day while monitoring closely
- Do not break or chew venlafaxine modified-release capsules, as this will alter controlled-release properties
* For patients with severe problems discontinuing venlafaxine, dosing may need to be tapered over many months (i.e. reduce dose by 1% every 3 days by crushing tablet and suspending or dissolving in 100 mL of fruit juice, and then disposing of 1 mL while drinking the rest; 3–7 days later, dispose of 2 mL, and so on). This is both a form of very slow biological tapering and a form of behavioural desensitisation (not for modified-release)
- For some patients with severe problems discontinuing venlafaxine, it may be useful to add an SSRI with a long half-life, especially fluoxetine, prior to taper of venlafaxine; while maintaining fluoxetine dosing, first slowly taper venlafaxine and then taper fluoxetine
- Be sure to differentiate between re-emergence of symptoms requiring reinstitution of treatment and withdrawal symptoms

Overdose

- Can be lethal; may cause no symptoms; possible symptoms include sedation, convulsions, rapid heartbeat
- Fatal toxicity index data from UK suggest a higher rate of deaths from overdose with venlafaxine than with SSRIs

- Unknown whether this is related to differences in patients who receive venlafaxine or to potential cardiovascular toxicity of venlafaxine

Long-Term Use
- See doctor regularly to monitor blood pressure, especially at doses >225 mg/day

Habit Forming
- No

How to Stop
- If taking venlafaxine for more than 6–8 weeks, it is not recommended to stop it suddenly due to the risk of withdrawal effects (headache, anxiety, tremor, dizziness, sleep disturbances, nausea, stomach cramps, sweating, tingling, dysaesthesias)
- Taper dose gradually over 4 weeks, or longer if withdrawal symptoms emerge
- Inform all patients of the risk of withdrawal symptoms
- If withdrawal symptoms emerge, raise dose to stop symptoms and then restart withdrawal much more slowly
- *Withdrawal effects can be more common or more severe with venlafaxine than with some other antidepressants

Pharmacokinetics
- Parent drug has 3–7-hour half-life
- Active metabolite has 9–13-hour half-life
- Food does not affect bioavailability

Drug Interactions
- Tramadol increases the risk of seizures in patients taking an antidepressant
- Can cause a fatal "serotonin syndrome" when combined with MAOIs, so do not use with MAOIs or for at least 14 days after MAOIs are stopped
- Do not start an MAOI for at least 5 half-lives (5 to 7 days for most drugs) after discontinuing venlafaxine
- Possible increased risk of bleeding, especially when combined with anticoagulants (e.g. warfarin, NSAIDs)
- Beware when using with concomitant drugs that increase the QT interval
- Concomitant use with cimetidine may reduce clearance of venlafaxine and raise venlafaxine levels
- Could theoretically interfere with the analgesic actions of codeine or possibly with triptans

- Be cautious when prescribing concomitantly with another serotonergic agent (e.g. SNRI, SSRI, St John's wort) as there may be an increased risk of serotonin syndrome

Other Warnings/Precautions
- Use with caution in patients with history of seizures
- Use with caution in patients with history of diabetes
- Use with caution in patients with history of bleeding disorders
- Use with caution in patients with susceptibility to angle-closure glaucoma
- Use with caution in patients with conditions associated with high risk of cardiac arrhythmia and heart disease, particularly those with long QT (monitor blood pressure)
- Use with caution in patients with a personal or family history of mania unless treated with concomitant mood-stabilising agent
- When treating children, carefully weigh the risks and benefits of pharmacological treatment against the risks and benefits of non-treatment with antidepressants and make sure to document this in the patient's chart
- Warn patients and their caregivers about the possibility of activating side effects and advise them to report such symptoms immediately
- Monitor patients for an increase in suicidal ideation, especially children and adolescents

Do Not Use
- If patient has uncontrolled angle-closure glaucoma
- In uncontrolled hypertension
- If patient is taking an MAOI
- If there is a proven allergy to venlafaxine

Renal Impairment
- Lower dose by 50% in patients with eGFR less than 30 mL/minute/1.73 m^2
- Patients on dialysis should not receive subsequent dose until dialysis is completed

Hepatic Impairment
- Lower dose by 50% in patients with mild to moderate hepatic impairment

Venlafaxine (Continued)

- Use with caution and reduce dose by at least 50% in patients with severe hepatic impairment

Cardiac Impairment

- Drug should be used with caution
- Hypertension should be controlled prior to initiation of venlafaxine and should be monitored regularly during treatment
- Venlafaxine has a dose-dependent effect on increasing blood pressure
- Venlafaxine is contraindicated in patients with uncontrolled hypertension
- Venlafaxine can block cardiac ion channels *in vitro* and cause prolongation of the QT interval
- Venlafaxine worsens (i.e. reduces) heart rate variability in depression, perhaps due to norepinephrine reuptake inhibition

Elderly

- Elderly patients tolerate lower doses better, and may benefit from monitoring of blood pressure upon initiation
- Risk of SIADH is higher in the elderly

Children and Adolescents

- Venlafaxine is not licensed for use in children and adolescents
- Venlafaxine not recommended by NICE for use as an antidepressant in children and adolescents
- Nevertheless short-term trials have shown efficacy over placebo in anxiety disorders

Pregnancy

- Controlled studies have not been conducted in pregnant women
- Not generally recommended for use during pregnancy, especially during first trimester
- Nonetheless, continuous treatment during pregnancy may be necessary and has not been proven to be harmful to the foetus
- Must weigh the risk of treatment (first trimester foetal development, third trimester newborn delivery) to the child against the risk of no treatment (recurrence of depression, maternal health, infant bonding) to the mother and child
- For many patients this may mean continuing treatment during pregnancy
- Although there is no data to substantiate, there is a theoretical risk that as with SSRIs when used beyond the 20th week of pregnancy there is increased risk of persistent pulmonary hypertension (PPHN) in newborns
- SSRI/SNRI antidepressant use in the month before delivery may result in a small increased risk of postpartum haemorrhage
- Small studies have reported an association between venlafaxine use during pregnancy and specific malformations including cardiac and respiratory malformations, cleft palate, hypospadias and gastroschisis. These findings have either not been confirmed or have not been replicated by larger studies
- Neonates exposed to SSRIs or SNRIs late in the third trimester have developed complications requiring prolonged hospitalisation, respiratory support, and tube feeding; reported symptoms are consistent with either a direct toxic effect of SSRIs and SNRIs or, possibly, a drug discontinuation syndrome, and include respiratory distress, cyanosis, apnoea, seizures, temperature instability, feeding difficulty, vomiting, hypoglycaemia, hypotonia, hypertonia, hyperreflexia, tremor, jitteriness, irritability, and constant crying

Breastfeeding

- Moderate to significant amounts found in mother's breast milk
- Small amounts may be present in nursing children whose mothers are on venlafaxine
- Case reports of reduced weight gain in the infant
- If child becomes irritable or sedated, breastfeeding or drug may need to be discontinued
- Immediate postpartum period is a high-risk time for depression, especially in women who have had prior depressive episodes, so drug may need to be reinstituted late in the third trimester or shortly after childbirth to prevent a recurrence during the postpartum period
- Must weigh benefits of breastfeeding with risks and benefits of antidepressant treatment versus nontreatment to both the infant and the mother
- For many patients, this may mean continuing treatment during breastfeeding
- Other antidepressants may be preferable, e.g. paroxetine, sertraline, imipramine, or nortriptyline

THE ART OF PSYCHOPHARMACOLOGY

Potential Advantages

- Patients with atypical depression
- Patients with psychomotor retardation
- Patients with co-morbid anxiety
- Some patients with depression may have higher remission rates on SNRIs than on SSRIs
- Depressed patients with somatic symptoms, fatigue, and pain
- Patients who do not respond or remit on treatment with SSRIs

Potential Disadvantages

- Patients sensitive to nausea
- Patients with borderline or uncontrolled hypertension
- Patients with cardiac disease
- Patients with post stroke depression (increased risk of new stroke)

Primary Target Symptoms

- Depressed mood
- Energy, motivation, and interest
- Sleep disturbance
- Anxiety

Pearls

* May be effective in patients who fail to respond to SSRIs, and may be one of the preferred treatments for treatment-resistant depression
* May be used in combination with other antidepressants for treatment-refractory cases
- Modified-release formulation improves tolerability, reduces nausea, and requires only once-daily dosing

- May be effective in a broad array of anxiety disorders
* Has greater potency for serotonin reuptake blockade than for norepinephrine reuptake blockade, but this is of unclear clinical significance as a differentiating feature from other SNRIs
* *In vitro* binding studies tend to underestimate *in vivo* potency for reuptake blockade, as they do not factor in the presence of high concentrations of an active metabolite, higher oral mg dosing, or the lower protein binding which can increase functional drug levels at receptor sites
- Effective dose range is broad (i.e. 75–375 mg in many difficult cases, and up to 600 mg or more in heroic cases)
* Preliminary studies in neuropathic pain and fibromyalgia suggest potential efficacy
- Efficacy as well as side effects (especially nausea and increased blood pressure) are dose-dependent
- Blood pressure increases rare for modified-release formulation in doses up to 225 mg
- More withdrawal reactions reported upon discontinuation than for some other antidepressants
- May be helpful for hot flushes in perimenopausal women
- May be associated with higher depression remission rates than SSRIs
* Contraindicated in uncontrolled hypertension and should only be used with extreme caution in conditions associated with high risk of cardiac arrhythmia
- Venlafaxine's toxicity in overdose is less than that for TCAs, nevertheless fatalities have been reported after mixed overdoses

 Suggested Reading

Buckley NA, McManus PR. Fatal toxicity of serotonergic and other antidepressant drugs: analysis of United Kingdom mortality data. BMJ 2002;325:1332–3.

Cheeta S, Schifano F, Oyefeso A, et al. Antidepressant-related deaths and antidepressant prescriptions in England and Wales, 1998–2000. Br J Psychiatry 2004;184:41–7.

Cipriani A, Furukawa TA, Salanti G, et al. Comparative efficacy and acceptability of 21 antidepressant drugs for the acute treatment of adults with major depressive disorder: a systematic review and network meta-analysis. Lancet 2018;391(10128):1357–66.

Davidson J, Watkins L, Owens M, et al. Effects of paroxetine and venlafaxine XR on heart rate variability in depression. J Clin Psychopharmacol 2005;25:480–4.

Venlafaxine (Continued)

Lassen D, Ennis ZN, Damkier P. First-trimester pregnancy exposure to venlafaxine or duloxetine and risk of major congenital malformations: a systematic review. Basic Clin Pharmacol Toxicol 2016 Jan;118(1):32–6.

Smith D, Dempster C, Glanville J, et al. Efficacy and tolerability of venlafaxine compared with selective serotonin reuptake inhibitors and other antidepressants: a meta-analysis. Br J Psychiatry 2002;180:396–404.

Wellington K, Perry CM. Venlafaxine extended-release: a review of its use in the management of major depression. CNS Drugs 2001;15:643–9.

Vortioxetine

Brands
- Brintellix

Generic?
No, not in UK

Class
- Neuroscience-based nomenclature: pharmacology domain – serotonin; mode of action – multimodal
- Multimodal antidepressant

Commonly Prescribed for
(Bold for BNF indication)
- **Major depression**
- Generalised anxiety disorder (GAD)
- Cognitive symptoms associated with depression
- Depression in the elderly

 How the Drug Works
- Increases release of several different neurotransmitters (serotonin, noradrenaline, dopamine, glutamate, acetylcholine, and histamine) and reduces the release of GABA through three different modes of action
- Mode 1: blocks serotonin reuptake pump (serotonin transporter)
- Mode 2: binds to G protein-linked receptors (full agonist at serotonin 1A receptors, partial agonist at serotonin 1B receptors, antagonist at serotonin 1D and serotonin 7 receptors)
- Mode 3: binds to ion channel-linked receptors (antagonist at serotonin 3 receptors)
- Full agonist actions at presynaptic somatodendritic serotonin 1A autoreceptors may theoretically enhance serotonergic activity and contribute to antidepressant actions
- Full agonist actions at postsynaptic serotonin 1A receptors may theoretically diminish sexual dysfunction caused by serotonin reuptake inhibition
- Antagonist actions at serotonin 3 receptors may theoretically enhance noradrenergic, cholinergic, and glutamatergic activity and contribute to antidepressant and pro-cognitive actions

- Antagonist actions at serotonin 3 receptors may theoretically reduce nausea and vomiting caused by serotonin reuptake inhibition
- Antagonist actions at serotonin 7 receptors may theoretically contribute to antidepressant and pro-cognitive actions as well as reduce insomnia caused by serotonin reuptake inhibition
- Partial agonist actions at serotonin 1B receptors may enhance not only serotonin release, but also acetylcholine and histamine release
- Antagonist actions at serotonin 1D receptors may enhance serotonin release and may also theoretically enhance the release of pro-cognitive neurotransmitters and thereby enhance pro-cognitive actions

How Long Until It Works
- Onset of therapeutic actions is usually not immediate, but often delayed 2–4 weeks
- However, vortioxetine has a specific claim of onset of action at week 2
- If it is not working within 3–4 weeks, it may require a dosage increase or it may not work at all
- May continue to work for many years to prevent relapse of symptoms

If It Works
- The goal of treatment is complete remission of current symptoms as well as prevention of future relapses
- Treatment most often reduces or even eliminates symptoms, but is not a cure since symptoms can recur after medicine is stopped
- Continue treatment until all symptoms are gone (remission), especially in depression and whenever possible in anxiety disorders
- Once symptoms are gone, continue treating for at least 6–9 months for the first episode of depression or >12 months if relapse indicators present
- If >5 episodes and/or 2 episodes in the last few years then need to continue for at least 2 years or indefinitely
- Use in anxiety disorders may also need to be indefinite

If It Doesn't Work
- Important to recognise non-response to treatment early on (3–4 weeks)
- Many patients have only a partial response where some symptoms are improved but

Vortioxetine (Continued)

others persist (especially insomnia, fatigue, and problems concentrating)
- Other patients may be non-responders, sometimes called treatment-resistant or treatment-refractory
- Some patients who have an initial response may relapse even though they continue treatment
- Consider increasing dose, switching to another agent, or adding an appropriate augmenting agent
- Lithium may be added for suicidal patients or those at high risk of relapse
- Consider psychotherapy
- Consider ECT
- Consider evaluation for another diagnosis or for a co-morbid condition (e.g. medical illness, substance abuse, etc.)
- Some patients may experience a switch into mania and so would require antidepressant discontinuation and initiation of a mood stabiliser

Best Augmenting Combos for Partial Response or Treatment Resistance

- Augmentation experience is limited compared to other antidepressants
- Use with caution with antidepressants that are CYP450 2D6 inhibitors (e.g. bupropion, duloxetine, fluoxetine, paroxetine), as these agents will increase vortioxetine levels and may require a dose reduction of vortioxetine
- Mood stabilisers or atypical antipsychotics for bipolar depression
- Atypical antipsychotics for psychotic depression
- Atypical antipsychotics as first-line augmenting agents (quetiapine MR 300 mg/day or aripiprazole at 2.5–10 mg/day) for treatment-resistant depression
- Atypical antipsychotics as second-line augmenting agents (risperidone 0.5–2 mg/day or olanzapine 2.5–10 mg/day) for treatment-resistant depression
- Mirtazapine at 30–45 mg/day as another second-line augmenting agent (a dual serotonin and noradrenaline combination, but observe for switch into mania, increase in suicidal ideation or rare risk of non-fatal serotonin syndrome)
- Although T3 (20–50 mg/day) is another second-line augmenting agent the evidence

suggests that it works best with tricyclic antidepressants
- Other augmenting agents but with less evidence include bupropion (up to 400 mg/day), buspirone (up to 60 mg/day) and lamotrigine (up to 400 mg/day)
- Benzodiazepines if agitation present
- Hypnotics or trazodone for insomnia (but there is a rare risk of non-fatal serotonin syndrome with trazodone)
- Augmenting agents reserved for specialist use include: modafinil for sleepiness, fatigue and lack of concentration; stimulants, oestrogens, testosterone
- Lithium is particularly useful for suicidal patients and those at high risk of relapse including with factors such as severe depression, psychomotor retardation, repeated episodes (>3), significant weight loss, or a family history of major depression (aim for lithium plasma levels 0.6–1.0 mmol/L)
- For elderly patients lithium is a very effective augmenting agent
- For severely ill patients other combinations may be tried especially in specialist centres
- Augmenting agents that may be tried include omega-3, SAM-e, L-methylfolate
- Additional non-pharmacological treatments such as exercise, mindfulness, CBT, and IPT can also be helpful
- If present after treatment response (4–8 weeks) or remission (6–12 weeks), the most common residual symptoms of depression include cognitive impairments, reduced energy and problems with sleep

Tests
- None for healthy individuals

SIDE EFFECTS
How Drug Causes Side Effects
- Theoretically due to increases in serotonin concentrations at serotonin receptors in parts of the brain and body other than those that cause therapeutic actions (e.g. unwanted actions of serotonin at central serotonin 1A receptors causing nausea, unwanted actions of serotonin in the CNS causing sexual dysfunction, etc.)
- Most side effects are immediate but often go away with time, in contrast to most therapeutic effects, which are delayed and are enhanced over time

Notable Side Effects
- Nausea, vomiting, constipation
- Sexual dysfunction

Common or very common
- CNS: abnormal dreams, dizziness
- GIT: constipation, diarrhoea, nausea, vomiting
- Other: skin reactions

Uncommon
- Flushing, night sweats

Frequency not known
- Angioedema, haemorrhage, hyponatraemia, neuroleptic malignant syndrome, serotonin syndrome

 Life-Threatening or Dangerous Side Effects
- Rare seizures
- Rare induction of mania
- Rare increase in suicidal ideation and behaviours in adolescents and young adults (up to age 25), hence patients should be warned of this potential adverse event

Weight Gain

- Reported but not expected

Sedation

- Reported but not expected

What to Do About Side Effects
- Wait
- Wait
- Wait
- In a few weeks, switch to another agent or add other drugs

Best Augmenting Agents for Side Effects
- Many side effects are dose-dependent (i.e. they increase as dose increases, or they re-emerge until tolerance redevelops)
- Many side effects are time-dependent (i.e. they start immediately upon dosing and upon each dose increase, but go away with time)
- Often best to try another antidepressant monotherapy prior to resorting to augmentation strategies to treat side effects
- Trazodone or a hypnotic for insomnia

- For sexual dysfunction: can augment with bupropion for women, sildenafil for men; or otherwise switch to another antidepressant
- Bupropion for emotional flattening, cognitive slowing, apathy, or sexual dysfunction (with caution, as bupropion can raise vortioxetine levels via CYP450 2D6 inhibition)
- Mirtazapine for insomnia, agitation, and gastrointestinal side effects
- Benzodiazepines for jitteriness and anxiety, especially at initiation of treatment and especially for anxious patients
- Increased activation or agitation may represent the induction of a bipolar state, especially a mixed dysphoric bipolar condition sometimes associated with suicidal ideation, and requires the addition of lithium, a mood stabiliser or an atypical antipsychotic, and/or discontinuation of vortioxetine

DOSING AND USE

Usual Dosage Range
- 5–20 mg/day

Dosage Forms
- Tablet 5 mg, 10 mg, 20 mg

How to Dose
- Adult: initial dose 10 mg/day; can decrease to 5 mg/day or increase to 20 mg/day depending on patient response; max recommended dose generally 20 mg/day
- Elderly: initial dose 5 mg/day; increased if necessary up to 20 mg/day

 Dosing Tips
- Can be taken with or without food
- Tablet should not be divided, crushed, or dissolved
- If intolerable anxiety, insomnia, agitation, akathisia, or activation occur either upon dosing initiation or discontinuation, consider the possibility of activating a bipolar disorder and switch to a mood stabiliser or an atypical antipsychotic

Overdose
- No fatalities have been reported; nausea, dizziness, diarrhoea, abdominal discomfort, generalised pruritus, somnolence, flushing

Long-Term Use
- Long-term treatment of major depressive disorder is generally necessary

Habit Forming

- No

How to Stop

- Taper not necessary with recommended doses

Pharmacokinetics

- Metabolised by CYP450 2D6, 3A4/5, 2C19, 2C9, 2A6, 2C8, and 2B6
- Mean terminal half-life about 66 hours
- Steady-state plasma concentrations are achieved in about 2 weeks

Drug Interactions

- Tramadol increases the risk of seizures in patients taking an antidepressant
- Can cause a fatal "serotonin syndrome" when combined with MAOIs, so do not use with MAOIs or for at least 14–21 days after MAOIs are stopped
- Do not start an MAOI for at least 5 half-lives (about 14 days for vortioxetine with a half-life of 66 hours) after discontinuing vortioxetine
- Strong CYP450 2D6 inhibitors can increase plasma levels of vortioxetine, possibly requiring its dose to be decreased
- Broad CYP450 2D6 inducers can decrease plasma levels of vortioxetine, possibly requiring its dose to be increased
- Could theoretically cause weakness, hyperreflexia, and incoordination when combined with sumatriptan or possibly other triptans, requiring careful monitoring of patient
- Possible increased risk of bleeding, especially when combined with anticoagulants (e.g. warfarin, NSAIDs)

⚠ Other Warnings/Precautions

- Use with caution in patients with history of seizures; discontinue use if patient develops seizures or if there is an increase in seizure frequency
- Use with caution in patients with a history of bleeding disorders
- Use with caution in patients with susceptibility to angle-closure glaucoma
- Use with caution in patients with cirrhosis of the liver (risk of hyponatraemia)
- Possible risk of hyponatraemia related to SIADH (syndrome of inappropriate antidiuretic hormone secretion) with serotonergic drugs
- Use with caution in patients with bipolar disorder unless treated with concomitant mood-stabilising agent
- Not approved in children, so when treating children off-label, carefully weigh the risks and benefits of pharmacological treatment against the risks and benefits of non-treatment with antidepressants and make sure to document this in the patient's chart
- Warn patients and their caregivers about the possibility of activating side effects and advise them to report such symptoms immediately
- Monitor patients for activation of suicidal ideation, especially children and adolescents

Do Not Use

- If patient is taking an MAOI
- If there is a proven allergy to vortioxetine

SPECIAL POPULATIONS

Renal Impairment

- Caution in severe impairment

Hepatic Impairment

- No dose adjustment necessary for mild to moderate impairment
- Caution in severe impairment

Cardiac Impairment

- Not systematically evaluated in patients with cardiac impairment
- Treating depression with SSRIs in patients with acute angina or following myocardial infarction may reduce cardiac events and improve survival as well as mood; not known for vortioxetine

Elderly

- Use more caution when treating elderly patients with doses over 10 mg/day
- Risk of SIADH with SSRIs is higher in the elderly
- Reduction in risk of suicidality with antidepressants compared to placebo in adults age 65 and older

Children and Adolescents

- Not licensed for use in children and adolescents
- Safety and efficacy have not been established

Pregnancy

- Controlled studies have not been conducted in pregnant women
- Not generally recommended for use during pregnancy, especially during first trimester
- Nonetheless, continuous treatment during pregnancy may be necessary and has not been proven to be harmful to the foetus
- At delivery there may be more bleeding in the mother and transient irritability or sedation in the newborn
- Must weigh the risk of treatment (first trimester foetal development, third trimester newborn delivery) to the child against the risk of no treatment (recurrence of depression, maternal health, infant bonding) to the mother and child
- For many patients, this may mean continuing treatment during pregnancy
- Exposure to serotonin reuptake inhibitors early in pregnancy may be associated with increased risk of septal heart defects (absolute risk is small)
- Use of serotonin reuptake inhibitors beyond the 20th week of pregnancy may be associated with increased risk of pulmonary hypertension (PPHN) in newborns, although this is not proven
- Exposure to serotonin reuptake inhibitors late in pregnancy may be associated with increased risk of gestational hypertension and pre-eclampsia
- Neonates exposed to SSRIs or SNRIs late in the third trimester have developed complications requiring prolonged hospitalisation, respiratory support, and tube feeding; reported symptoms are consistent with either a direct toxic effect of SSRIs and SNRIs or, possibly, a drug discontinuation syndrome, and include respiratory distress, cyanosis, apnoea, seizures, temperature instability, feeding difficulty, vomiting, hypoglycaemia, hypotonia, hypertonia, hyperreflexia, tremor, jitteriness, irritability, and constant crying
- Small increased risk of postpartum haemorrhage when used in the month before delivery

Breastfeeding

- Unknown if vortioxetine is secreted in human breast milk, but all psychotropics assumed to be secreted in breast milk

- If child becomes irritable or sedated, breastfeeding or drug may need to be discontinued
- Immediate postpartum period is a high-risk time for depression, especially in women who have had prior depressive episodes, so drug may need to be reinstituted late in the third trimester or shortly after childbirth to prevent a recurrence during the postpartum period
- Must weigh benefits of breastfeeding with risks and benefits of antidepressant treatment versus nontreatment to both the infant and the mother
- For many patients, this may mean continuing treatment during breastfeeding
- Other antidepressants may be preferable, e.g. paroxetine, sertraline, imipramine, or nortriptyline

THE ART OF PSYCHOPHARMACOLOGY

Potential Advantages

- Lower incidence of sexual dysfunction than SSRIs
- Patients with cognitive symptoms of depression
- Patients with residual cognitive symptoms after treatment with another antidepressant
- Elderly patients
- Patients who have not responded to other antidepressants
- Patients who do not want weight gain

Potential Disadvantages

- Cost

Primary Target Symptoms

- Depressed mood
- Cognitive symptoms
- Anxiety

Pearls

- Recommended for treating major depressive episodes in adults who within the current episode have not responded adequately to at least 2 antidepressants
- Consider for those who have experienced sexual dysfunction with SSRIs
- Multiple studies show pro-cognitive effects greater than a comparator antidepressant in patients with major depressive episodes

Vortioxetine (Continued)

- Patients who do not respond to antidepressants with other mechanisms of action may respond to vortioxetine
- Effective specifically in elderly patients with depression, with a positive trial showing improvement of cognition as well as mood
- Has a unique claim of preventing recurrences in major depression
- No weight gain in clinical trials
- Long half-life means vortioxetine can generally be abruptly discontinued, although some caution may be necessary

when stopping higher doses (i.e. 15 or 20 mg/day)
- Despite serotonin 3 antagonist actions, nausea is common, presumably due to full agonist actions at serotonin 1A receptors
- Dose response for efficacy in depression: higher doses are more effective
- Vortioxetine has a unique multimodal mechanism of action
- Non-response to vortioxetine in elderly may require consideration of mild cognitive impairment or Alzheimer's disease

 Suggested Reading

Bang-Anderson B, Ruhland T, Jorgensen M, et al. Discovery of 1-[2-(2,4-dimethylphenylsulfanyl) phenyl]piperazine (Lu AA21004): a novel multimodal compound for the treatment of major depressive disorder. J Med Chem 2011;54(9):3206–21.

Cipriani A, Furukawa TA, Salanti G, et al. Comparative efficacy and acceptability of 21 antidepressant drugs for the acute treatment of adults with major depressive disorder: a systematic review and network meta-analysis. Lancet 2018;391(10128):1357–66.

Mork A, Montezinho LP, Miller S, et al. Vortioxetine (LU AA21004), a novel multimodal antidepressant, enhanced memory in rats. Pharmacol Biochem Behav 2013;105:41–50.

Stahl SM, Lee-Zimmerman C, Cartwright S, et al. Serotonergic drugs for depression and beyond. Curr Drug Targets 2013;14(5):578–85.

Westrich I, Pehrson A, Zhong H, et al. In vitro and in vivo effects of the multimodal antidepressant vortioxetine (Lu AA21004) at human and rat targets. Int J Psychiatry Clin Pract 2012;5(Suppl 1):S47.

Zolpidem tartrate

Brands
• Non-proprietary

Generic?
Yes

Class
• Neuroscience-based nomenclature: pharmacology domain – GABA; mode of action – positive allosteric modulator (PAM)
• Non-benzodiazepine hypnotic; alpha 1 isoform selective agonist of GABA-A/ benzodiazepine receptors

Commonly Prescribed for
(bold for BNF indication)
• **Insomnia (short-term use)**
• Catatonia

How the Drug Works
• Binds selectively to a subtype of the benzodiazepine receptor, the alpha 1 isoform
• May enhance GABA inhibitory actions that provide sedative hypnotic effects more selectively than other actions of GABA
• Boosts chloride conductance through GABA-regulated channels
• Inhibitory actions in sleep centres may provide sedative hypnotic effects

How Long Until It Works
• Generally takes effect between 30 minutes and less than an hour

If It Works
• Improves sleep onset, sleep onset latency, and staying asleep and quality of sleep
• Short-term treatment for sleep initiation or sleep maintenance
• Effects on total wake-time and number of night time awakenings may be decreased over time

If It Doesn't Work
• If insomnia does not improve after 7–10 days, it may be a manifestation of a primary psychiatric or physical illness such as obstructive sleep apnoea or restless leg syndrome which requires independent evaluation
• Increase the dose
• Improve sleep hygiene

• Switch to another agent

 Best Augmenting Combos for Partial Response or Treatment Resistance
• RCTs support the effectiveness of Z-hypnotics over a period of at least 6 months
• Better to switch to another agent
• Trazodone
• Agents with antihistamine actions (e.g. promethazine, TCAs)
• Use melatonin and melatonin-related drugs (adults over the age of 55)

Tests
• None for healthy individuals

How Drug Causes Side Effects
• Actions at benzodiazepine receptors that carry over to the next day can cause daytime sedation, amnesia, and ataxia
• Studies on sustained-release preparations of zolpidem and other alpha 1 selective non-benzodiazepine hypnotics suggest lack of notable tolerance or dependence developing over time

Notable Side Effects
* Sedation, drowsiness
* Dizziness, ataxia
* Dose-dependent amnesia
* Hyperexcitability, nervousness
• Rare hallucinations
• Diarrhoea, nausea
• Headache
• Short-term: headache, drowsiness, dizziness, diarrhoea
• Long-term: drowsiness, dizziness, sinusitis, flu-like symptoms, diarrhoea, constipation, rash, allergy, abnormal dreams, loss of memory

Common or very common
• CNS: anterograde amnesia, anxiety, dizziness, hallucinations (visual), headache, sleep disorders
• GIT: abdominal pain, diarrhoea, nausea, vomiting
• Other: back pain, fall, fatigue, increased risk of infection

Zolpidem tartrate (Continued)

Uncommon
- Confusion, diplopia, irritability

Frequency not known
- CNS/PNS: abnormal behaviour, abnormal gait, decreased level of consciousness, delusions, depression, drug dependence, fall, impaired concentration, psychosis, speech disorder
- Other: angioedema, hepatic disorders, hyperhidrosis, libido disorder, muscle weakness, respiratory depression, skin reactions, withdrawal syndrome

 Life-Threatening or Dangerous Side Effects
- Respiratory depression, especially when taken with other CNS depressants in overdose
- Rare angioedema
- Drug tolerance and withdrawal with sudden discontinuation
- Cross-tolerance with alcohol and with benzodiazepines

Weight Gain

unusual · not unusual · common · problematic

- Reported but not expected

Sedation

unusual · not unusual · common · problematic

- Many experience and/or can be significant in amount

What to Do About Side Effects
- Wait
- To avoid problems with memory, only take zolpidem if planning to have a full night's sleep
- Lower the dose
- Switch to a shorter-acting sedative hypnotic
- Administer flumazenil if side effects are severe or life-threatening

Best Augmenting Agents for Side Effects
- Many side effects cannot be improved with an augmenting agent

DOSING AND USE

Usual Dosage Range
- 5–10 mg at bedtime (for up to 4 weeks)

Dosage Forms
- Tablet 5 mg, 10 mg

How to Dose
∗Insomnia (short-term use):
- Adult: 10 mg/day at bedtime for up to 4 weeks
- Elderly or debilitated patients: 5 mg/day at bedtime for up to 4 weeks

 Dosing Tips
- Adult: 10 mg/day for up to 4 weeks, dose to be taken at bedtime
- For debilitated patients or elderly patients: 5 mg/day for up to 4 weeks, dose to be taken at bedtime
- Zolpidem is not absorbed as quickly if taken with food, which could reduce onset of action
- Patients with lower body weight may require a reduced dose as per elderly
- Zolpidem should generally not be prescribed in quantities greater than a 1-month supply
- Risk of dependence may increase with dose and duration of treatment
- However, treatment with alpha 1 selective non-benzodiazepine hypnotics may cause less tolerance or dependence than benzodiazepine hypnotics

Overdose
- Fatalities reported with zolpidem monotherapy and combined with other substances; sedation, ataxia, confusion, hypotension, respiratory depression, coma
- Zolpidem overdose can be treated with the GABA-A receptor antagonist flumazenil, which displaces zolpidem from its binding site on the GABA-A receptor to rapidly reverse the effects of the zolpidem
- Blood or plasma zolpidem concentrations are usually in a range of 30–300 mcg/L in persons receiving the drug therapeutically, and 1000–7000 mcg/L in victims of acute overdose

Long-Term Use
- Original studies with zolpidem did not assess long-term use

- Increased wakefulness during the latter part of the night (wearing off) or an increase in daytime anxiety (rebound) may occur

Habit Forming

- Zolpidem is a Class C/Schedule 4 drug
- Some patients may develop dependence and/or tolerance; risk may be greater with higher doses
- History of drug addiction may increase risk of dependence

How to Stop

- Although rebound insomnia could occur, this effect has not generally been seen with therapeutic doses of zolpidem
- If taken for more than a few weeks, taper to reduce chances of withdrawal effects

Pharmacokinetics

- Onset < 30 minutes
- Peak 2–3 hours
- Mean elimination half-life of about 2.4 hours
- Metabolism: liver
- Excretion: kidneys 56%, faecal 34%
- Duration of action up to 6 hours

Drug Interactions

- Increased depressive side effects when taken with other CNS depressants (e.g. alcohol and opioids)
- Sertraline may increase plasma levels of zolpidem
- Rifampicin may decrease plasma levels of zolpidem
- Ketoconazole may increase plasma levels of zolpidem
- Use with imipramine or chlorpromazine may be associated with decreased alertness
- Increase in visual anomalous experiences when taken in combination with SSRIs

Other Warnings/Precautions

- Insomnia may be a symptom of a primary disorder rather than a primary disorder itself
- Some patients may exhibit abnormal thinking or behavioural changes similar to those caused by other CNS depressants (e.g. either depressant or disinhibiting actions)
- Some depressed patients may experience a worsening of suicidal ideation

- Rare angioedema has occurred with sedative hypnotic use and could potentially cause fatal airway obstruction if it involves the throat, glottis or larynx; thus if angioedema occurs, treatment should be discontinued
- Sleep walking and sleep driving and other complex behaviours such as eating and preparing food and making phone calls have been reported in patients taking sedative hypnotics
- Avoid prolonged use and abrupt cessation
- Use with caution in elderly patients
- Use only with caution in patients with a history of alcohol/drug abuse
- Use with caution in patients with muscle weakness
- Zolpidem should only be administered at bedtime
- Temporary memory loss may occur at doses above 10 mg/night
- Visual hallucinations are frequent if staying awake after zolpidem intake

Do Not Use

- If patient has significant neuromuscular respiratory weakness
- If patient is exhibiting acute or severe respiratory depression
- If patient has obstructive sleep apnoea
- If patient has myasthenia gravis
- If patient suffers from a psychotic illness
- If there is a proven allergy to zolpidem

SPECIAL POPULATIONS

Renal Impairment

- No dose adjustment necessary
- Patients should be monitored

Hepatic Impairment

- Recommended dose 5 mg in mild-moderate impairment
- Can precipitate coma due to impaired clearance
- Patients should be monitored
- Avoid in severe impairment

Cardiac Impairment

- No available data

Elderly

- Recommended dose: 5 mg at bedtime for up to 4 weeks

Children and Adolescents

- Safety and efficacy have not been established
- Long-term effects of zolpidem in children/adolescents are unknown
- Hallucinations in children 6–17 years have been reported
- Should generally receive lower doses and be more closely monitored

Pregnancy

- Human data is limited, one case report where zolpidem was found in cord blood at delivery
- Reports of increased risks of small for gestational age, low birth weight and preterm delivery
- Controlled studies do not show increased risk of overall congenital malformations
- Possible association with specific gastrointestinal malformations
- Several animal studies show adverse effects
- Infants whose mothers took sedative hypnotics during pregnancy may experience some withdrawal symptoms
- Neonatal flaccidity has been reported in infants whose mothers took sedative hypnotics during pregnancy

Breastfeeding

- Small amounts found in mother's breast milk
- If drug is continued while breastfeeding, infant should be monitored for possible sedation
- Mothers taking hypnotics should be warned about the risks of co-sleeping

THE ART OF PSYCHOPHARMACOLOGY

Potential Advantages

- Patients who may require longer-term treatment

Potential Disadvantages

- More expensive than some other sedative hypnotics

Primary Target Symptoms

- Time to sleep onset
- Total sleep time
- Night time awakenings

Pearls

- NICE Guidelines recommend medication for insomnia only as a second-line treatment after non-pharmacological treatment options have been tried (e.g. cognitive behavioural therapy for insomnia)
- Zolpidem is a popularly prescribed hypnotic in Europe and USA
- The use of secure prescription pads has reduced the exposure of the French population to zolpidem
- Zolpidem has been shown to increase the total time asleep and to reduce the amount of night time awakenings
- Improves sleep onset, sleep onset latency, staying asleep and quality of sleep
- May be preferred over benzodiazepines because of its rapid onset of action, short duration of effect and safety profile
- In some patients, zolpidem blood levels may be high enough the morning after use to impair activities that require alertness including driving – leave at least 8 hours between taking zolpidem and performing skilled tasks (e.g. driving or operating machinery)
- May not be ideal for patients who desire immediate hypnotic onset and eat just prior to bedtime
- Not a benzodiazepine itself, but binds to benzodiazepine receptors
- May have fewer hangover effects than some other sedative hypnotics
- May cause less dependence than some other sedative hypnotics, especially in those without a history of substance abuse
- Women may require lower doses of zolpidem
- Zolpidem has been used to treat catatonia
- Visual hallucinations are frequent if staying awake after zolpidem intake

Suggested Reading

aley C, McNiel DE, Binder RL. "I did what?" Zolpidem and the courts. J Am Acad Psychiatry aw 2011;39(4):535–42.

ock SB, Wong SH, Nuwayhid N, et al. Acute zolpidem overdose – report of two cases. J Anal oxicol 1999;23(6):559–62.

reenblatt DJ, Roth T. Zolpidem for insomnia. Expert Opin Pharmacother 2012;13(6):879–93.

unja N. The clinical and forensic toxicology of Z-drugs. J Med Toxicol 2013;9(2):155–62.

ush CR. Behavioral pharmacology of zolpidem relative to benzodiazepines: a review. harmacol Biochem Behav 1998;61:253–69.

oyka M, Bottlender R, Moller HJ. Epidemiological evidence for a low abuse potential of olpidem. Pharmacopsychiatry 2000;33:138–41.

oner LC, Tsambiras BM, Catalano G, et al. Central nervous system side effects associated with olpidem treatment. Clin Neuropharmacol 2000;23:54–8.

Zopiclone

Brands
- Zimovane

Generic?
Yes

Class
- Neuroscience-based nomenclature: pharmacology domain – GABA; mode of action – positive allosteric modulator (PAM)
- Non-benzodiazepine hypnotic; alpha 1 isoform selective agonist of GABA-A/ benzodiazepine receptors

Commonly Prescribed for
(bold for BNF indication)
- **Insomnia (short-term use)**
- **Insomnia (short-term use) in patients with chronic pulmonary insufficiency**

How the Drug Works
- Binds selectively to a subtype of the benzodiazepine receptor, the alpha 1 isoform
- May enhance GABA inhibitory actions that provide sedative hypnotic effects more selectively than other actions of GABA
- Boosts chloride conductance through GABA regulated channels
- Inhibitory actions in sleep centres may provide sedative hypnotic effects

How Long Until It Works
- Generally takes effect in less than an hour

If It Works
- Improves quality of sleep
- Effects on total wake-time and number of night time awakenings may be decreased over time
- Short-term treatment for sleep initiation or sleep maintenance

If It Doesn't Work
- If insomnia does not improve after 7–10 days, it may be a manifestation of a primary psychiatric or physical illness such as obstructive sleep apnoea or restless leg syndrome which requires independent evaluation
- Increase the dose
- Improve sleep hygiene
- Switch to another agent

Best Augmenting Combos for Partial Response or Treatment Resistance
- RCTs support the effectiveness of Z-hypnotics over a period of at least 6 months
- Better to switch to another agent
- Trazodone
- Agents with antihistamine actions (e.g. promethazine, TCAs)
- Use melatonin and melatonin-related drugs (adults over the age of 55)

Tests
- None for healthy individuals

SIDE EFFECTS

How Drug Causes Side Effects
- Actions at benzodiazepine receptors that carry over to the next day can cause daytime sedation, amnesia, and ataxia
- Long-term adaptations of zopiclone, a mixture of an active S enantiomer and an inactive R enantiomer, have not been well studied, but chronic studies of the active isomer eszopiclone and other alpha 1 selective non-benzodiazepine hypnotics suggest lack of notable tolerance or dependence developing over time

Notable Side Effects
* Sedation
* Dizziness, ataxia
* Dose-dependent amnesia
* Hyperexcitability, nervousness
- Dry mouth, loss of appetite, constipation, bitter taste
- Impaired vision

Common or very common
- Bitter/metallic taste, dry mouth

Uncommon
- Anxiety, dizziness, fatigue, headache, nausea, sleep disorders including nightmares, vomiting

Rare or very rare
- CNS: abnormal behaviour, hallucination, irritability, memory impairment
- Other: dyspnoea, fall, libido disorder, skin reactions

Frequency not known

- CNS/PNS: cognitive disorder, delusions, depressed mood, diplopia, drug dependence and tolerance, impaired concentration, movement disorders, paraesthesia, speech disorder
- Other: dyspepsia, muscle weakness, respiratory depression, withdrawal syndrome

 Life-Threatening or Dangerous Side Effects

- Respiratory depression, especially when taken with other CNS depressants in overdose
- Rare angioedema

Weight Gain

- Reported but not expected

Sedation

- Many experience and/or can be significant in amount

What to Do About Side Effects

- Wait
- To avoid problems with memory, only take zopiclone if planning to have a full night's sleep
- Lower the dose
- Switch to a shorter-acting sedative hypnotic
- Administer flumazenil if side effects are severe or life-threatening

Best Augmenting Agents for Side Effects

- Many side effects cannot be improved with an augmenting agent

DOSING AND USE

Usual Dosage Range

- 3.75–7.5 mg at bed time

Dosage Forms

- Tablet 3.75 mg, 7.5 mg

How to Dose

*Insomnia (short-term use):
- Adult: 7.5 mg/day at bedtime for up to 4 weeks
- Elderly: initial dose 3.75 mg/day at bedtime for up to 4 weeks, may be increased to 7.5 mg/day at bedtime

*Insomnia (short-term use) in patients with chronic pulmonary insufficiency:
- Adult: initial dose 3.75 mg/day at bedtime for up to 4 weeks, may be increased to 7.5 mg/day at bedtime

 Dosing Tips

- Adult: 7.5 mg/day at bedtime (up to 4 weeks)
- Elderly or in patients with chronic pulmonary insufficiency: 3.75 mg/day at bedtime, increased to 7.5 mg/day if necessary (up to 4 weeks)
- Zopiclone should generally not be prescribed in quantities greater than a 1-month supply
- Risk of dependence may increase with dose and duration of treatment
- However, treatment with alpha 1 selective non-benzodiazepine hypnotics may cause less tolerance or dependence than benzodiazepine hypnotics

Overdose

- Fatalities reported with zopiclone monotherapy and combined with other substances; clumsiness, mood changes, sedation, weakness, breathing trouble, unconsciousness

Long-Term Use

- Not generally intended for use past 4 weeks

Habit Forming

- Zopiclone is a Class C/Schedule 4 drug
- Some patients may develop dependence and/or tolerance; risk may be greater with higher doses
- History of drug addiction may increase risk of dependence

How to Stop

- Rebound insomnia may occur the first night after stopping
- If taken for more than a few weeks, taper to reduce chances of withdrawal effects

Pharmacokinetics
- Metabolised by CYP450 3A4 and 2E1
- Terminal elimination half-life is about 5 hours (3.5–6.5 hours)
- Excretion via kidneys 80%

 Drug Interactions
- Increased depressive side effects when taken with other CNS depressants
- Theoretically, inhibitors of CYP450 3A4 such as nefazodone and fluvoxamine could increase plasma levels of zopiclone

 Other Warnings/Precautions
- Insomnia may be a symptom of a primary disorder rather than a primary disorder itself
- Some patients may exhibit abnormal thinking or behavioural changes similar to those caused by other CNS depressants (e.g. either depressant or disinhibiting actions)
- Some depressed patients may experience a worsening of suicidal ideation
- Use with caution in patients with psychiatric illness
- Use with caution in patients with chronic pulmonary insufficiency; should only be administered at bedtime
- Rare angioedema has occurred with sedative hypnotic use and could potentially cause fatal airway obstruction if it involves the throat, glottis or larynx; thus if angioedema occurs, treatment should be discontinued
- Sleep walking and sleep driving and other complex behaviours such as eating and preparing food and making phone calls have been reported in patients taking sedative hypnotics
- Avoid prolonged use and abrupt cessation
- Use with caution in elderly patients
- Use only with caution in patients with a history of alcohol/drug abuse
- Use with caution in patients with muscle weakness
- Zopiclone should only be administered at bedtime

Do Not Use
- If patient has significant neuromuscular respiratory weakness
- If patient is in respiratory failure
- If patient has severe obstructive sleep apnoea
- If patient has myasthenia gravis
- If there is a proven allergy to zopiclone

Renal Impairment
- Increased cerebral sensitivity
- Increased plasma levels
- May need to lower dose

Hepatic Impairment
- Increased plasma levels
- Reduce dose to 3.75 mg in mild to moderate impairment
- Not recommended in patients with severe impairment

Cardiac Impairment
- Dosage adjustment may not be necessary

Elderly
- Initial dose 3.75 mg at bedtime for up to 4 weeks, increased if necessary to 7.5 mg/day

 Children and Adolescents
- Safety and efficacy have not been established
- Long-term effects of zopiclone in children/adolescents are unknown
- Should generally receive lower doses and be more closely monitored

 Pregnancy
- Human data is limited
- Reports of increased risks of small for gestational age and preterm delivery
- Controlled studies do not show increased risk of overall congenital malformations
- Possible association with specific gastrointestinal malformations
- Some animal studies show adverse effects
- Infants whose mothers took sedative hypnotics during pregnancy may experience some withdrawal symptoms

Zopiclone (Continued)

- Neonatal flaccidity has been reported in infants whose mothers took sedative hypnotics during pregnancy

Breastfeeding

- Small amounts found in mother's breast milk
- If drug is continued while breastfeeding, infant should be monitored for possible sedation
- Mothers taking hypnotics should be warned about the risks of co-sleeping

THE ART OF PSYCHOPHARMACOLOGY

Potential Advantages

- Patients who require long-term treatment

Potential Disadvantages

- More expensive than some other sedative hypnotics

Primary Target Symptoms

- Time to sleep onset
- Total sleep time
- Night time awakenings

Pearls

- NICE Guidelines recommend medication for insomnia only as a second-line treatment after non-pharmacological treatment options have been tried (e.g. cognitive behavioural therapy for insomnia)
- May be preferred over benzodiazepines because of its rapid onset of action, short duration of effect and safety profile
- Zopiclone does not appear to be a highly dependence-causing drug, at least not in patients without a history of drug abuse
- Rebound insomnia does not appear to be common
- Not a benzodiazepine itself, but binds to benzodiazepine receptors
- May have fewer hangover effects than some other sedative hypnotics
- Women may require lower doses

 Suggested Reading

Fernandez C, Martin C, Gimenez F, et al. Clinical pharmacokinetics of zopiclone. Clin Pharmacokinet 1995;29:431–41.

Hajak G. A comparative assessment of the risks and benefits of zopiclone: a review of 15 years' clinical experience. Drug Saf 1999;21:457–69.

Noble S, Langtry HD, Lamb HM. Zopiclone. An update of its pharmacology, clinical efficacy and tolerability in the treatment of insomnia. Drugs 1998;55:277–302.

Zuclopenthixol

Brands

- Clopixol (oral tablets)
- Ciatyl-Z (oral drops)
- Clopixol Acuphase (acetate, solution for injection)
- Clopixol (decanoate, solution for injection)
- Clopixol Conc (decanoate, solution for injection)

Generic?

Yes

Class

- Neuroscience-based nomenclature: pharmacology domain – dopamine; mode of action – antagonist
- Conventional antipsychotic (neuroleptic, thioxanthene, dopamine 2 antagonist); dopamine receptor antagonist

Commonly Prescribed for

(bold for BNF indication)

- **Schizophrenia and other psychoses (oral, acetate injection)**
- **Maintenance treatment of schizophrenia (oral, decanoate injection)**
- **Short-term management of acute psychosis (acetate injection)**
- **Short-term management of mania (acetate injection)**
- **Short-term management of exacerbation of chronic psychosis (acetate injection)**
- Bipolar disorder
- Aggression

How the Drug Works

- Blocks dopamine 2 receptors, reducing positive symptoms of psychosis

How Long Until It Works

- For injection, psychotic symptoms can improve within a few days, but it may take 1–2 weeks for notable improvement
- For oral formulation, psychotic symptoms can improve within 1 week, but may take several weeks for full effect on behaviour

If It Works

- Most often reduces positive symptoms in schizophrenia but does not eliminate them
- Most patients with schizophrenia do not have a total remission of symptoms but rather a reduction of symptoms by about a third
- Continue treatment in schizophrenia until reaching a plateau of improvement
- After reaching a satisfactory plateau, continue treatment for at least a year after first episode of psychosis in schizophrenia
- For second and subsequent episodes of psychosis in schizophrenia, treatment may need to be indefinite
- Reduces symptoms of acute psychotic mania but not proven as a mood stabiliser or as an effective maintenance treatment in bipolar disorder
- After reducing acute psychotic symptoms in mania, switch to a mood stabiliser and/ or an atypical antipsychotic for mood stabilisation and maintenance

If It Doesn't Work

- Consider trying one of the first-line atypical antipsychotics (risperidone, olanzapine, quetiapine, aripiprazole, paliperidone, amisulpride)
- Consider trying another conventional antipsychotic
- If 2 or more antipsychotic monotherapies do not work, consider clozapine

 Best Augmenting Combos for Partial Response or Treatment Resistance

- Augmentation of conventional antipsychotics has not been systematically studied
- Addition of a mood-stabilising anticonvulsant such as valproate, carbamazepine, or lamotrigine may be helpful in both schizophrenia and bipolar mania
- Augmentation with lithium in bipolar mania may be helpful
- Addition of a benzodiazepine, especially short-term for agitation

Tests

Baseline

- *Measure weight, BMI, and waist circumference
- Get baseline personal and family history of diabetes, obesity, dyslipidaemia, hypertension, and cardiovascular disease
- Check for personal history of drug-induced leucopenia/neutropenia

Zuclopenthixol (Continued)

*Check pulse and blood pressure, fasting plasma glucose or glycosylated haemoglobin (HbA1c), fasting lipid profile, and prolactin levels
- Full blood count (FBC)
- Assessment of nutritional status, diet, and level of physical activity
- Determine if the patient:
  - is overweight (BMI 25.0–29.9)
  - is obese (BMI ≥30)
  - has pre-diabetes – fasting plasma glucose: 5.5 mmol/L to 6.9 mmol/L or HbA1c: 42 to 47 mmol/mol (6.0 to 6.4%)
  - has diabetes – fasting plasma glucose: >7.0 mmol/L or HbA1c: ≥48 mmol/L (≥6.5%)
  - has hypertension (BP >140/90 mm Hg)
  - has dyslipidaemia (increased total cholesterol, LDL cholesterol, and triglycerides; decreased HDL cholesterol)
- Treat or refer such patients for treatment, including nutrition and weight management, physical activity counselling, smoking cessation, and medical management
- Baseline ECG for: inpatients; those with a personal history or risk factor for cardiac disease

Monitoring
- Monitor weight and BMI during treatment
- Consider monitoring fasting triglycerides monthly for several months in patients at high risk for metabolic complications and when initiating or switching antipsychotics
- While giving a drug to a patient who has gained >5% of initial weight, consider evaluating for the presence of pre-diabetes, diabetes, or dyslipidaemia, or consider switching to a different antipsychotic
- Patients with low white blood cell count (WBC) or history of drug-induced leucopenia/neutropenia should have full blood count (FBC) monitored frequently during the first few months and zuclopenthixol should be discontinued at the first sign of decline of WBC in the absence of other causative factors
- Monitor prolactin levels and for signs and symptoms of hyperprolactinaemia

How Drug Causes Side Effects
- By blocking dopamine 2 receptors in the striatum, it can cause motor side effects
- By blocking dopamine 2 receptors in the pituitary, it can cause elevations in prolactin
- By blocking dopamine 2 receptors excessively in the mesocortical and mesolimbic dopamine pathways, especially at high doses, it can cause worsening of negative and cognitive symptoms (neuroleptic-induced deficit syndrome)
- Antihistaminergic actions may cause sedation, blurred vision, constipation, dry mouth
- Antihistaminic actions may cause sedation, weight gain
- By blocking alpha 1 adrenergic receptors, it can cause dizziness, sedation, and hypotension
- Mechanism of weight gain and any possible increased incidence of diabetes or dyslipidaemia with conventional antipsychotics is unknown

Notable Side Effects
- Extrapyramidal symptoms
- Tardive dyskinesia (risk increases with duration of treatment and with dose)
- Priapism
- Galactorrhoea, amenorrhoea
- Rare lens opacity
- Sedation, dizziness
- Dry mouth, constipation, vision problems
- Hypotension
- Weight gain

Frequency not known
- CNS/PNS: abnormal gait, anxiety, depression, headaches, hyperacusis, impaired concentration, increased reflexes, memory loss, neuromuscular dysfunction, paraesthesia, sleep disorders, speech disorder, tinnitus, vertigo, vision disorders
- CVS: palpitations, syncope
- GIT: abnormal appetite, decreased weight, diarrhoea, flatulence, gastrointestinal discomfort, hepatic disorders, hypersalivation, nausea, thirst
- Other: asthenia, dyspnoea, eye disorders, fever, impaired glucose tolerance, hot flush, hyperhidrosis, hyperlipidaemia, hypothermia, malaise, muscle complaints, nasal congestion, pain, seborrhoea, sexual dysfunction, skin reactions,

thrombocytopenia, urinary disorders, vulvovaginal dryness, withdrawal syndrome

 Life-Threatening or Dangerous Side Effects

- Rare neuroleptic malignant syndrome
- Rare neutropenia
- Rare respiratory depression
- Rare agranulocytosis
- Rare seizures
- Increased risk of death and cerebrovascular events in elderly patients with dementia-related psychosis

Weight Gain

unusual   not unusual   common   problematic

- Many do experience weight gain, and this can be significant in amount
- Some people may lose weight

Sedation

unusual   not unusual   common   problematic

- Many do experience sedation, and this can be significant in amount
- Acetate formulation may be associated with an initial sedative response

What to Do About Side Effects

- Wait
- Wait
- Wait
- Reduce the dose
- Low-dose benzodiazepine or beta blocker may reduce akathisia
- Take more of the dose at bedtime to help reduce daytime sedation
- Weight loss, exercise programmes, and medical management for high BMIs, diabetes, and dyslipidaemia
- Switch to another antipsychotic (atypical) – quetiapine or clozapine are best in cases of tardive dyskinesia

Best Augmenting Agents for Side Effects

- Dystonia: antimuscarinic drugs (e.g. procyclidine) as oral or IM depending on the severity; botulinum toxin if antimuscarinics not effective
- Parkinsonism: antimuscarinic drugs (e.g. procyclidine)
- Akathisia: beta blocker propranolol (30–80 mg/day) or low-dose benzodiazepine (e.g. 0.5–3.0 mg/day of clonazepam) may help; other agents that may be tried include the 5HT2 antagonists such as cyproheptadine (16 mg/day) or mirtazapine (15 mg at night – caution in bipolar disorder); clonidine (0.2–0.8 mg/day) may be tried if the above ineffective
- Tardive dyskinesia: stop any antimuscarinic, consider tetrabenazine

DOSING AND USE

Usual Dosage Range

- **Oral for adults:** 20–50 mg/day (max per dose 40 mg), for debilitated patients, use elderly dose
- **Acetate for adults:** 50–150 mg every 2–3 days
- **Decanoate for adults:** 200–500 mg every 1–4 weeks

Dosage Forms

- **Oral tablets:** Clopixol 2 mg, 10 mg, 25 mg
- **Oral drops:** Ciatyl-Z 20 mg/mL
- **Acetate form: solution for injection –** Clopixol Acuphase 50 mg/mL
- **Decanoate form: solution for injection –** Clopixol 200 mg/mL, Clopixol Conc 500 mg/mL

How to Dose

- **Oral:** initial dose 20–30 mg/day in divided doses; can increase by 10–20 mg/day every 2–3 days; maintenance dose (usually 20–50 mg/day, max 40 mg per dose) can be administered as a single night time dose; max dose generally 150 mg/day
- **Injection** should be administered IM in gluteal region in the morning
- **Acetate** generally should be administered every 2–3 days if required; some patients may require a second dose 24–48 hours after the first injection; duration of treatment should not exceed 2 weeks; max cumulative dosage should not exceed 400 mg; max number of injections should not exceed four
- **Decanoate:** initial test dose 100 mg; followed by a second injection of

200–500 mg after at least 7 days; then maintenance treatment is generally 200–500 mg every 1–4 weeks, adjusted according to response, higher doses of more than 500 mg can be used; do not exceed 600 mg weekly

 Dosing Tips

- Onset of action of IM acetate formulation following a single injection is generally 2–4 hours; duration of action is generally 2–3 days
- Zuclopenthixol acetate is not intended for long-term use, and should not generally be used for longer than 2 weeks; patients requiring treatment longer than 2 weeks should be switched to a depot or oral formulation of zuclopenthixol or another antipsychotic
- When changing from zuclopenthixol acetate to maintenance treatment with zuclopenthixol decanoate, administer the last injection of acetate concomitantly with the initial injection of decanoate
- The peak of action for the decanoate is usually 4–9 days, and doses generally have to be administered every 2–3 weeks
- Stop treatment if neutrophils fall below 1.5×10^9/L and refer to specialist care if neutrophils fall below 0.5×10^9/L

Overdose

- Sedation, convulsions, extrapyramidal symptoms, coma, hypotension, shock, hypo/hyperthermia

Long-Term Use

- Zuclopenthixol decanoate is intended for maintenance treatment
- Some side effects may be irreversible (e.g. tardive dyskinesia)

Habit Forming

- No

How to Stop

- Slow down-titration of oral formulation (over 6–8 weeks), especially when simultaneously beginning a new antipsychotic while switching (i.e. cross-titration)
- Rapid oral discontinuation may lead to rebound psychosis and worsening of symptoms

- If anti-Parkinson agents are being used, they should be continued for a few weeks after zuclopenthixol is discontinued

Pharmacokinetics

- Metabolised by CYP450 2D6 and 3A4
- For oral formulation, elimination half-life about 20 hours
- For acetate, rate-limiting half-life about 32 hours
- For decanoate, rate-limiting half-life about 17–21 days with multiple doses

 Drug Interactions

- Zuclopenthixol may antagonise the effects of levodopa and dopamine agonists
- Theoretically, concomitant use with CYP450 2D6 inhibitors (such as paroxetine and fluoxetine) or with CYP450 3A4 inhibitors (such as fluoxetine and ketoconazole) could raise zuclopenthixol plasma levels and require dosage reduction
- Theoretically, concomitant use with CYP450 3A4 inducers (such as carbamazepine) could lower zuclopenthixol plasma levels and require dosage increase
- CNS effects may be increased if used with other CNS depressants
- If used with anticholinergic agents, may potentiate their effects
- Combined use with adrenaline may lower blood pressure
- Zuclopenthixol may block the antihypertensive effects of drugs such as guanethidine, but may enhance the actions of other antihypertensive drugs
- Using zuclopenthixol with metoclopramide may increase the risk of extrapyramidal symptoms
- Some patients taking a neuroleptic and lithium have developed an encephalopathic syndrome similar to neuroleptic malignant syndrome

 Other Warnings/Precautions

- All antipsychotics should be used with caution in patients with angle-closure glaucoma, blood disorders, cardiovascular disease, depression, diabetes, epilepsy and susceptibility to seizures, history of jaundice, myasthenia gravis, Parkinson's

disease, photosensitivity, prostatic hypertrophy, severe respiratory disorders
- If signs of neuroleptic malignant syndrome develop, treatment should be immediately discontinued
- Decanoate should not be used with clozapine because it cannot be withdrawn quickly in the event of serious adverse effects such as neutropenia
- Possible antiemetic effect of zuclopenthixol may mask signs of other disorders or overdose; suppression of cough reflex may cause asphyxia
- Use only with great caution, if at all, in Lewy body disease
- Observe for signs of ocular toxicity (pigmentary retinopathy and lenticular and corneal deposits)
- Avoid undue exposure to sunlight
- Avoid extreme heat exposure
- Do not use adrenaline in event of overdose as interaction with some pressor agents may lower blood pressure
- Use with caution in hyperthyroidism and hypothyroidism
- Risk of QT interval prolongation
- When transferring from oral to depot therapy, the dose by mouth should be reduced gradually

Do Not Use
- If patient is taking a large concomitant dose of a sedative hypnotic
- If patient is taking guanethidine or a similar-acting compound
- If patient has CNS depression, is comatosed, or has subcortical brain damage
- If patient has acute alcohol, barbiturate, or opiate intoxication
- If patient has angle-closure glaucoma
- If patient has phaeochromocytoma, circulatory collapse, or blood dyscrasias
- In case of pregnancy
- In apathetic states or withdrawn states
- In children
- If there is a proven allergy to zuclopenthixol

Renal Impairment
- Use with caution
- Halve dose in renal failure; smaller starting doses used in severe renal impairment because of increased cerebral sensitivity

Hepatic Impairment
- Use with caution
- Manufacturer advises 50% dose reduction of the recommended dose

Cardiac Impairment
- Use with caution – risk of QT interval prolongation

Elderly
- Some patients may tolerate lower doses better
- Oral: initial dose 5–15 mg/day in divided doses, increased if necessary up to 150 mg/day; usual maintenance 20–50 mg/day (max per dose 40 mg)
- Maximum acetate dose 100 mg
- Decanoate: a quarter to half usual starting dose to be used
- Although conventional antipsychotics are commonly used for behavioural disturbances in dementia, no agent has been approved for treatment of elderly patients with dementia-related psychosis
- Elderly patients with dementia-related psychosis treated with antipsychotics are at an increased risk of death compared to placebo, and also have an increased risk of cerebrovascular events

 Children and Adolescents
- Safety and efficacy have not been established in children under age 18
- Is currently not for use in children, but preliminary open-label data show that oral zuclopenthixol may be effective in reducing aggression in children with intellectual disabilities

 Pregnancy
- Controlled studies have not been conducted in pregnant women
- There is a risk of abnormal muscle movements and withdrawal symptoms in newborns whose mothers took an antipsychotic during the third trimester; symptoms may include agitation, abnormally increased or decreased muscle tone, tremor, sleepiness, severe difficulty breathing, and difficulty feeding

Zuclopenthixol (Continued)

- Psychotic symptoms may worsen during pregnancy and some form of treatment may be necessary
- Use in pregnancy may be justified if the benefit of continued treatment exceeds any associated risk
- Switching antipsychotics may increase the risk of relapse
- Antipsychotics may be preferable to anticonvulsant mood stabilisers if treatment is required for mania during pregnancy
- Effects of hyperprolactinaemia on the foetus are unknown
- Depot antipsychotics should only be used when there is a good response to the depot and a history of non-concordance with oral medication

Breastfeeding

- Small amounts in mother's breast milk
- Risk of accumulation in infant due to long half-life
- Haloperidol is considered to be the preferred first-generation antipsychotic, and quetiapine is the preferred second-generation antipsychotic
- Infants of women who choose to breastfeed should be monitored for possible adverse effects

systematically investigated for these properties at low doses
- Patients have similar antipsychotic responses to any conventional antipsychotic, but responses to atypicals can vary greatly from one atypical antipsychotic to another
- Patients with inadequate responses to atypical antipsychotics may benefit from a trial of augmentation with a conventional antipsychotic such as zuclopenthixol or from switching to a conventional antipsychotic such as zuclopenthixol
- However, long-term polypharmacy with a combination of a conventional antipsychotic such as zuclopenthixol with an atypical antipsychotic may cause more side effects rather than increased efficacy
- For treatment-resistant patients, especially those with impulsivity, aggression, violence, and self-harm, long-term polypharmacy with a combination of 2 atypical antipsychotics or with a combination of 1 atypical antipsychotic and 1 conventional antipsychotic may be useful with close monitoring
- In such cases, can combine 1 depot antipsychotic with 1 oral antipsychotic
- Adding 2 conventional antipsychotics together has little rationale and may reduce tolerability without clearly enhancing efficacy

THE ART OF PSYCHOPHARMACOLOGY

Potential Advantages

- Non-concordant patients (decanoate)
- Emergency use (acute injection)

Potential Disadvantages

- Children
- Elderly
- Patients with tardive dyskinesia

Primary Target Symptoms

- Positive symptoms of psychosis
- Negative symptoms of psychosis
- Aggressive symptoms

Pearls

- Zuclopenthixol depot may reduce risk of relapse more than some other depot conventional antipsychotics, but it may also be associated with more adverse effects
- Zuclopenthixol may have serotonin 2A antagonist properties, but has never been

ZUCLOPENTHIXOL DECANOATE

Zuclopenthixol Decanoate Properties

Vehicle	Thin vegetable oil (derived from coconuts)
Duration of action	2–4 weeks
Tmax	4–9 days
T1/2 with multiple dosing	17–21 days
Time to reach steady state	About 12 weeks
Dosing schedule (maintenance)	1–4 weeks
Injection site	Intramuscular (gluteal)
Needle gauge	21
Dosage forms	200 mg, 500 mg
Injection volume	200 mg/mL, 500 mg/mL; not to exceed 2 mL

Usual Dosage Range

- Maintenance in schizophrenia and paranoid psychoses

- Adult: usual maintenance dose 200–500 mg every 1–4 weeks; max 600 mg per week
- Elderly: dose is initially quarter to half adult dose

How to Dose

- Adult: test dose 100 mg, dose to be administered into the upper outer buttock or lateral thigh, followed by 200–500 mg after at least 7 days, then 200–500 mg every 1–4 weeks, adjusted according to response, higher doses of more than 500 mg can be used; do not exceed 600 mg every week
- Elderly: test dose 25–50 mg, dose to be administered into the upper outer buttock or lateral thigh, followed by 50–250 mg after at least 7 days, then 50–250 mg every 1–4 weeks, adjusted according to response, higher doses of more than 250 mg can be used; do not exceed 300 mg every week
- An interval of at least 1 week should be allowed before the second injection is given at a dose consistent with the patient's condition

 Dosing Tips

- Adequate control of severe psychotic symptoms may take up to 4 to 6 months at high enough dosage. Once stabilised lower maintenance doses may be considered, but must be sufficient to prevent relapse
- Injection volumes of greater than 2 mL should be distributed between two injection sites
- With depot injections, the absorption rate constant is slower than the elimination rate constant, thus resulting in "flip-flop" kinetics – i.e. time to steady state is a function of absorption rate, while concentration at steady state is a function of elimination rate
- The rate-limiting step for plasma drug levels for depot injections is not drug metabolism, but rather slow absorption from the injection site
- In general, 5 half-lives of any medication are needed to achieve 97% of steady-state levels
- Because plasma antipsychotic levels increase gradually over time, dose requirements may ultimately decrease from initial; if possible obtaining periodic plasma levels can be beneficial to prevent unnecessary plasma level creep
- The time to get a blood level for patients receiving depot is the morning of the day they will receive their next injection

THE ART OF SWITCHING

Switching from Oral Antipsychotics to Zuclopenthixol Decanoate

- Discontinuation of oral antipsychotic can begin immediately if adequate loading is pursued; however, oral coverage may still be necessary for the first week
- How to discontinue oral formulations:
  - Down-titration is not required for: amisulpride, aripiprazole, cariprazine, paliperidone
  - 1-week down-titration is required for: lurasidone, risperidone
  - 3–4-week down-titration is required for: asenapine, olanzapine, quetiapine
  - 4+-week down-titration is required for: clozapine
  - For patients taking benzodiazepine or anticholinergic medication, this can be continued during cross-titration to help alleviate side effects such as insomnia, agitation, and/or psychosis. Once the patient is stable on the depot, these can be tapered one at a time as appropriate

 Suggested Reading

Coutinho E, Fenton M, Adams C, et al. Zuclopenthixol acetate in psychiatric emergencies: looking for evidence from clinical trials. Schizophr Res 2000;46:111–18.

Coutinho E, Fenton M, Quraishi S. Zuclopenthixol decanoate for schizophrenia and other serious mental illnesses. Cochrane Database Syst Rev 2000;(2):CD001164.

Davies S, Westin A, Castberg I, et al. Characterisation of zuclopenthixol metabolism by in vitro and therapeutic drug monitoring studies. Acta Psychiatr Scand 2010;122(6):444–53.

Zuclopenthixol (Continued)

Fenton M, Coutinho ES, Campbell C. Zuclopenthixol acetate in the treatment of acute schizophrenia and similar serious mental illnesses. Cochrane Database Syst Rev 2000;(2):CD000525.

Huhn M, Nikolakopoulou A, Schneider-Thoma J, et al. Comparative efficacy and tolerability of 32 oral antipsychotics for the acute treatment of adults with multi-episode schizophrenia: a systematic review and network meta-analysis. Lancet 2019;394(10202):939–51.

Stahl SM. How to dose a psychotropic drug: beyond therapeutic drug monitoring to genotyping the patient. Acta Psychiatr Scand 2010;122(6):440–1.

Medicines and Driving

Prescribers should advise patients if their treatment could affect their ability to perform skilled tasks such as driving. This is particularly important with drugs that cause sedation. Patients should be alerted to the fact that alcohol can enhance the sedative effects of these drugs. Further general information about fitness to drive can be found on the Driver and Vehicle Licensing Agency (DVLA) website: www.gov.uk/government/organisations/driver-and-vehicle-licensing-agency

Since 2015 in the UK, it has been an offence for anyone to drive, attempt to drive, or be in charge of a vehicle, showing levels of certain controlled drugs in excess of specified limits. This is in addition to existing rules on drug-impaired driving and fitness to drive. The rules apply to two drug groups: certain drugs of abuse (amfetamines, cannabis, cocaine, ketamine) and medicines such as benzodiazepines and opioids.

A driver found to have blood levels above the specified limits for any of the drugs, including related drugs such as apomorphine hydrochloride, will be found guilty even if their driving was unimpaired. This includes prescribed drugs, such as selegiline, which metabolise to drugs included in the offence.

Patients should carry appropriate evidence to show that the drug was prescribed to treat a medical problem, and taken according to prescriber instructions or specific drug information (patient information leaflet or repeat prescription form). For further information, please check the Department for Transport website: www.gov.uk/government/collections/drug-driving

The British National Formulary (BNF) outlines advice relating to certain classes of psychotropics and specific individual drugs. A summary of the advice relating to some of the individual drugs and classes of drugs found in this prescriber's guide is found below.

Anticholinergics
- **Hyoscine hydrobromide:**
- Antimuscarinics can affect performance of skilled tasks (e.g. driving). With transdermal use - drowsiness may persist for up to 24 hours or longer after removal of patch; effects of alcohol enhanced
- **Procyclidine hydrochloride, trihexyphenidyl hydrochloride:**
- Antimuscarinics can affect performance of skilled tasks (e.g. driving)

Antidepressants
- **Esketamine:**
- Patients and carers should be counselled on effects on driving and performance of skilled tasks. These may include anxiety, dissociation, dizziness, perceptual abnormalities, sedation, somnolence, and vertigo
- **Monoamine Oxidase Inhibitors (MAOIs) – isocarboxazid, phenelzine, tranylcypromine:**
- Drowsiness may affect performance of skilled tasks (e.g. driving)
- **Selective serotonin reuptake inhibitors (SSRIs) – citalopram, escitalopram, fluoxetine, fluvoxamine maleate, paroxetine, sertraline:**
- May impair performance of skilled tasks (e.g. driving, operating machinery). Patients should be advised of effects on driving and skilled tasks
- **Trazodone hydrochloride:**
- Drowsiness may affect performance of skilled tasks (e.g. driving). Effects of alcohol enhanced

- **Tricyclic antidepressants – amitriptyline hydrochloride, clomipramine hydrochloride, dosulepin hydrochloride, doxepin, imipramine hydrochloride, lofepramine, mianserin hydrochloride, nortriptyline, trimipramine:**
- Drowsiness may affect performance of skilled tasks (e.g. driving or operating machinery), especially at start of treatment; effects of alcohol enhanced
- **Tryptophan:**
- Patients should be counselled on effects on driving and performance of skilled tasks – drowsiness
- **Venlafaxine:**
- May affect performance of skilled tasks (e.g. driving)
- **Vortioxetine:**
- Patients and carers should be counselled on effects on driving and performance of skilled tasks, especially when starting treatment or changing dose

Antihistamines
- **Hydroxyzine hydrochloride, promethazine hydrochloride:**
- Drowsiness may affect performance of skilled tasks (e.g. cycling or driving); alcohol can enhance sedating effects

Antipsychotics
- **Amisulpride, asenapine, benperidol, cariprazine, chlorpromazine hydrochloride, clozapine, flupentixol, haloperidol, levomepromazine, loxapine, lurasidone hydrochloride, olanzapine, paliperidone, pimozide, prochlorperazine, quetiapine, risperidone, sulpiride, trifluoperazine, zuclopenthixol:**
- Drowsiness may affect performance of skilled tasks (e.g. driving or operating machinery), especially at start of treatment; effects of alcohol enhanced

Anxiolytics
- **Benzodiazepines – chlordiazepoxide hydrochloride, diazepam, flurazepam, loprazolam, lorazepam, midazolam, nitrazepam, oxazepam, temazepam:**
- May cause drowsiness, impair judgement and increase reaction time, and thus affect ability to drive or perform skilled tasks; effects of alcohol enhanced. Hangover effects of a night dose may impair performance the following day
- **Buspirone hydrochloride:**
- May affect performance of skilled tasks (e.g. driving); effects of alcohol may be enhanced
- **Pregabalin:**
- Patients and carers should be counselled on effects on driving and performance of skilled tasks – dizziness or visual problems

Attention deficit hyperactivity treatments
- **Clonidine hydrochloride:**
- Drowsiness may affect performance of skilled tasks (e.g. driving); effects of alcohol may be enhanced
- **Guanfacine:**
- Patients and carers should be counselled about the effects on driving and performance of skilled tasks – dizziness and syncope
- **Stimulants – dexamfetamine sulfate, lisdexamfetamine mesilate, methylphenidate hydrochloride:**
- Prescribers should advise patients if treatment is likely to affect their ability to perform skilled tasks (e.g. driving), especially for drugs with sedative effects; patients should be warned that these effects are enhanced by alcohol

Hypnotics

- **Sodium oxybate:**
- Leave at least 6 hours between taking sodium oxybate and performing skilled tasks (e.g. driving or operating machinery); effects of alcohol and other CNS depressants enhanced
- **Zolpidem tartrate:**
- Drowsiness may persist the next day – leave at least 8 hours between taking zolpidem and performing skilled tasks (e.g. driving, or operating machinery); effects of alcohol and other CNS depressants enhanced
- **Zopiclone:**
- Drowsiness may persist the next day and affect performance of skilled tasks (e.g. driving); effects of alcohol enhanced

Mood stabilisers

- **Lithium:**
- May impair performance of skilled tasks (e.g. driving, operating machinery)

Substance use disorder treatments

- **Bupropion hydrochloride:**
- Patients and carers should be counselled on effects on driving and performance of skilled tasks – dizziness and light-headedness
- **Opioids:**
- **Buprenorphine:** Drowsiness may affect performance of skilled tasks (e.g. driving); effects of alcohol enhanced. Driving at start of therapy and following dose changes should be avoided. For subcutaneous implant, patients and carers should be counselled on the risk of somnolence which may last for up to 1 week after insertion
- **Methadone hydrochloride:** Drowsiness may affect performance of skilled tasks (e.g. driving); effects of alcohol enhanced. Driving at start of therapy and following dose changes should be avoided
- **Varenicline:**
- Patients and carers should be cautioned on effects on driving and performance of skilled tasks – dizziness, somnolence, and transient loss of consciousness

Other Drugs

- **Prazosin:**
- May affect performance of skilled tasks (e.g. driving)
- **Tetrabenazine:**
- May affect performance of skilled tasks (e.g. driving)

Index by Drug Name

Index by Use

Index by Class

Abbreviations

5HT	5-hydroxytryptamine
6-S-MT	6-sulphatoxy-melatonin
ACh	acetylcholine
AChE	acetylcholinesterase
ADHD	attention deficit hyperactivity disorder
AIMS	Abnormal Involuntary Movement Scale
AMPA	alpha-amino-3-hydroxy-5-methyl-4-isoxazolepropionic acid
ASD	autism spectrum disorder
AUC	area under the curve
AV	atrio-ventricular
BAR	behavioural activity rating
BDNF	brain-derived neurotrophic factor
BMI	body mass index
BNF	British national formulary
BP	blood pressure
BOLD	blood-oxygen-level-dependent
BuChE	butyrylcholinesterase
Ca	calcium
CBT	cognitive behavioural therapy
CGI	Clinical Global Impression
Cmax	maximum concentration
CRP	C-reactive protein
CSF	cerebrospinal fluid
CMI	clomipramine
CNS	central nervous system
COPD	chronic obstructive pulmonary disease
CYP450	cytochrome P450
CVS	cardiovascular system
DCAR	desmethyl cariprazine
DDCAR	didesmethyl cariprazine
De-CMI	desmethyl-clomipramine
DLB	dementia with Lewy bodies
DN-RIRe	dopamine and noradrenaline reuptake inhibitor and releaser
D-RAn	dopamine receptor antagonist
DRESS	drug reaction with eosinophilia and systemic symptoms
DS-Ran	dopamine and serotonin receptor antagonist
ECG	electrocardiogram
ECT	electroconvulsive therapy
EEG	electroencephalogram
eGFR	estimated glomerular filtration rate
EMS	eosinophilia-myalgia syndrome
EPS	extrapyramidal side effects

ERP	exposure response prevention
FBC	full blood count
FEP	first-episode psychosis
fMRI	functional magnetic resonance imaging
GABA	gamma-aminobutyric acid
GAD	generalized anxiety disorder
GHB	gamma hydroxybutyrate
GIT	gastrointestinal tract
Glu-CB	glutamate, voltage-gated sodium and calcium channel blocker
Glu-MM	glutamate multimodal
HDL	high-density lipoprotein
HbA1c	glycosylated haemoglobin
HIV	human immunodeficiency virus
HLA	human leucocyte antigen
HR	heart rate
HRT	habit reversal therapy
IM	intramuscular
IPT	interpersonal therapy
IR	immediate-release
IV	intravenous
K	potassium
kg	kilograms
LAAM	levomethadyl acetate hydrochloride
LAI	long-acting injection
LDL	low-density lipoprotein
LFTs	liver function tests
Li	lithium
MAO	monoamine oxidase
MAOI	monoamine oxidase inhibitor
mcg	microgram
MCI	mild cognitive impairment
MDD	major depressive disorder
MDMA	3,4-methylenedioxymethamphetamine (ecstasy)
mg	milligram
Mg	magnesium
MI	myocardial infarction
mL	milliliter
mmHg	millimeters of mercury
MR	modified release
MT	melatonin receptor
mTORC1	mammalian target of rapamycin complex 1
NaSSA	noradrenaline and specific serotonergic agent
NDRI	noradrenaline dopamine reuptake inhibitor

NET	norepinephrine transporter
ng	nanogram
NICE	national institute for health and care excellence
NMDA	N-methyl-D-aspartate
NMS	neuroleptic malignant syndrome
NNT	number needed to treat
nocte	nightly
NSAIDs	nonsteroidal anti-inflammatory drugs
NRI	noradrenaline reuptake inhibitor
NRT	nictotine replacement therapy
NT1	paediatric type 1 narcolepsy
OCD	obsessive-compulsive disorder
ODD	oppositional defiant disorder
ODV	O-desmethylvenlafaxine
OPITCS	eosinophilia-myalgia syndrome monitoring scheme
PAM	positive allosteric modulator
PCP	phencyclidine
PDE	phosphodiesterase
PET	positron emission tomography
PMDD	premenstrual dysphoric disorder
PNS	peripheral nervous system
PPHN	persistent pulmonary hypertension of the newborn
prn	as needed
PTSD	post-traumatic stress disorder
QTc	QT corrected
qds	4 times a day
RCT	randomised controlled trial
Resp	respiratory system
SAM-e	s-adenosyl methionine
SARI	serotonin 2 antagonist/reuptake inhibitor
SCARs	severe cutaneous adverse reactions
SCN	suprachiasmatic nucleus
SGA	second generation antipsychotic
SIADH	syndrome of inappropriate antidiuretic hormone secretion
SLE	systemic lupus erythematosus
SNRI	dual serotonin and norepinephrine reuptake inhibitor
SN-RAn	serotonin norepinephrine receptor antagonist
SR	sustained-release
SSRI	selective serotonin reuptake inhibitor
TCA	tricyclic antidepressant
tds	3 times a day
Tmax	time to reach maximum concentration
T3	triiodothyronine

TMN	tuberomammillary nucleus
UGT	uridine 5'-diphospho-glucuronosyltransferase
TSH	thyroid-stimulating hormone
VMA	vanillylmandelic acid
VMAT	vesicular monoamine transporter
WBC	white blood cell count